Manual of
Ocular
Diagnosis
and Therapy

1991

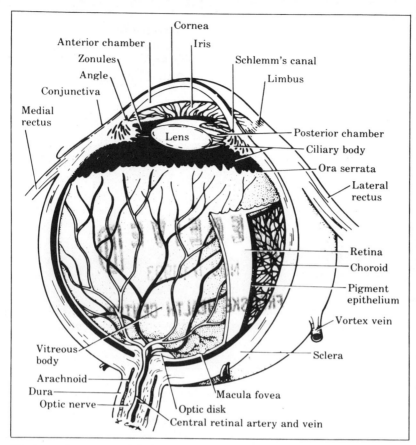

The internal structures of the human eye. (Adapted from the original drawing by Paul Peck, *Anatomy of the Eye*. Courtesy of Lederle Laboratories, Pearl River, N.Y.)

Manual of Ocular Diagnosis and Therapy

Third Edition

Edited by
Deborah Pavan-Langston,
M.D., F.A.C.S.

Associate Professor of Ophthalmology, Harvard Medical School; Surgeon in Ophthalmology, Massachusetts Eye and Ear Infirmary; Senior Scientist, Eye Research Institute, Boston

Little, Brown and Company
Boston/Toronto/London

Contents

Contributing Authors

William P. Boger III, M.D.

Clinical Instructor in Ophthalmology, Harvard Medical School and The Children's Hospital, Boston; Associate in Ophthalmology, The Children's Hospital, Boston, and Active Staff, Emerson Hospital, Concord, Massachusetts

David L. Epstein, M.D.

Associate Professor of Ophthalmology, Harvard Medical School; Surgeon in Ophthalmology, Massachusetts Eye and Ear Infirmary, Boston

Gary N. Foulks, M.D., F.A.C.S

Professor of Ophthalmology, Duke University School of Medicine; Cornea Service, Duke University Eye Center, Durham, North Carolina

George Edw. Garcia, M.D.

Assistant Professor of Ophthalmology, Harvard Medical School; Associate Chief of Ophthalmology, Massachusetts Eye and Ear Infirmary, Boston

Arthur S. Grove, Jr., M.D.

Assistant Professor of Ophthalmology, Harvard Medical School; Associate Surgeon, Massachusetts Eye and Ear Infirmary, Boston

Mohandas M. Kini, M.D., Ph.D.

Associate Professor of Ophthalmology, Boston University School of Medicine, and Assistant Clinical Professor of Ophthalmology, Harvard Medical School; Surgeon in Ophthalmology, Massachusetts Eye and Ear Infirmary, Boston

Deborah Pavan-Langston, M.D., F.A.C.S.

Associate Professor of Ophthalmology, Harvard Medical School; Surgeon in Ophthalmology, Massachusetts Eye and Ear Infirmary; Senior Scientist, Eye Research Institute, Boston

Robert A. Petersen, M.D.	Assistant Professor of Ophthalmology, Harvard Medical School; Senior Associate in Ophthalmology, The Children's Hospital, Boston
Shirley H. Wray, M.D., Ph.D., F.R.C.P.	Associate Professor of Neurology, Harvard Medical School; Director, Unit for Neuro-Visual Disorders, Massachusetts General Hospital, Boston
Gilbert K. Yamamoto, M.D., F.A.C.S.	Associate Clinical Professor of Surgery (Ophthalmology), John A. Burns School of Medicine, University of Hawaii; Staff Surgeon, The Queen's Medical Center, Honolulu

Preface

This third edition of the Manual has, in many areas, undergone extensive revision from previous editions—revision promoted by the gratifying advances made in clinical and laboratory diagnosis, high technology, and new approaches in drug development. The object of the original exercise, however, remains unchanged: to publish a highly practical and specific book on ocular diagnosis and therapy that will be of use to the doctor on "the front lines," the one sitting face to face with a patient. This updated book is written for the widest possible audience: practicing eye care specialists, emergency room physicians, internists, neurologists, pediatricians—that is, seasoned practitioners and house officers in virtually any discipline, as well as medical students first learning about ocular disease. It is for anyone involved in decisions concerning either care of the eyes or what the eyes can tell us about other care needed by the patient.

Each chapter covers the clinical findings of a multitude of ocular problems, diagnostic tests, differential diagnoses, and detailed treatments. The subject matter varies widely and includes the latest information on topics from the simple removal of corneal foreign bodies to new imaging techniques, management of chemical burns, infections (bacterial, viral, fungal, parasitic), the great variety of glaucomas, extraocular muscle imbalance, neuroophthalmic problems, and the use of corticosteroids, immunosuppressives, and numerous other therapeutic agents. The indications and techniques of laser therapy for the front and back of the eye and an expanded section on cataract extraction and intraocular lenses are presented in the light of today's knowledge. The ocular findings in systemic disease and the ocular toxicities of systemic drugs are thoroughly tabulated by disease and drug for easy reference. The straightforward outline form of the text, and the index, drug formulary, drawings, and tables are all designed so that information can be rapidly located and a pertinent review brought quickly to hand.

Each contributing author was selected primarily for his or her skill as a practicing physician or surgeon with expertise in the area covered. All are knowledgeable in clinical and laboratory research as well and are, therefore, up to date on new developments in the field. I am indebted to these fine physicians for their contributions to this book. Susan Pioli and Karen Oberheim of Little, Brown and Company have been encouraging and helpful. For countless hours of copyediting, typing and retyping, and encouragement when exasperation was the easier reaction, I thank my longtime administrative assistant, Mary Lou Moar. I acknowledge also the excellent drawings of Laurel Cook and Peter Mallen, and I am most appreciative of the assistance given me by Patricia Geary. Without the help of all these people and countless others too numerous to mention by name, this book might never have been published.

D.P.-L.

Manual of
Ocular
Diagnosis
and Therapy

Ocular Examination Techniques and Diagnostic Tests

Deborah Pavan-Langston

I. General principles

A. **Physical examination and evaluation of the ocular system** are greatly facilitated by a number of techniques that may be performed in the office, using equipment readily available through any optical or medical supply house. Some of the more complicated techniques, however, must be performed by a specialist in a hospital setting. These techniques are discussed with a view to (1) their indications, (2) how they are done, so that the referring examiner can explain to a patient what might be expected, and (3) the necessary information to aid the examiner in management of the patient.

B. **Order of examination.** Examination of the eye and its surrounding tissues with and without special aids may yield valuable information for the diagnosis and treatment of primary ocular disease or disease secondary to systemic problems. So that nothing is overlooked, a systematic routine should be adopted and particular attention given to those factors that brought the patient to testing in the first place. With time and increased experience, an examination that initially may take a somewhat prolonged period of time can be shortened significantly with no loss of accuracy and frequently with increased accuracy of perception. Individual chapters should be referred to for related detail.

C. **The general order for nonemergency examination** is as follows:

1. **History.** Present complaints, previous eye disorders, family eye problems, present and past general illnesses, medications, and allergies.

2. **Visual acuity.** Distant and near without and with glasses, if used, and with pinhole if less than 20/30 is obtained.

3. **Extraocular muscle function.** Range of action in all fields of gaze, stereopsis testing, and screening for strabismus and diplopia.

4. **Color vision testing.**

5. **Anterior segment examination** under some magnification if possible (loupe or slit lamp), with and without fluorescein or rose bengal dyes.

6. **Intraocular pressures (IOPs).**

7. **Ophthalmoscopy** of the fundi.

8. **Confrontation or other field testing.**

9. **Other tests** as indicated by history and prior examination:
   a. Tear film adequacy.
   b. Corneal sensation.
   c. Transillumination.
   d. Exophthalmometry.
   e. Keratoscopy.
   f. Keratometry.
   g. Tonography.
   h. Gonioscopy.
   i. Ultrasonography.
   j. Fluorescein angiography.
   k. Electroretinography and electrooculography.
   l. Radiology.

   Procedures **f** through **k** are done by specialists in eye care, and referral should be made if such testing is indicated.

II. Routine office examination techniques

A. Visual acuity. Determination of visual acuity is a test of macular function and should be part of any eye examination, regardless of symptomatology or lack thereof.

1. **Distant visual acuity.** Visual acuity is examined one eye at a time, the other eye being occluded. Pressure on the occluded eye should be avoided so that there will be no distortion of the image when that eye is tested subsequently. If the patient normally wears glasses, the test should be made both with and without corrected lenses and recorded as "uncorrected" (sc) and "corrected" (cc).

   a. **The chart** most commonly used for distance vision with literate patients is the Snellen chart, which is situated 20 feet (approximately 6 meters) away from the patient and diffusely illuminated without glare. At this distance the rays of light from the object in view are almost parallel, and no effort of accommodation (focusing) is necessary for the normal eye to see the subject clearly. The Snellen chart is made up of letters of graduated sizes; the distance at which each size subtends an angle of 5 minutes is indicated along the side of the chart. The farther one is from an object, the smaller the retinal image. By combining the two factors of size and distance, it is possible to determine the minimum visual angle, i.e., the smallest retinal image that can be seen by a given eye. A normal visual system can identify an entire letter subtending an angle of 5 minutes of arc and any components of the letter subtending 1 minute of arc at a distance of 20 feet. Some patients, however, may resolve letters subtending even smaller visual angles. The vision of a normal eye is recorded as 20/20, or 6/6 in metric measurement. If the patient is able to read down only to the 20/30 line, the vision is recorded as 20/30. If the patient is unable to read even the large E at the top, which subtends an arc of 400 degrees, he or she may be moved closer so that the distance measurement is changed. The visual acuity may then be recorded as 10/400, for instance, if the patient is able to read this letter at 10 feet from the chart.

   b. **Pinhole vision** is tested if the patient is unable to read the 20/30 line. A pinhole aperture is placed in front of the eye to ascertain any improvement in acuity. The use of a pinhole will correct for any uncorrected refractive error such as nearsightedness, farsightedness, and astigmatism (regular or irregular from corneal surface abnormalities) without the need for lenses. Through the pinhole a patient with a refractive error should read close to 20/20. If the pinhole fails to improve the patient's visual acuity score, the examiner must suspect another cause for the reduced vision, such as opacities in the ocular media or macular or optic nerve disease.

   c. **Preschool children** or **patients who are unable to read** should be shown the Illiterate E chart, which is made up entirely of the letter E facing in different directions. Patients are instructed to point their finger in the direction of the bars of the E. Children as young as 3 years of age may be able to cooperate in this testing. Another form of testing is with Allen cards, which are small cards with test pictures printed on each one; at a distance of 20 feet, a visual acuity of 20/30 may be tested. If the patient is unable to identify the pictures at that distance, the distance at which the picture is identified is recorded, e.g., 10/30, 5/30, and so on.

   d. **If a patient is unable to identify any letter** on the chart at any distance, visual acuity is recorded as counting fingers (CF) at whatever distance the patient is able to perform this function, e.g., CF 3. Vision less than counting fingers is recorded as hand motion (HM) or light perception (LP). If an eye is unable to perceive light, the examiner should record no light perception (NLP) rather than the misleading term *blind*.

e. **Tests of light projection** may demonstrate normal retinal function when vision is extremely poor and the **examiner is unable to see the retina,** as in the presence of mature cataract or severe corneal scarring. This test is done by covering the other eye completely and holding a light source in four different quadrants in front of the eye in question. The patient is asked to identify the direction from which the light is approaching the eye. A red lens is then held in front of the light and the patient is asked to differentiate the red from the white light. If all answers are correct, the examiner may be reasonably certain that retinal function is normal. It is important to note that normal retinal and macular function may be present despite abnormal light perception due to unusually dense anterior segment disease, which prevents light sufficient to give the retina proper stimulation from reaching it.

f. **The potential acuity meter (PAM)** is a useful device for differentiating between visual loss from anterior segment (corneal scarring, cataract) and macular disease. It allows a preoperative prediction for what the potential postoperative vision might be. For example, if the vision is 20/400 by routine testing but 20/40 with PAM, one can assume good macular function and good correction of vision once the anterior segment defect has been corrected. Conversely, if the vision is 20/400 both by regular and PAM testing, one can assume that almost all of the visual loss is due to macular disease and that anterior segment surgery or medical therapy will be to no avail. The PAM attaches easily to a standard slit lamp and projects a Snellen acuity chart into the eye using a 1.5-mm diameter pinhole aperture. In cases where the cornea is clear but cataract obstructs vision, the patient is tested at different points on the cornea in an attempt to project through clearer areas in the lens and allow the best possible reading.

g. **Macular photostress test.** Very early macular dysfunction, whether from spontaneous or toxic degeneration, may be detected by the macular photostress test. The patient looks at a flashlight held 2 cm from the eye for 10 seconds. The time it takes for visual recovery to one line less than the visual acuity determined prior to this test is measured. Normal time is about 55 seconds. Recovery taking longer than this indicates macular dysfunction, even though the area may appear anatomically normal.

h. **Macular function** may be tested in the presence of **opaque media** by gently massaging the globe through closed lids with the lighted end of a small flashlight. If the macula is functioning normally, the patient will usually see a red central area surrounded by retinal blood vessels. If macular function is abnormal, the central area will be dark rather than red and no blood vessels will be seen.

i. **Legal blindness.** Visual acuity correctable by glasses or contact lenses to 20/200 or less in both eyes, or visual fields of less than 10 degrees centrally, constitutes legal blindness in the United States. Its presence requires that the patient be reported to the Commission for the Blind in the patient's home state. Report forms are short and readily available from the Commission.

2. **Close visual acuity** is usually measured using a multipurpose reading card such as the Rosenbaum Pocket Vision Screener or the Lebensohn Chart. The patient holds the chart approximately 35 cm from the eye and, reading separately with each eye with and without glasses, reads the smallest print he or she is able to identify. This may then be recorded directly from the chart as 20/30, 20/25, or as Jaeger equivalents J-1, J-2. In patients older than the late thirties, the examiner should suspect uncorrected presbyopia if the patient is unable to read a normal visual acuity at 35 cm but is able to read it completely or at least better if the card is held further away. Abnormally low close vision in an elderly patient without reading glasses is meaningless per se except for comparative purposes in serial examinations of the severely ill.

B. Extraocular muscle function. The movement of the eyes in all fields of gaze should be examined (see also Chap. 11, secs. I and XI).

    1. In the primary position of gaze (i.e., straight ahead) the straightness, or orthophoria, of the eyes may be ascertained by observing the reflection of light on the central corneas. The patient is asked to look directly at a flashlight held 30 cm in front of the eye. Normally, the light reflection is symmetric and central in both corneas. The asymmetric positioning of a light reflex in one eye indicates deviation of that eye. Location of the reflex on the nasal side of the central cornea indicates that the eye is aimed outward, or exotropic; location of the reflex temporal to the central cornea indicates that the eye is deviated inward, or esotropic. Each millimeter of deviation is equivalent to 7 degrees or 15 diopters of turn. A paretic or paralytic extraocular muscle would be the cause of such ocular deviation. Vertical deviation may be determined by noting the location of a light reflex above or below the central cornea. In some patients, the light reflex will be slightly inside or outside the central cornea due to a normal difference between the visual axis and the anatomic axis between the central cornea and the fovea. This angle is referred to as the **angle kappa** and is positive if the eye appears to be deviating outward, negative if the eye appears to be deviating inward. No ocular movement will occur on cover-uncover testing if the apparent deviation is due to angle kappa alone (see also Chap. 11, sec. **IV.A**).

    2. Cardinal positions of gaze. The patient is asked to look in the six cardinal positions of gaze, i.e., left, right, up and right, up and left, down and right, down and left. **Congruity** (parallelism) of gaze between the two eyes should be noted as well as the extent of the excursion. The examiner should check for restriction of gaze in any direction or for double vision in any field of gaze due to restriction of one eye. Occasionally, involuntary movement may occur in normal patients at the extremes of gaze; this movement is referred to as *end-gaze* or *physiologic nystagmus*. **Nystagmus** is a short-excursion, back and forward movement of the eye that may be fine or coarse, slow or rapid. Occasionally, fine rotational nystagmus may also be observed. Except in end-gaze nystagmus, this rotational nystagmus may bear further investigation (see Chap. 11, secs. **XI** and **XIII**).

    3. The near point of conversion (NPC) is the point closest to the patient at which both eyes converge on an object as it is brought toward the eyes. This point is normally 50–70 mm in front of the eye. The moment one eye begins to deviate outward, the limit of conversion has been reached. An NPC greater than 10 cm is considered abnormal and may result in excessive tiring of the eyes on close work such as reading or sewing.

    4. Stereopsis is tested grossly by having the patient touch the end of one finger to the tip of the examiner's finger coming in horizontally end to end. Past pointing may indicate lack of depth perception in the absence of central nervous system (CNS) disease. More refined testing is done using the Wirt Test fly, circle, and animal figures with 3-D glasses. Stereopsis may be graded from the equivalent of 20/400 (large fly) to 20/20 (nine circle depth perception) using this commercially available test. Simultaneous perception of four red and green lights while wearing glasses with a red lens over one eye (eye sees only red) and a green over the other (eye sees only green) indicates a more gross but significant form of fusion. This test is the Worth Four-Dot test and is also available commercially.

C. Color vision testing

    1. Purpose. Demonstration of adequate color vision is mandatory for certain jobs in a number of states and for obtaining a driver's license. Jobs affected are armed services trainees, transportation workers, and others whose occupations require accurate color perception. Color vision may be disturbed in early macular disease, whether toxic or idiopathic degenerative, and in optic nerve disease, particularly in nutritional deficiencies such as avitaminosis A. Some of the earliest and reversible drug toxicities, such as that from chloroquine, are detected by repeated color vision testing; regression and progression may also be documented. These tests are designed for

   a. **Screening defective color vision from normal.**
   b. **Qualitative classification** as to type of defect. Protans and deutans are red-green deficient and are found in 4.0% of all males and 0.4% of all females; tritans and tetartans are very rare and are blue-yellow deficient.
   c. **Quantitative analysis** of degree of deficiency: mild, medium, or marked.
2. **Technique.** The most commonly used tests are the polychromatic plates of Ishihara, Stilling, or Hardy-Rand-Ritler. The progressively more subtle and difficult plates are made up of dots of primary colors printed on a background of similar dots in a confusion of colors or grays. These dots are set in patterns, shapes, numbers, or letters that would be recognized by a normal individual but not perceived by those with color perception defects. Patients are shown a series of plates, the number of correct answers totaled in various color test areas, and the type and severity of any deficiency thus defined.

D. **Anterior segment examination** (see frontispiece)
   1. **Magnifying loupes.** The external examination of the eye itself is greatly facilitated by the use of a bright light source, such as a flashlight or trans-illuminator, and a magnifying loupe. Many different kinds of loupes are available, but basically they may be divided into two categories. One form is worn as a spectacle loupe and has magnification ranging from $2\times$ to $5\times$, with working distances ranging between 20 and 35 cm. These magnifying spectacles may be mounted on the normal prescription glasses if these are worn by the examining physician. The second form of loupe is a headband loupe, which can range in power from $1.75\times$ to $5.25\times$, with working distances ranging between 20 and 50 cm. Loupes are of great help in evaluating not only local tissue changes and location of corneal abrasions and staining but also in minor surgical procedures and the removal of corneal foreign bodies. Handheld magnifiers do not leave both hands free for other purposes.
   2. **Eyelids and palpebral fissures.** Under good lighting conditions the lashes and eyebrows should be inspected for the presence of inflammation, scaling, or dandruff, and the lashes also for orientation, i.e., being turned in or out, misdirected, missing, or present as more than one row. Focal changes in pigmentation are also important to note. The observer should inspect the general appearance of the lid margins as to color, texture, swelling, position, and motility. Note should be made of signs of inflammation, pouting of the meibomian gland openings, rash, unusual vascularity, or old scars. The normal lid margins should overlie the corneal limbus by 1-2 mm above and below with no exposure of sclera. Voluntary lid closure should be complete with no inferior exposure. Involuntary blinking should occur every 3-6 seconds with complete closure of the lids. Both upper lids should elevate well on upward gaze and drop on downward gaze. The space between the upper and lower lid margin ranges normally between 9 and 13 mm. This measurement is not so critical as is a disparity in the size of this measurement between the two eyes in a given patient. The lid margins should follow the globe synchronously on downward and upward gaze without evidence of lid lag. The borders should have good anatomic apposition to the globe with the tear puncta (upper and lower punctal openings are located 2-4 mm temporal to the medial canthus in contact with the tear film that they drain).
   3. **Lid eversion.** The upper lid may easily be everted for inspection of the palpebral conjunctiva by having the patient look down while the examiner grasps the lashes with one hand, pulling out and down, pressing on the lid with a cotton-tipped applicator stick 1 cm above the edge of the lid margin, i.e., at the superior border of the tarsal plate, and flipping the lid over the stick (Fig. 1-1). In the presence of pain, a topical anesthetic may assist in

Fig. 1-1. A. Technique of lid eversion. **B.** Foreign body easily located with everted lid held against upper orbital rim.

this part of the examination. To restore the everted upper lid, the examiner simply asks the patient to look up and simultaneously pulls the lashes down gently. The lower palpebral conjunctiva is easily seen by pressing down over the bony maxilla to pull the lid down with a finger and asking the patient to look up.

4. **The main lacrimal gland** is situated at the superotemporal quadrant of the orbit. It may be seen as a globulated pink mass under the upper eyelid when the patient is asked to look down and nasally and traction is placed on the upper outer eyelid. Tears are carried from this gland as well as from the accessory lacrimal glands in the conjunctiva from the superotemporal quadrant of the eye down toward the infranasal area, where tears pass through the lacrimal canaliculi via the puncta and down into the lacrimal sac. From there they enter the nasolacrimal duct opening under the inferior turbinate of the nose. Tears flow down the back of the throat, occasionally giving patients the taste of medication instilled into the conjunctival cul-de-sac.

5. **The bulbar (eyeball) conjunctiva** is examined by gently separating the lids and asking the patient to look in all directions of gaze—up, down, right, and left. The normal conjunctiva is a thin membrane almost entirely transparent and appearing white, although a few patients may normally have hyperemic (red) eyes due to dilation of the many fine conjunctival vessels running throughout the membrane. In general, the examiner should be able to observe the white sclera through the transparent bulbar conjunctiva without difficulty, although occasionally deposits of pigment may be seen. On either side of the limbus a slightly raised yellow area (pinguecula) may normally be seen and may with age turn slightly yellow, due to benign degeneration of elastic tissue. Benign pigmented nevi may be present; these are flat and often translucent under magnification.

6. **The palpebral conjunctiva** is seen by lid eversion and varies in appearance with age. Above and below the tarsal plate it has many shallow folds; frequently, small bumps that represent follicles or lymphoid tissue formation are present. Follicles are normally absent in infants, prominent in children, and less notable in adults. Over the tarsal plate the conjunctiva is firmly bound to the fibrous plate and normally shows no follicles. The examiner may see faint yellow lines of the meibomian gland running vertically in the tarsal plate through the translucent overlying tissue. **Conjunctival lacerations or abrasions** are easily detected with a drop of sterile fluorescein solution or the application of a sterile fluorescein paper strip to the tear film. A white light will show the injured area as a yellow-green. A cobalt blue light will show the area as bright green.

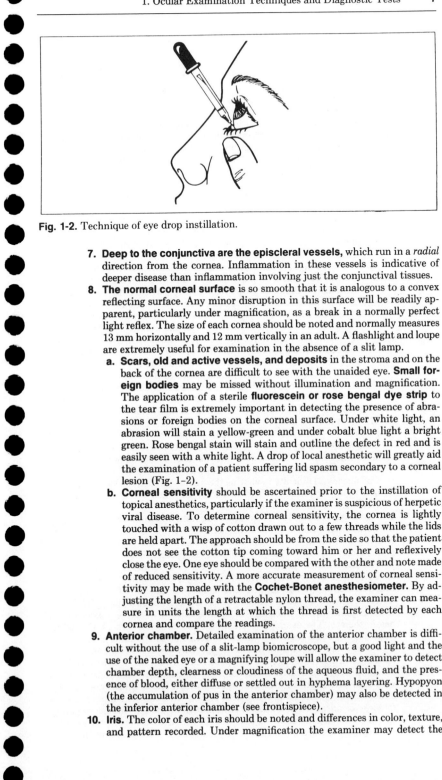

Fig. 1-2. Technique of eye drop instillation.

7. **Deep to the conjunctiva are the episcleral vessels,** which run in a *radial* direction from the cornea. Inflammation in these vessels is indicative of deeper disease than inflammation involving just the conjunctival tissues.

8. **The normal corneal surface** is so smooth that it is analogous to a convex reflecting surface. Any minor disruption in this surface will be readily apparent, particularly under magnification, as a break in a normally perfect light reflex. The size of each cornea should be noted and normally measures 13 mm horizontally and 12 mm vertically in an adult. A flashlight and loupe are extremely useful for examination in the absence of a slit lamp.

   a. **Scars, old and active vessels, and deposits** in the stroma and on the back of the cornea are difficult to see with the unaided eye. **Small foreign bodies** may be missed without illumination and magnification. The application of a sterile **fluorescein or rose bengal dye strip** to the tear film is extremely important in detecting the presence of abrasions or foreign bodies on the corneal surface. Under white light, an abrasion will stain a yellow-green and under cobalt blue light a bright green. Rose bengal stain will stain and outline the defect in red and is easily seen with a white light. A drop of local anesthetic will greatly aid the examination of a patient suffering lid spasm secondary to a corneal lesion (Fig. 1-2).

   b. **Corneal sensitivity** should be ascertained prior to the instillation of topical anesthetics, particularly if the examiner is suspicious of herpetic viral disease. To determine corneal sensitivity, the cornea is lightly touched with a wisp of cotton drawn out to a few threads while the lids are held apart. The approach should be from the side so that the patient does not see the cotton tip coming toward him or her and reflexively close the eye. One eye should be compared with the other and note made of reduced sensitivity. A more accurate measurement of corneal sensitivity may be made with the **Cochet-Bonet anesthesiometer.** By adjusting the length of a retractable nylon thread, the examiner can measure in units the length at which the thread is first detected by each cornea and compare the readings.

9. **Anterior chamber.** Detailed examination of the anterior chamber is difficult without the use of a slit-lamp biomicroscope, but a good light and the use of the naked eye or a magnifying loupe will allow the examiner to detect chamber depth, clearness or cloudiness of the aqueous fluid, and the presence of blood, either diffuse or settled out in hyphema layering. Hypopyon (the accumulation of pus in the anterior chamber) may also be detected in the inferior anterior chamber (see frontispiece).

10. **Iris.** The color of each iris should be noted and differences in color, texture, and pattern recorded. Under magnification the examiner may detect the

presence of nevi, abnormal areas of very dark pigmentation, new vessels, atrophy, tears, or surgical openings. Transillumination is useful here, as abnormalities will show up against the red pupillary-iris reflex (see sec. **L.2**).

11. **The pupils** should be inspected for size, shape, and reaction to direct and consensual (in the opposite pupil) light as well as the accommodation reflex. All of these reflexes involve decrease in pupil size on exposure to light or on attempted near focus.

   a. **Normal pupils** are equal in size, although in blue-eyed patients there may be a 0.5-mm difference under normal conditions. The range of normal pupils is 3-5 mm in room light. Pupils smaller than 3 mm in diameter are miotic; pupils larger than 7 mm are mydriatic. Pupils may be miotic if the patient is taking certain drugs for glaucoma or is on heroin. They may be abnormally large in cases of ocular contusion, systemic poisoning, and neurologic disease of the midbrain (see Chap. 12, sec. **III**).

   b. **The pupil is normally** round in shape. In the absence of surgical manipulation, irregularity is almost always pathologic. The shape may be affected by congenital abnormality, scarring down from iritis, syphilis, trauma, or the presence of surgically placed intraocular lenses (IOLs).

   c. **The direct light reflex** is tested in a semidark room with a light brought in from the side. The pupil should contract to direct light as well as when light is shined in the pupil of the opposite side; this latter response is the **consensual** reaction to light. Reaction to accommodation is tested by holding a finger approximately 10 cm away from the eye being tested. The patient is asked to look at the finger and then at the far wall directly beyond it. The pupil normally constricts when looking at the near object and dilates when looking at the far object. Under normal conditions, if the pupil reacts to light, it will react to accommodation as well. The Argyll Robertson pupil is a condition due to CNS lues and occasionally to herpes zoster in which there is a failure of direct and consensual light response but a normal reaction to accommodation. Adie's tonic pupil responds to either stimulation but abnormally slowly.

12. **The lens** may be observed under magnification for opacity using either a loupe or the plus lenses of an ophthalmoscope. This procedure is more easily done with the pupil dilated so that as much of the lens as possible may be seen. The examiner should also note the central location of the lens and its stability in position (partially dislocated lenses are tremulous) as well as its translucency. Difficulty in viewing the fundus through the lens is indicative of a significant cataract. The hazier the view into the eye, the hazier the view out of it for the patient.

E. **Slit-lamp biomicroscopy of anterior segment and fundus.** Biomicroscopy involves examination of the external ocular structures and the front of the eye to a depth of the anterior vitreous using a specially designed microscope and light source. Use of a slit lamp is indicated in any condition where examination is facilitated and made more accurate by a well-illuminated and highly magnified view of the anterior segment of the eye, e.g., corneal ulcerations, iris tumors, cataract evaluation. The fundi are seen by placing a Goldmann three-mirror lens with a central fundus lens on the cornea, swinging a Hruby lens (−40 diopters [d]) into position, or hand holding a 78- or 90-d aspheric lens before the eye. The examiner then shines the slit beam through the **dilated pupil** slightly at an angle to focus on the retina, thus obtaining a stereoscopic view under high magnification. This is especially useful for evaluating macular edema, optic nerve lesions, or other posterior pole lesions. It is less useful for the peripheral retina but is useful out to the equator. One should note that the view is inverted with the aspheric lenses. Patient and examiner are seated on either side of the slit lamp, the patient placing the chin on a chin rest and the *forehead against a frame* while the examiner views the eye through the microscope. By moving the microscope in and out with a hand control, the examiner can adjust the depth of focus so that the object of interest is brought clearly into view. The general order of examination is to start with the lid and then progress to conjunctiva, cornea, anterior chamber, iris and pupil, lens, and anterior vitreous. Techniques for views of the deeper vitreous, retina, and optic nerve are described above.

1. **Special dyes** such as fluorescein to detect ulcerations or rose bengal to detect dead and dying cells on the ocular surface may be used. With fluorescein, a cobalt filter is swung into place to delineate clearly the areas of epithelial absence. A white light is used for rose bengal staining.

2. **The slit-lamp beam** may be widened to a full circle to illuminate the entire front of the eye or narrowed to a tiny slit that will assist the examiner in determining the thickness of various anterior segment structures. The tissue illuminated by the narrow beam is referred to as an *optical section* and represents an optical cut through the various depths of tissue. The cornea and lens under magnification and illuminated by the intense narrow beam of focal light passing from the slit lamp may be seen to be made up of multiple layers of different optical densities. Layers seen in a normal cornea are epithelium, stroma, and endothelium; those in a normal lens are cortex and nucleus. Opacities and other local pathologic processes can be located with great accuracy in the anterior segment using the slit lamp.

3. **The slit-lamp beam may also be narrowed to a single fine point of light** that can be focused through the front of the eye to reveal changes in the density of the **aqueous fluid** in the anterior chamber. Such changes are particularly significant in the presence of intraocular inflammation or trauma. Cells or increased protein in the aqueous or cells in the vitreous, invisible with ordinary illumination and magnification, may be seen using the narrow beam of the slit lamp (the Tyndall phenomenon). In a normal person the aqueous humor is clear or optically empty, but with increased protein content, as in intraocular inflammation, the beam is visible and referred to as aqueous flare. Its intensity may be measured by a subjective rating used by the observer, ranging from 0–4+. (See also Chap. 8.)

F. **Intraocular pressure (IOP) measurements for glaucoma or hypotony**

1. **Finger tension.** A rough but reasonably accurate determination of IOP may be made by palpation of the eyeball through closed lids. The patient is asked to look down (but not close the eyes) and the examiner places two forefingers on the upper lid over the globe, exerting pressure alternately with each forefinger while the other rests on the globe. Pressure just sufficient to indent the globe slightly should be applied. In the absence of inflammation this is a painless procedure, but it should be avoided if rupture of the globe is suspected. After experience with palpating a number of normal eyeballs, the examiner will learn what normal resistance is and by comparison may determine whether an eyeball is either too hard or too soft. With increased experience the examiner may estimate within 3–5 mm Hg the actual IOP.

2. **Tonometry.** Accurate IOP may be determined by use of tonometers. If the IOP is between 22 and 25 mm Hg or more, glaucoma must be considered. Visual field and ophthalmoscopic study of the nerve head should be performed and tonometry readings repeated at different hours of the day to determine diurnal curve, or tonography should be performed (or both) (see sec. **3**). Pressures greater than 25 mm Hg are generally accepted as being ocular hypertensive. In the presence of a visual field defect or asymmetric or marked cupping of the optic nerve head, the diagnosis of glaucoma may be definitely established.

   a. **The Schiötz tonometer** is the device most commonly used by the general physician for measuring IOP. It consists of a foot plate curved to fit the average normal cornea, with a metal plunger in the center for holding various weights. On top of the plunger is a short, curved arm with a lever whose long arm is a pointer for reading positions on a scale. The 0 reading on the scale is seen when the ocular end of the plunger fits flush with the curved foot plate. As the plunger indents the cornea, the scale reading increases according to the resistance encountered. Each

A **B**

Fig. 1-3. A. Technique of Schiötz tonometry. Digital pressure on the globe is avoided.
B. Applanation tonometry. The applanation tonometer may be handheld or mounted
on a slit-lamp biomicroscope. (Adapted from D. Paton and J. Craig, *Glaucomas:
Diagnosis and Management.* Clinical Symposia. Summit, N.J.: Ciba Pharmaceutical
Co., 1976, with permission.)

instrument is accompanied by a graph that expresses the scale readings
in millimeters of mercury of internal pressure within the eye.
  b. **Technique of Schiötz tonometry.** After the instillation of local anesthesia, such as one drop of proparacaine or tetracaine, the patient is
placed in a supine position and asked to look directly upward, fixing on
some object such as his or her extended hand. The physician separates
the lids to keep them from contacting the eyeball, taking care not to
exert pressure on the globe (Fig. 1–3A). The instrument is placed gently
in a vertical position over the cornea, and the plunger is allowed
to exert its full weight. With the instrument held steady the pointer
will stay fixed at a single scale, with slight oscillations 0.5 mm in either
direction because of alterations in the internal pressure caused by the
arterial pulse in the eye. If the reading with the 5.5-gm weight is between 3 and 6 on the scale, this reading may be used. Readings below
3 are inaccurate with this instrument, and a 7.5-gm weight should be
added and the reading taken again. If the reading is still below 3, the
10-gm weight should be used. If the patient squeezes his or her lids, this
will raise the IOP; note should be made of this, as a falsely high pressure
may be recorded. Schiötz tonometry tends to be less accurate in myopic
patients or patients with thyroid ocular disease. Applanation tonometry
is more accurate in these patients.

c. **Applanation tonometry.** This very accurate method for measuring IOP may be performed with an applanation tonometer mounted on a routine slit-lamp biomicroscope or with a handheld applanation tonometer (Fig. 1–3B). After local anesthesia is induced as with Schiötz tonometry, fluorescein paper strips are inserted into the lower cul-de-sac to place dye in the tear film. The tonometer scale is set at 0 and the head is then brought gently against the anterior corneal surface with the patient looking straight ahead. On contact and with the cobalt blue light in place, two fluorescein semicircles are seen through the microscope, one higher than the other; the top with the outer curve up and the bottom with the outer curve down. The semicircles should be equal in size and in the middle of the field of view. Their steady pulsation indicates that the instrument is in the correct position. Pressure on the eye is increased by turning the calibrated dial of the tonometer until the inner border of each semicircle just touches and overlaps with each pulsation. The pressure reading is determined directly by reading from the measuring drum. This reading is multiplied by 10 and is the measurement of the IOP in millimeters of mercury. This machine is more accurate than Schiötz tonometry in patients with altered scleral rigidity (myopia, thyroid disease). The flow of volumetric displacement of 9.56 nm increases the IOPs by only 2.5% as compared with the much greater volumetric displacement encountered with Schiötz tonometry.

d. **The pneumotonometer** is an electronic tonometer that has its greatest use in patients with corneal scarring or altered corneal shape such that conventional Schiötz or applanation tonometers cannot be employed with any accuracy. The tip of a blunt pencil-like device connected by wire to an electronic recorder is momentarily touched to the anesthetized cornea. Pressure is calculated by the jump in scale readings from baseline noncontact curve to that of the momentary touch flattening the cornea or indicated directly on a digital screen.

e. **The air puff noncontact tonometer** is an accurate electronic tonometer that has the advantage of use without topical anesthetic. The patient sits with the head in a slit-lamp-like device, and a 3-msec puff of air (a blink takes 10 msec) is blown against the cornea. The indentation pattern is detected by the tonometer eye. The pressure is calculated by the amount of corneal flattening by the fixed air puff pressure and displayed on digital readout. This machine is ideal for use in mass glaucoma-screening programs.

3. **Tonography (aqueous outflow studies).** Tonography is the indirect measurement of the rate of aqueous outflow from the anterior chamber.

a. **Purpose.** This technique is of particular use in those patients who run high normal IOPs, but in whom the actual diagnosis of glaucoma is difficult despite multiple office visits and determinations of IOP. It is useful in distinguishing those patients who are at the high end of a bell-shaped curve of normal IOPs from those who actually have glaucoma.

b. **Techniques.** Tonography is based on change in IOP occurring while an electronic Schiötz-type tonometer is applied to the eye for 4 continuous minutes. The instrument is generally used only by specialists in the field, as precise technique is necessary for accurate interpretation of the findings. After instillation of local anesthetic drops, the patient lies on a table and fixes his or her gaze on a spot directly above the head. The tonometer is then allowed to rest on the patient's cornea for 4 minutes. The IOP is read in millimeters of mercury from the electronic scale. The procedure is then repeated on the other eye. The graph continuously records the decrease in intraocular tension, and the difference between the first and last readings is correlated with this graph to determine the facility of aqueous outflow.

c. **Interpretation.** The normal coefficient of outflow factor is greater than 0.2. If it is less than this, the patient is suspected of having glaucoma.

In the absence of other clinical evidence of glaucoma, such as asymmetric or abnormal cupping of the nerve head or abnormal visual field defects, the patient should be reexamined every 6 months, as he or she is a high-risk candidate for glaucoma.

G. Direct ophthalmoscopy

   1. **Examination of the posterior segment of the eye** (vitreous, optic nerve head or disk, vessels, retina, choroid) is performed with the aid of an ophthalmoscope. A satisfactory examination of the posterior pole can usually be made through an undilated pupil, provided that the media (aqueous, lens, vitreous) are clear; however, a greater extent of the peripheral posterior segment can be examined through a dilated pupil. Ophthalmoscopy is best done in a darkened room.

   2. **For optimum dilated fundus examination,** mydriatic agents in common use are cyclopentolate 0.5% or tropicamide 1%; phenylephrine 2.5% may be used, but with caution in any patient with a history of cardiovascular disease. No mydriatic agent should be instilled in an eye in which a shallow anterior chamber is suspected. An estimate of the anterior chamber depth can be made by illuminating it from the side with a penlight. **If the iris seems abnormally close to the cornea, dilation should be foregone because of the risk of inducing acute angle-closure glaucoma** (see Chap. 9, sec. III). A slit-lamp beam depth of less than four corneal thicknesses is also indicative of possible shallow chamber and is a relative contraindication to dilation.

   3. **Ophthalmoscopes.** There are many forms of ophthalmoscopes, the most commonly used being handheld ophthalmoscopes designed for direct magnified (14×) view. The source of illumination is projected by means of a mirror or prism coinciding with the observer's line of vision through the aperture.

   4. **Technique of ophthalmoscopy.** The ophthalmoscope is held close to the observer's eye and approximately 15 cm from the patient's eye in the observer's right hand to examine the patient's right eye and in the observer's left hand to examine the patient's left eye. The observer uses his or her right eye for the patient's right eye and his or her left eye for the patient's left eye. The patient should not be wearing glasses and should be fixating on a distant target with the eye as steady as possible. From time to time the patient may have to be reminded to refixate on a distant target to avoid accommodation from interfering with the observer's level of focus within the eye. The physician may have to adjust the ophthalmoscope power setting to accommodate for the patient's refractive error or his or her own—red numbered minus lenses for nearsighted errors, black numbered plus lenses for farsighted errors. Eyes that have had cataracts removed (aphakia) should be examined with a +8 to +12 lens for view of the fundus, with the ophthalmoscope held close to the patient's eye. If both patient and examiner have normal eyes and the lens is set at 0, a red reflex will be seen and is considered normal. Moving the ophthalmoscope as close to the patient's eye as possible, the observer uses black or positive lenses. Lens settings of +4 to +8 will focus the ophthalmoscope on the anterior segment to reveal corneal opacities or changes in the iris and lens. The retina in a normal eye will focus at 0, provided that no refractive error is present. By decreasing the power of the lens from + toward −, the depth of focus will become greater so that the examiner may move from the anterior segment progressively through structures until the vitreous and retina are reached.

   5. **Vitreous opacities** such as hemorrhages and floaters should be localized and noted, and changes in the posterior segment structures focused and studied.

   6. **The optic nerve head** should be brought into focus and examined. This structure is generally circular to oval with vertical orientation and pink in color. The temporal side is usually lighter pink than the nasal side. The center of the disk may have some depression, which is referred to as the

physiologic cup, the bottom of which may be fibrous in appearance and represents the fibers of the lamina cribrosa of the sclera. Normal cupping may vary from absence to 80% involvement of the nerve head. In the presence of extensive or asymmetric cupping, glaucoma should be suspected. In optic atrophy the entire nerve head will be pale; in papilledema or papillitis it will be swollen and congested. The size of the normal nerve head may vary with the refractive error of the patient, being small in farsighted patients and large in myopic patients. The border of the nerve head is usually discretely demarcated from the retina, but may merge gradually into the surrounding tissue without any clear-cut edge. A white border representing a scleral ring or crescent is often present and formed by exposure of sclera between the choroidal vasculature and the opening for the optic nerve. There may be excessive pigment in this area due to the presence of choroidal pigment.

7. **Fundic lesions** should be measured using the disk diameter (dd) as a reference size. For example, a retinal scar may be described as being 3 dd in size and located 5 dd nasal to the nerve head at 1 o'clock. Elevation of this lesion may also be measured by noting the difference between lens powers that clearly focus the top of the lesion and an adjacent normal area of the fundus. Elevation of 3-d lens change would be equivalent to approximately 1 mm in actual elevation. Multiples of this may be made according to the size and height of the lesion.

8. **Retinal arteries and veins (AV).** The arteries are red and smaller than the veins in about a 4:5 ratio. Because of a thicker wall, the arteries have a shiny central reflex stripe. The column of blood traversing these vessels may be seen through the transparent walls. Branching is variable. The examiner should evaluate the transparency of the vessels, the presence of pressure effects such as AV compression (nicking) where vessels cross each other, and presence of focal narrowing of arterioles, as well as increased tortuosity and widening of venules, hemorrhages, and exudates around the vessels. Round hemorrhages may occur in patients with diabetes mellitus and are generally located between the posterior vitreous face and the retina. Flame-shaped hemorrhages are usually intraretinal and are commonly found in patients with high blood pressure and blood dyscrasias.

9. **The macular area** located about 2 dd temporal to the optic nerve head is darker than the surrounding retina and in a young person will have a lustrous central yellow point called the fovea centralis (see frontispiece). This appears as a small area of dark red with a tiny yellow light reflex at the center of the fovea. The foveal reflex dulls with age or certain drug-induced retinal toxicities.

10. **The periphery of the fundus** may be examined by the movement of the ophthalmoscope in various directions as well as by having the patient move the eye in various quadrants horizontal and vertical. Through a dilated pupil, the periphery can be seen directly with a direct ophthalmoscope up to 1.5 mm from the peripheral retinal attachment (ora serrata).

11. **Normal variations of the fundus.** With increased experience the observer will become acquainted with a wide range of normal variations. Vasculature is particularly variable. Vessels may appear from the temporal half of the nerve head and run to the macular area. These cilioretinal vessels originate from the vascular circle of Zinn behind the nerve head in the sclera and are formed by branches from the short posterior ciliary arteries. They represent anastomosis between the choroidal (ciliary) and retinal circulation. Occasionally, a tuft of connective tissue arises from the nerve head on its nasal side and projects forward into the vitreous. This embryonic remnant of the hyaloid artery is located in the surrounding canal of Cloquet. If located near the edge of the nerve head, the disk margin may appear blurred or even elevated. Such persistent hyaloid remnants do not interfere with vision unless associated with other ocular defects. Medullated nerve fibers are another normal variation and may be seen as striking projections of white feathery tissue originating near the optic disk and extending for variable

distances into the peripheral retina. Visual field defects may be present in the area of myelination of the nerve fibers running in this area. Drusen, small round hyaline excrescences formed on Bruch's membrane, may create variations in elevation of the nerve head or scalloping of its border, or they may more commonly occur as scattered small yellow lesions in the peripheral fundus. They may occasionally produce pseudopapilledema of the nerve head, but no visual field defect will be present except for enlargement of the blind spot.

H. Indirect ophthalmoscopy is a technique generally used by specialists and involves the use of a head-mounted, prism-directed light source coupled with use of a high (+14, +20, or +30) diopter condensing lens to see the retinal image.

   1. Optics. Several designs of indirect ophthalmoscopes are available, but all produce an image that is inverted, real, and capable of being seen on a semitransparent film held at the focal plane of the lens. Although most indirect ophthalmoscopes are designed for use through dilated pupils, some may be used through a miotic or undilated pupil; this is a great advantage in patients who cannot be dilated either because they do not respond to topical drugs, are angle-closure glaucoma risks, or have scarring of the pupil to the lens.

   2. The image seen with the indirect ophthalmoscope is a brilliantly illuminated, binocular, stereoscopic one that covers approximately 10 times the area usually seen in the field of the direct ophthalmoscope. The image, however, is smaller than a direct ophthalmoscope ($3\times$), although the larger field of view gives great perspective to the entire fundus and is helpful in locating multiple lesions or in evaluating retinal detachment. Another advantage is stronger illumination, which allows light to pass through opacities of the vitreous obstructive to a direct ophthalmoscope. See sec. **E** for the use of lenses for magnified stereoscopic view of the posterior pole.

I. Visual field testing (see also Chap. 12, sec. I)

   1. The purpose of visual field testing is to determine both the outer limits of visual perception by the peripheral retina as well as the varying qualities of vision within that area. Visual field interpretation is important for diagnosing disease, localizing it in the visual pathway between the retina and the occipital cortex in the brain, and noting its progress, stability, or remission. As a result, repeated tests of the visual field are important both diagnostically and in ascertaining the effects of therapy. Each eye is tested separately. With one eye fixing on a given distant test object, the sensitivity of various areas of the visual field may be tested with varying size and color test objects moved throughout that field. The greatest sensitivity, of course, is at the fovea and represents the highest visual acuity of central fixation. This visual acuity drops off rapidly as the test objects are moved away from central fixation. Colored objects offer less stimulus to the retina than white objects of similar size. Therefore, an object may be too small to be detected by peripheral retinal receptors but quite effective in mapping out central visual field within 10–15 degrees of foveal fixation.

   2. Techniques. Visual fields are examined most frequently by four methods: Amsler grid, confrontation, perimetry, and tangent screen.

      a. Amsler charts for qualitative vision evaluation make it possible to analyze the earliest maculopathies and their progression as well as to detect any scotomatous defects encroaching on the central 10 degrees of vision.

         (1) Technique. The small book of six charts contains diffusely dotted or lined square grids 10 cm on the side, the latter with smaller 5-mm squares within. With the chart held at 30 cm from the patient's eye, the linear measurements correspond to visual angles of 20 degrees and 1 degree, respectively. The patient stares at the center of the squares one eye at a time. Alterations in perception of the regular patterns indicate various field defects.

         (2) Purpose. The examiner may find central scotomas as in macular scarring, cecocentral scotomas as in toxic amblyopias, paracentral scotomas as in chorioretinitis, and metamorphopsia (distortion of vision) as in very early maculopathies. The edge of a glaucomatous Bjerrum scotoma, a peripheral field defect secondary to central nervous system, or peripheral retinal disease encroaching on the central 10 degrees of vision will also be detected.

b. **Confrontation.** No special instruments are required for this form of visual field testing, which provides a rough estimate of the patient's visual field by comparing it with the examiner's visual field. It is assumed that the examiner's visual field is normal.

(1) **Technique.** The patient and examiner face each other at a distance of 1 m. With the left eye covered, the patient is instructed to look with the right eye at the left eye of the examiner, whose own right eye is covered. A small object such as a pencil or a larger one such as a wiggling finger may be used as a target. The examiner places her hand midway between the patient and herself and initially beyond the limits of field of vision of either in a given meridian, e.g., far temporal to both patient and examiner. As the test object is moved slowly toward the line of vision between patient and examiner, the patient is asked to respond as soon as he is able to see the target. The physician compares this to the time when she is able to perceive the target. This is repeated at eight to ten equally spaced meridians at approximately 360 degrees. The visual field is considered normal if the patient sees the target 90 degrees temporally, 50 degrees nasally, 50 degrees upward, and 65 degrees downward. The test is then repeated on the other eye. With careful testing the blind spot and focal scotomas may be picked up.

(2) **Purpose.** This test may also pick up gross alteration in field defects due to ocular disease such as chorioretinitis or advanced glaucoma or to intracranial disease such as brain tumor or hemorrhage.

c. **Perimetry.** For accurate examination of the peripheral extent of the visual field, special equipment such as a Goldmann perimeter or automated perimeter, such as the Humphrey or Octopus, is needed. In addition to varying target size, most perimeters can vary target brightness as well. Goldmann perimetry is **kinetic** testing and involves moving a constantly suprathreshold test object from nonseeing to seeing areas of vision. Size I is 0.25 mm^2 and size V is 64 mm^2 with gradations in between. Luminance varies from 32 apostilbs (1 e) to 1000 apostilbs (4 e) with 10 gradations in between. Automated perimeters are **static** (nonmoving) test targets flashed at different locations. Most provide normal values and compare the patient to normal in the printout of the results. The Humphrey will also give a probability that any test location is not normal dependent on patient age and location in the visual field. The **Octopus** detects threshold sensitivity to a light stimulus at 72 points in the visual field. The intensity of the stimulus is carried to below threshold and worked up to suprathreshold. Its advantages are that the Octopus picks up the earliest, most subtle field defects, the results are reproducible, and progression of subtle or gross defects may easily be documented. The disadvantages of all automated perimeters are subjective patient fatigue, the expense of the machines, and the need for trained personnel to run them.

Visual field examination is indicated when the physician detects or suspects a disorder that has constricted the side, paracentral, or central vision. In uncooperative patients the results of this test are unreliable.

(1) **Technique.** The patient is seated at the perimeter with one eye covered and the chin on the chin rest. The patient must fix his or her vision on the central target of the perimeter and a test target, static or kinetic as just described, is presented at some location in the field. The patient is asked to signal immediately when he or she

sees the target, indicate when it disappears, and indicate again when it reappears. By the end of the test, the entire 360 degrees of field have been mapped out.

(2) Purpose. The examiner may accurately map defects in the peripheral vision all the way from the far extent of the field into central or foveal fixation. The smaller the test target used, the greater the possibility of discovering scotomas in the field.

d. Tangent screen. Up to 90% of all visual field defects in the central 30 degrees may be picked up using this second method of kinetic perimetry (a suprathreshold stimulus moving from nonseeing to seeing areas of vision). It is not as sensitive in picking up early defects as the Goldmann or automated perimeters.

(1) Technique. The patient is seated 1 m from a 2-m² black screen with a direct line of fixation on the central object in the tangent screen. One eye is tested at a time. A 3- to 50-mm white test object is brought in from the periphery, exploring 8–10 meridians from periphery to central fixation, as in perimetry. The patient indicates immediately perception of the object, when it disappears, and when it reappears so that the examiner may map areas of decreased or absent vision. The blind spot should be outlined carefully and early in the examination to show the patient the nature of scotoma mapping. The findings, including the size and color of the test object and the distance from the screen, are charted. *Color fields* with red and blue test objects are most useful in the central 10–15 degrees of vision and may be the test that picks up early toxic retinopathy soonest.

(2) Purpose. The results of this uncomplicated but fairly accurate central field test are charted for present disease detection, future reference, and comparison with earlier tests.

J. Tear film adequacy: clinical tests. The testing of tear film adequacy may be divided into three separate areas: (1) tear quantity, (2) tear quality, and (3) tear secretion. Each is of importance in determining the role of the tear film in the symptomatology and pathologic changes noted in dry eye syndromes.

1. Tear quantity test. Tear secretion may be divided into basal and reflex secretion. Basal secretion is maintained by the accessory conjunctival lacrimal glands of Krause and Wolfring. Reflex secretion is a product of the main lacrimal gland. Accurate interpretation of tests requires assessment of the role that reflex tearing played during the test. The average basal tear volume is from 5–9 µl with a flow rate of 0.5–2.2 µl/minute. Unlike reflex tearing, this parameter is not age dependent, and basal volume or flow rate does not normally decrease in elderly persons. The majority of clinical complications of tear volume, however, result from hyposecretion. The epithelium, cornea, and conjunctiva are extremely sensitive to decreased tear volume, especially in the exposed interpalpebral area. The early effects of dryness are degeneration and death of epithelial cells, which may progress in severe cases to keratinization of the cornea and conjunctiva.

a. Schirmer test I. The purpose of this test is the measurement of the **total (reflex and basal) tear secretion.** To minimize reflex tearing, the eyes should not be manipulated before starting this test. There is no contraindication to this test. The materials used are commercially available Whatman No. 41 filter paper strips 5 mm wide × 30 mm in length, known as Schirmer tear test filter strips. The patient is seated in a dimly lit room, and the filter paper strips are folded 5 mm from the end. The folded end is placed gently over the lower palpebral conjunctiva at its lateral one-third. The patient keeps the eyes open and looks upward. Blinking is permissible. After 5 minutes the strips are removed and the amount of wetting is measured from the folded end. If the strips are completely wetted before 5 minutes, they may be removed prematurely. A normal patient will wet from 10–30 mm in 5 minutes; this is age dependent and decreases after the age of 60 but is rarely less than 10 mm in 5 minutes. Measurements greater than 30 mm at 5 minutes indicate that reflex tearing is intact but not controlled and, therefore, are of little diagnostic value. Between 10 and 30 mm of tear secretion may be normal, or basal secretion may be low but compensated for by reflex secretion. Values less than 5 mm on repeated testing indicate hyposecretion of basic tearing. There is a 15% chance of diagnostic error in this test.

b. **Basic secretion test.** The purpose of this test is to measure the basal secretion by eliminating reflex tearing. Topical anesthetic is instilled into the conjunctiva and a few minutes allowed to pass until reactive hyperemia has subsided. The room is darkened and the procedure is the same as in the Schirmer test I. Interpretation of the results is also similar. The difference between the results of this test and those of the Schirmer test I is a measurement of reflex secretion contraindications and any contraindication to the local anesthetic. Materials used are the Schirmer strip and proparacaine 0.5%.

c. **Schirmer test II.** The purpose of this test is to ascertain **reflex secretion.** The procedure is similar to the basal secretion test, but after the strips are installed, the unanesthetized nasal mucosa is irritated by rubbing with a dry cotton-tipped applicator. The amount of wetting of the filter paper is measured after 2 minutes. Less than 15 mm of wetting indicates failure of reflex secretion. Since this failure is not of major clinical consequence, the test is seldom used. Contraindications are the same as for the basal secretion test or the presence of nasal pathologic conditions. Materials used are the same as for basal secretion test.

d. **Rose bengal staining.** The purpose of this test is to ascertain indirectly the presence of reduced tear volume through **detection of damaged epithelial cells.** The eye is anesthetized topically with proparacaine 0.5%. Tetracaine or cocaine may give false-positive tests because of their softening effect on corneal epithelium. One drop of 1% rose bengal solution is instilled in each conjunctival sac. Rose bengal is a vital stain taken up by dead and degenerating cells that have been damaged by the reduced tear volume, particularly in the exposed interpalpebral area. This test is particularly useful in early stages of conjunctivitis sicca and keratoconjunctivitis sicca syndrome. A positive test will show triangular stipple staining of the nasal and temporal bulbar conjunctiva in the interpalpebral area and possible punctate staining of the cornea, especially in the lower two-thirds. False-positive staining may occur in conditions such as chronic conjunctivitis, acute chemical conjunctivitis secondary to hair spray use and drugs such as tetracaine and cocaine, exposure keratitis, superficial punctate keratitis secondary to toxic or idiopathic phenomena, and foreign bodies in the conjunctiva. The stain will also color mucus and epithelial debris, which may mask the results. Certain patients who are normal will show some positive staining to rose bengal on the cornea. Because of this, conjunctival as well as corneal staining should be present before the diagnosis of keratoconjunctivitis sicca is made.

2. **Tear quality test** involves tests for the presence of mucus, protein, and tear film stability. Mucin lowers the surface tension of the tears and converts the hydrophobic corneal epithelial surface to a wettable hydrophilic surface. Mucin is produced by conjunctival goblet cells and spread by the action of the lids over the corneal epithelium. Mucin-deficient diseases such as Stevens-Johnson syndrome and pemphigus result in corneal dessication despite normal tear volume, due to the lack of mucus as a wetting agent.

a. **A conjunctival biopsy** may be done to ascertain the presence or absence of mucin-producing goblet cells. Four percent cocaine solution on a cotton-tipped swab is applied directly to the lower nasal fornix, an area containing the highest population of goblet cells. After 60 seconds a Vannas scissors and a jeweler's forceps are used to excise a conjunctival

sample 5 mm long × 2 mm deep. The tissue is spread gently on a 2- ×
2-cm cardboard, epithelial side up until it is flat. The cardboard is placed
in 95% alcohol and sent to the pathology laboratory with a request for
periodic acid Schiff (PAS) stain. Histologically, the normal lower nasal
fornix contains from 10–14 goblet cells/field at 200×. In a mucin-deficient state this population is markedly diminished or absent. This
procedure is extremely simple and painless. The conjunctiva heals rapidly over a 24- to 48-hour period. Local antibiotic ointment such as
erythromycin or bacitracin should be instilled.

   b. A qualitative mucous assay may be performed to determine the presence of mucus. Cotton strips 3 × 10 mm are placed in the inferior cul-
   de-sac of the unanesthetized eye for 5 minutes. Each strip is then placed
   on a glass slide and stained with PAS reagent. Color change is noted 1
   minute later and compared with a sample from a known normal subject.
   If adequate mucus is present the strip will show a positive PAS reaction,
   turning dark purple. In the absence of mucus the reaction is negative.
   This test may be meaningful only in those eyes containing at least some
   tear film.

3. **Tear film stability.** After a certain time interval following blinking, the tear
   film normally ruptures and forms dry spots. Increased meibomian gland
   secretion possibly may act to decrease tear film stability. Deficiency of mucin and aqueous tears will also decrease the tear film stability and shorten
   the time interval between the opening of the eye and the appearance of dry
   spots.

   a. The technique of tear film break-up time (BUT). No anesthesia is
   used. A small amount of fluorescein is instilled in the lower cul-de-sac,
   and a blue cobalt filtered light from flashlight source or the slit lamp is
   used to observe the tear film over the cornea with the eyes kept wide
   open. The time of appearance of the dry spot formation (small black
   spots within the blue-green field) from the last blink measures the tear
   BUT.

   b. Interpretation of BUT. A wetting time greater than 20 seconds reflects
   a normal tear film stability. BUT less than 10 seconds indicates significant tear film instability. The greater the number of dry spots, the more
   unstable the tear film. The consistent appearance of dry spots in one
   area indicates an anatomic surface abnormality in that area. Abnormal
   BUT is invariably seen in clinically significant sicca and mucin-deficient syndromes. Local anesthetic or tonometry prior to testing or holding the lids apart with the fingers will give false-positive testing.

K. **Tear secretion tests.** Tests of tear secretion are important in ascertaining the
   etiology of chronic tearing (epiphora). The causes of epiphora can be divided
   into (1) partial or complete obstruction of the excretory canal, (2) increased
   lacrimal secretion (see sec. **J.1**), and (3) decreased basal lacrimal secretion with
   secondary reflex tearing (see sec. **J.1**). Tear excretion involves the pumping
   action of the lids and good anatomic apposition of the patent punctal openings
   against the globe. Any lid abnormality such as entropion, ectropion, or punctal
   occlusion may be associated with chronic tearing. Examination of the eyelids
   prior to the test may reveal an anatomic etiology for chronic tearing rather
   than a deficiency of the deeper nasolacrimal canal drainage system.

   1. **Regurgitation test** is the test of the excretory patency medial to the lac-
      rimal sac (canalicular canals running in the lid margin). The examiner gently
      compresses the skin over and around the medial canthal ligament while
      observing the punctum under magnification. Obstruction medial to the lac-
      rimal sac, i.e., in the canal, results in regurgitation of fluid, often mucoid
      or purulent, through the punctum when pressure is applied over the lacrimal
      sac. This obstruction is almost always complete and is usually associated
      with inflammation in the sac (dacryocystitis).

   2. **The primary dye test** is used to test the patency of the entire excretory
      system (the nasolacrimal drainage system into the back of the nose). Fluo-

rescein is instilled into the lower cul-de-sac. A small wisp of cotton on the end of a wire cotton applicator or a sterile cotton tip is placed 3.8 cm into the nose under the inferior meatus. (This is along the floor of the nasal canal.) After 2 minutes the cotton is removed and examined. If the cotton is fluorescein-stained, the test is positive and the system is patent and functioning. If there is no dye on the cotton, either the cotton was misplaced or the excretory mechanism is obstructed. There is no localizing value regarding the site of obstruction within the nasolacrimal canal.

3. **The secondary dye test** (lacrimal irrigation test) is another test of the excretory patency and is used if the primary dye test is negative. A 2-ml syringe is filled with saline and a lacrimal cannula attached to it. This cannula is placed in the lower canaliculus, entering through the lower punctum, and the saline is injected. The patient leans forward and the naris on the ipsilateral side is observed. If the patient tastes the saline in his or her throat or if fluorescein fluid comes from the naris, the test is positive. If the primary dye test is negative and the secondary dye test positive, the system is partially blocked. If both tests are negative, the excretory system is totally blocked. There is no localizing value to this test for lesions within the nasolacrimal system. As the pressure of the injection may open a partially obstructed system, lacrimal irrigation without performing the primary dye test may be misleading.

4. **Canaliculus testing** is a test for the patency of the canaliculi or canals running in the lid margin. Clear saline is injected through the punctum of one canaliculus using a 2-ml syringe and lacrimal cannula. The opposite punctum on the same eye is observed. If saline returns through the other canaliculus, both are patent and the obstruction is in or beyond the common canaliculus beyond the medial canthus. If no fluid comes from the opposite punctum, at least one of the canaliculi is obstructed. This test is contraindicated in the presence of acute inflammation of the lacrimal sac.

5. **Dacryocystography** for localization of obstruction site is discussed under radiographic techniques (see sec. III.F.6).

L. **Transillumination**

1. **Intraocular tumors** may often be detected by transillumination of the globe. Intense light, such as that from a small handheld flashlight, placed on the sclera in successive quadrants behind the ciliary body will be transmitted inside the eye, where it produces a red reflex in the pupil. Intraocular masses, such as malignant melanoma containing pigment, will block the light when it is placed over the tumor, thus diminishing or preventing the red reflex. The presence of tumor under a retinal detachment (detachments are commonly caused by intraocular tumors) may be detected in this manner; the test is also useful for distinguishing a retinal detachment due to other causes than tumor. Normally, retinal detachment will not interfere with the normal red reflex so produced.

2. **Atrophy of the iris pigment layer** or ciliary body may also be revealed by transillumination. Such atrophy is frequently seen in patients with chronic intraocular inflammation. This test should be performed in a completely darkened room, with the examiner dark adapted and the instrument placed 8 mm posterior to the limbus to avoid the ciliary body, which would normally cut off light entering the eye.

M. **Exophthalmometry.** The exophthalmometer **(Hertel)** is used to determine the degree of anterior projection or prominence of the eyes. This instrument is helpful in diagnosing and in following the course of exophthalmus.

1. **Technique.** The patient holds the head straight and looks directly at the examiner's eyes. Two small concave attachments of the exophthalmometer are placed against the lateral orbital margins, and the distance between these two points is recorded from the central bar. This distance must be constant for all successive examinations in order to judge accurately the status of ocular protrusion. The examiner views the cornea of the patient's

right eye in the mirror while the patient fixes the right eye on the examiner's left eye. Simultaneously, the cornea is lined up in the mirror with the scale, which reads directly in millimeters. A similar reading is then taken from the left eye with the patient fixing on the examiner's right eye. The bar reading and the degree of exophthalmus are then recorded in millimeters; e.g., a bar reading of 100 might have right eye 17 mm, left eye 18 mm.

2. **Interpretation.** The normal range of exophthalmometry readings is 12–20 mm. The readings are normally within 2 mm of each other and indicate the anterior distances from the corneas to the lateral orbital margins. Exophthalmus is present if the reading is greater than 20 mm in one eye and indicates a search for an underlying cause such as thyroid ocular disease or orbital tumor. A disparity of 3 mm or greater between readings taken from each eye during a test is also an indication for further investigation, even though both readings may fall within the normal range.

N. **Placido disk and Klein keratoscope.** These simple instruments are useful in the diagnosis of corneal reflex regularity and irregular astigmatism. The presence of a pathologic state, such as subtle or gross scarring or early keratoconus, will cause the normally regular concentric circles viewed through the keratoscope or disk to be asymmetric or frankly distorted and irregular. The examiner holds the disk or keratoscope to his or her eye and observes the illuminated cornea of the patient through the aperture. Distortion or roughening of the rings may account for marked decrease in vision through a cornea that may appear normal on initial examination. A focally indented area in the rings indicates a shortening of that meridian such as from a tight suture that may need to be cut to relieve astigmatism.

O. **Keratometry.** The keratometer is an instrument generally used by specialists for measuring corneal astigmatism in two main meridians. It is particularly useful in the fitting of corneal contact lenses but may also be used to detect irregular astigmatism and early pathologic states such as keratoconus. Successive readings several months apart will indicate progression or stability of corneal disease. The device is similar to a slit lamp in use. The corneal reflex is evaluated for regularity and measured at 90-degree axes in the two meridians of greatest difference, i.e., the flattest and steepest planes.

P. **Gonioscopy.** The visually inaccessible **anterior chamber angle** may be viewed directly with gonioscopic techniques that involve the use of a contact lens, focal illumination, and magnification. The contact lens eliminates the corneal curve and allows light to be reflected from the angle so that its structures may be seen in detail.

1. **Technique.** This procedure may be performed with topical anesthetic drops at the slit lamp and such lenses as the Alan-Thorpe, Goldmann, or Zeiss lenses, all of which have periscopic mirrors by which the angle is examined with reflected light. The patient may also have gonioscopy without slit lamp while in the supine position when the Koeppe contact lens is used. The angle is viewed through a handheld microscope with the Barkan light held in the other hand giving bright focal illumination. Greater magnification is achieved with the Koeppe lens than with lenses on the slit lamp, thereby allowing greater magnification of details of the angle, but this technique is used less frequently than lenses applied with the patient at the slit lamp due to relative inconvenience.

2. **Purpose.** This technique is most useful in determining various **forms of glaucoma,** such as open-angle, narrow-angle, angle-closure, and secondary angle-closure glaucoma, by allowing evaluation of the angle width (distance of the iris root from the trabecular meshwork) and study of the tissues in the angle of the glaucomatous eyes at various stages. Gonioscopy is also of great use in examining **other problems** within the anterior chambers such as retained intraocular foreign bodies hidden in the recess of the angle. It is useful in the study of iris tumors and cysts as well as in the evaluation of trauma to the tissues in the area of the angle. With wide pupillary dilation

the area behind the iris (posterior chamber), including ciliary processes, zonules, lens, and equator, may be seen in many patients.

III. Hospital or highly specialized office techniques

A. Fluorescein angiography of the fundus

1. **Purpose.** Fluorescein angiography has proved to be a valuable tool in the diagnosis and management of a large number of retinal disorders that affect either the retinal vascular system or the choriocapillaris, Bruch's membrane, or the pigment epithelial layers. Disease states particularly amenable to evaluation by angiography include diabetic retinopathy, ocular histoplasmosis, macular edema and idiopathic preretinal macular fibrosis, retrolental fibroplasia, vascular occlusive disease, flecked retina syndrome, sickle cell retinopathy, retinal telangiectasis, Lindau-von Hippel disease, Eales's disease, and choroidal tumor, both primary melanoma and metastatic carcinoma, as well as benign hemangioma. The fundic fluorescein angiogram may provide three kinds of information to the clinician:

   a. **Documentation of the fine anatomic detail** of the fundus.

   b. **Physiologic information** pertinent to the index of flow of blood to the eye and flow through the retinal circulation.

   c. **Documentation of fundic pathology** when dye is seen passing vascular barriers ordinarily impermeable.

2. **Technique.** After the patient's pupils have been dilated, he or she is seated at a slit lamp mounted with a fundus camera and equipped with both exciter and barrier interference filters. These filters will allow only green light from the fluorescent dye passing through the vessels to be recorded on the film, thus exclusively outlining the vascular pattern and pathologic structures contained therein. Five milliliters of sodium fluorescein 10%, a harmless and painless dye, is injected into the antecubital vein. Photographs of one eye are taken at 5 seconds and then every second thereafter for 15 more seconds. Photographs will then be taken for up to 1 minute at 3- to 5-second intervals and then repeated at 20 minutes in both eyes. Occasionally, in patients with sensory epithelial detachments or diffuse retinal edema, photographs will be taken at 1 hour or more.

3. **Side effects.** Normally, the patient will have some afterimage effect and a yellowish discoloration of the skin, both of which will disappear within a matter of a few hours. The urine will also be discolored for approximately 1 day. Transient episodes of nausea may occur, and rarely there may be transient vomiting. Fainting is uncommon but may be seen, particularly in young male patients. Such patients should be held in the office for 1 hour to ascertain that there is no more severe reaction following. Severe allergic reactions such as anaphylaxis or cardiorespiratory problems are extremely rare and should be handled by a competent medical team.

4. **Stages of the normal angiogram.** Dye is visible in the choroidal circulation approximately 1 second before its appearance in the retinal arterioles (arterial phase). It lasts until the retinal arteries are completely filled. The AV phase of the transit involves complete filling of both retinal arteries and capillaries and the early stages of laminar flow in the veins. The venous phase of the dye transit includes initial laminar flow along the walls of the veins and then complete venous filling. The transit time in the macula is the most rapid, and the retinal capillary bed is best resolved in the macula because of increased pigmentation in the retinal pigment epithelium, which will block out underlying choroidal fluorescence.

5. **In interpreting the angiogram** the examiner may refer to a few terms that need definition.

   a. **Pseudofluorescence** results from fluorescein leakage into the vitreous and is a reflected illumination from this body.

   b. **Autofluorescence** pertains to true fluorescence of structures in the retinal area such as drusen of the optic nerve head.

   c. **A window defect** is a localized deficiency of pigment granules in the retinal pigment epithelium through which choroidal fluorescence is seen.

    d. Pooling is an accumulation of dye in a tissue space such as that between retinal pigment epithelium and Bruch's membrane.

    e. Staining is an increased accumulation of dye within tissue substance such as the sensory retinal capillary bed.

    f. Blocked fluorescence is interference with visualization of the normal underlying choroidal fluorescence, as in increased retinal pigment epithelium thickness, increased choroidal pigmentation as in a nevus, or the presence of retinal hemorrhages or exudates in the sensory retina beneath the pigment epithelium.

    g. A filling defect is an area of decreased fluorescence where circulation is occluded. It occurs in either the choroidal or retinal vascular bed. The rate of filling, emptying, and configuration assists the examiner in diagnosis and evaluation of various disease states of the fundus such as ischemic diabetic retinopathy.

B. Fluorescein angiography of the iris is performed to document abnormal vascular patterns, tumors, ischemia, and inflammatory patterns. Unfortunately the iris pigment often absorbs emitted fluorescein enough to make this test worthwhile only in light to medium (hazel) pigmented eyes. It may be performed on the fundus fluorescein camera by dialing a plus lens into the optical system, pulling the camera further back and focusing on the iris. Photography is delayed a few seconds longer than retinal angiography because of the longer arm-to-iris circulation time for the injected fluorescein.

C. Electroretinography (ERG)

    1. Purpose. The ERG is an important instrument in the detection and evaluation of hereditary and constitutional disorders of the retina. These disorders include partial and total color blindness, night blindness, retinal degeneration such as retinitis pigmentosa, chorioretinal degenerations or inflammations including choroideremia, Spielmeyer-Vogt disease, leutic chorioretinitis, Leber's congenital amaurosis, retinal ischemia secondary to arteriosclerosis, giant-cell arteritis, central retinal artery or vein occlusion, and carotid artery insufficiency. Toxicity secondary to administration of drugs such as hydroxychloroquine, chloroquine, and quinine may be detected and quantitated by the ERG. Siderosis, whether from local iron deposit or systemic disease, will also produce abnormal changes in the recording. Frequently, the ERG will not distinguish among these but will indicate the presence of diffuse abnormalities. Retinal detachment will reduce the recording levels of the ERG, although ultrasonography is probably a better way to detect such detachment in the presence of an opacity of the ocular media. Systemic diseases associated with low-voltage ERG include hypovitaminosis A, mucopolysaccharidosis, hypothyroidism, and anemia. The ERG may also be used to rule out the retina as the level of blindness in certain conditions such as cortical blindness, dyslexia, and hysteria.

    2. ERG is a technique of placing an ocular fitted contact lens electrode on the patient's eye so that recordings of electrical responses from various parts of the retina to external stimulation by light of varying intensity may be made. The A and B waves originate in the outer retinal layers, the A wave being produced by the photoreceptor cells and the B wave by the interconnecting Müller cells.

    3. Disadvantages. The ganglion cells do not contribute to the ERG as their electrical signals are in the former spike, which cannot be recorded externally. Therefore, a normal ERG may be recorded in the absence of ganglion cells and in the presence of total optic nerve atrophy or advanced retinal diseases, such as Tay-Sachs disease, in which the metabolic defect is located in the ganglion cells. In addition, as the ERG is a mass response from the retina, diseases of the macula that represent only a small part of the retina will not be recorded on the ERG.

D. Electrooculography (EOG) is an electrical recording based on the standing potential of the eye.

1. **Use in retinal disease.** The EOG is useful in situations in which the ERG is not sufficiently sensitive to pick up macular degeneration. This includes Best's disease (vitelliform macular degeneration), in which the ERG is abnormal even in carriers, and early toxic retinopathies such as those due to chloroquine or other antimalarial drugs. Supranormal EOGs have been found in albinism and aniridia, in which chronic excessive light exposure appears to have resulted in attendant peripheral retinal damage. The EOG records metabolic changes in the retinal pigment epithelium as well as in the neuroretina. Therefore, it serves as a test that is supplemental and complementary to the ERG and, in certain disease states, more sensitive than the ERG.

2. **Use in eye movements.** By placing the skin electrodes around the eye and using the cornea as the positive electrode with respect to the retina, eye movements of both eyes may be recorded either separately or together, using bitemporal electrodes. This technique is most useful in recording various forms of nystagmus and is particularly useful for clinicians who desire objective recordings of spontaneous and caloric-induced nystagmus. The technique is highly specialized, and the information produced therefrom is of use to only a fairly small number of clinicians.

E. **Ultrasonography.** Diagnostic ocular ultrasonography has made possible the detection of intraocular abnormalities not visualized clinically because of opacification of the cornea, anterior chamber, lens, or vitreous, as well as pathologic processes involving the periorbital tissues. It provides much the same information as a CT scan. Ultrasonography is analogous in many ways to soft tissue x ray and consists of the propagation of high-frequency sound waves through soft tissue, with the differential reflection of these waves from objects in the beam pathway. The reflected waves create echoes that are displayed on an oscilloscope screen as in sonar or radar systems, producing a picture that is amenable to clinical interpretation. This technique has an advantage over x rays or CT scans in being a dynamic examination allowing innumerable views including studies of the moving globe. The main disadvantage is need for direct contact with the globe or lid. Because of the highly sophisticated and expensive equipment involved and the necessity of dynamic interpretation of data, this technique is performed only by specialists within the field.

1. **Two forms of ultrasonic testing** are commonly used: A-mode and B-mode. A-mode is a one-dimensional time-amplitude representation of echoes received along the beam path. The distance between the echo spikes recorded on the oscilloscope screen provides an indirect measurement of tissue such as globe length or lens thickness. The height of the spike is indicative of the strength of the tissue sending back the echo; e.g., cornea, lens, retina, or sclera produce very high amplitude spikes while vitreous membranes or hemorrhage produces lower spikes. In B-mode ultrasound the same echoes produced in A-mode may be presented as dots instead of spikes. By use of scanning technique these dots may be integrated to produce an echo representation of a two-dimensional section of the eye rather than the one-dimension seen with A-mode. The location, size, and configuration of structures are rapidly apparent with this technique. The combination of both A-mode and B-mode techniques simultaneously produces the most successful results in ultrasonic testing.

2. **Technique.** Both types of ultrasound may be performed by either contact or immersion methods, both with the patient lying on a table.

   a. **In the contact method,** a transducer probe shaped like a pencil is held in direct contact with the eye or closed lid, using a topical anesthetic with a viscous coupling agent. In A-mode ultrasound the examiner moves the probe around the eyes systematically until abnormal areas are found. These abnormal echoes are then tested with electronic variables to characterize them in terms of location, density, thickness, and shape. Since this equipment is portable, the examination may be done at the patient's bedside or in the operating room. In uncooperative young children the contact method may be the only practicable method. The major drawback is obscuration of the first few millimeters of the anterior segment and ciliary body.

B-scan contact techniques are similar to those employed with A-mode instruments. Without immersion, echo characterization is limited to determining tissue configuration and density, and resolution suffers somewhat due to the continuous rapid display on the oscilloscope. The anterior segment and adjacent areas are obscured by electronic artifact, as with the A-mode. B-scan using the contact method is satisfactory for detecting most kinds of intraocular pathologies but is of limited value in the orbit.

b. Immersion. The most successful use of ultrasound is with immersion methods, where the eye is in direct contact with a water bath with the transducer tip held just beneath the water surface but not against the eye. Anterior segment examination as well as examination of the deeper ocular and orbital structures is very successful under these conditions. Although untoward experience is unlikely, immersion techniques are not used on recently traumatized or postoperative eyes unless the information derived will influence treatment.

3. Interpretation. Ultrasonic techniques may be used to ascertain the size, shape, and integrity of the wall of the globe and are frequently useful in picking up hidden anterior as well as posterior penetrating wounds. Collapse of the globe would be obvious on ultrasound as is phthisis bulbi (end-stage shrinkage of the globe).

a. Anterior segment examination reveals chamber depth and configuration as well as debris. Cataractous changes and subluxation of the lens may be identified most easily by B-scan techniques. Iris abnormalities such as iris bombé, recession of the root, cysts, and tumors may be shown if they are sufficiently large. Ultrasonography does not determine the functional status of the angle relative to outflow of aqueous in glaucoma, only its physical status.

b. Examination of the posterior segment by either A- or B-scan ultrasound may pick up subtle vitreous changes such as asteroid hyalosis or synchysis scintillans. Membrane opacities such as retinal detachment, choroidal detachment, vitreous membranes, diffuse debris, and organized tissue are also easily detected. In cases of penetrating injury the path followed by a foreign body may be detected on ultrasound as a track of moderate amplitude echoes from hemorrhage or debris. An echo track may indicate the location of a foreign body exiting from the eye posteriorly. Intraocular tumors may be located, and configuration and degree of choroidal excavation may be helpful clues to differentiating melanomas from metastatic tumors and benign hemangiomas; however, these criteria are not highly reliable with present techniques. Other masses such as subretinal hemorrhage and diskiform chorioretinopathy may simulate the tumor pattern. Vitreous membranes, retinal detachments, and choroidal detachments all produce distinctive pictures that may differentiate one from the other.

c. The localization of foreign bodies is most accurately detected and located by a combination of A- and B-scan ultrasound. Radiographic techniques, however, have long been in use and also provide very accurate information as to the localization and nature of most intraocular foreign bodies. Radiologically there is no way to differentiate among iron, copper, stone, or leaded glass fragments. Foreign bodies such as vegetable matter, nonleaded glass, or plastic, however, may not be sufficiently radiopaque to show up on film where they would show up on ultrasound. Not only may the foreign body be located within the globe, but the amount and density of tissue damage or tissue reactions surrounding it may also be determined. Ultrasound is superior to CT scan if the foreign body is localized near the ocular wall, as a foreign body

CT artifact may obscure whether the object is inside or outside of the eye. The magnetic character of a foreign body may be ascertained by pulsing a weak magnet over the eye and observing the behavior of the foreign body echo on the oscilloscope. Orbital foreign bodies, unlike intraocular ones, are much more difficult to locate with ultrasound because of the high reflection from the surrounding fat, muscle, and associated bony structures. Although in theory there is no limit to the size of foreign bodies that may be detected, practically speaking, small foreign bodies may be missed because the examiner may search randomly with the probe, not passing the beam through the exact area of the foreign body. Consequently, a negative report does not exclude foreign body in the eye, whereas the positive finding of foreign body is usually quite definite and highly localizing.

   d. Orbital ultrasonography is most useful in evaluation of soft tissue lesions causing exophthalmus. Pseudoproptosis due to a large globe or a shallow orbit may be detected, and cystic, solid, angiomatous, and infiltrative mass lesions may be differentiated from each other. Inflammatory disease such as pseudotumor oculi, Graves' disease, neuritis, and cellulitis are also amenable to localization and differentiation, as is retrobulbar hemorrhage. Fractures of orbital walls are not amenable to ultrasonic evaluation; radiographic study should be used in such situations.

   e. Surgical implications. Ultrasonography has been an invaluable technique for determining the potential functional status of an eye where the ocular media has made impossible ordinary clinical examination. Electroretinography is frequently unreliable in the presence of opaque media; under such circumstances ultrasound may be the sole means of determining the integrity of intraocular contents. Ascertaining of normal posterior segment will allow a surgeon to proceed with keratoplasty or cataract extraction with greater confidence of good results than when forced to operate on an eye with no knowledge of the status of the posterior segment. This technique is a noninvasive, well-tolerated, safe procedure with no known toxicity.

   f. Intraocular lenses. A very frequent use of ultrasonography is the determination of certain ocular measurements such as anterior chamber depth and global length. This, coupled with keratometry readings, will allow a surgeon to determine which implant power will make a cataract patient emmetropic, hyperopic, or myopic postoperatively (see Chap. 6, **VII.C**).

F. Radiologic studies of the eye and orbit. Radiologic examination of the eye and orbit is useful in evaluating trauma, foreign bodies, and tumors.

   1. Anatomy. Each orbit is a four-sided pyramidal cavity with the apex aimed posteromedially and the base opening onto the face. It is made up of seven bones and divided into the roof, lateral wall, medial wall, and the floor.

      a. The roof separates the orbital cavity from the anterior fossa of the skull. Anteriorly it is formed by the orbital segment of the frontal bone and posteriorly by the lesser wing of the sphenoid. The trochlea of the superior oblique muscle is located anteromedially on the roof.

      b. The lateral side of the roof slants inferiorly to join the greater wing of the sphenoid, and these two form the major part of the lateral wall. The anterior one-third of the lateral wall is formed by the zygomatic bone. The lateral wall is oblique and runs lateral medially proceeding from the anterolateral to posteromedial angle.

      c. The medial wall is nearly vertical and is formed by the frontal process of the maxilla, which is followed by the lacrimal bone, the extremely delicate laminal papyracea of the ethmoid, and most posteriorly by a small part of the body of the sphenoid.

      d. The floor is formed primarily by the orbital plate of the maxilla, the orbital process of the zygomatic bone, and most posteriorly by the orbital process of the palatine bone. Located in the middle of the floor is the infraorbital groove leading into the infraorbital canal, which transmits the infraorbital artery and vein and the infraorbital nerve (V2). These surface through the infraorbital foramina immediately beneath the inferior rim of the orbit. The floor of the orbit is extremely thin, occasionally only 1 mm thick and, therefore, the frequent site of fractures secondary to contusions. Located between the floor and lateral wall is the inferior orbital fissure. The **superior orbital fissure** (SOF) is located between the lateral wall and the roof near the apex. Through the SOF run the third, fourth, fifth, and sixth cranial nerves, sympathetic nerves, arteries, and veins. The optic foramen is located at the orbital apex and transmits the optic nerve. The base is boarded by the orbital rim formed by the frontal, zygomatic, and maxillary bones.

2. **Routine radiologic views** in many cases, will reveal as much information as a CT scan and are indispensable in cases where a patient cannot cooperate for the longer scanning procedure. They are of little use in soft tissue injuries of the eye. X-ray studies of the orbits are more difficult than x rays of other sites of the body because of the superimposition of other bones of the skull. The patient is placed on the radiographic table, usually in the prone position. The head may be adequately adjusted and immobilized by a clamp device, headband, or sandbags. Several variations of position may be used as well as tomographic techniques to localize at a particular depth.

   a. **Caldwell's view** is a PA projection of the orbit. The patient is in prone position with the forehead and nose resting on the table. This position offers the following **advantages:** (1) the petrous ridges are projected downward and there is a clear visualization of the **orbital rim and roof,** (2) the **greater wing of the sphenoid** is easily detected as it forms the large part of the lateral wall, (3) the **orbital section of the lesser wing of the sphenoid** is projected close to the medial wall, (4) the **SOF** is clearly seen between the greater and lesser wings of the sphenoid, and (5) the **foramen rotundum** is projected under the inferior rim of the orbit.

   b. **Waters' view.** This PA film allows additional visualization of the orbital and periorbital structures. The patient is again prone with the head extended so that the chin lies on the table and the tip of the nose is approximately 4 cm above the table. The Waters' view allows a clear **view of the maxillary antrum** separate from the superimposed petrous bones; the petrous ridges are projected downward while the antral contours are complete and not deformed. Visualization of the maxillary antrum is of use in revealing orbital pathology. The **inferior orbital rim, the lateral wall, the zygomatic arch, and frontal and ethmoidal sinuses** are all demonstrated in this view.

   c. **The oblique view** is used for visualization of the outer wall of the orbit and should be taken from both sides. The patient rests with cheek, nose, and brow of the side of interest resting on the table. The x rays are projected through the occiput and exit through the center of the orbit. This technique obtains better visualization of the **outer rim of the orbit** and is of particular interest if orbital rim fracture is suspected.

   d. **The Rheese position** is useful for demonstration of the **optic canal.** The patient is prone with head adjusted so that the zygoma, nose, and chin rest on the table. The structures that are visualized are the optic canal (appearing in the lateral quadrant of the orbit), the ethmoid cells, the lesser wing of the sphenoid, and the superior orbital fissure. If the patient is unable to lie prone, this film may be taken in the supine position as well.

   e. **The lateral view** is useful for localization of **foreign bodies.** The patient lies on the side, and the outer canthus of the orbit of interest is placed against the film. The x rays are directed vertically through the canthus.

3. **Orbital tomography.** Body section radiography **(polytomograms)** is a method whereby the examiner may blur the superimposed surrounding structures and clearly visualize a given spot at a given depth. During exposure the x-ray tube is moved in one direction above the object and the film in the opposite direction with the tube adjusted so that the fulcrum point is at the level of anatomic interest. This plane will then be shot focused against the blurred anatomic structures around it. Tomography is of particular use in **localizing small fractures** as well as in determining the **extent of linear fractures** and the presence of **orbital tumors.** In conjunction with specialized routine views, polytomograms are felt by most radiologists to be as informative as a CT scan.

4. **Computerized tomography (CT scan).** The CT scan's ability to delineate tissues of varying density make it an invaluable diagnostic tool. Routine CT scans are usually multiple axial or transverse "cuts," 8, 2, or even 1 mm apart depending on the lesions being evaluated, starting at the skull vertex and going to the skull base. As such, the orbital walls, eye, and extraocular muscles are sectioned longitudinally in the horizontal plane. Orbital and extraocular examinations are enhanced by coronal and sagittal sections. Radiopaque medium may be injected during the scan to demonstrate vascular abnormalities. The CT is the study of choice in soft tissue inquiries. Spatial resolution of better than $1 \times 1 \times 1.5$ mm³ provides fine detail. Cuts 1–2 mm should be used especially for injuries such as potential optic nerve damage or localization of ocular or orbital foreign bodies of varying composition and density. Blow-out fractures with muscle incarceration are best seen with coronal sections through the orbital floor and maxillary antrum. Incarceration of muscle may be distinguished from that of fat. Other diagnoses possible with CT scanning include tumors or hematomas of the lids, extraocular muscles, orbit, or optic sheath, transected muscle or optic nerve, incarcerated muscle, ruptured globe, dislocated lens, vitreous hemorrhage, choroidal or retinal detachment, fractures of the optic canal, fracture of any wall, and secondary sinus involvement. The main disadvantages of CT scanning are poor contrast between some different soft tissues, possible radiation hazards (orbital CT scan = 2–3 rad, similar to an orbital series of skull x rays), beam-hardening artifacts created by metallic objects or cortical bone, and lack of direct scanning in the sagittal plane. Indicated uses of CT versus NMR imaging is discussed under sec. **5.**

5. **Nuclear magnetic resonance (NMR)** imaging is being used with increasing frequency in ophthalmology for the detailed imaging of global, orbital, and neuroophthalmic structures from the orbit through the brain.

    a. **Advantages and disadvantages.** The patient is in a magnetic field and not exposed to ionizing radiation. The technique is therefore extremely safe as long as the area examined is **free of foreign magnetic metal** and the patient has **no cardiac pacemaker,** which may be turned off or on by the NMR. Other advantages of NMR are that the technique is not hampered by bone, which, because of low molecular mobility, is relatively invisible on the images. Soft tissues are thus seen in an unobstructed fashion; anatomic delineation of normal and abnormal structures as well as a metabolic profile of those structures is obtained. Better resolution is obtained with 3-D isotropic images where thinner slices (2.0 mm) are taken, and better contrast is obtained on 2-D images with their thicker slices (3–5 mm), which give greater signal to noise. Lesions smaller than 2 mm are best seen on 3-D images, as they do not blend into their surrounding tissues, while larger lesions can be demonstrated on either 2-D or 3-D imaging. NMR is capable of differentiating hemorrhages, ischemia, multiple sclerosis, and tumors of the brain as well as virtually all ocular and orbital structures.

    b. **Ocular indications** for use of NMR (usually 3-D imaging) and/or CT include ocular trauma, tumors within opaque media when ultrasound is equivocal, and suspected intraocular foreign bodies. **NMR should not**

be used if the intraocular foreign body is thought to be ferromagnetic (e.g., BB's, iron, unknown composition) however, and CT and ultrasound should be used for such evaluations. IOL haptics of titanium or platinum are not a contraindication to NMR. NMR can distinguish retinoblastoma (low-intensity mass) from hemorrhage or exudate, which appears brighter, and from Coats' disease or toxocariasis because of the latter two having bright T2 based signals. NMR will distinguish choroidal melanotic melanomas from nonpigmented tumors and effusions but not from fat.

   c. Orbital indications for CT and/or NMR imaging are proptosis, papilledema, and orbital inflammatory, infectious, or neoplastic disease. Two-dimensional imaging is commonly used. Excellent contrast is provided between fine cortical bone, orbital fat, extraocular muscles, optic nerve, the globe, and the numerous disease processes that may involve these structures. Dye-contrasted CT and NMR resolve vascular lesions with excellent delineation, e.g., hemangiomas, carotid-cavernous sinus fistulas, and thrombosed ophthalmic veins.

   d. Neuroophthalmic indications for CT and/or NMR include the above orbital disorders if unexplained after orbital evaluation plus unexplained optic and cranial neuropathies, eye movement disorders, visual field defects, or any other signs or symptoms of intracranial disease. NMR images are generally superior to CT in delineating vascular or solid lesions in the sella turcica, cavernous sinus, optic chiasm, posterior fossa, and brain stem. NMR also shows multiple sclerosis plaques and hemorrhages better than CT, but CT is superior if a calcified lesion is under evaluation.

   The election of CT, NMR, or both must be based on clinical suspicion of the nature of the disease but with faster scan time, finer resolution use of paramagnetic contrast agents, increased availability, lack of radiation exposure, and decreasing cost taken into consideration. NMR may progressively become the procedure of first choice over CT scanning.

  6. Dacryocystography is the radiographic evaluation of the excretory system in an attempt to localize the precise **site of obstruction.** The procedure will vary with the radiologist. Water-soluble contrast medium such as cyanographin or salpix is used. The lacrimal irrigation test (secondary dye test) with the patient at an x-ray machine is performed and 1 ml of contrast solution is injected through the lower canaliculus. AP Waters' and lateral projections are taken of the excretory system. If both sides are injected simultaneously, a back view should be taken in case the lateral views overlap. The results of radiographic examination will reveal the site of obstruction. This is of particular value in partial or intermittent obstruction, obstruction secondary to trauma, or obstruction associated with diverticulum or fistula. **Contraindications** to the test are radiologic contraindications as determined by the radiologist, acute dacrycystitis, and allergy to iodine.

G. Anterior chamber aspiration (keratocentesis)

  1. Indications. Diagnostic aspiration of aqueous from the anterior chamber is indicated for (1) specific identification of intraocular microbes, (2) identification of inflammatory cell types indicative of disease type, and (3) determination of specific antibodies in the aqueous and comparison of these to serum antibodies against the same antigen in an attempt to localize antigens to the eye.

  2. Technique. Keratocentesis may be carried out on an outpatient basis in the minor surgery room. A lid speculum is applied and, after a single proparacaine drop is instilled, a cotton-tipped applicator moistened with cocaine 4% is applied for approximately 15 seconds to an area of conjunctiva near the inferior limbus. This area is thereby anesthetized so that it may be grasped firmly with a toothed forceps. A 30-gauge disposable needle attached to a disposable tuberculin syringe is then inserted into the cornea near the forceps with minimum pressure while the examiner slowly turns the syringe barrel back and forth in his or her finger. As the bevel of the needle enters the anterior chamber, the examiner's assistant withdraws the plunger, thereby aspirating 0.1–0.2 ml of aqueous. The needle tip is kept over the iris at all times to avoid hitting deeper ocular structures. If the chamber shallows so that the anterior surface of the iris approaches the site of needle penetration, the bevel should be withdrawn and the procedure halted regardless of the amount of fluid withdrawn. At the end of the procedure, antibiotic ointment and cycloplegic drops should be applied and a light patch put over the eye for a few hours. Keratocentesis is basically painless although hyphema may develop in patients with neurovascularization of the iris; it is, therefore, not recommended in such a clinical situation. There may be a transient rise in IOP for 12 hours after paracentesis, particularly in patients with Behçet's syndrome. The etiology of this pressure rise is unknown.

3. **Diagnostic tests.** The aqueous fluid so withdrawn is very limited in quantity; consequently, the clinician should have a clear idea of which tests are desired at the time of the tap so that no fluid is wasted. Tests include bacterial cultures, parasitic or cytologic examination using conventional stains, or fluorescent antibody stains for viruses and dark-field examination for treponemas. Aqueous may be concentrated on the millipore filter disk for electron microscopic examination or prepared by wet fixation for Papanicolaou testing for malignancy. Serologic examination of the aqueous humor is of value if specific antibody is present in the aqueous in higher concentration than in the circulating serum. This finding is indicative of the presence of antigen within the eye; such antigen is most likely the cause of a given disease state, e.g., toxoplasma. Serologic examination must be done in a hospital university research laboratory or by the state laboratory. In cases of **endophthalmitis,** aqueous cultures and smears are of **limited use.** Vitrectomy is the diagnostic procedure of choice (see Chap. 8).

Burns and Trauma

Deborah Pavan-Langston

I. **Anterior segment burns** may be chemical, thermal, radiation, or electrical.
   A. **Chemical burns** are the most urgent and are caused usually by **alkali** or **acid**. Other forms of anterior segment burns that should be managed as chemical burns are those due to **tear gas** and **mace**. These are generally thought not to cause permanent ocular damage; however, there have been reports of eyes lost after such burns. Ocular injury from **sparklers** and **flares** containing magnesium hydroxide should also be managed as chemical rather than as thermal burns.
   B. **Pathology of chemical burns.** The most serious chemical burns are produced by alkali material such as lye (NaOH); caustic potash (KOH); fresh lime [$Ca(OH)_2$], i.e., plaster, cement, whitewash; and ammonia (NH_4), which is present in household cleaner, fertilizers, and refrigerant.
      1. **Alkali burns** are more severe than acid burns because of their rapid penetration, often less than 1 minute, through the cornea and anterior chamber combining with cell membrane lipids, thereby resulting in disruption of the cells and stromal mucopolysaccharide with concomitant tissue softening. Damage from alkali burns is related more to the degree of alkalinity (pH) than to the actual cation. Permanent injury is determined by the nature and concentration of the chemical as well as by the time lapsed before irrigation.
      2. **Acid burns,** such as those caused by battery acid (H_2SO_4), laboratory glacial acetic acid, fruit and vegetable preservatives, bleach, refrigerant (H_2SO_3), and industrial solvents and glass etching agents (HFl), cause their maximum damage within the first few minutes to hours and are less progressive and less penetrating. Acids precipitate tissue proteins that rapidly set up barriers against deep penetration by the chemical. Damage is therefore localized to the area of contact, with the exception of burns from hydrofluoric acid or from acids containing heavy metals, both of which tend to penetrate the cornea and anterior chamber, ultimately giving rise to intraocular scarring and membrane formation.
      3. **Mace** (chloroacetophenone) and other **tear gas** compounds are not under government regulation and therefore variable in their toxic contents and clinical effects. If sprayed, as recommended, from more than 6 feet away, not directed at the eyes, and at a conscious individual, only minor chemical conjunctivitis occurs. More direct and concentrated spray toward the eyes in a person whose defensive reflexes are compromised will result in severe injury clinically similar to an alkali burn. Mace and other lacrimator ocular burns should be managed like alkali burns.
   C. **Classification and prognosis** of the chemically burned eye is most useful for alkali burns but also extends to acid and toxic chemical injuries of the eye.
      1. **Mild injury** involves erosion of corneal epithelium, faint haziness of the cornea, and no ischemic necrosis of conjunctiva or sclera (no blanching). A mild alkali burn will exhibit sluggish reepithelialization and mild corneal haze with ultimate minimum visual handicap regardless of treatment.
      2. **Moderately severe burns** involve corneal opacity, blurring iris detail, and minimum ischemic necrosis of conjunctiva and sclera (partial blanching).

Moderately severe burns take variable courses, depending on the extent of the injury. There may be moderate stromal opacification with increased corneal thickness and heavy proteinaceous aqueous exudation in a markedly hyperemic eye. Superficial neovascularization of the cornea may follow the advancing edge of regenerating epithelium, and there may be persistent epithelial defects that ultimately lead to stromal thinning and perforation. A scarred and vascularized cornea will result in permanent visual impairment.

   3. **Very severe burns** involve marked corneal edema and haze, with blurring of the pupillary outline, and blanching of conjunctiva and sclera (marked whitening of the external eye). The most severe alkali burns present with an opalescent cornea, absent epithelium, and ischemic necrosis of more than two-thirds of the perilimbal conjunctiva and sclera. For the first 2 weeks, the corneal integrity is undisturbed although anterior iritis may be severe and go undetected. As epithelium begins to heal back across the stroma, ulceration begins and perforation may ensue secondary to the release of collagenases, elastases and other enzymes from epithelium, polymorphonuclear neutrophil leukocytes, and keratocytes, and decreased collagen synthesis due to severe ascorbate deficiency in alkali burned eyes.

D. **Therapy** is classified by time postinjury.
   1. **Immediate treatment** for chemical burns is copious irrigation using the most readily available source of water (shower, faucet, drinking fountain, hose, or bathtub). The greater the time between injury and decontamination, the worse the prognosis. The victim should not wait for sterile physiologic or chemical neutralizing solutions. The lids should be held apart and water irrigated continuously over the injured globe(s). The initial lavage at the site of the injury should continue for several minutes, so that both eyes receive copious irrigation. Orbicularis spasm may make this difficult. Use of a cloth material on the lids will help the irrigator to hold otherwise slippery spastic lids. Skin irrigation may be started simultaneously by pouring water over the affected area but is unquestionably secondary to ocular lavage.
   2. **After the initial lavage** the patient should be taken immediately to an emergency room with a phone call made ahead so that treatment is waiting by the time the patient arrives. In the emergency room, lavage is continued with at least 2000 ml of normal saline 0.9% over a minimum period of 1 hour. Lid retractors should be used if necessary and **topical anesthetic** instilled q20min to relieve some of the considerable pain. The conjunctival fornices and palpebral conjunctiva should be swept with sterile cotton-tipped applicators to remove any foreign matter that may have been retained at the time of injury. If eversion of upper or lower lids reveals chemical still embedded in the tissue, 0.01- to 0.05-mol ethylenediaminetetraacetic acid (EDTA) solution should be used as irrigant or the fornices further swabbed with cotton-tipped applicators soaked in EDTA. Careful examination after lavage for perforating ocular injury should be made. *Direct pressure on the globe during lavage should be avoided if ocular global laceration is at all suspected* (see also sec. **VI**).
   3. **Irrigation should be continued** until pH paper reveals that the conjunctival readings are close to normal (pH between 7.3 and 7.7). Once a relatively normal pH is achieved the patient should be checked again in 5 minutes to ascertain that the pH is not changing again in the direction of acidity or alkalinity, depending on the nature of the burn.
   4. **Medications.** While the pH is being stabilized near normal, the **mydriatic-cycloplegics** cyclopentolate 1.0% or scopolamine 0.1% and phenylephrine 2.5% should be instilled to dilate the pupil and prevent massive iris adhesions to the lens (posterior synechiae) as well as to reduce the pain secondary to iridociliary spasm. After irrigation is complete, **antibiotics** such as gentamicin, tobramycin, erythromycin, or chloramphenicol ointment should be started to protect against infection. In the case of alkali burns there is

frequently an **immediate rapid rise in intraocular pressure** (IOP) secondary to shrinkage of the collagen fibers of the sclera. Carbonic anhydrase
inhibitors such as acetazolamide, 500 mg IV or PO stat, should be given.

5. **For pain** systemic analgesics should be administered. Percocet, 1 tablet PO
   q3h, or meperidine, 50–75 mg IM or PO q4h, is effective.

6. **An emergency complete physical examination** should be done not only
   by the ophthalmologist but also by an otolaryngologist and an internist,
   since many toxic chemicals are aspirated or swallowed at the time of original injury and there may be concomitant chemical burns of the respiratory
   or upper gastrointestinal tract. During irrigation the examiner should always be aware of the possibility of an **acute obstruction of the airway**
   secondary to chemical burn, inducing laryngeal edema.

7. **Once the immediate emergency situation is controlled** the burned eye(s)
   is patched and the patient admitted unless the burn is mild, in which case
   therapy may be done on an outpatient basis with initial frequent office
   visits. Topical antibiotic ointments and drops should be continued q4–6h
   along with the mydriatic-cycloplegics.

E. **Midterm therapy** is used for several days to weeks immediately postburn.

   1. **Elevation of IOP** may be noted and is probably due to prostaglandin release.
      Long-term elevation of pressure is secondary to scarring of outflow chan-
      nels. Carbonic anhydrase inhibitors such as acetazolamide, 250 mg PO qid,
      ethoxzolamide, 50 mg PO tid, or dichlorphenamide, 50 mg PO tid, are usu-
      ally effective in reducing this pressure and should be continued as long as
      it is elevated more than 22–25 mm Hg. Timolol, 0.25 or 0.50%, betaxolol
      0.5%, or levobunolol 0.5% drops bid may be added and, if needed, glycerol,
      40–60 ml PO q12h, may be used as an oral hyperosmotic agent for a few
      days in severely elevated pressure. Mannitol 20% solution IV, 2.5 ml/kg,
      may be given for short-term pressure control in those patients who cannot
      take oral medication. **Cardiac status** should be ascertained before use of
      any hyperosmotic agent, and long-term carbonic anhydrase inhibitors (with
      the exception of ethoxzolamide) should be avoided in patients with a his-
      tory of **renal stones.**

   2. **Topical steroids** such as dexamethasone 0.1% q4h should be used but only
      during the first 7–10 days after injury to control secondary iridocyclitis.
      After this period, if the corneal epithelium is not 100% intact, particularly
      in alkali burns, steroids should be withdrawn because of the increased chance
      of corneal melting and perforation due to collagenolytic enzyme release.
      Systemic steroids such as prednisone, 30 mg PO bid, may be substituted
      if iridocyclitis is still uncontrolled. **Collagenase inhibitors** such as acetyl-
      cysteine are rarely used now because of equivocal efficacy.

   3. **Therapeutic soft contact lenses** with high water content (Sauflon, Per-
      malens) may be of great benefit in assisting epithelial healing, which in turn
      will inhibit enzyme release and stromal melting. The lenses should be fitted
      as soon as possible after injury and are generally left in place for 6–8 weeks.

   4. **Topical antibiotics** (drops if a soft contact lens is in place) should be used
      several times daily initially and then tapered to qid and **cycloplegia** main-
      tained as long as there is more than mild cells and flare in the anterior
      chamber.

   5. **Ascorbate or citrate supplement** appears to be important in alkali burned
      eyes. These eyes become rapidly scorbutic, thus interfering with collagen
      synthesis and leading to ulceration. In mild to moderate burns, ciliary body
      aqueous secretion is sufficient to use the oral route, and ascorbate (vitamin
      C), 2 gm PO, is given qid for 3–4 weeks. In more severe burns, aqueous
      secretion is usually very diminished and topical 10% ascorbate in artificial
      tears should be given qlh for 14 hours/day starting within hours of the
      injury for 1–2 weeks and then tapered as warranted. Ascorbate should **never**
      be used in **nonalkali burn** situations, as ciliary body concentration of the
      drug will enhance rather than inhibit corneal melting. Topical 10% sodium

citrate used on a similar schedule may be even more beneficial than ascorbate, as the former inhibits accumulation of leukocytes in the cornea.

6. **Appropriate therapy for concomitant dermal injury** should be undertaken with the guidance of a dermatologist.

F. **Long-term therapy** depends on the severity of the burn and may vary from an antibiotic and artificial tears to surgical reconstruction of the eye with conjunctival flaps or transplants, mucous membrane transplants, patch grafts, and penetrating keratoplasty.

II. **Thermal injuries** usually involve injury to the lids. Their treatment is similar to that of thermal injury elsewhere in the body.

A. **A contact burn** of the globe may be mild, such as one due to tobacco ash, or severe, such as one seen with molten metal, which may produce severe permanent burns of the globe itself. Burns caused by glass and iron have caused the most severe injury because of their high melting points of 1200°C. Lead, tin, and zinc melt below 1000°C and therefore do less damage, although it is not infrequent that after an external cast of the eye has been removed from under the lid a permanently opacified globe is found underneath regardless of the type of metal.

B. **Therapy.** For partial-thickness lid burn, topical antibiotic ointment with sterile dressings is used, but with minimum burns no dressing is needed. Frequent saline or lubricated dressing, avoidance of early debridement, topical antibiotic qid, prevention of secondary infection, and protection of the globe are critical factors in successful management. Topical steroids such as dexamethasone 0.1% or prednisolone 1% qid may be used to decrease scarring between the lids and globe (symblepharon formation) if the corneal epithelium is intact. Secondary steroid glaucoma should be checked for periodically. Systemic steroids may be used to control secondary iridocyclitis if topical steroids are contraindicated because of the severity of the corneal burn.

C. **Exposure therapy.** If the eyelids are burned so severely that there is exposure of the globe, topical antibiotic ointment tid should be placed on the lid and globe and a piece of sterile plastic wrap placed over this to protect the globe from exposure by forming a moist chamber. This same technique of a plastic wrap moist chamber may be used to protect patients with exposure secondary to marked exophthalmus, severe conjunctival hemorrhage or chemosis, or traumatic avulsion of the eyelid. The covering film is cut in 10- × 15-cm rectangular pieces and may be gas autoclaved in individual packages. These pieces are large enough to cover the entire orbit from forehead to cheek. When the plastic wrap is applied, antibiotic ointment is applied to the skin around the orbit, and the sterile film is placed over the area to be protected. The film will adhere to the skin by static charge and by adherence to the ointment.

In mild burn cases where **exposure is minimum** and Bell's reflex is good so that only the inferior conjunctiva is exposed, antibiotic ophthalmic ointments q4h should suffice to protect the globe until surgical repair, if needed, is possible.

III. **Radiation burns: ultraviolet and infrared**

A. **Ultraviolet radiation** is the most common cause of light-induced ocular injury. Sources are welding arcs, sun lamps, and carbon arcs. Ultraviolet burns may be prevented by use of ordinary crown glass or regular glass lenses, as they absorb the rays.

1. **After exposure** there is a delay of 6–10 hours before the burn becomes symptomatically manifest. **Symptoms** may range from mild irritation and foreign body sensation to severe photophobia, pain, and spasm of the lid.

2. **Examination** will reveal varying lid edema, conjunctival hyperemia, and punctate roughening of the corneal epithelium. This punctate staining is easily seen with fluorescein staining. Because of high absorption in the cornea, ultraviolet light rarely damages the lens and does so only if intensity has been extremely high. This radiation does not reach the retina and therefore produces no deep changes within the eye.

3. Therapy is a short-acting cycloplegic drop such as cyclopentolate 1% to relieve ciliary spasm and topical antibiotic ointment or drop. A semipressure dressing with the eyes well closed underneath is left on for 24 hours. The patient in pain may need sedatives and analgesics. The patient should be reassured that damage is transient and that all symptomatology will be gone within 24–48 hours.

B. Infrared burns are also usually of little consequence and produce only temporary lid edema and erythema but little or no damage to the globe. Therapy is antibiotic ointment twice daily for 4–5 days after injury. Chronic exposure to infrared light is seen in glass blowers and metal furnace stokers improperly protected by industrial goggles. These workers develop cataracts after many years of exposure, but no other anterior segment changes are found, and the posterior segment is not affected. The mechanization of furnaces has made this problem relatively rare.

C. Ionizing radiation from cyclotron exposure and beta-irradiation from periorbital therapy of malignancy are the most common causes of radiation burns. The cornea, lens, uvea, retina, and optic nerve may suffer from injury but also may be protected from it by use of lead screens and leaded glass to absorb x, gamma, and neutron radiation.

1. Signs and symptoms are conjunctival hyperemia, circumcorneal injection, and watery or mucopurulent discharge. The earliest sign of corneal damage is hypesthesia. Radiation keratitis ranges from a punctuate epithelial staining to sloughing of large areas of epithelium and stromal edema with interstitial keratitis and aseptic corneal necrosis. The minimum cataractogenic dose from x ray is approximately 500–800 rad. The younger the lens the greater the vulnerability to x ray. A latency period of 6 months to 12 years exists, depending on dosage but independent of whether gamma rays or neutrons were the source of injury. The uveal tract may undergo vascular dilation with subsequent boggy edema. Intraretinal hemorrhages, papilledema, and central retinal vein thrombosis may rarely be seen after radiation injury.

2. Therapy of radiation injury is symptomatic. Cycloplegics such as cyclopentolate 1% or scopolamine 0.1% bid, and topical antibiotic ointments or drops such as tobramycin or gentamicin qid, should be used to reduce the pain of ciliary spasm, to prevent synechia formation, and to protect against infection. Steroids topically are rarely indicated and should not be used in the presence of epithelial ulceration. A **therapeutic soft contact lens** with antibiotic eye drops (ointments dislodge the lens) may assist healing of an epithelial defect. The lens should not be applied prophylactically because it may create an epithelial defect in a borderline situation.

D. Solar viewing. Unprotected viewing of the sun as in a solar eclipse or psychotic state can cause irreversible macular burns via focusing of visible and short infrared rays on this retinal area. An immediate loss of visual acuity may become permanent, or there may be return of vision toward normal. There is no specific treatment, and prophylaxis is the key to prevention, e.g., viewing through treated photographic film or indirect viewing via a series of mirrors in combination with treated photographic film.

E. Laser burns of an accidental nature are being seen with increasing frequency with industrial use of these machines. The burns are almost always macular, with instantaneous and usually permanent loss of central vision. Prophylactic wearing of absorbing goggles will protect against indirect laser beam scatter, but only avoidance of direct viewing of the beam will prevent the tragic irreversible and untreatable macular burns.

IV. Electric shock cataract. After electrical injury is sustained, particularly around the head, a periodic check for cataract formation through dilated pupils should be made, starting a few weeks after injury. The appearance of characteristic vacuoles is a key prognostic factor. Latency period for cataract formation ranges from months to years.

V. Corneal abrasions and foreign bodies

A. **Traumatic corneal abrasions** result in the partial or complete removal of a focal area of epithelium on the cornea, producing severe pain, lacrimation, and blepharospasm. Motion of the eyeball and blinking increase the pain and foreign body sensation.

1. **Examination** should be made after a drop of topical anesthetic is instilled. The cornea is inspected under magnification, if possible, using a bright hand light and oblique illumination. Even without fluorescein dye a corneal abrasion may be detected by noting that an obvious shadow is cast on the iris from a surface defect illuminated with incident light. Identification of these abrasions, however, is infinitely easier if sterile fluorescein strips or drops are used to dye the tear film. A green dye will be seen wherever corneal epithelial cells have been damaged or lost. The presence of a **foreign body under the upper lid** should always be looked for in the presence of a corneal abrasion (see Chap. 1, sec. **II.D**).

2. **Differential diagnosis.** Viral keratitis, particularly that due to either herpes simplex or herpes zoster, may produce a foreign body sensation associated with lacrimation and blepharospasm. Fluorescein staining of the corneal ulcer, however, will usually reveal a diagnostic branching dendritic ulcer, although a nondescript ovoid or map-shaped ulcer similar to that seen after traumatic abrasion may also be secondary to herpetic infection.

3. **Treatment** involves the instillation of antibiotic ointment such as erythromycin or gentamicin and a short-acting cycloplegic such as cyclopentolate 1%. A moderate, two-pad pressure dressing is then placed over the closed lids of the affected eye for 24–48 hours. After removal of the dressing, topical antibiotic ointment or drops 2–3 times a day should be continued for 4 days after the injury as protection against infection.

B. **Contact lens abrasion.** Acute discomfort caused by a contact lens may be due to a foreign body between the lens and the cornea, improper fit, overwear with secondary corneal edema, or damage to the corneal epithelium on inserting or removing the lens.

1. **Removal of lens.** If the lens is still in place at the time the patient is seen, **topical anesthesia** should be instilled. A **hard contact lens** is removed with a suction cup apparatus or by sliding the lens to the nasal portion of the bulbar conjunctiva by gently pressing two fingers on the globe through the upper lid just lateral to the contact lens, with the patient looking horizontally toward the side of the affected eye. Once the lens has slid over the nasal conjunctiva, finger pressure is applied through the lids at the lower margin of the contact lens so that the upper lens margin is flipped off the globe. The upper lid margin is then slid beneath the contact lens and the lids allowed to close behind the lens. If the lens slides into the upper or lower fornix, the edge of the lid is simply grasped and the patient asked to look in the direction opposite from that where the lens is located. The edge of the lid is then slipped under the edge of the contact lens nearest it and the lens flipped out of the eye. **Soft lenses** are pinched off the eye between the thumb and index finger.

2. **The type of fluorescein staining** of the cornea seen after removal of the contact lens may determine the cause of the abrasion. Diffuse mild central staining and haziness indicate contact lens overwear, that the lens fitting is too tight, or that the lens chemical cleaners were not well washed off before insertion of the lens. Small irregular abrasions, usually near the limbus, may indicate difficulties with inserting or removing the lens. Irregular linear scratches on the corneal epithelium are indicative of foreign body trapped between the lens and the cornea. The lens should be examined to see if there are defective edges, cracks, or foreign bodies on the posterior surface.

3. **Treatment** of **hard contact lens** abrasion is the same as for other forms of corneal abrasions. Contact lens wear may begin again 2 days after the cornea has healed. For **soft contact lens** abrasion, a potential *Pseudomonas* infection must be suspected until proved otherwise. The abrasion should

be cultured and treated with tobramycin drops qlh for 6 hours and then q3h until seen by the physician again the next day. If there is an infiltrate present on first or follow-up examination, the patient should be managed as in central microbial ulcers (bacterial, fungal, *Acanthamoeba*) (see Chap. 5).

C. **Spontaneous corneal ulceration (recurrent erosion)** (see also Chap. 5, **VIII.B.4**). Fingernail or paper cut injuries to the cornea may lead many months to years later to spontaneous ulceration of the cornea secondary to imperfect healing of basement membrane. Such recurrent erosions may occur, however, without a past history of injury and be due to trophic changes spontaneously developing within the patient's basement membrane.

1. **Symptoms.** The patient usually awakens in early morning with severe pain, redness, and lacrimation in the affected eye. Fluorescein staining will reveal a nondescript ovoid or triangular ulcer, frequently with a filament of detached epithelium still clinging to it. There may be superficial corneal edema and haze at the site of the abrasion.

2. **Treatment** of the acute erosion is antibiotic ointment and semipressure patching for 24 hours. Over the ensuing 2–3 months copious use of artificial tears q2–3h and antibiotic or artificial tear ointment at bedtime should be used in an effort to prevent another erosion by lubricating the interface between lid and corneal epithelium. In severe recurrent cases, constant-wear therapeutic soft contact lenses with artificial tears may prove successful in resolving and permanently healing the condition.

D. **Corneal foreign bodies.** Foreign bodies embedded in the corneal epithelium may be single or multiple, easily seen without magnification or barely detectable with slit-lamp examination.

1. **Types.** Bits of rust, windblown dirt, glass fragments, caterpillar hairs, and vegetable matter are the most commonly found foreign bodies.

2. **History.** While taking a history of the origin of the foreign body, it is important to note **if the object was propelled** toward the eye with a force that might cause the examiner to suspect intraocular foreign bodies as well. Hammering steel on steel is one such typical situation. The examiner should also note whether or not the **accident** occurred during the **course of employment.**

3. **Iron foreign bodies** will frequently form **rust rings,** ring-shaped orange stains in the anterior stroma that will wash out spontaneously with time leaving a white, nebulous telltale scar.

4. **Treatment.** After topical anesthetic has been instilled, the corneal foreign body may often be removed with a gentle wipe with a moistened applicator. Foreign bodies embedded somewhat more firmly may often be picked off the cornea with the side of the beveled edge of a No. 18 needle attached to a handle or syringe (Fig. 2–1). Alternatively, a "golf stick" instrument may be obtained from a commercial medical supply house. The physician should not be unduly concerned about perforating the cornea when using the side of a needle or a golf stick to remove the corneal foreign body, as it takes considerable pressure to penetrate the stroma; nonetheless, direct pressure on the cornea with the end of a sharp instrument is contraindicated. Rust rings may be removed either at the time of the initial scraping or, **if healing does not occur** over the rust ring within a few days, it may be removed with a handheld, battery-driven rust ring removal burr. If possible, these procedures should be done under magnification with a loupe or slit lamp.

a. **If multiple foreign bodies** are present in the corneal epithelium, such as after an explosion, undue scarring may occur from attempted removal of every particle. It is advisable in this situation to put in topical anesthetic and to denude the entire epithelium to within 1 or 2 mm of the limbus with an alcohol- or ether-soaked cotton-tipped applicator. Bowman's membrane is thereby spared additional scarring and the superficial foreign bodies will be removed. Those located along the limbus may be removed individually, thereby leaving a semi-intact rim of cor-

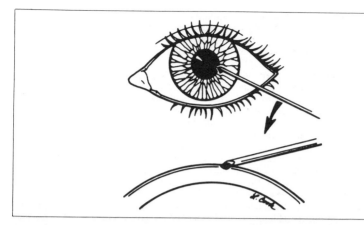

Fig. 2-1. Removal of superficial corneal foreign body. Front and side views illustrate thickness of cornea relative to beveled needle edge. Needle should be moved in a sideways motion to lift or gently scrape off foreign body.

neal epithelium that will provide the source of cells from which reepithelialization of the cornea will take place over the next several days.

b. **After removal of the foreign body or bodies,** a short-acting cycloplegic such as cyclopentolate 1% and broad-spectrum antibiotic ointment such as tobramycin or gentamicin should be instilled in the lower cul-de-sac and a moderate pressure patch placed over the closed lids for 24–48 hours. More extensive reepithelialization may take longer to heal, thereby requiring another few days of antibiotic and pressure patching. If penetrating injury of the eye is suspected, ointment should not be instilled as the injury may allow it access to the anterior chamber. In this case a protective metal shield and cotton pads should be placed over the eye and the patient referred for surgical management.

c. **Contraindicated therapy.** It is important to note that **no patient with a corneal abrasion or foreign body should be maintained on topical anesthetics.** Topical anesthetics will not only prevent healing but also will ultimately cause total breakdown of the epithelium, stromal edema, and severe pain, as the anesthetic loses its ability to prevent pain in an eye that has had multiple applications of the drug. Similarly, no eye that has had an epithelial abrasion or foreign body should be treated with a medication containing topical steroids because of the greatly increased chance of secondary bacterial, viral, or fungal infection.

5. **Deep corneal foreign bodies** that are suspected of partially penetrating into the anterior chamber should be removed only by an ophthalmologist as there is great danger that an **aqueous leak** will result, with collapse of the anterior chamber. A patch and protective shield should be placed over such an eye and the patient referred for surgical management.

Certain deep corneal foreign bodies need not be removed because of their nontoxic nature and because their removal may result in greater scarring than if they were left in situ. These foreign bodies should be buried sufficiently deeply (but not protruding into the anterior chamber) that the epithelium over them heals without difficulty and the nature of the foreign body should be such that it is inert. An excellent example of this is nonleaded glass, which may be found when a patient has been struck in the glasses, resulting in multiple pieces of shattered glass fragments entering the cornea. Only accessible foreign bodies on the surface should be removed in such a situation. Many such eyes have excellent vision despite an array of inert foreign material scattered throughout the mid- and deep stromal layers of the cornea.

VI. **Corneoscleral lacerations** (see also sec. **VIII.H** and Chap. 10, sec. **XVI**). If the cornea or sclera has been lacerated anteriorly, the eye frequently but not always will be extremely soft. Intraocular contents may protrude from the wound, making the extent of the injury quite obvious.

  A. **History.** When a perforation or intraocular foreign body is suspected, a careful history should be taken to ascertain an exact description of the accident, which may indicate the extent and seriousness of the injury. In children, the most common causes of perforating global injuries are knives, pens, pencils, needles, and sharp toys. In adults, industrial accidents are the most common cause of intraocular foreign bodies or global laceration and include glass fragments, sharp instruments and tools, and small flying metallic and nonmetallic foreign bodies.

  B. **The examination** of the globe should be done most cautiously, with great care taken not to apply pressure that might rupture a partial-thickness laceration or herniate intraocular contents through a full-thickness laceration. If blepharospasm is marked and prevents examination or threatens to herniate intraocular contents, akinesia of the lids may be induced with a **50 : 50 2% xylocaine–0.75% bupivacaine block.** SQ and IM anesthetic should be infiltrated lateral to the lateral canthus and just above and below the lateral two-thirds of the orbital rim. Under no circumstances should any further part of the examination take place without ascertaining visual acuity in the affected eye, especially for medicolegal reasons.

  C. **If the wound is large** and if any manipulation in the emergency area may threaten the entire integrity of the globe, **no further examination should be done at this time.** A cotton pad and a metallic shield should be placed over the eye and the patient sent to the operating room where, after primary temporary repair, further investigation such as x-ray examination for intraocular foreign body may be carried out.

  D. **Signs of global perforation.** Any one or combination of the following suggest possible perforation of the globe:
    1. Decreased visual acuity.
    2. Hypotony (markedly decreased IOP).
    3. Shallowing or flattening of the anterior chamber or hyphema.
    4. Alteration in pupil size, shape, or location.
    5. Focal iris transillumination.
    6. Corneal, lens, or vitreal track.
    7. Marked conjunctival edema (chemosis) or subconjunctival hemorrhage.

  E. **Perforation may be present even though the eye appears entirely normal.** Any patient with a high index of suspicion for perforating injury should be referred for further evaluation. Similarly, presence of some of the preceding signs, such as lowered IOP, may be present after ocular **contusion without any perforation.** Conjunctival chemosis may also occur without perforation. Anterior chamber shallowing, however, is indicative of an **aqueous leak** through a perforation in the absence of any previous history of disease that might have shallowed the chamber at an earlier time. The instillation of a sterile **fluorescein paper strip** in the lower cul-de-sac will stain the tear film, and any aqueous flow through the cornea will be seen as a bright green stream. Alteration in pupillary shape and location indicates uveal extrusion through a wound that may not be visible because of its posterior location or because subconjunctival hemorrhage and chemosis mask the laceration.

  F. **Immediate management of global perforation.** After any lifesaving measures necessary to stabilize the patient have been performed, the immediate management of the global injury is as follows:
    1. **Determine visual acuity,** even if only to ascertain light perception or hand motion.
    2. **Gently culture** for bacteria and fungus from the lower conjunctival cul-de-

sac, **only if possible without pressure on the globe.** More definitive cultures may be done in the operating room.

3. Place a light patch and metal shield over the eye for protection. Cycloplegic or miotic eye drops should **not** be used prior to surgery, as their use may make subsequent repair more difficult or may pull out iris incarcerated in a corneal laceration where it is serving as a plug against a direct opening into the anterior chamber. Topical antibiotics may interfere with cultures taken in the operating room. **No ointments** should be instilled in any eye suspected of having an open wound because ointment may enter the open globe and be irretrievable.

4. **Nausea or vomiting** should be suppressed by immediate administration of antiemetics. Any Valsalva maneuver will raise the IOP and thus threaten prolapse of intraocular tissue through the wound.

5. **The patient should be put on NPO status** in anticipation of administration of general anesthesia in the immediate future.

6. **Appropriate sedatives and analgesics** as well as **tetanus antitoxin** should be administered.

7. **Obtain appropriate x rays, ultrasound, CT scan,** or **NMR** (see Chap. 1).

G. **Ultimate therapy is surgical repair** under general anesthesia. **Systemic antibiotic treatment** IV should be started as in endophthalmitis (see Chap. 8, sec. **XV,** and Appendix B) using an aminoglycoside (tobramycin, amikacin) and cephalosporin (cefazolin, ceftriaxone) or, in penicillin-allergic patients, vancomycin may be substituted for the cephalosporin.

VII. **Intraocular foreign bodies** must always be ruled out whenever periorbital ocular tissue damage or wounds are apparent (see also Chap. 10).

A. **History.** At the time the patient first comes to the emergency area, the physician should ascertain the circumstances of the injury, particularly how it occurred: Was the patient at work? Were safety glasses in place? Had the patient been drinking? The timing of events is important in that the physician must know the exact time of injury and what activities occurred after the injury, particularly those that might have resulted in increased IOP, such as the lifting of heavy objects. It is also important to note when the patient last ate, since general anesthesia may be anticipated if a perforation is present. The last time the patient had tetanus immunization must be ascertained as well as allergy to tetanus antitoxin in anticipation of the administration of tetanus immunization for injury. The condition of the eye prior to the injury, particularly visual acuity, is critical information, as is the status of the uninjured eye. Questions pertinent to the foreign body include whether it was shot as a missile or simply fell or blew gently into the eye, what its composition is, if known, and if metallic, its magnetic properties. It is also important to ascertain if the foreign body hit the eye as a highly driven missile, what materials were being used at the time, e.g., steel on steel, concrete, wood, brass. Intracranial extension of the injury must also be considered.

B. **Foreign bodies are either metallic or nonmetallic,** with the metallic being divided into magnetic and nonmagnetic foreign bodies. It is extremely important to note if the foreign body is magnetic as this not only indicates the presence of toxic iron content but also means that the foreign body is amenable to removal from the eye using magnetic devices. The following indicates the most commonly seen metallic (in order of decreasing toxicity) and nonmetallic foreign bodies and their toxicities:

Metallic		Nonmetallic	
Toxic	*Nontoxic*	*Toxic*	*Nontoxic*
Iron	Gold	Vegetable matter	Stone
Copper (bronze, brass)	Silver	Cloth particles	Glass
	Platinum	Cilia	Porcelain
Mercury	Tantalum	Eyelid particle	Carbon
Aluminum			Some plastics
Nickel			
Zinc			
Lead			

It is obvious that every effort should be made to locate and remove those intraocular foreign bodies that have toxic potential. Iron and copper (bronze and brass alloys) can cause electroretinogram changes and consequent siderosis (iron deposition in intraocular epithelial cells such as retinal pigment epithelium) or chalcosis (copper deposition in basement membranes such as lens capsule or Descemet's membrane). Foreign bodies that are nontoxic may be left in place if their removal would be so difficult that damage to the eye would be greater from surgical manipulation than from leaving them in place.

C. **Techniques by which foreign bodies may be located** include magnified view of the anterior segment, ophthalmoscopy of the posterior segment, x ray, ultrasound, CT scan, and NMR **(if metal is nonmagnetic).** The first three may be carried out by the emergency room physician. Radiologic views most useful for intraocular foreign body location are the Waters' view, which moves the shadow of the petrous pyramid away from the region of the eyeball, and Bellow's modified lateral view, which superimposes only the shadow of the lateral orbital wall onto the area of the eyeball. Bone-free projections of the anterior segment should be taken using dental x-ray film if anterior segment foreign body is suspected. (See Chap. 1 for the roles of ultrasound, CT scan, and NMR.) The responsible physician should be present during any radiologic procedures because a radiologist or a radiologic technician might be unaware of the potential dangers involved in certain manipulations of the patient that might produce undue pressure on the globe.

D. **The size of retained foreign bodies** varies, with the smallest foreign body that may enter an eye being 0.25 mm × 1 mm × 1 mm in size and the largest being 3 mm × 3 mm × 3 mm and 500 mg in weight. Any foreign body larger than this will usually destroy the globe. Frequently, direct visualization of the foreign body by slit lamp or ophthalmoscopy may be successful; however, hemorrhage or cataract formation may obscure the examiner's view, leaving x-ray, CT, or NMR techniques (see Chap. 1) the only alternatives for locating the foreign body. The decision as to whether a foreign body should be removed from the globe should be made before the particle becomes encapsulated by fibrous tissue. This process of encapsulation takes a few days, however, thereby giving the physician sufficient time to perform necessary diagnostic tests.

E. **Intraocular foreign bodies are retained at different sites** with varying frequencies: in the anterior chamber, 15%; in the lens, 8%; in the posterior segment, 70%; and in the orbit (double perforation), 7%. The presence of more than one foreign body must always be looked for, and the examiner should not be satisfied with the detection of a single foreign body in any one of these sites, although a single foreign body is certainly sufficient grounds for immediate referral for surgical management.

F. **Immediate management** is the same as for global perforation (see sec. **VI.F**).

VIII. **Contusion injuries of the anterior segment.** A direct blow to the eye by a blunt missile such as a clenched fist, squash ball, or champagne cork may produce any one or a combination of the following injuries: hyphema (blood in the anterior chamber), dislocation of the crystalline lens, blowout fracture of the orbital floor or nasal wall, iridodialysis (rupture or tear of the iris from its base on the ciliary body), traumatic pupillary mydriasis (dilation), or traumatic iritis. The most common finding, **subconjunctival hemorrhage** is the only one of little to no consequence. It requires no treatment and will resolve over one to several weeks.

A. **Traumatic hyphema** may be very mild and detectable only with slit-lamp examination, revealing multiple red cells floating in the aqueous, or may be severe, with filling of the entire anterior chamber with blood to produce the "eight ball hemorrhage." Approximately 20% of all hyphemas rebleed. These are usually in eyes that have had moderately severe to severe hyphemas at the time of the original injury. Microscopic hyphemas rarely rebleed. Of those eyes that do have a secondary or initial total hyphema, 20-50% will end up with visual acuity of 20/40 or less. Approximately 5-10% of traumatic hyphemas require surgical intervention, and 7% of patients with a history of such hyphema develop glaucoma in later years, particularly if there has been a recession or partial rupture and posterior dislocation of the iris angle. In approximately 8% of cases dislocation of the lens and vitreous hemorrhage occur. Retinal hemorrhage, although usually less ominous, occurs in more than 50% of cases.

1. **Signs and symptoms.** The patient will frequently present with a history of trauma to the eye. Examination may reveal marked decrease in vision with a reddish haze present diffusely throughout the anterior chamber, a settled layer of blood present inferiorly, or a complete filling of the anterior chamber so that no posterior segment structures may be seen with the ophthalmoscope. IOP may be raised due to interference with aqueous drainage by the blood, or the eye may be soft due to decreased aqueous production secondary to ciliary body trauma. The pupil is often irregular and poorly reactive. Traumatic hyphemas, regardless of severity, are frequently accompanied by such marked **somnolence**, particularly in children, that the examining physician may suspect neurologic complication. The hyphema alone may be sufficient cause for this somnolence although the presence of concussion or more severe neurologic damage must always be considered.

2. **Therapy.** Patients, other than reliable adults who have minimum hyphema (less than one-third of the anterior chamber) and who may rest quietly at home with no young children to care for, should be hospitalized for 5 days after the initial bleed. Daily examination under magnification and determination of IOP are important for detecting rebleeding or rise in IOP that may result in iron staining of the cornea. The patient should be allowed quiet activity. Current studies indicate that strict bed rest, sedation, and bilateral patching or steroids are not significantly more effective in preventing complications or rebleeds than are ambulation, no sedation, and patching only on the traumatized eye. Atropine cycloplegia of the affected eye, however, will prevent contraction of the ciliary body and pupil with subsequent disruption of recently diffusely damaged vessels. There is little evidence that pupillary constriction or use of topical or systemic steroids has any constructive effect in the management of traumatic hyphema.

3. **Rebleeding** occurs in up to one-third of patients, usually between 3 and 5 days after the initial trauma and almost invariably before the seventh day posttrauma. Rebleeding is more frequent in black than white patients. A rebleed is almost invariably more severe than the original hemorrhage and the prognosis for reduced vision, **corneal blood staining,** and **secondary glaucoma** is worse. If there is not immediate resorption of the blood, iron pigment will enter the cornea, particularly if IOP is raised. If the corneal endothelium is unhealthy, blood staining will occur even without raised IOP. It will take many months for this pigment to clear. Clearing occurs from the periphery toward the center so that the visual axis is the last to resorb. It may be a cause of **deprivation amblyopia** in a very young child, and patching the other eye may be necessary after clearing of corneal staining. Elevated IOP is managed by carbonic anhydrase inhibitors such as acetazolamide, 250 mg PO qid, or ethazolamide, 50 mg PO tid, and systemic hyperosmotic agents such as glycerol in juice q12h. **Aminocaproic acid,** an antifibrinolytic agent, in dosage of 50 mg/kg PO or IV q4h to a maximum dose of 30 gm/24 hours, may reduce rebleeding.

   If rebleeding does occur during hospitalization, the physician should start counting time again from day zero at the time of the rebleed and keep the patient hospitalized until the hyphema has totally cleared and there has been **no further rebleeding for at least 7 days.**

4. **Surgical intervention** is indicated in 5–10% of patients in order to prevent secondary glaucoma, optic atrophy, and peripheral anterior synechia formation. Blood staining of the cornea occurs in almost all cases of total hyphema if IOP exceeds 25 mm Hg for at least 6 days. Optic nerve damage may be expected with IOPs of 50 mm Hg or more for at least 5 days or 35 mm Hg for 7 days. Patients with sclerotic vascular disease of hemoglobinopathies are at even greater risk, due to reduced ocular tolerance of blood

flow impairment. Peripheral anterior synechia formation is usually found in total hyphemas lasting 9 days or more.

B. **Iridodialysis** is the disinsertion of the iris base from the ciliary body. It is frequently associated with hyphema. Its presence and location should be noted at the time of initial examination. **No treatment is immediately necessary** for this condition. Whether or not surgical repair will be necessary may be decided when the effect and extent of the iridodialysis on visual acuity are determined after a suitable recovery period.

C. **Traumatic pupillary mydriasis and miosis.** At the time of the initial examination after blunt contusion of the eye, an abnormal mydriasis (dilation) or miosis (constriction) of the pupil may be present. Additionally, the pupil may react only minimally or not at all to light and have an irregular shape. In the absence of a global rupture or perforation, this deformity is indicative of partial or complete rupture of the iris sphincter, and its presence may be permanent or transient, as is the mydriasis or miosis.

D. **Posttraumatic iridocyclitis** is a mild inflammatory reaction of the iris or ciliary body or both frequently seen after blunt trauma to the eye. The patient complains of an aching in the eye, and IOP is low normal in the early posttraumatic period. Cells and flare may be seen in the anterior chamber. Great relief is achieved by dilation with cycloplegics such as cyclopentolate 1% tid and topical corticosteroids such as prednisolone 1% qid for 5-10 days.

E. **Traumatic angle recession** is a separation or posterior displacement of the tissue at the anterior chamber angle at the site of the trabecular meshwork (area of aqueous drainage from the eye). At least 20% of eyes with a history of traumatic hyphema have some chamber angle recession and therefore should be followed periodically for the development of secondary glaucoma. There is no emergency care needed for angle recession (see also Chap. 9, sec. **XVII.B**).

F. **Luxation and subluxation of the lens.** Traumatic rupture of the zonular fibers holding the lens to the ciliary body may occur after blunt trauma.

1. **If more than 25% of these fibers are ruptured,** the lens is no longer securely held behind the iris. There may be deepening of the anterior chamber uniformly or locally due to tilting of the lens posteriorly, or the anterior chamber may shallow if the lens moves anteriorly, particularly if **pupillary block** develops because the lens entirely occludes the pupil, thereby blocking escape of aqueous humor from the posterior chamber. Additionally, the **iris becomes tremulous (iridodonesis).** This may be easily detected with the handheld flashlight while the patient moves the eye back and forth.

2. **Subluxation** of the lens should be particularly suspected in patients who have Marfan's syndrome, lues, Marchesani's syndrome, or homocystinuria.

3. **Emergency treatment** for luxation is necessary only if there is shallowing of the anterior chamber with pupillary block and secondary glaucoma. Treatment is dilation of the pupil with a strong mydriatic cycloplegic such as atropine 4% to break the pupillary block and allow aqueous to escape from the posterior chamber. The patient should then be referred for evaluation for surgical management.

4. **Surgery** is indicated if the lens is entirely dislocated into the anterior chamber where it may compromise the corneal endothelium by direct abrasion. Miotics such as pilocarpine 2% qid will prevent the lens from falling back into the vitreous cavity. Dislocation of the lens into the **vitreous cavity** is **not** an indication for **emergency therapy,** either medical or surgical. As relief of secondary open-angle glaucoma associated with a vitreous dislocated lens is unreliable using surgical techniques, surgery should be reserved for those cases where a phacolytic glaucoma from hypermaturation of the cataract will predictably relieve the secondary inflammatory glaucoma.

G. **Contusion cataract.** The presence on the anterior lens capsule of a **circle of iris pigment (Vossius ring)** may be noted after pupillary dilation. A Vossius ring is benign in itself but is diagnostic of previous blunt trauma. Contusion cataracts in the form of anterior cortical vacuoles, anterior nodular plaques, posterior cortical opacification, wedge-shaped and generalized opacification, and total lens swelling may occur as an immediate or long-term result of blunt injury to the eye. Treatment is surgical removal when visual impairment becomes significant.

H. **Scleral rupture.** Intact conjunctiva may mask a significant scleral rupture. The most **common sites of rupture** after blunt trauma are in a circumferential arc parallel to the corneal limbus at the insertion of the rectus muscle opposite the site of impact, or at the equator of the globe. The most common site to be ruptured is the supranasal quadrant near the limbus.

1. **Rupture should be suspected** if the anterior chamber is filled with blood and the eye is soft or if there is marked hemorrhagic chemosis of the conjunctiva out of proportion to other evidence of injury.

2. **Management** is the same as corneoscleral laceration in terms of immediate management, with ultimate therapy being surgical repair.

IX. **Contusion injuries of the posterior segment** (see also Chap. 7, sec. **IX,** and Chap. 8, sec. **XVII**)

A. **Trauma to the choroid.** A typical small choroidal hemorrhage is a round, dark red-blue mound with pinkish edges, located at the equator or adjacent to the disk. It takes many weeks to resorb and leaves areas of pigmentary alteration. Massive subchoroidal hemorrhage is often associated with profound secondary glaucoma. If it is recognized early enough, sclerotomy may be attempted. Choroidal tears appear to result from contrecoup mechanisms producing a yellow-white crescentic scar concentric with the optic disk and usually temporal to it. There may be multiple scars parallel to each other.

B. **Traumatic choroiditis.** Chorioretinitis sclopetaria refers to direct choroidal and retinal trauma from a propelled object wound in the orbital area. A peculiar syndrome secondary to trauma, usually of the perforating type that involves the lens, is **pseudoretinitis pigmentosa.** There is a selective loss of the photoreceptor layer, extinguished electroretinogram (ERG), and migration of pigment into the retina.

C. **Ciliochoroidal (uveal) effusion.** There is a collection of fluid in the potential space of the suprachoroid that is external to the main layers of the choroid and ciliary body and internal to the sclera. *Effusion* is considered a better term than *edema* or *detachment* because the fluid is contained within the expansion zone of the uveal tract. Fluid collection is limited anteriorly by the scleral spur and posteriorly by the attachment of the choroid at the optic disk. Where large veins, arteries, or nerves course through the suprachoroid, the lamellae are compacted. Significant landmarks are the vortex veins and the anterior ciliary arteries. There are three types of collections of suprachoroidal fluid according to the clinical appearance: annular, lobular, and flat.

1. **The annular type** involves the ciliary body and peripheral choroid.

2. **Lobular effusions** are hemispheric. Valleys separating them superiorly and inferiorly are created by the vortex veins.

3. **Flat detachments** are most often in isolated peripheral choroidal areas.

4. **A ciliochoroidal effusion** is likely to occur after surgery or trauma and is the second most common lesion of the ciliary body to be confused with malignant melanoma. It is difficult to differentiate ring malignant melanoma from annular choroidal detachment. Acute myopia may develop from ciliary body effusion. Whenever suprachoroidal edema develops without clear traumatic or surgical antecedent, a systemic or focal vascular disease, inflammatory focus, or malignancy must be considered. Scleritis sufficient to produce suprachoroidal edema need not cause signs of choroidal inflammation. Suprachoroidal effusion has been seen in toxemia of pregnancy and can be treated by treating the general disorder. A positive phosphorus-32 test may be obtained. Provided that retinal detachment does not eventuate, the prognosis in suprachoroidal effusion from inflammation is good.

5. **The uveal effusion syndrome** usually presents in uninflamed eyes of middle-aged males as an insidious, progressive, usually bilateral, nonrhegmatogenous retinal detachment with dependent fluid, flat peripheral effusion,

occasional retinal exudates, and localized areas of retinal pigment epithelial hypertrophy and hyperplasia. The process responds poorly to steroids. Prostaglandin inhibitors, indomethacin, aspirin, diflunisal, or naproxen may be tried once or twice daily with some success.

Eyelids and Lacrimal System

Arthur S. Grove, Jr.

I. Eyelids. The eyelids protect the eye by preventing contact with foreign materials and by preventing excessive drying of the cornea and conjunctiva. The palpebral fissure must be wide enough to allow light to enter the pupil and should close sufficiently to provide protection and moisture to the globe. The lid contours and palpebral fissures should be symmetric in order to avoid cosmetic deformity.

A. Eyelid anatomy. The eyelids are lamellar structures covered on their outer surfaces by skin and on their inner surfaces by conjunctiva. Between the skin and conjunctiva are the fibrous tarsal plates, the orbital septum, the upper lid elevators (levator muscle, levator aponeurosis, and Müller's muscle), and the lower lid retractors (inferior rectus fascia and inferior tarsal muscle). The levator muscle is innervated by the third cranial nerve, whereas Müller's muscle and the inferior tarsal muscle are innervated by sympathetic nerves. The lids and palpebral fissures are maintained in a stable position by periosteal attachments provided by the medial and lateral canthal tendons. The palpebral fissure is closed by the orbicularis muscle, which is innervated by the seventh cranial nerve.

B. Congenital and developmental eyelid anomalies

1. **Ptosis.** Most ptosis is congenital and is caused by a deficiency of the striated fibers in the levator muscle. Many cases of congenital ptosis are associated with other developmental abnormalities such as blepharophimosis and epicanthus. Congenital ptosis will be discussed with other eyelid malpositions (see sec. **C.1**).

2. **Blepharophimosis and epicanthus.** Blepharophimosis is a generalized narrowing of the palpebral fissure. This abnormality is frequently associated with congenital ptosis and epicanthus. Epicanthus is a semilunar fold of skin that crosses the medial canthus. Blepharophimosis and epicanthus should usually be repaired prior to surgical correction of ptosis.

3. **Colobomas** are usually full-thickness defects in the medial portions of the upper lids. Colobomas are often associated with other congenital defects such as facial dermoids. Unless exposure keratopathy occurs, surgical repair of most colobomas can be delayed until the child is several years old.

4. **Ankyloblepharon** is an abnormal fusion of the upper and lower eyelid margins, usually near the lateral canthus. The fused lids may be surgically divided if the attachment is cosmetically disfiguring.

5. **Ectropion and entropion** are both uncommon congenital disorders (see secs. **D** and **E**). Congenital ectropion is usually minimum and may be associated with blepharophimosis. Congenital entropion is quite unusual but is frequently confused with epiblepharon.

6. **Epiblepharon** is a condition in which a prominent skin fold is present in front of the tarsus, usually near the medial margin of the lower lid. The lashes may be rotated inward without actual entropion. Surgical correction is seldom required, since epiblepharon usually resolves spontaneously.

C. Ptosis is a malposition of the upper eyelid in which the lid margin is abnormally low because of insufficient upper eyelid retraction. Evaluation of a patient with ptosis should include measurement of palpebral fissure heights and levator functions. The positions of the eyelid folds and any abnormalities of the extraocular muscles should be documented. The type of ptosis should be carefully established by history, since the treatment of congenital ptosis is usually different from that for acquired ptosis. It is much more common to overcorrect acquired ptosis than congenital ptosis. Both congenital and acquired ptosis must be distinguished from pseudoptosis, a condition in which the upper eyelid appears to be low but lid elevation is adequate.

1. **Congenital ptosis** is usually unilateral, although approximately one-fourth of the cases involve both upper eyelids. It may be associated with other abnormalities:

   a. **Blepharophimosis-epicanthus inversus-ptosis syndrome.**

   b. **Marcus Gunn "jaw-winking" syndrome,** a synkinesis in which the ptotic eyelid is elevated with movement of the mandible.

   c. **Extraocular muscle palsies,** particularly those involving the superior rectus and inferior oblique muscles ipsilateral to the ptosis.

   d. **Treatment** of congenital ptosis usually requires resection of part of the weak levator muscle and aponeurosis, or suspension of the lids from the frontalis muscle.

2. **Acquired ptosis** is frequently associated with good levator muscle function and may be categorized according to etiology.

   a. **Involutional** (senile) ptosis often involves both upper lids of older patients and may occur following cataract extraction. This is the most common form of acquired ptosis and is caused by degeneration of the levator aponeurosis.

   b. **Myogenic** ptosis may be associated with a variety of muscular disorders, including myasthenia gravis, oculopharyngeal muscular dystrophy, and progressive external ophthalmoplegia.

   c. **Neurogenic** ptosis can be caused by deficient innervation of the third cranial nerve to the levator muscle or deficient sympathetic innervation to Müller's muscle.

   d. **Traumatic** ptosis may result from lacerations of the levator muscle or aponeurosis and may sometimes follow severe blunt trauma with eyelid edema.

   e. **Mechanical** ptosis may be associated with lid tumors such as neurofibromas and may result from scars or foreign bodies.

   f. **Treatment** of acquired ptosis involves correcting the cause of the ptosis, if possible. When this is not possible, the eyelid can be vertically shortened if levator function is good or may be suspended from the frontalis muscle if levator function is poor.

3. **Pseudoptosis** is a condition in which the upper eyelid appears to be abnormally low without insufficiency of the lid retractors. Causes of pseudoptosis include:

   a. Epicanthus and facial asymmetry.

   b. Excessive upper eyelid skin, as found in dermatochalasis.

   c. Contralateral palpebral fissure widening.

   d. Palpebral fissure narrowing associated with adduction in Duane's retraction syndrome.

   e. Hypertropia or contralateral hypotropia.

   f. Enophthalmos or contralateral exophthalmus.

D. **Ectropion** is a malposition of the eyelid in which the lid margin is turned away from the globe. The lower lid is involved much more commonly than the upper lid. Ectropion sometimes leads to exposure keratopathy and conjunctival hypertrophy. Tearing may result from eversion of the lacrimal punctum if the ectropion involves the medial lid.

1. **Congenital ectropion** is quite uncommon, although it may be found with blepharophimosis. Treatment is rarely required because the eversion is usually minimum.

2. **Acquired ectropion** is categorized on the basis of etiology.

   a. **Involutional** (senile) ectropion is relatively common and is a frequent cause of tearing **(epiphora).** This abnormality is caused by attenuation of the lower eyelid retractors, the orbicularis muscle, and the canthal tendons. Treatment involves horizontal eyelid shortening and canthal suspension. If punctal eversion is the most significant feature, conjunctival shortening and a punctaplasty may reduce tearing.

  b. **Paralytic** ectropion usually results from seventh nerve injury, with resulting drooping of the lower lid and widening of the palpebral fissure. Treatment may require tarsorrhaphy, horizontal lid shortening, canthoplasty, or the use of prostheses such as plastic bands. A flaccid brow and upper lid may be surgically elevated if they partially cover the palpebral fissure.

  c. **Mechanical** ectropion may be caused by abnormalities that push or pull the lid away from the eye. Treatment usually involves treatment of the underlying abnormality.

  d. **Cicatricial** ectropion is caused by scarring associated with skin traction and tissue loss. Linear and circumscribed scars may respond to massage or relaxing operations. More extensive cicatricial ectropion usually requires a skin graft.

E. **Entropion** is a malposition of the eyelid in which the lid margin is turned toward the globe. Entropion is functionally important because inturned lid margins may damage the cornea and produce keratitis or ulceration. Related conditions that should be differentiated from entropion are epiblepharon, trichiasis, and distichia.

  1. **Congenital entropion** is rare and is usually associated with other abnormalities such as tarsal hypoplasia or microophthalmia. It may be confused with epiblepharon, a mild deformity that usually resolves spontaneously. Depending on severity, this condition may be treated similarly to acquired entropion.

  2. **Acquired entropion** is a common disorder that is usually either involutional, as a result of aging, or cicatricial, resulting from tarsoconjunctival shrinkage.

   a. **Involutional** (senile) entropion usually involves the lower lid and is caused by degenerative changes similar to those that cause involutional ectropion. With aging, atrophy of the orbital tissues can lead to a relative enophthalmos and a tendency for inward rotation of already attenuated eyelid structures. Treatment should be directed toward correction of those abnormalities that are most prominent. Penetrating pretarsal cautery or three Quickert lid eversion sutures may temporarily correct a moderate entropion, but may be followed by recurrence. Many operations have been devised for correction of involutional entropion. The most physiologic procedures are those that restore the action of attenuated eyelid retractors and that tighten a lax lower lid.

   b. **Spastic** entropion is a temporary or intermittent accentuation of involutional changes caused by irritation and vigorous lid closure. Treatment can be directed toward removing the cause of irritation or toward treating the underlying involutional abnormalities.

   c. **Cicatricial** entropion is usually the result of tarsoconjunctival shrinkage. This may be caused by a wide variety of disorders, including trachoma, Stevens-Johnson syndrome, pemphigus, ocular pemphigoid, and mechanical, thermal, or chemical injury. Cicatricial changes are often accompanied by trichiasis, reduced tear production, mucosal epidermalization, and punctal occlusion. Treatment may consist of marginal rotation of the lid margin and grafts of mucosa or other tissue to replace contracted tarsus and conjunctiva.

F. **Blepharospasm** is a disorder of unknown cause that involves involuntary closure of the eyelids. The severity of this closure ranges from mild increased frequency of blinking to severe spasms that completely occlude the eyes. Essential blepharospasm, in which the eyelids are chiefly involved, is distinguished from conditions such as Meige's disease, where lower face and neck muscles also spasm, and hemifacial spasm, which may be caused by facial nerve compression. Excision of facial muscles (myectomy) and nerves (neurectomy) has been used in the past as treatment for severe cases of essential blepharospasm. Currently **botulinum toxin injections** are considered the most effective treatment for the majority of patients with this condition. Multiple small amounts of the toxin are injected into the muscles around the eyelids. Blepharospasm is usually relieved within several days, but the effect is temporary and additional injections are often necessary within 3 months. Side effects include ptosis, double vision, and drying of the eyes from inability to close the lids (see Chap. 11, sec. **XII**).

G. **Eyelash disorders.** The eyelashes normally emerge from the lid margin anterior to the mucocutaneous junction and are directed away from the surface of the eye. In a number of conditions the lashes either arise abnormally posterior or are directed toward the eye.

1. **Distichiasis** is an abnormality in which extra lashes arise from the lid margin behind the mucocutaneous junction, frequently from the meibomian gland orifices. These lashes are usually small and cause few symptoms, but occasionally they may produce severe corneal damage. Treatment is not required in mild cases. If the eye is being injured, the lashes may be destroyed with cryotherapy, electrolysis, or surgery.

2. **Trichiasis** is an acquired condition in which the lashes are directed posteriorly, toward the surface of the eye. Although the lid margin is not necessarily inverted, trichiasis can occur in association with entropion. Trichiasis often accompanies chronic blepharoconjunctivitis or cicatricial conjunctivitis. **Cryotherapy** is probably the best method of permanently treating most cases of trichiasis. Electrolysis is usually ineffective in treating large numbers of abnormal lashes. Surgical excision of the lashes and replacement with a mucous membrane graft may be used to treat severe cases of trichiasis in which it is desired to retain some normal lashes.

H. **Eyelid tumors.** The first priority in treating any tumor of the eyelids is to establish the diagnosis. Except for inflammatory lesions such as chalazions, any tissue removed from the eyelids should be examined histologically. Treatments such as cauterization that destroy tissue and make histologic evaluation impossible should not be used. In the case of a small skin lesion, excisional biopsy can be performed with removal of all clinical evidence of the tumor. If a benign tumor is suspected, the margins of the incision may be within 1 or 2 mm of the lesion. If a malignant tumor is suspected, 3–5 mm of clinically uninvolved tissue should be removed with the lesion. When a tumor is histologically malignant, the pathologist should be asked to examine all margins of the specimen, including the deep surface, for evidence of tumor that has been cut across. If the tumor is found to have been transected, additional tissue should usually be removed. The management of each kind of tumor should obviously depend on its individual growth characteristics and on the requirements for reconstructing functional eyelids. The most common benign and malignant tumors of the eyelids are listed below:

Benign tumors	Malignant tumors
Keratoses	Basal cell carcinomas
Nevi	Squamous cell carcinomas
Epithelial, sebaceous, and sudoriferous cysts	Malignant melanomas
	Sebaceous cell carcinomas

1. **Basal cell carcinomas** are by far the most common malignant tumors of the eyelids. These tumors most frequently arise on the sun-exposed lower lids and medial canthal areas. Most basal cell carcinomas are nodular with a pearly surface and telangiectatic vessels. Some are flat and leathery and are described as morpheaform or sclerosing basal cell carcinomas. This latter type of tumor is particularly likely to be infiltrative. Treatment usually consists of histologically confirmed surgical excision. Although cryotherapy and radiation are sometimes used to destroy basal cell carcinomas, their

use does not provide microscopic confirmation of complete tumor excision. Radiation of smaller ($<$ 3 mm) biopsy-proved primary growths may be preferable to more extensive plastic surgery in older patients. Any recurrence should be treated surgically. These regrowths after irradiation are rare, however. Metastatic spread of basal cell carcinomas is exceedingly uncommon.

2. **Squamous cell carcinomas** usually arise among older patients and commonly develop from actinic keratoses. Differentiation from benign keratoacanthomas is sometimes difficult. Treatment of these potentially metastasizing tumors should consist of wide surgical excision that is histologically confirmed to be adequate by careful examination of all margins.

3. **Malignant melanomas** of the eyelids are uncommon and usually arise from melanomas of the conjunctiva. These potentially metastasizing tumors may occur de novo or may evolve from preexisting nevi or from areas of acquired melanosis. The histologic feature of greatest prognostic importance seems to be the tendency toward vertical growth (deep invasion below the epithelial surface). Conjunctival melanomas that grow deeply tend to be more lethal than those that grow peripherally. Treatment of eyelid melanomas is controversial, since some patients die from these tumors despite any treatment. Complete wide excision is the most common therapy, and radical surgery such as exenteration is frequently advised.

4. **Sebaceous cell carcinomas** arise most often from the meibomian glands within the tarsal plates. These highly malignant tumors may also develop from the sebaceous glands of the eyelashes, the caruncle, and the eyebrow. Their growth may mimic **chalazions** and the contents of a presumably recurrent chalazion should always be examined histologically. Fat stains should be performed on fresh tissue whenever sebaceous carcinoma is suspected. These tumors may be multifocal and can spread peripherally by intraepithelial or pagetoid growth. Metastasis and orbital extension frequently occur. Treatment consists of wide surgical excision, with histologic confirmation of complete removal. Because of insidious intraepithelial growth, multiple areas of excision or exenteration may be required.

I. **Eyelid inflammation and degeneration.** The most common inflammations of the eyelids are those involving the lashes and the lid margins (blepharitis) and those that arise within the meibomian glands as an acute lesion (hordeolum) or evolve into a chronic lesion (chalazion). Diffuse inflammatory eyelid atrophy (blepharochalasis) should be distinguished from involutional degeneration of the eyelids (dermatochalasis).

1. **Blepharitis** is the most common inflammation of the eyelids. It usually involves the lid margins and frequently is associated with conjunctivitis. Bacterial infection by *Staphylococcus* is frequently responsible for chronic blepharoconjunctivitis and may be associated with superficial punctate keratitis. Severe cases may produce purulent discharge and permanent changes in eyelid structure. Treatment of staphylococcal blepharoconjunctivitis usually involves mechanical debridement of the lid margins with scrubs using cotton-tipped applicators. Warm moist compresses help to reduce discomfort and increase blood flow. Topical antibiotics should be used to control the infection (see Chap. 5, sec. **III.B** and **D**).

2. **Hordeolum** is a focal acute infection arising within the meibomian glands or other glands at the eyelid margins. These lesions are commonly caused by *Staphylococcus* and usually respond to conservative therapy. Treatment by warm, moist compresses and topical antibiotics usually produces resolution of the inflammation (see Chap. 5, sec. **III.B** and **D**).

3. **Chalazion** is a focal chronic inflammation of a meibomian gland. It is a common disorder that may occur as the chronic result of a resolved hordeolum. If a presumed chalazion recurs after initial treatment, the possible diagnosis of **sebaceous cell carcinoma** should be considered. Treatment by warm compresses is effective in most cases, with topical antibiotics used

to prevent secondary spread of infection. **Injection of the lesion** with 0.1 ml aqueous dexamethasone 24 mg/ml will usually resolve the mass, but incision and curettage through the conjunctiva may be necessary in some instances. Recurrent lesions should be examined histologically (see Chap. 5, sec. III).

4. **Blepharochalasis** is a rare condition that results from repeated idiopathic episodes of eyelid edema and inflammation. These acute attacks occur most frequently among younger individuals and are more common among women than men. The inflammation often results in wrinkling of the skin, atrophy of fat, and ptosis. Treatment of acute attacks is usually not necessary because they are self-limited, although systemic steroids may be of some value. The chronic atrophic changes may respond to blepharoplasty and to repair of the acquired ptosis.

5. **Dermatochalasis** is a redundancy of the skin of the eyelids that is often accompanied by herniation of fat through the orbital septum. This condition usually occurs as an involutional change among older or middle-aged people. A familial predisposition is common, although there is no sex predilection. The excessive skin may cause a pseudoptosis, although a true involutional ptosis may be present. Treatment is blepharoplasty with optional fat excision and repair of acquired ptosis, if present.

J. **Eyelid trauma.** Injuries to the globe may be relatively occult and may be overshadowed by obvious lid damage. Therefore, the eye should be carefully examined and the visual acuity should be documented before injured eyelids are treated. During lid repairs the globe should be protected to prevent additional injury. The possible occurrence of orbital fractures or of embedded foreign bodies should always be considered. If necessary, x rays and computerized tomography may be used to evaluate these possibilities.

1. **Burns** of the lids may be chemical, thermal, or electrical (see Chap. 2, secs. I and II). The first priority is to treat associated ocular injury. Lid retraction and cicatricial ectropion may result from burns and require skin grafting or other surgical repair after a period of time.

2. **Lacerations** of the eyelids may be repaired primarily even as long as 12–24 hours after injury, because of their rich vascular supply and the rarity of infections. Treatment should involve minimum debridement and retention of as much tissue as possible. The wound should be explored to rule out foreign bodies, and all tissues should be replaced in their anatomic positions. The tarsus should be separately approximated by sutures tied away from the surface of the eye. Tissue loss can be replaced by lid advancement or a skin graft. When the deep tissues of the upper eyelid are involved by a laceration, the levator aponeurosis should be examined and repaired if it is damaged.

II. **Lacrimal system.** The tear film is composed of mucin, oil, and watery lacrimal fluid. The mucin component is the product of the conjunctival goblet cells, while oil is secreted by the sebaceous meibomian glands within the tarsal plates and by the glands of Zeis and Moll, which lie near the lid margins. The bulk of the tear film is made up of lacrimal fluid from the main lacrimal gland and from the accessory lacrimal glands of Krause and Wolfring (see Chap. 1, secs. II.J and K for the **clinical tests** used to measure tear film adequacy, including tests of secretion). The lacrimal secretions are distributed over the surface of the eye by gravity, capillary action, and the eyelids. Tears leave the eye by evaporation and by flow through the lacrimal excretory system, composed of the puncta, the canaliculi, the lacrimal sac, and the nasolacrimal duct.

A. **Lacrimal excretory anatomy and physiology**

1. **Puncta.** The puncta are small openings approximately 0.3 mm in diameter that lie at the edge of each eyelid. Each upper punctum is approximately 6 mm temporal to the medial canthal angle among adults, while the lower punctum is slightly more temporal than the upper.

2. **Canaliculi.** The canaliculi are composed of short vertical segments that begin at the puncta and of horizontal segments approximately 8 mm long

that empty into the lacrimal sac. The upper and lower canaliculi usually empty into a common canaliculus (sinus of Maier) before communicating with the sac. In approximately 10% of patients the upper and lower canaliculi each open separately into the lacrimal sac.

3. **Lacrimal sac.** The sac is a cystic structure lined with columnar epithelium. The medial canthal tendon passes in front of the sac, and the lacrimal diaphragm and Horner's muscle (the deep head of the pretarsal muscle) pass behind the sac.

4. **Nasolacrimal duct.** This duct is a vertically oriented tube that is continuous with the lower end of the sac. It passes through the bony nasolacrimal canal to drain into the nose beneath the inferior turbinate via the nasal ostium. At the junction between the duct and the nasal fossa, a mucosal fold (valve of Hasner) may be found.

5. **Lacrimal excretion.** Passage of tear fluid from the surface of the eye through the excretory system depends on the anatomic patency of each segment of the pathways. In order for fluid to enter the system, the puncta must be in anatomic apposition to the tear film meniscus on the surface of the eye. Entrance of tears into the canaliculi is aided by capillary action. Movement of fluid through the pathways is aided by a **lacrimal pump** mechanism. This pumping action results from eyelid blinking, during which the muscles and diaphragm around the lacrimal sac move to create internal pressure changes and propel tears. The patency and function of the excretory system can be evaluated by dye tests, irrigation, and dacryocystography.

B. **Congenital and developmental lacrimal anomalies**

1. **Nasolacrimal duct obstruction** is the most common congenital abnormality of the lacrimal system. As many as 30% of newborn infants are believed to have closure of the duct at birth. This obstruction is usually located at the nasal mucoperiosteum, near the site of the valve of Hasner. In most cases, this obstruction is transient, and patency occurs within 3 weeks of birth. Tears and mucus may accumulate in the lacrimal sac, causing distention of the sac and sometimes leading to dacryocystitis. Treatment of a distended sac in an infant consists of sac massage and application of topical antibiotics. If the obstruction is not relieved within 4–8 weeks, irrigation, and probing into the nose can usually be performed on a young infant without general anesthesia. In most instances, a single probing will relieve the obstruction.

2. **Punctal and canalicular** abnormalities include absence, stenosis, duplication, and fistulization. Imperforate or absent puncta can sometimes be opened by a sharply pointed dilator and a microscope. Fistulas can be surgically excised. Absent canaliculi can be bypassed by performing a conjunctivodacryocystorhinostomy with insertion of a glass or plastic tube into the nose.

3. **Diverticula** may arise from the lacrimal sac, the canaliculi, or the nasolacrimal duct. These cystic outpouchings may accumulate fluid and therefore simulate a mucocele of the lacrimal sac. They may become infected and mimic dacryocystitis. Chronic epiphora, however, is usually not a prominent symptom of diverticula. Treatment is surgical excision.

C. **Lacrimal sac tumors.** Neoplasms of the lacrimal sac are unusual and therefore may go undiagnosed for a long time because they are confused with inflammations and other causes of nasolacrimal obstruction. Tumors of the sac typically cause **epiphora** with a subcutaneous mass superior to the medial canthal tendon. Blood may reflux from the puncta and saline irrigation may pass into the nose, despite a history suggestive of dacryocystitis. Squamous papillomas are the most common benign tumors of the sac, while epidermoid carcinomas are the most frequent malignancies. Treatment of lacrimal sac tumors usually requires dacryocystectomy. Removal of the medial canthal tissues and adjacent bone may be necessary to eradicate malignant epithelial lesions. Lymphoid tumors frequently respond to radiation therapy.

D. Lacrimal inflammations and degenerations. Acquired obstructions of the lacrimal excretory system may result from infections, other inflammations, and involutional changes.

   1. Dacryocystitis usually follows a mucocele of the lacrimal sac, which in turn results from obstruction of the nasolacrimal duct. Dacryocystitis usually produces localized pain, edema, and erythema over the lacrimal sac. This clinical pattern must be distinguished from acute ethmoid sinusitis, although purulent discharge from the puncta almost always indicates an infection within the sac. Irrigation and probing should usually not be performed during an acute infection. This disorder usually responds to warm moist compresses, together with topically and systemically administered antibiotics. A distended lacrimal sac should be incised and drained only if the infection does not respond to conservative therapy and if an abscess becomes localized.

   2. Lacrimal sac obstructions are uncommon and generally result from dacryoliths. Solid concretions within the sac may be caused by infection with *Actinomyces israelii (Streptothrix).* Although such infections sometimes respond to irrigation with antibiotics, the sac must frequently be opened and a dacryocystorhinostomy performed.

   3. Nasolacrimal duct obstruction usually occurs among older individuals and is commonly idiopathic. Most such involutional cases are probably the result of mucosal degeneration with stenosis. The most common sequelae of duct obstruction are epiphora and a mucocele of the sac. Dacryocystitis often follows a chronic mucocele. Probing of obstructed nasolacrimal ducts among adults rarely restores patency. Partial obstruction may respond to intubation of the entire excretory system with Silastic tubing. A dacryocystorhinostomy may be considered in cases when the canaliculi are patent. Such an operation is usually not indicated unless tearing and mucous discharge are extremely bothersome or unless the patient suffers repeated attacks of dacryocystitis. It is possible that a duct obstruction may result from a mass within the nose. Therefore, the nasal fossa should always be examined before a dacryocystorhinostomy is performed.

   4. Punctal and canalicular obstructions may occur in association with conjunctival disorders such as Stevens-Johnson syndrome, pemphigus, ocular pemphigoid, and mechanical, thermal, or chemical injury. Canaliculitis may sometimes result from infections caused by *A. israelii.* Stenotic or obstructed puncta can be dilated and incised if necessary. If canalicular stenosis can be opened by probing, Silastic tubing can sometimes be passed through the entire excretory system into the nose to maintain patency. In cases of complete and irreversible punctal or canalicular stenosis when epiphora is severe, the obstruction can be bypassed by performing a conjunctivodacryocystorhinostomy with insertion of a glass or plastic tube into the nose.

E. Lacrimal trauma. Although the lacrimal excretory system may be obstructed by trauma to any of its components, the most common injuries are lacerations of the canaliculi or puncta and nasolacrimal duct obstructions associated with medial orbital fractures (see Chap. 4, sec. **VIII**).

   1. Lacerations of the canaliculi usually need not be repaired as emergencies. Because of the rich vascular supply and the infrequency of infections near the eyelids and medial canthus, primary repair can sometimes be delayed for as long as 12–24 hours after injury. Such a delay may actually be beneficial because transected canaliculi can occasionally be better identified after a period of time and because nighttime surgery may be avoided. If only one canaliculus is severed, it should be repaired, but unnecessary damage to the uninjured canaliculus should be carefully avoided. In many individuals no significant tearing occurs even after complete obstruction or loss of a single canaliculus. A wide variety of sutures, wires, and tubes have been described for the support of lacerated canaliculi during surgical approximation and healing. If possible, these supports should remain within the canaliculus until 4–6 weeks after injury.

2. **Avulsions** of both canaliculi will in most cases result in complete obstruction of tear flow into the lacrimal sac. If no canalicular tissue is present for reapproximation, a conjunctivodacryocystorhinostomy can be performed with insertion of a glass or plastic tube into the nose at the time of original repair of the wounds.

Orbital Disorders

Arthur S. Grove, Jr.

The orbits are bony cavities located on each side of the nose. Each orbit contains a complex structure of soft tissues including the globe, optic nerve, extraocular muscles, fat, fascia, and vessels. Orbital disorders are associated with a wide variety of local and systemic diseases, and their treatment requires a thorough knowledge of regional anatomy, radiology, neurology, and endocrinology.

I. **Orbital anatomy.** Each bony orbit is pear shaped, tapering posteriorly toward the apex and the optic canal. The medial orbital walls are nearly parallel and are approximately 25 mm apart in the average adult.

A. **Orbital walls.** The surfaces of each orbit (roof, lateral wall, medial wall, and floor) are composed of seven bones: ethmoid, frontal, lacrimal, maxillary, palatine, sphenoid, and zygomatic. The thinnest of these surfaces are the lamina papyracea over the ethmoid sinuses (along the medial wall) and the maxillary bone over the infraorbital canal (along the orbital floor).

B. **Orbital apertures**

1. **The ethmoidal foramen** is located in the medial orbital wall, through which pass the anterior and posterior ethmoidal arteries.

2. **The superior orbital fissure** is located between the greater and lesser wings of the sphenoid, through which pass most of the orbital veins, some sympathetic fibers, the third, fourth, and sixth cranial nerves, and the ophthalmic division of the fifth cranial nerve.

3. **The inferior orbital fissure** is located at the lower portion of the orbital apex, through which pass some orbital veins, the zygomatic nerve, and the maxillary division of the fifth cranial nerve.

4. **The zygomaticofacial and zygomaticotemporal canals** are located in the lateral orbital wall, through which pass vessels and branches of the maxillary nerve.

5. **The nasolacrimal canal** is formed by the maxilla and lacrimal bone, through which passes the nasolacrimal duct between the lacrimal sac and the inferior nasal meatus.

6. **The optic canal** is located in the lesser wing of the sphenoid, through which pass the optic nerve, the ophthalmic artery, and sympathetic nerves. This canal is 5-10 mm long and is separated from the superior orbital fissure by the bony optic strut. The orbital end of the canal is the optic foramen, which normally measures 6.5 mm or smaller in diameter. In young children the **sizes of both foramens should be compared.** A foramen that is at least 1.5 mm larger than the contralateral foramen is commonly considered abnormal and suggests the presence of an **optic nerve glioma.**

II. **Orbital evaluation** (see also Chap. 1). The evaluation and diagnosis of an orbital abnormality is guided by considering the most common disorders that occur among children and adults (see sec. **III**). A clinical history should include questions about the presence of malignant tumors or thyroid disease that might involve the orbit. Evaluation of the orbits should be preceded by a careful ophthalmic examination.

A. **X rays** provide a simple method of studying the orbital bones, but their use is limited because of poor soft tissue definition.

B. **Ultrasonography** is a sensitive technique for evaluating intraocular details and for visualizing many orbital lesions. However, the sound waves cannot penetrate bone, and some orbital masses may not be detected unless the waves strike a perpendicular surface.

C. **Computed tomography** (CT) uses thin x-ray beams to obtain tissue density values, from which detailed cross-sectional images of the body are produced by a computer. CT simultaneously visualizes orbital and intracranial structures including soft tissues, bones, and many foreign bodies. Vessels may be seen most clearly after intravenous injection of contrast material. CT is the most useful single imaging technique for orbital evaluation.

D. **Magnetic resonance imaging** (MRI) is a method of visualizing thin anatomic sections by exposing patients to a magnetic field and then recording the radiofrequency emissions from protons (which are the nuclei of hydrogen atoms). Advantages of MRI include the lack of ionizing radiation (as used in x rays and CT) and the ability to distinguish among certain vascular and neurologic abnormalities. A disadvantage is that bone does not give magnetic resonance signals; therefore some lesions may be better evaluated by CT scans.

E. **Arteriography** is performed by injection of radiopaque dye into the carotids to visualize the orbital and intracranial arteries. It has a low, but significant, risk of serious neurologic and vascular complications. Maximum information can be obtained from arteriography through use of selective internal and external carotid injections, magnification, and radiographic subtraction.

III. **Incidence of orbital abnormalities.** It is useful to group orbital disorders into those that most commonly occur during childhood through the second decade of life and those that are found predominately among adults.

A. **Common orbital abnormalities among children**
   1. Orbital cellulitis.
   2. Pseudotumor.
   3. Dermoid and epidermoid cysts.
   4. Capillary hemangioma.
   5. Lymphangioma.
   6. Rhabdomyosarcoma.
   7. Optic nerve glioma.
   8. Neurofibroma.
   9. Leukemia.
   10. Metastatic neuroblastoma.

B. **Common orbital abnormalities among adults**
   1. Ophthalmic Graves' disease.
   2. Pseudotumor.
   3. Metastatic neoplasms.
   4. Secondary neoplasms.
   5. Cavernous hemangioma.
   6. Lymphangioma.
   7. Lacrimal gland tumors.
   8. Lymphoma.
   9. Meningioma.
   10. Dermoid and epidermoid cysts.

IV. **Exophthalmus** is one of the most common clinical manifestations of an orbital abnormality. *Exophthalmus* is defined as an abnormal prominence of one or both eyes, usually resulting from a mass, a vascular abnormality, or an inflammatory process. Among adults, the usual distance from the lateral orbital rim to the corneal apex is approximately 16 mm; it is uncommon for a cornea to protrude more than 21 mm beyond the orbital rim. **An asymmetry of more than 2 mm between the eyes is suggestive of unilateral exophthalmus.**

A. **Unilateral exophthalmus** among children is most commonly caused by orbital cellulitis as a complication of either ethmoid sinus disease or a respiratory infection. Among adults, prominence of one eye is most commonly due to ophthalmic Graves' disease.

B. **Bilateral exophthalmus** among children may be caused by leukemia or by metastatic neuroblastoma. Among adults, bilateral exophthalmus is most often caused by ophthalmic Graves' disease and less often by other inflammations such as pseudotumor or Wegener's granulomatosis.

C. Pseudoexophthalmus is either the simulation of abnormal prominence of the eye or a true asymmetry that is not due to a mass, a vascular abnormality, or an inflammatory process. Causes of pseudoexophthalmus are as follows:

1. Enlarged globe:
   a. Myopia.
   b. Trauma.
   c. Glaucoma.
2. Asymmetric orbital size:
   a. Congenital.
   b. Postradiation.
   c. Postsurgical.
3. Asymmetric palpebral fissures:
   a. Contralateral ptosis.
   b. Lid retraction.
   c. Facial nerve paralysis.
   d. Lid scar, ectropion, entropion.
4. Extraocular muscle abnormalities:
   a. Postsurgical muscle recession.
   b. Paralysis or paresis.
5. Contralateral enophthalmos:
   a. Contralateral orbital fracture.
   b. Contralateral small globe.
   c. Contralateral cicatricial tumor (especially metastatic breast carcinoma).

Even if a patient is found to have pseudoexophthalmus, it is appropriate to examine the orbits carefully and to obtain orbital x rays to serve as a reference for future examinations.

V. **Orbital inflammations.** Inflammations of the orbit are probably responsible for more cases of exophthalmus than are neoplasms. Among adults, ophthalmic Graves' disease causes more unilateral and bilateral exophthalmus than any other disorder. Among children, orbital cellulitis probably produces exophthalmus more often than any neoplasm. Pseudotumors are idiopathic inflammations that resemble neoplasms and are often associated with exophthalmus and pain. The orbit is a common site of occurrence for a wide variety of other inflammatory disorders related to infections, trauma, and systemic disease.

A. **Graves' disease.** *Ophthalmic Graves' disease* has been defined as a multisystem disease of unknown etiology characterized by one or more of three pathognomonic clinical entities: hyperthyroidism with diffuse thyroid hyperplasia, infiltrative dermopathy, and infiltrative ophthalmology. Ophthalmic Graves' disease includes any of the orbital manifestations of this disorder.

1. **Key clinical signs and their eponyms**
   a. Lid retraction (Dalrymple).
   b. Upper lid "lag" on down gaze (von Graefe).
   c. Upper lid resistance to downward traction (Grove).
   d. Tremor of closed lids (Rosenbach).
   e. Infrequent blink (Stellwag).
   f. Increased lid pigmentation (Jellinek).
   g. Poor convergence (Möbius).
   h. Extraocular muscle palsies (Ballet).
   i. Weak lateral gaze fixation (Suker).
   j. Unequal pupillary dilation (Knie).
   k. Jerky pupillary consensual light contraction (Cowen).
   l. Poor forehead wrinkling on up gaze (Joffroy).
   m. Audible bruit over closed eye (Riesman).
2. **Werner's classification of ocular signs of Graves' disease**
   a. **Class 0.** No abnormalities.
   b. **Class 1.** No symptoms. Signs are lid retraction, stare, and proptosis.

   c. **Class 2.** Soft tissues involved. Symptoms are lacrimation, photophobia, foreign body sensation, and retrobulbar discomfort. Signs are lid and conjunctival edema and hyperemia, extrusion of orbital fat, and palpable main lacrimal gland and inferior extraocular muscles.

   d. **Class 3.** Proptosis (classes 2–6): minimum, 21–33 mm; moderate, 24–27 mm; marked, 28 mm or more.

   e. **Class 4.** Extraocular muscle palsy ranges from mild restriction to total fixation of globe. Diplopia is often due to inferior and medial rectus contraction and fibrosis.

   f. **Class 5.** Corneal involvement is minimum, with stippled stain, moderate epithelial ulceration, marked corneal scarring, necrosis, or perforation.

   g. **Class 6.** There is visual loss secondary to optic nerve involvement, with disk pallor, papilledema, and visual field defects. Mild loss, 20/20 to 20/60; moderate loss, 20/70 to 20/200; severe loss, 20/200 or less.

3. **Thyroid tests** are usually abnormal among patients with ophthalmic Graves' disease. Some patients, however, will have only abnormal thyroid suppressibility and others will be euthyroid by all tests, so that the diagnosis of Graves' disease is established by clinical features alone.

   a. **Initial screening tests.** Thyroxin levels (total T_4 and free T_4) and triiodothyronine level (T_3).

   b. **Thyroid suppressibility tests.** T_3 suppression test (Werner test) and thyrotropin-releasing hormone (TRH) test should be considered if screening tests are normal or equivocal and Graves' disease is still suspected.

4. **Anatomic tests** visualize characteristic but not pathognomonic changes in orbital anatomy in association with Graves' disease.

   a. **Ultrasound B scans** show enlarged extraocular muscles and inflammatory changes in the orbital fat.

   b. **CT scans** show enlarged extraocular muscles and congestive changes at the orbital apex.

   c. **Radionuclide scans** show increased uptake of technetium-labeled compounds within inflamed extraocular muscles.

5. **Treatment.** Since ophthalmic Graves' disease often produces symptoms because of corneal drying, initial treatment usually consists of topical ophthalmic lubricants. If corneal damage becomes severe because of exophthalmus and lid retraction, emergency high-dose systemic steroids should be given and the palpebral fissure may be narrowed by a simple lateral tarsorrhaphy of the acute one-third lid margin or by scleral grafts to raise the inferior lid and lower the upper lid (see Chap. 5, sec. **V.A**). If orbital congestion becomes more severe and optic neuropathy occurs, systemic steroids may be given. Surgical decompression or local radiation may be considered if vision progressively declines. Surgical treatment of extraocular muscle abnormalities should usually be performed only after eye movement restriction has been stable for 6 months.

B. **Pseudotumors (pseudotumor oculi).** Orbital inflammations of unknown etiology are collectively described as pseudotumors. Patients with pseudotumors typically have orbital pain, exophthalmus, restricted eye movement, and impaired vision.

1. **Painful ophthalmoplegia (Tolosa-Hunt syndrome)** is a variant of pseudotumor in which the inflammation is localized either near the superior orbital fissure and optic canal or to the cavernous sinus. Bilateral orbital inflammation among adults raises the likelihood of a systemic vasculitis or lymphoproliferative disorder. Among children, however, nearly one-half of the cases of orbital pseudotumor are bilateral and few are associated with systemic disease.

2. **Treatment.** Oral steroids usually produce rapid and dramatic resolution of pseudotumor symptoms. Although pseudotumors can simulate neoplasms,

secondary inflammatory responses caused by actual tumors can also subside after steroid therapy.

C. **Cellulitis.** Orbital cellulitis is probably the most common cause of exophthalmus in early childhood and is usually the result of extension of infection from the ethmoid sinuses.

1. **Clinical signs** of orbital cellulitis include fever, pain, soft tissue edema, and restricted eye movements. Orbital x rays usually show opacification of the involved sinus without bone destruction.

2. **The most common organisms** that cause orbital cellulitis are *Staphylococcus aureus, Streptococcus,* and *Haemophilus influenzae.* Cavernous sinus thrombosis can result from cellulitis and is usually manifested by ophthalmoplegia with pupillary abnormalities and by the development of diffuse neurologic disturbances.

3. **Treatment.** Cultures should be obtained from the nasopharynx and conjunctiva. Initial treatment consists of systemic administration of penicillinase-resistant drugs such as methicillin or of other appropriate antibiotics (see Appendix B). Surgical drainage of the affected sinus should be deferred if possible until the acute inflammation has subsided. Orbital surgery is not necessary unless an abscess cavity is present. If cavernous sinus involvement is suspected, a lumbar puncture may reveal acute inflammatory cells and may yield a positive (CSF) culture.

D. **Phycomycosis.** The most common and most virulent fungal diseases involving the orbit are caused by organisms of the class *Phycomycetes.*

1. **The most common fungal genera** causing phycomycosis are *Mucor* (mucormycosis) and *Rhizopus.* These fungi usually extend from the sinuses or the nasal cavity and commonly grow among patients with metabolic acidosis and disabling systemic illness. The most common factors that predispose to such infections are diabetes, renal failure, malignant tumors, and therapy with antimetabolites or steroids.

2. **Treatment.** Diagnosis is made by biopsy of the involved tissues and the finding of nonseptate branching hyphae. Any underlying metabolic abnormality should be corrected, if possible. Infected tissues should be surgically excised and amphotericin B used to control growth of the fungi (see Appendix A).

VI. **Orbital tumors**

A. **Dermoids, epidermoids,** and **teratomas.** These tumors, most of which are benign, are usually considered to be developmental growths (choristomas) rather than neoplasms. Although choristomas are usually cystic, a solid component is often present and the lesions may be completely solid.

1. **Dermoids** contain one or more dermal adnexal structures such as hair follicles and sebaceous glands. The cystic component is lined with keratinizing epidermis. Treatment is surgical excision, with special care to avoid leaving potentially irritating cyst contents within the orbit.

2. **Lipodermoids** are solid tumors usually found beneath the conjunctiva adjacent to the superior temporal quadrant of the globe. Unless these lesions enlarge dramatically, they should be observed without surgery, since excision may be complicated by ptosis, restricted ocular motility, or damage to the globe.

3. **Epidermoids** contain epidermal tissues without adnexal structures. These lesions are almost always cystic, in which case the cavity may contain cholesterol crystals and epithelial debris such as keratin. Treatment is surgical excision.

4. **Teratomas** are rare tumors that arise from multiple germinal tissues including ectoderm and either endoderm or mesenchyme or both. Although exenteration is sometimes performed because of fear of malignancy, cystic teratomas can sometimes be removed with preservation of the eye.

B. **Vascular tumors.** Hemangiomas and lymphangiomas are usually considered to be developmental growths (hamartomas) rather than neoplasms. Hemangiomas are among the most common benign tumors of the orbit and can be grouped into two major types: capillary hemangiomas (occurring among children) and cavernous hemangiomas (occurring among adults).

1. **Capillary hemangiomas** usually arise as enlarging red nodules during the first month after birth. The skin near the eyelids is often dimpled and elevated, accounting for the description of "strawberry birthmark." Since spontaneous regression and disappearance usually follows initial growth, treatment is usually not necessary. Marked refractive errors may be associated with eyelid and orbital hemangiomas among children, and efforts should be made to combat amblyopia. If significant ocular dysfunction or cosmetic deformity occurs, tumor size may be reduced by systemic steroids, low-dose superficial radiation therapy, and surgery or cryotherapy in severe cases.

2. **Cavernous hemangiomas** are the most common benign tumors of the orbit among adults, although they are rarely clinically evident during childhood. Symptoms usually result from a retrobulbar mass within the muscle cone that appears during the second to fourth decades of life. Complete surgical excision by a lateral orbitotomy is usually possible because of the thick capsule around the cavernous hemangioma.

3. **Lymphangiomas** are uncommon tumors that often enlarge because of spontaneous internal hemorrhage into delicate vascular spaces. Exophthalmus may be caused by blood-filled "chocolate cysts," which must be distinguished from a malignancy such as rhabdomyosarcoma. Treatment is usually not necessary since blood-filled cysts commonly resolve spontaneously. Aspiration and drainage of blood may be required if the optic nerve or eye is severely compressed.

C. **Neural tumors and meningiomas.** The most common tumors of neural origin involving the orbit are optic nerve gliomas and plexiform neurofibromas. Both of these abnormalities frequently occur in the neurofibromatosis syndrome (von Recklinghausen's disease) and are sometimes considered to be developmental lesions (hamartomas) rather than neoplasms.

1. **Optic nerve gliomas** are well-differentiated tumors, approximately one-fourth of which are found among patients with neurofibromatosis. Therefore, the presence of café au lait spots in a child with exophthalmus and optic nerve abnormalities should raise the likelihood that an optic nerve glioma is present. These findings, together with an enlarged optic canal on plain-film and tomographic x rays, are virtually pathognomonic of this tumor. CT and pneumoencephalography are usually performed if intracranial extension is suspected. Treatment is controversial, but it is reasonable to biopsy a suspected optic glioma and to excise the tumor when the optic canal is enlarged and vision is poor.

2. **Neurofibromas** are usually plexiform, highly vascular, infiltrative tumors that involve the lateral portion of the upper eyelid and the anterior orbit. Progressive ptosis and sphenoid dysplasia frequently accompany plexiform neurofibromas. Since complete excision of plexiform tumors is usually impossible, surgery should usually be limited to debulking, to eyelid reconstruction, and to ptosis correction.

3. **Meningiomas** arise from arachnoidal villi and usually originate intracranially, in which case they may secondarily extend into the orbit through bone or along the optic canal. Primary orbital meningiomas that arise from the optic nerve sheath are less common than intracranial meningiomas. Complete excision should be attempted, although this is seldom possible in the case of intracranial tumors because of their extensive growth.

D. **Rhabdomyosarcomas** are the most common primary orbital malignant tumors among children. Approximately 90% of these lesions occur in patients under 15 years of age. X rays may demonstrate bone destruction, which would help to establish the diagnosis of rhabdomyosarcoma, since other primary orbital tumors seldom destroy the orbital walls. The neck should be examined to rule out lymph node metastases, and chest x rays as well as bone marrow aspirates should be obtained to rule out distant metastases. The diagnosis should be established by biopsy. High-dose radiation therapy combined with systemic chemotherapy has replaced exenteration and may cure more than one-half of patients with rhabdomyosarcomas.

E. Lacrimal gland tumors. Approximately one-half of all lacrimal gland tumors arise from epithelial tissue, and most of these are nonmetastasizing benign mixed tumors. Most nonepithelial tumors are inflammatory and lymphoid lesions.

   1. Benign mixed tumors are nonmetastasizing epithelial tumors that tend to recur and may undergo frankly malignant degeneration unless they are completely removed. Symptoms usually occur during the fourth and fifth decades of life. The tumors usually grow slowly and may produce smooth deformities in the adjacent orbital bones. When a benign mixed tumor is suspected, the entire lesion should be excised if possible. Incisional biopsy may allow tumor cells to spill into the orbit and can lead to infiltrative recurrent tumor, which requires extensive surgery for removal.

   2. Malignant epithelial tumors are all highly aggressive and frequently lethal. Adenoid cystic carcinomas (cylindromas) are the most common malignant tumors of the lacrimal gland. Most malignant epithelial tumors arise de novo, but occasionally benign mixed tumors may undergo malignant transformation. All of these malignant tumors should be treated by radical surgery (exenteration and removal of involved bone) unless they have already metastasized or have invaded beyond possible excision.

   3. Nonepithelial tumors of the lacrimal gland are usually inflammatory, in which case they may be idiopathic pseudotumors, lymphoepithelial lesions, or sarcoid granulomas. Malignant lymphomas and lymphosarcomas occasionally involve the lacrimal gland. Malignant lymphoid tumors are usually treated by local radiation or by systemic chemotherapy.

F. Lymphoproliferative tumors. Both benign and malignant lymphoid tumors of the orbit occur much more frequently among adults than among children. Reactive lymphoid hyperplasia is an idiopathic benign process that must be distinguished from malignant lymphoma. Biopsy is almost always necessary to establish the diagnosis of these lesions. Evaluation of patients with orbital lymphoid tumors should include a general physical examination to detect manifestations of systemic lymphoma. The treatment of malignant lymphoid tumors is usually radiation therapy, although systemic chemotherapy may be used if disseminated disease is present.

G. Metastatic tumors. Among children, neuroblastoma and Ewing's sarcoma are the most common distant tumors that metastasize to the orbit. Most neuroblastomas occur among patients younger than 7 years of age and may produce bilateral exophthalmus with eyelid ecchymosis. Among adults, breast and lung malignancies metastasize to the orbit much more commonly than any other lesions. Metastatic breast carcinoma may arise in the orbit many years after primary cancer surgery. Rarely, breast metastases to the orbit elicit fibrosis that causes cicatricial enophthalmos. Treatment of metastatic tumors is usually palliative, using radiation and sometimes chemotherapy. Breast tumors should be assayed for estrogen receptor activity, so that the possible usefulness of adjunctive hormone therapy can be determined. Some metastatic tumors such as carcinoids should be treated by wide excision, since patients with slowly growing primary lesions may survive for long periods of time.

VII. Congenital and developmental orbital anomalies. Most nonneoplastic congenital and developmental orbital abnormalities are uncommon and are so obvious that they do not present a diagnostic problem. Some disorders, such as meningoencephaloceles, may resemble enlarging neoplasms. Other conditions, such as neurofibromatosis, may be associated with true neoplasms. Although choristomas (e.g., dermoids) and hamartomas (e.g., hemangiomas) are believed to be developmental in origin, they often produce initial symptoms during adult life and are usually grouped with the general category of orbital tumors.

A. Microphthalmus and anophthalmos. In most cases in which a child is born with a unilateral small orbit and no visible eye, a small microphthalmic globe is present within the orbital soft tissues. Microphthalmus is sometimes associated with an orbital cyst. All children with congenitally small or absent eyes have hypoplastic orbits. If possible, surgery should be avoided and the socket should be expanded using progressively larger conformers.

B. Craniostenosis. Premature closure of the cranial sutures results in craniostenosis. The most common facial-orbital syndromes associated with craniostenosis are Crouzon's disease (frequently including hypertelorism and exophthalmus) and Apert's syndrome.

C. Meningocele and encephalocele. Congenital dehiscences of the skull may permit herniation of intracranial contents into the orbit. A meningocele consists of herniated meninges and CSF. If brain is also found within the herniated meninges, the defect is an encephalocele. Defects in the greater wing of the sphenoid may occur in patients with neurofibromatosis and may produce **pulsating exophthalmus.**

D. Choristomas are developmental growths that arise from tissues **not normally found** at the involved location, such as dermoids, epidermoids, and teratomas.

E. Hamartomas are developmental growths that arise from tissues usually **found** at the involved location, such as hemangiomas, lymphangiomas, and many neurofibromas. Some investigators consider optic nerve gliomas to be hamartomas; others consider them to be true neoplasms. Neurofibromatosis (von Recklinghausen's disease) is a disseminated hamartoma syndrome or phakomatosis, of which the orbital manifestations may include plexiform neurofibromas, dysplasia of the orbital walls, and optic nerve gliomas.

VIII. Orbital trauma. Facial trauma can damage the orbital bones and adjacent soft tissues. Fractures may be associated with injuries to the orbital contents and brain, paranasal sinus injuries, nasolacrimal damage, CSF leaks, carotid-cavernous sinus fistulas, and embedded foreign bodies (see Chap. 2, secs. **VIII** and **IX**).

A. Soft tissue injuries. Because the eye may be seriously damaged even without actual penetration, the visual acuity should be measured and a thorough ophthalmic examination conducted in any patient who has suffered orbital trauma. Partial or complete visual loss may result from direct damage or secondary compression to the optic nerve or from interruption of its vascular supply. Injuries to the motor nerves or to the levator and extraocular muscles may cause ptosis and limitation of ocular motility. The eyelids, canthi, and lacrimal system may be lacerated or avulsed. Exophthalmus may be caused by orbital hemorrhage following trauma. Injuries to the eye should be treated as the first priority, after which damage to the eyelids and lacrimal apparatus can be repaired. Drainage or aspiration of an orbital hemorrhage is seldom necessary, unless visual function is compromised by compression of the optic nerve or globe.

B. Orbital fractures. Fractures of the orbital **roof** may involve the paranasal sinuses or cause cerebrospinal rhinorrhea. Fractures at the orbital **apex** may injure the optic nerve. They should be evaluated by tomography of the optic canal if there is no significant acute visual loss. **Emergency surgical decompression** of the optic canal should be performed if there is an acute visual loss. This decompression is done without undue extensive radiologic evaluation, because delay may result in irreversible damage to the nerve. Carotid-cavernous sinus fistulas should be suspected if prolonged conjunctival vascular congestion or bruits are found after orbital injury. Other important fractures, because of their possible effect on ocular and orbital function, are those that involve the medial wall and floor of the orbit.

1. Medial orbital fractures usually result from trauma to the nose or medial orbital rim. The lacrimal secretory system (especially the nasolacrimal duct) may be damaged, and the medial rectus muscle may be entrapped within fractures of the lamina papyracea. Dacryocystorhinostomy may be required if the nasolacrimal duct is obstructed. Surgical exploration of the medial orbit may be indicated if mechanical restriction of ocular motility is present.

2. **Orbital floor fractures** may be direct, in which the inferior orbital rim is involved, or indirect, in which the rim remains intact. Indirect fractures are frequently referred to as **blowout fractures** because they are produced by the transmission of forces through the orbital soft tissues by a nonpenetrating object such as a fist or ball. These fractures generally occur in the thin bone over the infraorbital canal and may be complicated by entrapment of the inferior rectus or inferior oblique muscles. Such fractures are usually evident on plain-film x rays, although radiographic tomographs may be needed to show their full extent. CT may demonstrate soft tissue injuries and entrapped extraocular muscles. Surgery is usually indicated only if the eye becomes severely enophthalmic or sinks into the maxillary sinus (lowering or ptosis of the globe), or if muscle entrapment is present and severe vertical diplopia persists in a functionally important position of gaze. *Most orbital floor fractures do not require surgical repair.*

C. **Intraorbital foreign bodies** can usually be localized by conventional x rays if they are radiopaque. Many wooden or vegetable matter foreign bodies, however, cannot be visualized by x rays. CT may sometimes localize such objects. If an infection occurs after a penetrating injury, a retained foreign body should be suspected. A fistula tract may be produced that can be surgically followed into the orbit. Wounds caused by intraorbital foreign bodies should be cultured and antibiotics administered. Foreign bodies should be removed if they are composed of vegetable matter, if they have sharp edges, or if they are anterior in the orbit. They can often be left in place if they are inert with smooth edges and located in the posterior orbit (see Chap. 2, sec. **VII**).

Cornea and External Disease

Deborah Pavan-Langston and
Gary N. Foulks

I. **Normal anatomy and physiology**
  A. **Conjunctiva: anatomy**
    1. **Gross anatomy.** The conjunctiva is a thin, transparent mucous membrane lining the inner surface of the eyelid (palpebral conjunctiva) and covering the anterior sclera (bulbar conjunctiva). The palpebral portion is designated as marginal, tarsal, and orbital and merges with the conjunctiva of the superior and inferior fornices in loose folds. The bulbar conjunctiva is adherent to the underlying Tenon's capsule and therefore to sclera, with the tightest adhesion occurring in a narrow band at the corneoscleral limbus. A delicate vertical crescent, the semilunar fold (plica semilunaris), separates the bulbar conjunctiva from the lacrimal caruncle at the medial canthus. The conjunctiva tends to be a mobile tissue and is capable of great distention with edema fluid, as is often seen with trauma or inflammation.
    2. **Microscopically,** the conjunctiva is composed of (1) an anterior stratified columnar epithelium that is continuous with the corneal epithelium, and (2) a lamina propria composed of adenoid and fibrous layers. The epithelium is from two to seven layers thick and contains numerous unicellular mucous glands (goblet cells) that secrete the inner mucoid layer of the tear film. Although the epithelium is never keratinized in health, it may become keratinized in certain disease states. The lamina propria is composed of connective tissue housing blood vessels, nerves, and glands. The accessory lacrimal glands of Krause are located deep in the substantia propria in the superior and inferior fornices. The accessory lacrimal glands of Wolfring are situated near the upper margin of the superior tarsal plate. The adenoid layer of the lamina propria, which develops particularly after 3 months of age, contains lymphocytes enmeshed in a fine reticular network without the presence of true lymphoid follicles. The fibrous layer of the lamina propria surrounds the smooth palpebral muscle of Müller.
    3. The **blood supply** of the palpebral conjunctiva originates from peripheral (bulbar and fornix) and marginal arterial arcades of the eyelid. Within 4 mm of the limbus the vascular supply is derived from the anterior conjunctival branches of the anterior ciliary arteries (superficial plexus), which anastomose with the posterior conjunctival vessels from the peripheral arcade. Conjunctival vessels move with the conjunctiva and constrict with instillation of 1:1000 epinephrine—a point of differentiation from the deeper episcleral and ciliary vessels.
    4. **Innervation** of the bulbar conjunctiva is via the sensory and sympathetic nerves from the ciliary nerves. The remaining palpebral and fornix conjunctiva is innervated by the ophthalmic and maxillary divisions of the trigeminal nerve (cranial nerve V).
    5. **Lymphatic** drainage of the conjunctiva parallels that of the lid, with lateral drainage to the preauricular nodes and medial drainage to the submandibular nodes.
  B. **Cornea**
    1. **Gross anatomy.** The cornea represents the anterior 1.3 cm² of the globe and is the main refracting surface of the eye. Although the cornea is continuous with the sclera at the limbus, the anterior cornea curvature (radius

equal to 7.8 mm) is greater than that of the sclera, with the central 4-mm optical zone almost spherical and the periphery gradually flattening toward the scleral curve. The horizontal diameter of the anterior surface of the cornea (11.6 mm) is longer than the vertical diameter (10.6 mm), so that the anterior aspect of the cornea forms a horizontal ovoid. Viewed from the posterior surface, the cornea is circular (with a diameter of 11.6 mm). A corneal diameter greater than 12.5 mm is termed *megalocornea;* a corneal diameter less than 11.0 mm is termed *microcornea.* The height of the cornea from the basal plane of the visible limbus to the apex is 2.7 mm. The central thickness of the cornea is 0.52 mm, which increases to 0.70 mm in the far periphery.

2. **Microscopically,** the cornea consists of five strata: the epithelium and its basement membrane, Bowman's layer, stroma, Descemet's membrane, and endothelium.

   a. The corneal **epithelium** is a uniform five- to six-layer structure 50–100 μ thick and is composed of (1) a basal cell layer of replicating cylindric cells, 18 μ high and 10 μ wide, (2) a wing cell layer with superior convex-inferior scalloped cells interdigitating between the apices of the basal cells, and (3) surface cells composed of flat cells in two or three layers culminating in a smooth corneal surface that is studded with ultrastructural microplicae and microvilli. Corneal **nerves** passing from the corneal stroma through Bowman's layer terminate freely between the epithelial cells, thus accounting for the great sensitivity of the cornea. The epithelium is firmly attached to the underlying Bowman's layer by a continuous basement membrane that is a very important source of firm epithelial adhesion.

   b. **Bowman's layer** is a homogeneous condensation of the anterior stromal lamellae continuous with the corneal stroma. Its termination at the corneal periphery marks the anterior margin of the corneoscleral limbus.

   c. The **stroma** represents 90% of the corneal thickness, with bundles of collagen fibrils of uniform thickness enmeshed in mucopolysaccharide ground substance. These bundles form 200 lamellae arranged parallel to the corneal surface but with alternate layers crisscrossing at right angles. This regular lattice structure, coupled with the deturgescent state of the stroma, has been credited with providing the extreme transparency of the cornea necessary for optical clarity.

   d. **Descemet's membrane** is the basement membrane of the endothelial cells and can be easily stripped from the stroma. When torn or traumatized, the ends will tend to retract, indicating an inherent elasticity. Gradual thickening of this layer with age is noted, with the thickness approximately 3–4 μm at birth but increasing to 10–12 μm as an adult. Peripheral dome-shaped excrescences of Descemet's membrane (Hassall-Henle warts) occur in persons over age 20. Histologically, the membrane is a homogeneous glasslike structure but ultrastructurally is composed of stratified layers of very fine collagenous filaments in the anterior layer (anterior banded layer) with an amorphous posterior layer that increases with age.

   e. The **endothelium** is a single layer of approximately 500,000 polygonal cells, 5 × 18 μ in size, which spread uniformly across the posterior surface of the cornea. Although mitotic activity can be seen in very young endothelial cells in the adult, repair most often occurs by amitotic enlargement of the central endothelial cells. These cells maintain deturgescence and contribute to the formation of Descemet's membrane.

3. The **blood supply** of the cornea arises predominantly from the conjunctival, episcleral, and scleral vessels that arborize about the corneoscleral limbus. The cornea itself is avascular.

4. The **innervation** of the cornea is that of a rich sensory supply mostly via the ophthalmic division of the trigeminal nerve. This innervation is via the

long ciliary nerves that branch in the outer choroid near the ora serrata region. These nerves pass via the sclera into the middle third of the cornea as 70–80 large nerve trunks that lose their myelin sheaths approximately 2–3 mm from the limbus but can be visualized as fine filaments beyond. There is significant dichotomous and trichotomous branching, and the subsequent passage of nerve fibers through Bowman's layer ends freely between the epithelial cells.

C. Physiology: precorneal tear film

1. The **physiology** of the cornea and conjunctiva is best introduced in a discussion of the **precorneal tear film**. This film, which is 6–10 μm thick, is composed of three layers: (1) superficial lipid layer, (2) middle aqueous layer, and (3) inner mucous layer. The normal tear volume in the conjunctival sac is about 3–7 μl and can increase to the conjunctival sac capacity of 25 μl before overflow occurs. Tear flow rate is approximately 1 μl/minute and comes from the secretion of the main and accessory lacrimal glands. After their release in the superotemporal region, the tears are distributed by the blinking action of the lids with the tear meniscus forming superior and inferior marginal tear strips before draining into the lacrimal puncta located near the medial canthus. With a pH of 7.6 and an osmolarity comparable to sodium chloride 0.9%, there is a low glucose concentration and an electrolyte distribution similar to plasma, with the exception of a slightly greater potassium content. Oxygen dissolves readily in the tear film, and the dissolved protein content of the tear film includes immunoglobulins and lysozyme. These characteristics allow the tear film to provide a smooth surface for refraction, to mechanically wash and protect the cornea and conjunctiva, to provide oxygen exchange for the epithelium, to lubricate the surface during a blink, and to provide bacteriostasis.

2. **Corneal function.** The primary physiologic function of the **cornea** is to maintain an **optically smooth surface** and a **transparent medium** while protecting the intraocular contents of the eye. This duty is fulfilled by an effective interaction of the epithelium, stroma, and endothelium. The epithelium, endothelium, and Descemet's membrane are transparent because of the uniformity of their refractive indices. The transparency of the stroma is conferred by the special physical arrangement of the component fibrils. Although the refractive index of collagen fibrils differs from that of the interfibrillar substance, the small diameter of the fibril (300 Å) and the small distance between them (300 Å) provide a separation and regularity that causes little scattering of light despite the optical inhomogeneity. The relative state of deturgescence is provided by the barrier functions of the epithelium and endothelium as well as by the dehydrating function of the endothelium. Disturbance of this equilibrium, such as occurs in corneal edema, will increase light scattering and the opacity of the stroma.

   a. The **anterior epithelial surface** with its microplicae and microvilli provides the necessary scaffold for a smooth and continuous precorneal tear film. In addition, the epithelium serves as a relatively impermeable barrier to water-soluble materials. The epithelium also provides an effective barrier to many infectious agents. The epithelium is the most mitotically active layer of the cornea, and because of its high cellular density consumes considerable glucose and oxygen. The major source of oxygen for the epithelium is atmospheric oxygen dissolved in the tear film when the eye is open and oxygen diffusing from palpebral conjunctival vessels when the eye is closed. The dependence on dissolved oxygen in the tear film explains the sensitivity to hypoxia that occurs in improperly fitted or overworn contact lenses. Glucose for the epithelium is obtained from the aqueous humor by diffusion through the corneal stroma. This substance is either used or stored as glycogen. Epithelial metabolism occurs through the hexose monophosphate shunt or tricarboxylic acid cycle in the presence of oxygen or via the anaerobic glycolysis pathway in the absence of oxygen. With these metabolic capabilities the turnover of the epithelium is rapid, occurring approximately once every 7 days, and explains the ability of the epithelium to heal itself rapidly.

b. Stroma. There is little turnover of the **stromal matrix,** and the keratocytes may survive as long as 2 years under normal conditions. Glucose is obtained from the aqueous humor and oxidized via the Embden-Meyerhof tricarboxylic acid cycle. Interaction of the interfibrillar substances, particularly the acid mucopolysaccharides, generates a swelling pressure for the stroma both in vivo and in vitro. This tendency to imbibe fluid results in light scattering if it is not kept in check by the dehydrating function of the endothelium.

c. Endothelium. The major function of the **endothelium** is the maintenance of proper corneal hydration. The endothelium requires oxygen and glucose to maintain the metabolically active process, but the exact nature of the endothelial pump is not completely clear. Impairment of the pump function can occur in dystrophic conditions (Fuchs's dystrophy), injury (postsurgical or traumatic), and in some inflammatory conditions (anterior segment necrosis).

II. Acute traumatic conditions

A. Abrasions and Lacerations. See Chap. 2, secs. **V** and **VI.**

B. Perforations

1. **Etiologically,** corneal perforation can result from any corneal ulceration, either infectious (bacterial, fungal, viral), inflammatory (rheumatoid arthritis, collagen disease), posttraumatic (burn), or trophic defects of degenerations, neurotrophic ulcer, or postherpetic ulcer.

2. **Treatment.** Occasionally, these perforations will seal with a small knuckle of iris and rarely can be self-sealing, but they usually result in partial or complete loss of the anterior chamber. Thus, they represent an urgent situation to be treated in most cases. Small, noninfectious perforations can often be splinted by use of a **soft contact bandage lens.** Such treatment will sometimes allow healing of the perforation but often is a stabilizing or interim treatment that requires further definitive therapy. Of great use in helping to seal small perforations is **medical adhesive. Cyanoacrylate tissue adhesive,** under FDA Investigational New Drug (IND) study **for ocular use,*** can successfully seal a perforation without excess ocular toxicity. It is essential that epithelium and necrotic stroma be debrided in order to allow firm adhesion of the cyanoacrylate glue to surrounding healthy basement membrane. A thin application of this glue will often remain intact for several months and is tolerated by the patient if covered with a continuously worn soft contact lens. Healing of the corneal defect will often occur beneath the glue. Even if spontaneous healing of the abnormality is not expected, the glue will provide adequate time to obtain corneal donor material if keratoplasty becomes necessary. It is essential to observe the patient closely to be sure the anterior chamber has reformed and there is no associated superinfection. Topical antibiotic coverage is advisable after gluing and with the use of a soft contact lens. When contact lens or adhesive therapy is inadequate, **surgical patch grafting** will usually be successful. For moderate size perforations a small lamellar button may be sutured into the debrided defect. In the event of large central perforations, it may be preferable to perform penetrating keratoplasty.

C. Burns. Anterior segment burns may be chemical, thermal, radiation, or electric (see Chap. 2, secs. **I–IV**).

D. Subconjunctival hemorrhage may be induced with major, minor, or no detectable trauma to the front of the eye. Occasionally, a patient will wake up with a "spontaneous" hemorrhage. Clinically, it presents as a striking flat, deep-red hemorrhage under the conjunctiva and may become sufficiently se-

---

* Nexacryl cyanoacrylate tissue adhesive, CRX Medical, Raleigh, N.C.

vere to cause a dramatic chemotic "bag of blood" to protrude over the lid margin. Occasionally, pneumococcal or adenoviral conjunctivitis may be associated, in which case there will be discomfort and discharge. In the absence of infection or significant trauma to the eye, **treatment** is unnecessary. The patient should be reassured that the blood will clear over a 2- or 3-week period.

III. **Conjunctival infection and inflammation**

A. **Conjunctivitis** is an inflammation of the conjunctiva characterized by vascular dilation, cellular infiltration, and exudation. The differential features of bacterial conjunctivitis versus that due to virus, allergy, or toxic factors are listed in Table 5-1.

B. **Bacterial conjunctivitis** can be acute or chronic. The **acute** stage classically is recognized by vascular engorgement and mucopurulent discharge, with the associated symptoms of irritation, foreign body sensation, and sticking together of the lids. Occasionally, a severe reaction with purulent conjunctivitis and corneal involvement can occur. The **chronic** infection is more innocuous in its onset, runs a protracted course, and is often associated with involvement of the lids or lacrimal system by low-grade inflammatory reaction. A wide variety of bacterial organisms can infect the conjunctiva. Although the bacterial etiology is often clinically apparent, the identity of the causative organism may not be obvious. Certain clinical features determined by the pathogenicity of the infectious agent, however, may provide an accurate clinical diagnosis.

1. **Acute bacterial conjunctivitis**

a. *Staphylococcus aureus* is probably the single most common cause of bacterial conjunctivitis and blepharoconjunctivitis in the Western world. The aerobic gram-positive coccus is often harbored elsewhere on the skin or in the nares. It may affect any age group. Although usually not aggressively invasive, the organism is very toxigenic and can provide corneal infiltrates, eczematous blepharitis, phlyctenular keratitis, and angular blepharitis.

b. *Staphylococcus epidermidis* is usually considered an innocuous inhabitant of the lids and conjunctiva, but in some instances it can cause blepharoconjunctivitis. The organism is capable of producing necrotic exotoxin and has been shown to colonize eye cosmetics, with subsequent production of blepharoconjunctivitis.

c. *Streptococcus pneumoniae* **(pneumococcus)** is an aerobic encapsulated gram-positive diplococcus that is often present in the respiratory tracts of asymptomatic carriers. This organism more commonly affects the conjunctiva of children and can run a self-limiting course of 9–10 days.

d. *Streptococcus pyogenes* is an aerobic gram-positive coccus. Although an infrequent cause of conjunctivitis, the organism is invasive and toxigenic and thus is capable of producing a pseudomembranous conjunctivitis. The pseudomembrane consists of a fibrinous layer entrapping inflammatory cells and is attached to the conjunctival surface. Removal of this pseudomembrane is possible with minimum bleeding of the underlying tissue.

e. *Haemophilus influenzae (Haemophilus aegyptius,* **Koch-Weeks bacillus)** is a fastidious aerobic gram-negative pleomorphic organism often seen as a slender rod or a coccobacillary form. It is frequently isolated from upper respiratory tracts of healthy carriers and most commonly causes conjunctivitis in children rather than in adults. It is a toxigenic organism and can be accompanied by patchy conjunctival hemorrhages during an acute infection. An untreated case can last for 9–12 days, occurring as a self-limited infection, but occasionally can be part of a more ominous periorbital cellulitis associated with respiratory infection that can lead to bacteremia in young children. Accompanying the acute infection and probably a manifestation of the toxigenic potential is the presence of **inferior corneal limbal infiltrates.**

Table 5-1. Clinical features of conjunctivitis

Sign	Bacterial	Viral	Allergic	Toxic	TRIC
Injection	Marked	Moderate	Mild to moderate	Mild to moderate	Moderate
Hemorrhage	+	+	−	−	−
Chemosis	++	±	++	±	±
Exudate	Purulent or mucopurulent	Scant, watery	Stringy, white	−	Scant
Pseudomembrane	± (Streptococcus, Corynebacterium diphtheria)	±	−	−	−
Papillae	±	−	+	−	±
Follicles	−	+	−	+ (medication)	+
Preauricular node	+ (purulent)	++	−	−	±
Pannus	−	−	− (except vernal)	−	+

Key: TRIC = trachoma-inclusion conjunctivitis (group); + + = strongly positive; + = positive; ± = sometimes positive; − = negative.

Table 5-2. Neonatal conjunctivitis

Agent	Onset	Cytology	Culture
Neisseria	2–4 days	Gram-negative intracel-lular diplococci	Blood agar, chocolate agar (37°, 10% CO_2)
Other bacteria	1–30 days	Gram-positive or gram-negative organisms	Blood agar
Inclusion blenorrhea	2–14 days	Giemsa-positive intra-cytoplasmic inclusions	Negative
Chemical	1–2 days	Negative	Negative or normal flora

    f. *Moraxella lacunata* is an aerobic gram-negative diplobacillus once considered the most common cause of **angular blepharoconjunctivitis.** While angular blepharoconjunctivitis is more commonly due nowadays to staphylococcal infection, *Moraxella* species can produce an acute conjunctivitis that occasionally results in a chronic conjunctivitis with follicular reaction.

2. Hyperacute conjunctivitis (acute purulent conjunctivitis)

    a. *Neisseria* species (gonococcus, meningococcus) of gram-negative diplococci, *Haemophilus* species, *Streptococcus* species, and *Corynebacterium diphtheria* are aggressively invasive bacteria that can produce a severe conjunctivitis that is often bilateral. Occurring in the child as an infection from the maternal genital tract, in adolescents via fomite transmission, or in adults from inoculation of infected genitalia, the conjunctivitis can start as a routine mucopurulent conjunctivitis that rapidly evolves into a severe inflammation with copious exudate and marked chemosis and lid edema. This clinical appearance demands laboratory confirmation, immediate therapy, and often hospitalization.

    b. Neonatal conjunctivitis (ophthalmia neonatorum). Conjunctivitis of the newborn deserves special mention because of the severity and threatening potential of this condition. Conjunctivitis caused by *Neisseria* species usually becomes symptomatic in the newborn 2–4 days following inoculation of the conjunctival mucosa at the time of birth. Clinically, a yellow purulent discharge with prominent lid edema and conjunctival chemosis appears. This condition needs to be distinguished from the neonatal conjunctivitis caused by inclusion conjunctivitis agents, chemical keratoconjunctivitis, nasolacrimal obstruction with other bacterial superinfection, or trauma. The differential points in diagnosis are tabulated in Table 5-2. (See also sec. **C.2** and Chap. 10, sec. **II.B.**)

3. Chronic bacterial blepharoconjunctivitis

    a. *S. aureus* is the most common cause of chronic bacterial conjunctivitis or blepharoconjunctivitis, with *S. epidermidis, Propionibacterium acnes, Corynebacterium* species, and the yeast *Pityrosporon* being other etiologic agents. Often this conjunctivitis is associated with a low-grade inflammation of the lid margins and colonization of the meibomian orifices and lash follicles with *Staphylococcus. Staphylococcus* can produce a variety of exotoxins, which probably accounts for the clinical manifestations. An ulcerative blepharitis can occur as well as an eczematoid scaling and sometimes weeping inflammation of the lids. Eczematoid **blepharitis** is usually distinguishable from the less severe seborrheic blepharitis, which is often accompanied by scaling and greasy deposits on the eyelid, as well as from frequently associated seborrheic dermatitis. An **angular blepharoconjunctivitis** with maceration of the tissue at the lateral canthus, at one time most commonly associated with *Moraxella* species, is now most commonly produced by *Staphylococcus.* The cornea also can be involved, with an inferior superficial punctate keratitis or by limbal infiltrates. **Marginal corneal ulcers** can be produced by chronic staphylococcal blepharoconjunctivitis.

   b. Chronic conjunctivitis can also be produced by gram-negative rods including *Proteus mirabilis, Klebsiella pneumoniae, Serratia marcescens,* and *Escherichia coli.* Gram-negative diplobacilli *(M. lacunata)* can produce a chronic blepharoconjunctivitis (angular conjunctivitis) as previously mentioned and may be present with a chronic follicular reaction.

C. Laboratory diagnosis in bacterial conjunctivitis. When clinical findings are insufficient to diagnose confidently the etiology of an infection, or in those situations where the reaction is severe or has not responded to routine therapy, conjunctival scrapings for microscopic examination and routine culture techniques are indicated. Scrapings should also be performed in cases of neonatal conjunctivitis, hyperacute conjunctivitis, and chronic recalcitrant conjunctivitis.

   1. Conjunctival cultures should be taken prior to the use of topical anesthetics, as these agents and their preservatives will markedly reduce the recovery of certain bacteria. Cultures are taken by moistening the sterile tip applicator with sterile saline and wiping the lid margin or conjunctival cul-de-sac with the swab. The culture medium is then inoculated directly with the swab tip. Inoculation of solid media can be made in the shape of the letter *R* for the right lid and *L* for the left lid margin. On the same plate, a conjunctival culture may be inoculated at a different site using a zigzag pattern. In this way, the site of culture may be distinguished by the pattern of growth on the plate. After inoculating solid media, the tip of the applicator may be broken off and dropped into a tube of liquid culture medium if it is available.

   2. For **bacterial isolation** and **identification,** the most widely used and generally available **media** are blood agar and chocolate agar. Brain heart infusion broth has a significantly higher growth rate for most common organisms but may not be readily available and must be secondarily plated for identification. Chocolate agar is well suited for growth of any organism that can be isolated on blood agar and has the added advantage of isolating *Haemophilus* and the fastidious *Neisseria* organisms. Thayer-Martin medium is a chocolate agar medium containing vancomycin, colistimethate, and nystatin and is of use in culture and isolation of gonococcus. Thioglycolate medium is a commonly used medium in cultivating anaerobic organisms from ocular infection. Liquid Sabouraud's medium may be useful in isolating organisms where solid agar medium has failed. Table 5-3 summarizes the culture media of use in specific ocular infectious states.

   3. Scrapings for microscopic examination are made after cultures have been taken. Local anesthetic is instilled. A platinum spatula is flamed and allowed to cool to room temperature. The spatula can then be used to scrape gently the involved conjunctival surface, and the material obtained can be spread in a thin layer on a precleaned glass slide. Two or three such slides should be made and stained for microscopic examination (Table 5-4).

   4. Stains most useful for identifying organisms and inflammatory cell type are the Gram and the Giemsa stain. If Giemsa stain is unavailable, Wright stain may be used. The Hansel stain is also a useful technique for rapid identification of any eosinophilic response. The Giemsa and Wright stains are most useful in revealing the condition and character of epithelial cells and inflammatory cells. The Giemsa stain is most effective in showing the presence or absence of viral cytoplasmic or intranuclear inclusion bodies and in outlining the morphology of bacteria. The Gram stain is useful in revealing whether an organism is gram-positive or negative; it also provides some information as to the morphology of the organism.

   5. The **cytologic features** of each type of conjunctivitis are helpful in diagnosis. As a rule, a **polymorphonuclear leukocyte** response occurs with

Table 5-3. Culture media

General media	Bacterial	Fungal
Blood agar plate	Good recovery (37°C)	Good recovery (room temperature)
Chocolate agar plate	Especially *Haemophilus* and *Neisseria*	
Sabouraud's		Good recovery (broth or agar)
Brain heart infusion (meat tube)	Good recovery (37°C)	Good recovery
Thioglycolate broth	Microaerophilic species	
Special media		
Lowenstein-Jensen	Mycobacteria	
Thayer-Martin	*Neisseria*	

Table 5-4. Cytologic features of conjunctivitis

Cell	Bacterial	Viral	Allergic	TRIC
Polymorph				
Neutrophil	+	+ (early)	−	+
Basoeosinophil	−	−	+	(occasional)
Mononuclear				
Lymphocyte	−	+	−	+
Plasma cell	−	−	−	+
Multinuclear	−	+	−	−
Inclusion				
Cytoplasm	−	+ (pox)	−	+
Nucleus	−	+ (Herpes)	−	−
Organism	+	−	−	−

Key: TRIC = trachoma-inclusion conjunctivitis (group); + = present; − = absent.

bacterial conjunctivitis (with the exception of diplobacillus). Acute Stevens-Johnson syndrome may produce a polymorphonuclear response, as will the early stages of a viral infection. A mixed outpouring of polymorphonuclear leukocytes and lymphocytes is commonly noted with adult and neonatal inclusion conjunctivitis. Such a mixed response with the added presence of plasma cells and macrophages (Leber cells) are almost diagnostic of trachoma. Chemical conjunctivitis can also produce a polymorphonuclear response. A predominantly **lymphocytic** response is most commonly seen in viral infections but can also be seen in toxic follicular conjunctivitis that is drug induced. Numerous **eosinophils** are indicative of vernal conjunctivitis or allergic conjunctivitis. The appearance of eosinophils and polymorphonuclear leukocytes in conjunction with a hyperacute conjunctivitis may be indicative of early erythema multiforme, particularly if associated with systemic symptoms. **Basophils,** rarely seen in conjunctival scrapings, are equivalent in interpretation to eosinophilic reaction. **Epithelial cells** may demonstrate cytoplasmic **inclusions** that, if basophilic, suggest inclusion conjunctivitis and, if eosinophilic, suggest pox virus. Pink intranuclear inclusions on Giemsa stain are diagnostic of herpesvirus infection (either simplex or zoster). Multinucleate giant cells are suggestive of a viral disorder.

6. When **organisms** are identified, gram-positive cocci in pairs or chains may indicate *S. pyogenes*. The gram-negative diplococci, appearing within polymorphonuclear leukocytes and having the "coffee bean" shape, indicate *Neisseria* species. Large gram-negative diplobacilli characterize *Moraxella* species. *H. influenzae* is a pleomorphic organism variably appearing as gram-negative coccobacillus or slender rods. Gram-negative rods may also be noted but are difficult to differentiate as to species.

D. **Treatment of bacterial conjunctivitis and blepharoconjunctivitis** (see also Chap. 3, sec. I.I)

1. **Acute mucopurulent conjunctivitis**

    a. **Topical therapy.** Acute mucopurulent conjunctivitis will typically respond to topical antimicrobial therapy in solution or ointment form. If treatment is based on clinical diagnosis alone, topical antimicrobials such as erythromycin or bacitracin ointment or sodium sulfacetamide 10–15% solution should be considered, as they cover the more common gram-positive infections. About 50% of staphylococci are now resistant to the sulfonamides, however. Neomycin-polymyxin-bacitracin (Neosporin, AK-spore) is an effective broad-spectrum antimicrobial (gram-positive and negative organisms covered) but suffers the disadvantage of a high incidence (6–8%) of sensitivity due to neomycin. Chloramphenicol is an equally effective broad-spectrum topical antimicrobial and is particularly useful where *Haemophilus* and *Moraxella* are the cause. Short-term use (4 weeks or less) with topical chloramphenicol has **not** been reported to cause adverse systemic reactions. Polymyxin B-bacitracin (Polysporin) ointment, polymyxin B-trimethoprim (Polytrim), and gentamicin (Garamycin, AKGent) or tobramycin (Tobrex) drops or ointment are all excellent broad-spectrum agents. The last two are usually reserved for suspected gram-negative organisms. If culture and antimicrobial sensitivity results are available, they should guide the rational selection of an antimicrobial agent. Drops instilled q3–4h, with ointment at bedtime, or ointment instilled qid for 7–10 days should, in most cases, shorten the course of the disease.

    b. **Systemic therapy.** For particularly acute staphylococcal blepharitis, oral cloxacillin or dicloxacillin or, if penicillin allergy exists, erythromycin or clindamycin is a very effective adjunct (see Appendix B).

    c. **Local measures** are of great value in treatment, particularly when blepharitis is present. **Warm wet compresses** improve circulation, mobilize meibomian secretions, and help cleanse crusting deposits of the lashes. Thick or inspissated lid secretions may require the physician to **express the lids** between cotton-tipped applicators after topical anesthesia, followed by daily lid massage performed by the patient. Seborrheic blepharitis is often improved by use of sebulytic or **dandruff shampoo** to the scalp and eyebrows. Daily application of steroid ointment (0.1% fluorometholone) **to lid margins** for 10–14 days often controls the pronounced lid inflammation.

2. **Hyperacute bacterial conjunctivitis** (acute purulent conjunctivitis) is a more serious situation and demands more vigorous therapy. After examining the patient and obtaining the necessary cultures and scrapings, it is important to institute treatment prior to obtaining the culture results.

    a. **Topical** tetracycline or bacitracin ointment or penicillin G drops 100,000 units/ml should be instilled every 2 hours for the first 2–3 days for *Neisseria gonorrhoeae*, *Neisseria meningitidis*, *Streptococcus* species, and *Corynebacterium diphtheria* in the neonate, child, or adult and then 5 times daily for 7 days. For **penicillin-resistant gonococcus,** gentamicin, erythromycin, or bacitracin ointment q2–3h is given as adjunct to systemic therapy. *Haemophilus* or *Moraxella* infections are treated with 0.5% chloramphenicol and gram-negative bacilli with 0.3% gentamicin or tobramycin in the same dosage schedule as for *Neisseria*. Hourly irrigation of the eyes with sterile saline is very therapeutic in washing away infected debris.

b. Systemic therapy is indicated for *N. gonorrhoeae, N. meningitidis,* and *H. influenzae* and is far **more critical than topical therapy.** The 1989 Centers for Disease Control-recommended therapy that covers penicillin-resistant strains is ceftriaxone, 1 gm or 50 mg/kg IV once on an outpatient basis or, for more severe cases, 1 gm IV bid for 3-5 days as an inpatient. Neonatal dosage is 125 mg IM qd for 1-2 days as an inpatient (see also Chap. 10, **II.B.2**). **Prophylactic** therapy for intimate contacts of *N. gonorrhoeae* patients is 1 gm of ceftriaxone IV once or for *N. meningitidis*, rifampin, 600 mg PO q12h for 4 days. If there is no corneal involvement, adult neisserial infections due to non-penicillin-resistant strains are treated on an inpatient basis with 10 million units/day of aqueous penicillin G IV plus 1 gm of probenecid PO qd for 5 days or, in neonates, 50,000 units/kg IV in 2 divided doses for 7 days. **Penicillin-allergic** patients may be effectively treated with norfloxacin 1200 mg PO once, spectinomycin 2 gm IM once, or erythromycin 500 mg PO qd for 7 days as an outpatient if there is no corneal infection. For more severe cases (corneal involvement—see sec. **IV** for keratitis), 2 gm IM bid for 3-5 days as an inpatient along with the topical therapy described above. Norfloxacin and spectinomycin are also effective against penicillin-resistant strains. Isolation of *H. influenzae* in children warrants therapy with ampicillin, 100-200 mg/kg IM or IV for 7-10 days or 50-100 mg/kg q6-8h PO for 10-14 days; neonates receive 50-200 mg/kg q12h IM or IV for 10 days (see Appendix B). Adult dosage is 2-4 gm PO, IM, or IV q6-8h for 10-14 days. If the *Haemophilus* strain is **ampicillin-resistant** or the patient **penicillin allergic,** chloramphenicol in the dosages described in Appendix B are given for 10-14 days. Children and neonates should be treated in consultation with a pediatrician.

3. Chronic conjunctivitis and **blepharitis** is especially common in patients with acne rosacea. It is usually cultured only if there is no response to standard treatment and then retreated in accordance with the sensitivities obtained after culturing the pathogen. The presence of recalcitrant blepharitis or meibomitis in association with chronic staphylococcal conjunctivitis requires not only topical treatment with bacitracin or erythromycin but also intensive **hygiene of the lid margins.** This hygiene must frequently be initiated in the office by expression of the lids (topical anesthesia) with cotton-tipped applicators. Daily lid hygiene with 5-minute hot compresses and lid massage by the patient are essential in completely eradicating the inflammation. Daily hand and face scrubs with pHisoHex for 2-3 weeks and then 3-4 times weekly will lower the facial germ count and reduce acneiform eruptions and styes. Tetracycline, 250 mg PO qd on an empty stomach, erythromycin, 250 mg PO qd, or doxycycline, 100 mg PO qd for 3-6 months, is often useful in controlling abnormal fatty acid metabolism, which invites lid margin inflammation. Infectious **eczematoid dermatitis** occurring with staphylococcal blepharitis is an indication for antimicrobial-steroid combination. Sulfacetamide-prednisolone combinations are particularly effective. These preparations are available in suspension and ointment form but should not be used daily longer than 3-4 weeks during any 3-month period. Sterile marginal infiltrates and ulcerations that occur with chronic staphylococcal blepharoconjunctivitis also respond to topical steroids, usually within 4 or 5 days. Phlyctenular lesions of the cornea will also decrease after treatment with steroids. **Acne rosacea** patients should use steroids infrequently, in very low concentrations, and under close supervision (see sec. **VII.G**; for chalazia, see Chap. 3, sec. **III.I.3**).

IV. Corneal infections and inflammation (keratitis and keratoconjunctivitis)

A. Superficial keratitis includes inflammatory lesions of the corneal epithelium and adjacent superficial stroma. Although some of the changes described in this section can be produced by noninflammatory conditions and therefore would more appropriately be considered keratopathy, they are considered here because of their diagnostic importance. The etiologies of this clinical condition include numerous **infective, toxic, degenerative, and allergic** conditions that can often be characterized by the morphology and distribution of the lesions produced. These conditions may occur with bacterial, viral, and fungal infections. Degenerative states due to dry eye, neurotrophic defects or in association with systemic disease can also produce ulceration of the cornea. When accompanied by infiltration or significant ocular anterior chamber reaction, infection must be excluded or diagnosed and treated.

1. **Morphologically,** the lesions include punctate **epithelial erosions** that are focal defects in the corneal epithelium, best visualized by rose bengal and fluorescein staining and slit-lamp biomicroscopy. Punctate **epithelial keratitis** is characterized by focal inflammatory infiltration of the epithelium, resulting in minute opaque epithelial lesions observed in focal illumination or with the slit lamp. Although they may occur without staining, they often do stain with rose bengal or fluorescein due to associated punctate epithelial erosion. Punctate **subepithelial infiltrates** are focal areas of infiltration that occur as opaque spots in the superficial stroma.

2. **Identification** of the morphology and distribution of the lesions are greatly enhanced by the use of vital **clinical stains,** most notably rose bengal and fluorescein. **Rose bengal** stains dead or degenerating cells and presently is available as sterile paper strips. Prior instillation of proparacaine 0.5% will relieve the smarting sensation produced by rose bengal, but tetracaine and cocaine should be avoided, as they will often produce an artifactual rose bengal staining pattern. Rose bengal is also an excellent stain for mucus and filaments. Fluorescein from a 2% solution or from a moistened Fluristrip will stain epithelial defects or bared basement membrane and is also used when highlighting corneal filaments.

3. The **distribution** of the epithelial and subepithelial lesions is of **diagnostic value.** Figure 5-1 summarizes the **six** clinical patterns and their respective etiologies. **Diffuse** and nonspecific **punctate epithelial erosions** may occur with early bacterial or viral infections of many types. Breakdown of microcystic areas of epithelial edema can also produce this pattern, and such areas of edema will also demonstrate areas of negative staining in the fluorescein film corresponding to intact epithelial microcysts. Any toxic reaction to topical medications or chemicals or aerosol sprays can produce this pattern. Mechanical trauma from a foreign body or eye rubbing must also be considered. The epithelial erosions secondary to molluscum contagiosum of the lids will occur in areas **contiguous** to the lesion. **Inferior** punctate epithelial erosions frequently are due to staphylococcal blepharitis or blepharoconjunctivitis and are often accompanied by epithelial keratitis and subepithelial infiltrates. Trichiasis or incomplete lid closure can produce this distribution of erosion, and the pattern is also occasionally seen in dry eye patients. The **interpalpebral** distribution is typical of keratitis sicca, ultraviolet radiation exposure, chronic exposure, or incomplete blinking. Conjunctival staining usually will accompany the corneal lesion. Episodic recurrent erosions frequently will occur in the inferior area or interpalpebral area. The **superior** distribution of epithelial erosion is typical of superior limbic keratoconjunctivitis but can also be seen in vernal conjunctivitis and with trachoma. Corneal epithelial filaments consisting of coiled epithelial remnants and adherent mucous strands may be associated with any of these patterns, but most typically appear with superolimbic keratoconjunctivitis or keratoconjunctivitis sicca.

4. The **etiology** of **punctate epithelial erosion** is often local desiccation. Instability of the tear film results in focal dry spots and epithelial breakdown. Epithelial membrane damage due to detergent chemicals, liquid solvents, quaternary amines, and a variety of drugs also results in erosions. Super-

Diffuse
Early bacterial
Viral
Medicamentosa

Inferior
Staphylococcal blepharoconjunctivitis
Trichiasis

Interpalpebral
Keratitis sicca
Photokeratopathy
Exposure
Inadequate blink

Superior
Superior limbic keratitis
Vernal conjunctivitis
TRIC

Contact lens overwear

Mechanical abrasion
Trichiasis

Fig. 5-1. Staining patterns of the cornea and conjunctiva in various disease states.
TRIC = trachoma-inclusion conjunctivitis (group).

ficial viral and chlamydial infections can produce focal erosions, as can the epithelial hypoxia of contact lens overwear. **Punctate epithelial keratitis** with minute focal opacities is typical of viral keratitis, especially that associated with epidemic keratoconjunctivitis of adenovirus, but may also be seen with staphylococcal and chlamydial infections as well. The infiltrates also occur with vaccinia, Reiter's syndrome, and acne rosacea. The coarse, granular infiltrates of punctate epithelial keratitis are quite characteristic of Thygeson's superficial punctate keratitis.

5. **Nonstaining punctate subepithelial infiltrates** in the superficial stroma are sometimes seen as sequelae of punctate epithelial keratitis after adenoviral, herpes simplex, herpes zoster, Epstein-Barr viral, vaccinial, chlamydial, Reiter's, and rosacea involvement. Staphylococcal infection must

be considered when this pattern appears in a marginal infiltrate distribution. Inferior peripheral limbal infiltrates can accompany acute *H. influenzae* conjunctivitis.

B. Bacterial corneal ulcers

1. **Central ulcer.** *S. aureus, S. pneumococcus, Pseudomonas,* and *Moraxella* are predominant causes of bacterial keratitis. *S. epidermidis,* streptococcal species, and Enterobacteriaceae *(Proteus, Serratia, E. coli,* and *Klebsiella)* are less common causes. Gram-negative diplococci are an uncommon cause of corneal ulceration except in inadequately treated cases of hyperacute conjunctivitis. Infection of the cornea usually tends to occur after injury to the epithelium or in compromised hosts. Stromal infiltration in an area of epithelial defect with surrounding edema and folds associated with endothelial fibrin plaques or anterior chamber reaction is usually indicative of microbial infection. Staphylococcal ulcers are often more localized while pneumococcus may produce a shaggy undermined edge of an ulcer that is associated with a hypopyon. A highly destructive keratitis with rapid necrosis and adherent mucopurulent discharge is highly suggestive of *Pseudomonas* or anaerobic infection. **Infectious crystalline keratopathy** is an indolent, noninflammatory branching crystalline growth commonly associated with *Streptococcus viridans* but also reported with *Peptostreptococcus* species, *S. epidermidis, H. influenzae,* and two fungal species. There is also often a history of local ocular trauma, contact lenses, steroids, and/ or chronic antibiotic administration.

2. **Marginal ulcers.** Ulceration of the corneal periphery is seen most commonly in association with staphylococcal bacterial disease. There is concurrent blepharoconjunctivitis. The ulceration may be due to hypersensitivity reaction since culture of the ulcer is often sterile. The ulceration must be distinguished from Mooren's ulcer and the peripheral ulceration seen with collagen vascular diseases such as rheumatoid arthritis. *Moraxella* species have been described as producing ulcers that extend to the limbus, especially inferiorly.

3. **Laboratory tests** for conjunctival diagnosis (see sec. III.C) apply also to bacterial corneal disease. Corneal scrapings must be taken after routine lid and conjunctival culture for bacteria and fungi. This scraping is performed after instillation of topical proparacaine 0.5% (tetracaine, benoxinate, and cocaine are more likely to interfere with recovery of the organisms) and should obtain as much material as feasible, particularly from the deeper areas and the margin of the ulcer. Scrapings should be examined microscopically with Gram and Giemsa stains. Cultures should be done on blood agar plates (at room temperature and 38°C), chocolate agar, brain heart infusion, thioglycolate broth, and Sabouraud's agar or broth (fungal cultures).

4. **Initial treatment** is based on clinical impression and results of the scraping. Coverage should be broad, intensive, and amenable to change when final culture and sensitivity reports are available. Antibiotic treatment of infectious corneal ulcers must be aggressive using fortified solutions and under close observation to prevent serious scarring or frank perforation. Initial antibiotic therapy should be guided by the results of the Gram stain of the corneal scraping (see Tables 5-5, 5-6, and 5-7 and Appendix B for detailed list of drug indications, dosage, and routes of administration).

    a. **Gram-positive cocci.** Unless the morphology of the organism from the scraping is unquestionably pneumococcus (lancet-shaped, encapsulated diplococci), it is best to assume that penicillin-resistant species may be present. In mild infections, frequent topical therapy alone may be considered, but it may be advisable to give subconjunctival therapy as well in severe infections.

        (1) Topical cefazolin solution, 133 mg/ml, should be used q30-60 min. Bacitracin, 10,000 units/ml, may be used hourly and may be supplemented with gentamicin topical ophthalmic solution. Genta-

Table 5-5. Initial topical antibiotic therapy of bacterial keratitis based on Gram stain findings[a]

Bacterial type	Drugs of choice (fortified)	Alternative drugs (fortified and nonfortified)
Gram-positive cocci	Cefazolin, 133 mg/ ml Bacitracin, 10,000 units/ml, Penicillin G, 100,000 units/ml	Vancomycin, 25–50 mg/ml Chloramphenicol, 5 mg/ml[b]
Gram-positive bacilli (filaments)	Penicillin G, 100,000 units/ml	Vancomycin, 25–50 mg/ml Bacitracin, 10,000 units/ml
Gram-positive rods	Gentamicin, 14 mg/ ml	Tobramycin, 14 mg/ml
Gram-negative cocci	Penicillin G, 100,000 units/ml Ceftriaxone, 50 mg/ ml Bacitracin, 10,000 units/ml	Erythromycin[c] Neomycin[c] Tetracycline[c] Chloramphenicol, 5 mg/ml[b]
Gram-negative bacilli	Gentamicin, 14 mg/ ml Tobramycin, 14 mg/ml Ticarcillin, 6 mg/ml	Amikacin, 10 mg/ml Polymyxin B, 50,000 units/ml
No organisms seen, but bacteria suspected	Cefazolin, 133 mg/ ml, plus tobramycin, 14 mg/ml	Gentamicin, 14 mg/ml, or amikacin, 10 mg/ml, plus vancomycin, 25 mg/ml, cefamandole, 50 mg/ml, or bacitracin, 10,000 units/ml

[a] See also Table 5-7 for dosage and preparation of fortified drops and subconjunctival doses and Appendix B for expanded drug dosage list and organism-susceptibility guide. Subconjunctival and systemic therapy use is based on extent of disease (see Table 5-7).
[b] Fortified drop available as commercial ophthalmic preparation.
[c] Not available in fortified form. Commercial strength only. Parenteral therapy should be used in addition to local treatment for *Neisseria* or *Haemophilus* infections.

micin is often effective against *Staphylococcus* but usually ineffective against pneumococcus or *Streptococcus*. Vancomycin, 14–25 mg/ml, is effective in gram-positive coccal and bacillus infections, especially methicillin-resistant *Staphylococcus*. Drops are tapered over a 1- to 2-week period to qid for 2 weeks more as indicated.

(2) **Subconjunctival** therapy is usually used only in uncooperative or unreliable patients as q30–60min drops are as effective. If used, a common combination is cefazolin, 100 mg, and tobramycin, 40 mg, q24h for 2 days (see Table 5-7 for other drugs). Although 10% **cross sensitivity between cephalosporins and penicillin** has been reported in **penicillin-allergic patients,** it is usually safe to proceed with cephalosporin therapy. Subconjunctival injections are **painful** and are best preceded by topical or local anesthetic or preinjection oral narcotic.

b. **Gram-negative cocci *(N. meningitidis, N. gonorrhoeae)*. Topical** and **systemic** therapy are required and are discussed under hyperacute con-

Table 5-6. Subsequent therapy for culture-identified bacterial ulcers*

Organism	Topical	Subconjunctival
Pseudomonas	Tobramycin, 14 mg/ml, or ticarcillin, 6 mg/ml	Tobramycin, 40 mg (1 ml), or ticarcillin, 100 mg
Staphylococcus	Cefazolin, 133 mg/ml, or bacitracin, 10,000 units/ml, or vancomycin, 25–50 mg/ml	Cefazolin, 100 mg, oxacillin, 100 mg, or vancomycin, 25 mg
Proteus	Gentamicin, 14 mg/ml, tobramycin, 14 mg/ml, or ceftriaxone, 50 mg/ml	Gentamicin, 20–40 mg, or carbenicillin, 100 mg
Enterobacter, Escherichia coli, Klebsiella, Acinetobacter	Gentamicin, 14 mg/ml, tobramycin, 14 mg/ml, or amikacin, 10 mg/ml	Tobramycin, 40 mg, or gentamicin, 40 mg

* See Appendix B for parenteral use of these and other drugs and organism-susceptibility guide. Table 5-7 shows method of preparational fortified drops and subconjunctival doses.

junctivitis (see sec. **III.D.2**). Topical drops are increased to q30–60min for the first 2–3 days, however, and tapered more slowly.

  c. Gram-positive rods. These uncommon agents of ocular infection usually respond to penicillin. *Bacillus* species are susceptible to moderate doses of penicillin; clostridial organisms require higher doses. *Bacillus cereus* infections may be extremely hard to treat, even using gentamicin or clindamycin. **Topical** and **subconjunctival** injections may be employed. Tetracycline topically and orally is a useful alternative drug.

  d. Gram-negative rods.

    (1) Topical therapy initially should be gentamicin or tobramycin ophthalmic solution q30–60min. If *Pseudomonas* is suspected, topical ticarcillin, 6 mg/ml, or carbenicillin, 4 mg/ml, should also be instituted q30min.

    (2) Subconjunctival therapy, if used, should include tobramycin, 40 mg, and carbenicillin, 100 mg, each injected in a different area of the conjunctiva for 1 or 2 injections.

  e. Anaerobic gram-positive filaments (*Actinomyces, Streptothrix*) are sensitive to penicillins and tetracyclines.

  f. When no organisms are identified but bacterial etiology is strongly suspected on clinical grounds:

    (1) Topical therapy should be with cefazolin q30–60min (vancomycin in penicillin-allergic patients) on an alternate basis with gentamicin or tobramycin 14 mg/ml solution instillation.

    (2) Subconjunctival therapy should be cefazolin, 100 mg, plus tobramycin, 40 mg, until culture results are available.

  g. Systemic antibiotics, a cephalosporin and an aminoglycoside, are given as in Appendix B if there is scleral extension of the infection or a threatened perforation. Therapy may be refined when culture and sensitivities return.

  h. The **antibiotic regimen** is **altered** if necessary when final culture and sensitivity information is available. Fortified vancomycin and bacitracin are used if **methicillin-resistant staphylococci** are recovered. In the event that a suspected gram-negative coccus infection was initially treated with penicillin and the subsequent culture results disclose *Acinetobacter* species, penicillin should be discontinued as these organisms

Table 5-7. Preparation of antibiotics for fortified topical and subconjunctival use

Antibiotic (IM or IV formulation)	Commercial solution	Fortified topical drops				Subconjunctival	
		Diluent[a] (ml) added to 1.0 ml commercial solution	Final concentration	Shelf life (4°C)[b]	Volume of diluent (ml) added to 1.0 ml commercial solution	Final concentration	Final dose
Amikacin	100 mg/1 ml	9.0	10 mg/ml	30 days	1.0	50 mg/ml	25–50 mg
Bacitracin	50,000 units/ 5 ml	—	10,000 units/ml	7 days	—	10,000 units/ml	5000 units
Carbenicillin	1.0 gm/10 ml	24.0	4 mg/ml	3 days	—	100 mg/ml	100 mg
Cefamandole	1.0 gm/7.5 ml	—	133 mg/ml	4 days	0.3	100 mg/ml	100 mg
Cefazolin	1.0 gm/10 ml	2.0	33 mg/ml	10 days	—	—	—
Cefazolin	1.0 gm/7.5 ml	—	133 mg/ml	10 days	0.3	100 mg/ml	100 mg
Ceftriaxone	1.0 gm/7.5 ml	—	133 mg/ml	10 days	0.3	100 mg/ml	100 mg
Chloramphenicol	1.0 gm/10 ml	19.0	5 mg/ml	7 days	—	100 mg/ml	100 mg
Gentamicin	80 mg/2 ml	1.8	14 mg/ml	30 days	—	40 mg/ml	20–40 mg
Penicillin G potassium	1 million units/ml	9.0	100,000 units/ml	7 days	—	1 million units/ml	1 million units
Polymyxin B	500,000 units/20–50 ml	—	10–25,000 units/ml	3 days	—	10,000 units/ml	10,000 units/ml
Ticarcillin	1.0 gm/10 ml	16.0	6 mg/ml	14 days	—	—	—
Tobramycin	80 mg/2 ml	1.8	14 mg/ml	30 days	—	40 mg/ml	20–40 mg
Vancomycin	500 mg/10 ml	1.0	25 mg/ml	14 days	—	50 mg/ml	25 mg

[a] With the exception of carbenicillin and vancomycin (sterile water for injection only) and bacitracin (normal saline for injection only), diluent may be sterile water or saline for injection (USP), or sterile artificial tears using the original tears bottle to administer the reconstituted drug solution.
[b] Frozen extends expiration time to 12 weeks for aminoglycosides, cephalosporins, and vancomycin; 4 weeks for ticarcillin.
Source: Adapted from D. Pavan-Langston and E. Dunkel, *Handbook of Ocular Drug Therapy and Ocular Side Effects of Systemic Drugs*, Boston: Little, Brown, 1991.

are often not sensitive to penicillin. Tables 5-5, 5-6, and 5-7, and Appendix B summarize the recommended therapy.

5. **Other treatment modalities**
   a. **Dilation.** Long-acting cycloplegics such as atropine 1% or scopolamine 0.25% should be used if significant anterior chamber reaction is present. Initial instillation is usually required at least 3 times a day. If significant synechiae are forming at the pupillary margin, 1 or 2 doses of topical 2.5% phenyephrine are often indicated to ensure mobility of the pupil.
   b. **Corticosteroid** use in treatment of infectious corneal ulcers is less controversial than in past years. It is probably unwise to use steroids until at least 24–48 hours of antibacterial treatment has been completed or until the etiologic agent has been identified and shown to be sensitive to the antibiotics being used. They are contraindicated if fungus is at all suspected. Low-dose topical corticosteroids (e.g., prednisolone 0.12% qid) may have a place in limiting the inflammatory reaction once the clinician is satisfied that the antibiotic treatment is effective.

6. **Collagen shields** (bovine—Chiron, porcine—Bausch and Lomb), initially developed to enhance corneal epithelial healing after surgery, trauma, or dystrophic erosions and filaments, are now being used as effective high-dose drug delivery systems. The lenses dissolve spontaneously and are available in 24-, 48-, or 72-hour dissolution times. One size fits all. Soaking the lenses in antibiotics such as tobramycin, 40- or 200-mg solutions, results in a 30-fold increase in antibiotic penetration into the aqueous compared to subconjunctival injection or to a regular therapeutic soft contact lens and q1h drops. The high level of drug may be maintained with q4h drops using the collagen shields. Antibiotic-soaked shields are being evaluated as substitutes for postoperative conjunctival injection and in treatment of corneal ulcers, and cyclosporine-containing shields (4 mg) in treatment of corneal allograft rejections. Adverse side effects and potential drug toxicity with use of shields have not been reported. Use of the shields as drug delivery systems has not been approved by the FDA.

7. **Special pediatric considerations.** Topical therapy remains the mainstay in treating keratitis in the pediatric age group and is often best accomplished with ointment medication q2–3h in lieu of topical drops q30min. **Subconjunctival** therapy is usually not feasible unless the child is anesthetized with general anesthesia at the time of corneal scraping. Should systemic medication be considered necessary, it is best done with the consultation of a pediatrician or internist. See Appendix B for dosages and organism indications.

C. **Chlamydial (trachoma-inclusion conjunctivitis [TRIC]) organisms** are intracellular "parasites" but not true viruses, having enzyme systems similar to bacteria. They can produce acute inflammatory diseases of the conjunctiva and cornea that will often progress to a more chronic follicular conjunctivitis. Infection with inclusion conjunctivitis usually takes different forms in children and adults.

1. **Neonatal inclusion conjunctivitis (inclusion blennorrhea)** has an acute onset 5–12 days after birth, presenting as an acute conjunctivitis with purulent discharge.
   a. **Diagnosis** of this *Chlamydia trachomatis* infection is facilitated by the presence of **intracytoplasmic inclusion bodies** apparent in epithelial cells obtained by conjunctival scraping. Giemsa stain is the most effective method for demonstrating the individual elementary bodies or larger initial bodies as basophilic inclusions with, at times, small eosinophilic opacities. It is obviously important to **distinguish** this infection from **Neisseria gonorrhoeae.** Although the infection can resolve without sequelae, a membranous conjunctivitis may develop and result in conjunctival scarring, and a definite keratitis may supervene with superficial corneal vascularization.

b. Treatment is **systemic antibiotics** with the topical route used only if a patient cannot tolerate full systemic doses. Erythromycin, 40 mg/kg PO daily in 4 divided doses for 3–4 weeks is the preferred therapy in newborns. Sulfisoxazole is the alternative drug. Dosages for children and newborns are given in Appendix B. Children under 8 years of age should not receive systemic tetracycline unless there is no alternative. In infants the usual topical treatment is sulfacetamide 10% or tetracycline 1% ointment qid for at least 3 weeks. Since the condition is acquired by the presence of *Chlamydia* in the birth canal, it should be assumed that the parents are infected and probably require treatment with systemic tetracycline to eliminate the source of the infection. If the mother is breast-feeding, erythromycin, 250 mg PO qid, or sulfonamides, 500 mg PO qid, should be used for 21 days (see sec. **2.b**).

2. Adult inclusion conjunctivitis usually presents as an acute follicular conjunctivitis with mucopurulent discharge occurring after an incubation period of 4–12 days. The disease usually occurs in sexually active young adults but may occur in senior citizens as well, often after having acquired a new sexual partner in the preceding 2 months. The acute conjunctivitis often evolves into a chronic follicular conjunctivitis. An epithelial keratitis may develop, as well as marginal and more central corneal infiltrates accompanied by superficial vascularization as an **inferior** limbal pannus. Iritis has been reported later in the condition, as well as Reiter's syndrome.

a. Diagnosis by Giemsa-stained scraping of the epithelium is less likely to show inclusion bodies, but these may be seen in a number of patients with the acute disease. Microtrak assay of scrapings is far more reliable diagnostically, but any culture or immune laboratory test may still have false-positives or false-negatives.

b. Treatment. Since the condition is often associated with an asymptomatic venereal infection, doxycycline, 100 mg PO bid, or tetracycline, 250–500 mg PO qid 30 min before meals or 2 hrs after for 21 days, is indicated. Erythromycin or sulfonamides are also effective. Topical antibiotics are relatively ineffective in treating the eye disease but may modify a conjunctivitis. The possibility of other venereal disease must be excluded. The usual precautions in the use of tetracycline should be observed; it should not be used in women who are pregnant or breast-feeding. Erythromycin base, 250 mg PO qid, erythromycin ethylsuccinate, 800 mg PO qid for 7 days or 400 mg PO qid for 21 days, or sulfisoxazole, 500 mg PO qid for 21 days, are effective alternatives.

3. Trachoma. The initial manifestation of trachoma is a chronic follicular conjunctivitis that is classically more marked on the upper tarsal plate, with progressive disease scarring of the conjunctiva occurring on the superior tarsal conjunctiva as fine linear scars and often as a transverse band of scar **(Arlt's line).** When marked, this scarring can lead to entropion and trichiasis, with secondary ocular surface breakdown, including corneal ulceration. Primary corneal involvement occurring with the conjunctivitis can include an epithelial keratitis, marginal and central corneal infiltrates, and superficial vascularization. This is usually more pronounced on the upper half of the cornea and can appear as a fibrovascular pannus. Follicle formation at the limbus regresses to sharply defined depressions **(Herbert's pits)** at the base of the pannus.

a. The disease as classically described by **MacCallan*** considers the **conjunctival changes** according to the following **classification:**

(1) Trachoma I. Immature follicles on the upper tarsal plate including the central area but without scarring.

(2) Trachoma II. Mature (necrotic or soft) follicles on the upper tarsus obscuring tarsal vessels but without scarring.

---

* MacCallan, A.F. The epidemiology of trachoma. *Br. J. Ophthalmol.* 15:369, 1931.

(3) Trachoma III. Follicles present on the tarsus and definite scarring of the conjunctiva.

(4) Trachoma IV. No follicles on the tarsal plate but definite scarring on the conjunctiva.

This infection is not commonly seen in developed countries, but only the United Kingdom and some parts of Europe are totally free of endemic disease.

b. Treatment. Individual patients with trachoma respond usually to a 3-week course of either tetracycline or erythromycin given orally in full dosages (250 mg tid). Clinical response may be slow, and prolonged treatment may be required. When large groups are treated, topical tetracycline or erythromycin ointments may be given twice daily for 2 months. When systemic treatment is used, tetracycline should be used in preference to oral sulfonamides due to the lower incidence of side effects with tetracycline.

D. Herpes simplex virus (HSV) keratoconjunctivitis and iritis. Ocular infections with herpesvirus represent a challenge to diagnosis and treatment. **Primary ocular herpes** usually occurs as an acute follicular keratoconjunctivitis with regional lymphadenitis, with or without vesicular ulcerative blepharitis or cutaneous involvement. The keratitis can occur as a coarse punctate or diffuse branching epithelial keratitis that does not usually involve the stroma. The condition is self-limited, but the virus establishes a latent infection in the trigeminal ganglion. It periodically reactivates under various forms of patient stress (fever, flu, emotional or physical exhaustion) and causes recurrence of the disease in a host who has both competent cellular and humoral immunity. **Recurrent disease** may occur as one or a combination of the following: epithelial infectious ulcers, epithelial trophic ulcers, stromal interstitial keratitis, stromal immune disciform keratitis, and iridocyclitis. Management of this disease, with its chronic recurring and often progressive nature, can be difficult and must be tailored to minimize permanent ocular damage from each recurrence and to avoid iatrogenic complications.

1. Epithelial infections. Dendritis or geographic ulceration of the cornea is caused by live virus present in intracellular and extracellular locations, particularly in the basal epithelium. The use of steroids in purely infectious epithelial disease serves only to make the ulceration spread and to prolong the infectious phase of the disease.

a. When the fluorescein or rose bengal staining dendritic figure is seen, **mechanical debridement** of the involved area plus a rim of normal epithelium is best performed under slit-lamp or loupe magnified visualization with a sterile cotton-tipped applicator.

b. Antiviral chemotherapy with topical **vidarabine 3%** or **idoxuridine 0.5%** ointment 5 times a day or **trifluridine 1%** solution 9 times a day for 14–21 days arrests viral replication until infected cells slough from the eye. Idoxuridine 0.1% drops must be given hourly by day and q2h at night or just ointment hs. With treatment, the infectious epithelial disease resolves 80–90% of time without complication and without the need for anti-inflammatory drugs. **Limbal ulcers** are more resistant to healing but eventually close without much scarring. HSV infections in **AIDS** patients show a predilection for peripheral versus central involvement, moderately prolonged course with mean healing time of 3 weeks with topical antivirals, rare stromal involvement, and tendency to frequent recurrence (1–3 times over 1½ years). With prolonged treatment, the antivirals can produce a **toxic** punctate keratopathy, retardation of epithelial healing, superficial stromal opacification, follicular conjunctivitis, or lacrimal punctate occlusion.

c. Acyclovir 3% ophthalmic ointment, applied 5 times a day, is available only on compassionate plea from Burroughs Wellcome in the United States. There is **no proven role for systemic acyclovir** in epithelial or stromal herpes. Past studies have used a dosage of 200 mg PO 5 times a day for 14–21 days with taper to bid for up to 18 months with some success in preventing recurrent infections. Formal study is under way now concerning a possible effect on stromal keratouveitis. Viral resistance and drug withdrawal rebound are possible adverse effects.

2. **Epithelial sterile trophic ulceration (metaherpetic, postinfectious).** An indolent linear or ovoid epithelial defect with heaped-up borders can occur at the site of a previous herpetic ulcer and be confused with infectious geographic ulcer. These defects are mechanical healing problems similar to recurrent traumatic erosion and are caused by damage to the basement membrane sustained during the acute infectious epithelial stage. Damaged basement membrane heals extremely slowly over 8–12 weeks. During this period, epithelial cells are unable to maintain their position after migrating across the bed of the ulcer.

   a. Because of the mechanical nature of the problem, **treatment** is designed to protect the damaged basement membrane by use of a high-water-content **therapeutic** (Permalens, Sauflon) **soft contact lens** worn for 2–3 months, patching, lid taping, partial tarsorrhaphy, or, infrequently, a surgically placed conjunctival flap. In the presence of underlying stromal inflammatory disease that may interfere with the healing of the basement membrane, mild corticosteroid such as ⅛% prednisolone bid is indicated. Antibiotic solution once or twice a day should be used when treatment includes continuously worn therapeutic contact lenses along with frequent lubrication with artificial tears for several months even after the lens has been removed.

   b. If active **corneal thinning** (melting) occurs, sealing off the ulcer with **cyanoacrylate tissue adhesive** (Nexacryl from Tri-Point Medical L.P., Raleigh, N.C.; now under FDA-IND study) should be considered. Under topical anaesthesia the physician debrides and dries the ulcer and peri-ulcer area of debris and loose cells with Weckcell sponges and scraping with the side of a No. 15 Bard Parker blade and applies the liquid adhesive in short strokes or concentric spots. It polymerizes almost instantly to the tissue. Sterile saline is dripped on the eye, a therapeutic soft contact lens is applied, and antibiotic drops given bid. If needed for inflammation, steroids may now be used with greater safety. The cornea should heal and dislodge the glue in 1–3 months, usually leaving the eye quiet but scarred and hopefully amenable to transplant if vision is significantly compromised.

3. **Stromal interstitial keratitis, immune rings, and limbal vasculitis.** Viral interstitial keratitis presents as necrotic, blotchy, cheesy-white infiltrates that may lie under ulcers or may appear independently. Immune rings are gray anterior stromal Wessley rings and limbal vasculitis a local Arthus reaction. All are believed due to antigen-antibody-complement–mediated immune reaction. These lesions must be distinguished from secondary bacterial or fungal infections, which are usually much less indolent. After several weeks of smoldering inflammation, dense leashes of stromal vascularization may begin to advance into the cornea.

   a. Whether steroids are used for **therapy** depends on the surgical plans for the eye and the severity of the general ocular reaction and associated corneal edema. If the inflammatory infiltrates do not involve the visual axis or there is no active neovascularization, steroid therapy is usually not indicated, since the process often burns itself out spontaneously in weeks to months and, with the exception of limbal vasculitis, leaves scarring even after steroid therapy. The vascularization regresses to leave ghost vessels. Generally, if **steroids** have never been used in an eye, the clinician should try to do without them, as it may be difficult to wean the eye off these drugs. Treatment in this situation is probably best confined to **cycloplegics** (if needed for associated iridocyclitis) and **lubricants.**

    b. If the inflammatory reaction becomes severe however, if steroids have been previously used, if the visual axis is threatened, or if there is active neovascularization, the use of steroids will control the inflammatory reaction and decrease formation of scar tissue and deep vessel invasion that could later compromise success of surgery. The minimum **corticosteroid dosage** needed to control the disease ranges from dexamethasone 0.1% q3h to prednisolone 0.12% every other day. Once hyperemia and edema begin to decrease, steroids should be tapered downward over several weeks to several months. While steroids are used, concomitant prophylactic antiviral agents such as trifluridine qid or vidarabine ointment bid should be used, and antibiotics such as erythromycin daily should be continued until steroid dose is reduced to the equivalent of prednisolone 1% once daily or less.

    c. Keratoplasty should be deferred until the eye has been quiet with little or no steroid treatment for several months, because viral interstitial keratitis is the form of herpes most likely to recur in a new graft.

4. Disciform keratitis is due to a delayed hypersensitivity reaction characterized by sensitized T lymphocytes and macrophages reacting to viral antigen in the cornea. The clinical appearance is that of a focal disk-shaped patch of stromal edema without necrosis or vascularization but occasionally accompanied by focal keratic precipitates. With progressive severity, more diffuse edema and folds in Descemet's membrane are seen and vessels may appear. In its most advanced stage, diffuse edema with ulcerating bullous keratopathy and necrotic stromal thinning accompanied by severe iritis supervene.

Therapeutically, the same rules apply to treatment of disciform keratitis as to viral interstitial keratitis (see sec. **3**).

5. If disciform stromal disease is present with an **infected epithelial ulcer,** gentle debridement of the epithelium and full antiviral therapy should be started at least a day or two before steroids. If the ulcer progresses despite topical antiviral therapy, the frequency and strength of steroid dosage should be reduced until the ulcer is under control and is healing. If disciform keratitis is combined with **trophic ulceration,** control of underlying stromal edema with low-dose topical steroids and the application of a thin soft contact lens will aid healing. A **persistent epithelial defect** carries the added risk of collagenase release, and steroids may enhance **melting,** with ultimate corneal perforation. Cyanoacrylate adhesives (see sec. **II.B**) or surgical intervention by conjunctival flap or penetrating keratoplasty may be necessary before perforation actually occurs.

6. Iridocyclitis, retinitis and occasionally **panuveitis** may occur with herpes simplex infection. Intraocular inflammation may occur without concomitant keratitis but almost invariably accompanies active keratitis. Uveitis in an eye with previous herpetic keratitis should be considered herpetic until proved otherwise. Therapy is discussed in Chap. 8, sec. **X.B.3.** Prophylactic antivirals and antibiotic agents should be used with the steroids. If ulcerative keratitis supervenes, particularly if the cornea is **melting, systemic steroids** such as oral prednisone, 60–80 mg/day may be substituted for part or all of the topical steroid regimen.

7. Steroid tapering. Special comment should be made regarding the gradual reduction and termination of steroid treatment. Since too rapid a steroid taper or abrupt cessation of treatment can often be accompanied by recrudescence of the inflammation, it is essential to control carefully the steroid dose. The rule of thumb is **never taper steroids by more than 50% at any given time.** Each level should be maintained for several days or, at lower doses, for several weeks depending on the severity of inflammation at the initiation of treatment and the therapeutic response. One method uses progressively decreasing strengths of glucocorticoid such that, from the dexamethasone 0.1% or prednisolone 1% daily, tapered from 4 times down to once, prednisolone 0.12% solution can be used 4 times a day with gradual reduction to 3 times a day, 2 times a day, once a day, every 2 days, and so forth, until cessation of treatment. Occasionally, patients will require chronic low-dose (once or twice weekly) prednisolone to maintain a quiet eye. Coverage with antiviral medication need not be continued after reduction to less than 1% prednisolone bid.

8. **Keratoplasty** (transplantation) of the herpes simplex scarred eye is now about 85% successful on first procedure in the quiet eye. Emergency surgery on inflamed eyes is less successful and ranges between 40 and 60% success. Intensive topical steroids are required postoperatively. Topical antivirals are generally indicated if steroids are being used to treat an **allograft rejection** but not as routine postoperative therapy.

E. **Herpes zoster ophthalmicus.** Herpes zoster is an acute infection of a dorsal root ganglion by the virus of chickenpox characterized by vesicular skin lesions distributed over the sensory dermatome innervated by the affected ganglion. Regional lymphadenopathy with associated pain is common. The ophthalmic (trigeminal ganglion) form of the disease usually presents as a combination of two or more of the following: conjunctivitis, episcleritis, scleritis, keratitis, iridocyclitis, and glaucoma. Chorioretinitis, V^1 dermatomal vesicular dermatitis, extraocular muscle palsies, and optic neuritis may also be seen (see Chap. 8, sec. **X.C**). Herpes zoster is increasing in frequency due to the AIDS epidemic.

1. **Conjunctivitis, episcleritis,** and **scleritis** occur in about one-half of the cases. Conjunctival involvement is common and may occur as watery hyperemia with petechial hemorrhages, follicular conjunctivitis with regional adenopathy, or severe necrotizing membranous inflammation. Scleritis or episcleritis may be diffuse or focal nodular. On resolution scleritis can leave scleral thinning and staphyloma.

2. **Keratitis** occurs in about 40% of all patients and may precede the neuralgia or skin lesions. It may occur as a fine or coarse punctate epithelial keratitis with or without stromal edema, or as actual vesicle formation with ulceration in a **dendritic** pattern that can be mistaken for herpes simplex keratitis. **Corneal sensation** is usually greatly reduced in herpes zoster keratitis. Rarely, chronic serpiginous ulceration may occur with slough of the entire epithelial surface. Melting and corneal perforation may supervene if persistent epithelial defect is present. Stromal keratitis, either immune disciform or white necrotic interstitial keratitis, may occur with or independently of epithelial disease. Neuroparalytic ulceration may occur as a sequela of the acute infection and ganglionic destruction.

3. **Iridocyclitis** is a frequent occurrence and may appear independent of corneal activity. After resolution of the acute perineuritis and vasculitis, there may be focal or sector atrophy of the iris. Hypopyon, hemorrhage into the anterior chamber (anterior segment necrosis, and phthisis bulbi may all result from zoster vasculitis and ischemia.

4. **Glaucoma** may occur acutely due to trabeculitis. In later stages synechial closure of the angle occurs (see Chap. 9, sec. **XVIII**).

5. **Therapy.** Because herpes zoster may cause such devastating disease, it is reasonable that the therapeutic approach be vigorous to prevent the more severe complications. Systemic antiviral acyclovir (Zovirax) decreases pain, stops viral progression, and significantly reduces the incidence and severity of keratitis and iritis. It has no effect on posthepertic neuralgia. **Systemic steroids** appear to be the only drugs to inhibit development of postherpetic neuralgia, and this is not totally confirmed. Fortunately 85% of neuralgias resolve spontaneously over several months. The elderly (older than 60 years) are at greatest risk for severe or permanent pain. **Cimetidine** (Tagamet), for 2–3 weeks starting within 48–72 hours of disease onset, has also been shown to reduce pain and pruritus in acute zoster presumably by histamine blockade in the periocular tissues. The following regimen is presently recommended for ocular management:

   a. **Acyclovir** (Zovirax), four 200-mg tablets PO 5 times a day (4000 mg/ day total) for 10 days in the immunocompetent patient or, in the immunosuppressed patient, 5–10 mg/kg or 500 mg/m^2 IV q8h for 5–7 days. Therapy is most effective if started within 72 hours of onset of disease.

b. Cimetidine (Tagamet), 300 mg PO qid if periocular edema and pruritus are excessive.

c. Topical steroids only if needed for corneal disciform immune edema or iritis, e.g., 1%–⅛% prednisolone qd–qid with gradual taper; **cycloplegia** (homatropine) for iritis.

d. Vidarabine ointment or **trifluridine antiviral** therapy if diagnosis of corneal ulcers is not definitely zoster as opposed to herpes simplex. Infectious (dentriform) zoster ulcers heal without therapy.

e. Topical antibiotic if epithelium is ulcerated or topical steroids are in use.

f. Lateral tarsorrhaphy if cornea is anesthetic, with frequent artificial tear lubrication to prevent neurotrophic ulceration.

g. Therapeutic high-water-content **soft contact lens** if epithelium is ulcerated; antibiotic drops bid for prophylaxis and artificial tears for lubrication. **Avoid soft contact lens** if the epithelium is rough but not ulcerated, as the lens may induce ulcer (see sec. **f**). Tape lid shut (Transpore, Transderm) if the patient is soft contact lens intolerant. A neovascular pannus will heal these eyes and should not be blocked with steroid therapy.

h. Cyanoacrylate **tissue adhesive** (glue, Nexacryl) if there is corneal ulcer melting (thinning). Cover with a soft contact lens, and administer prophylactic antibiotics and lubricants. Glue is under FDA-IND study.

i. Beta blockers (timolol, betaxolol, levobunalol) and/or **epinephrine** or its prodrug (Propine) or **carbonic anhydrase inhibitors** for secondary glaucoma; mydriatic cycloplegia to prevent synechiae; no miotics.

j. Nonnarcotic or narcotic analgesics for neuralgia during the first 10 days should be used to control pain. If relief is not obtained and the patient is immunocompetent (i.e., no AIDS, organ transplant immunosuppression), start prednisone, 60 mg daily for 7 days, followed by prednisone, 30 mg once daily for 7 days. Patients over 55 years are at greatest risk for permanent or prolonged neuralgia. Young patients rarely have sustained pain.

k. Postherpetic neuralgia is often markedly relieved by tricyclic **antidepressants** such as amitriptyline hydrochloride (25–150 mg PO qd). Other useful agents are desipramine, 25–75 mg PO qd, imipramine, 150 mg PO qd, or combinations such as Triavil 2–10 PO, 3–4 tablets/day. **Capsaicin** 0.025% (Zostrix) topical skin cream depletes substance P, a tachykinin involved in pain transmission, from the sensory peripheral neurons. It must be used a minimum of 3–6 times daily for relief of pain in the involved dermatome after the skin has healed. Use in the eyes is to be avoided, and the skin may burn temporarily after use. Pain relief will be noted in two to six weeks in 75% of patients. In middle-aged patients therapy is for usually three to five months, but may be restarted if pain returns. In older patients daily treatment may be required for several years.

6. Keratoplasty. Corneas sufficiently scarred by herpes zoster to warrant keratoplasty for restoration of sight are usually sufficiently anesthetic and susceptible to repeated inflammatory reaction that they are a poor risk for surgical rehabilitation. If done, a lateral tarsorrhaphy should also be done. Epithelial defects, melting, superinfection, and secondary iritis with glaucoma may complicate any surgical procedure. Although not visually effective, the **conjunctival flap** is often a safer procedure to perform against progressive melting defects if tissue glue has not aided healing.

F. Varicella or **chickenpox virus** is the same organism as that causes herpes zoster (VZV) and is morphologically indistinguishable from herpes simplex virus.

1. The most common clinical manifestation of the virus, **chickenpox**, is a contagious disease, predominantly of children, transmitted by droplet infection and characterized by fever and papulovesicular rash that is usually self-limiting and uncomplicated. **Vesicular lesions** may appear along the lid margin and **eyelids** during an episode of chickenpox and rarely may appear on the conjunctiva. Usually unilateral, small, papular lesions that can be contiguous with the lid margin, commonly occurring at the **limbus,** these lesions may resolve or may form a punched-out dark-red ulcer with swollen margins, causing pain and inflammation in the eye. More rarely, the cornea may become involved, with superficial punctate **keratitis** or a more serious stromal disciform keratitis accompanied by plastic **iridocyclitis** that can in the most severe cases destroy the eye. A late keratitis, occurring 1-6 months after the illness, has been reported and may be a late immune reaction or recurrent infectious VZV dendritic ulcerations. Intraocular penetration by the virus may produce uveitis, **retinitis,** and **optic neuritis,** as well as **cataract,** but this is unusual. Bell's palsy and ophthalmoplegia may occur.

2. **Therapy** includes
   a. **Good hygiene,** cool compresses, low illumination.
   b. **Cycloplegics** for iritis or keratitis.
   c. **Topical** vidarabine antiviral ointment 5 times a day for 10-14 days for surface vesicles or ulcers and antibiotic bid prophylaxis.
   d. **Cautious use of mild topical steroid** for nonulcerative interstitial or disciform stromal keratitis. Dissemination of varicella in children from exogenous systemic steroids is a well-recognized hazard.

G. **Adenoviral** infections are frequent and classic causes of acute follicular conjunctivitis. Clinically, they are usually encountered as epidemic keratoconjunctivitis (EKC), usually associated with adenovirus types 8 and 19, and pharyngoconjunctival fever (PCF), usually associated with adenovirus type 3. After an incubation period of 5-12 days following droplet or fomite inoculation onto the conjunctival surface, symptoms of irritation and watery discharge are accompanied by hyperemia of the conjunctiva and follicle formation, often in association with preauricular adenopathy. Patients are **contagious for 10-12 days** and should avoid close contact or sharing towels with others during this time (take sick leave from work).

1. **Epidemic keratoconjunctivitis** usually is **not** accompanied by systemic symptoms, and one eye is often involved prior to the other. The conjunctivitis runs a course of 7-14 days, at which time a superficial diffuse epithelial keratitis may develop and be superceded by slightly focal elevated epithelial lesions that stain with fluorescein. About the eleventh to fourteenth day round, focal subepithelial opacities develop. There may be petechial hemorrhages of the conjunctiva, conjunctival membrane formation, and marked lid swelling. Medical personnel examining or treating patients with this condition should be very vigilant about handwashing and cleansing of instruments.

2. **Pharyngoconjunctival fever** is characterized by pharyngitis, fever, and follicular conjunctivitis. The highly contagious (10-12 days) condition is usually unilateral and self-limited over 5-14 days. In the early stages, the condition can be confused with herpes conjunctivitis, acute inclusion conjunctivitis, and acute hemorrhagic conjunctivitis. The keratitis is similar to EKC but usually bilateral and much milder.

3. **Treatment** is primarily supportive management, using astringent drops and cool compresses. The antiviral drugs have been ineffective in limiting the severity or course of the condition, and topical antibiotics serve only to prevent secondary bacterial infection. Most patients are not so severely symptomatic to require corticosteroid anti-inflammatory drops; however, some patients may be so immobilized by the symptoms that they will require mild topical steroids tid-qid, e.g., ⅛% prednisolone. Topical steroids will inhibit the appearance of subepithelial corneal infiltrates in EKC and PCF, but on discontinuation of the steroids infiltrates will recur. Unfortunately, there are a large number of patients who require a long and gradual

tapering of the steroid dose due to recurrence of the symptoms. With time, all infiltrates will clear spontaneously.

H. Acquired immunodeficiency syndrome (AIDS), caused by the human immunodeficiency virus or HIV-1, causes a progressive, profound T-lymphocyte cellular immunodeficiency characterized by multiple opportunistic infections and malignancies (especially Kaposi's sarcoma). Over 60% of patients have ocular lesions; however, most involvement is chorioretinal. The virus has been isolated from the tear film and almost all ocular structures including cornea, vitreous, and chorioretinal tissues. Anterior ocular lesions include follicular conjunctivitis, Kaposi's sarcoma of the conjunctiva (a deep purple-red soft tumor), a punctate or geographic ulcerative keratitis that may mimic herpes infection, and nongranulomatous iritis. These are HIV-1 induced and occur independently of any opportunistic infection. Opportunistic anterior infections include herpes simplex, herpes zoster, and fungal and bacterial ulcers. **Therapy** of AIDS is systemic and is discussed in Chap. 8, sec. **X.E.** Opportunistic infections are discussed in their respective sections by diagnosis.

I. Molluscum contagiosum virus is a large member of the pox group that causes epithelial tumorlike eruptions involving the skin.

   1. Ophthalmic interest centers around the lesions that affect the brow area, eyelids (particularly the eyelid margins), and, rarely, the conjunctiva. The skin lesion often starts as a discrete papule that eventually becomes multiple pale nodules up to 2 mm in size with umbilicated centers from which a cheesy mass can be expressed. When one of the pearly umbilicated lesions affects the lid margin, a follicular conjunctivitis and an epithelial keratitis can result that is thought to be due to toxicity to products released by the lesion into the cul-de-sac. The conjunctivitis tends to be of the chronic follicular type with seromucous secretion or scant discharge. The keratitis tends to be a fine diffuse or focal epithelial keratitis that can, if chronic and untreated, lead to subepithelial infiltration and vascularization from the periphery that resembles a trachomatous pannus. The lid lesion must be differentiated from other eyelid tumors, including sebaceous cyst, verruca, chalazia, keratoacanthoma, and small fibroma.

   2. Treatment consists of complete eradication of the lesion. Following removal of the skin lesion, the conjunctivitis and keratitis rapidly clear. Cauterization and cryotherapy have been successful, but simple superficial excision or curettage is easily accomplished.

J. Ocular vaccinia occurs following an accidental inoculation to the eye after contact with a recent vaccinee.

   1. The **skin** of the eyelids becomes involved with a purulent ulceration and reaction that resembles the course of a primary vaccination as seen in the lid margin but can extend to the adjacent conjunctiva. In a previously vaccinated individual with a good level of immunity, little more than an acute focal purulent blepharoconjunctivitis can be seen; in the unvaccinated or weakly immune individual, a severe reaction may occur.

   2. Corneal involvement is seen in 30% of cases and varies from a mild superficial punctate keratitis to a severe stromal keratitis producing a disciform opacity, with occasional frank necrosis and rare perforation.

   3. Treatment

      a. Hyperimmune vaccinial gamma globulin (VIG), 0.25–0.5 ml/kg body weight IM, repeated in 48 hours if there is no improvement.

      b. Topical vidarabine or **idoxuriaine** ointment q4h.

      c. Topical antibiotic to prevent superinfection and cycloplegia for iritis.

      d. Topical steroids for disciform keratitis if the epithelium is healed and the infection is resolved.

K. Other viral causes of interstitial keratitis

   1. An evanescent interstitial keratitis can accompany **mumps** but usually clears very rapidly.

   2. Epstein-Barr virus (mononucleosis) may cause a prolonged nebulous interstitial keratitis (see Chap. 8, sec. **X.F**).

3. **Lymphogranuloma venereum** can produce a segmental and highly vascularized interstitial keratitis.

4. **Treatment.** Specific antiviral treatment is usually not effective, but control of the interstitial keratitis with atropine and topical steroids may be of benefit.

L. **Spirochetal infections**

1. **Syphilis *(Treponema pallidum).*** In past years syphilis has been responsible for more than 90% of the cases of diffuse interstitial keratitis, most commonly of the **congenital** form. Syphilis provokes a keratitis of widespread infiltrative inflammation of the corneal stroma, especially in the deeper layers, with a chronic course associated with inflammation of the anterior uveal tract. **Acquired** syphilis can produce interstitial keratitis much less frequently. It is usually uniocular, while the congenital variant is most often bilateral. Despite the congenital nature of the disease, manifestations of keratitis are usually not apparent until after age 10, with the greatest frequency between the ages of 10 and 20. The clinical course begins with an edema in the area of endothelium and deep stroma associated with pain, lacrimation, photophobia, and blepharospasm that progresses to a circumcorneal injection followed by a diffuse corneal haze. The clouding of the cornea often obscures an anterior uveitis. The acute inflammation resolves with the progressive appearance of vascular invasion from the periphery. Resolution of the edema leaves deep opacities and ghost vessels with hyaline excrescences on Descemet's membrane as secondary guttata. Hearing impairment and chorioretinal scarring (bone corpuscle or salt and pepper fundus) are often associated with the congenital variety of lues and interstitial keratitis. Neurosyphilis and cardiovascular syphilis are late forms of the systemic disease. Any patient with syphilis should be evaluated for AIDS and other sexually transmitted diseases (see Chap. 8, sec. **XI.B**).

a. **Systemic treatment** of the newborn for **congenital syphilis** is indicated if the mother's serology (FTA-ABS) is positive or becomes positive during pregnancy, even if the infant remains seronegative (not uncommon). Aqueous penicillin G potassium, 50,000 units/kg IM or IV, or procaine penicillin IM daily for 10 days is the therapy for such infants. Even this therapy may be insufficient for congenital ocular or neurosyphilis and retreatment may be required later. Children or adults with acute syphilitic interstitial keratitis are usually treated with ampicillin, 1.5 gm PO, in combination with probenecid, 500 mg PO q6h, on an empty stomach for 1 month. **Penicillin-allergic** patients may be treated effectively with erythromycin or, in children older than 8 years, erythromycin or tetracycline PO (see Appendix B for dosage). **Topical** steroids such as 0.1% dexamethasone q2-4h and cycloplegics (homatropine tid) are initiated and gradually tapered off as the disease responds. For severe interstitial keratitis, **subconjunctival** decadron, 4-12 mg qd for 3-4 days, may be necessary as initial steroid therapy along with steroid drops.

b. **Treatment of acquired primary, secondary, or latent syphilis** of less than 1 year's duration is 2.4 million units of benzathine penicillin G IM once or, for **penicillin-allergic** patients, erythromycin, 500 mg with meals, or tetracycline, 500 mg on an empty stomach, PO qid for 15 days. For **active syphilis** of over 1 year's duration, 2.4 million units of crystalline penicillin G is given IV q4h for 10 days followed by 2.4 million units of IM benzathine penicillin G qd for 3 weeks. Alternatives are 24-36 million units of IV crystalline penicillin G daily for 10 days or 1.5 gm of ampicillin and 0.5 gm of probenecid PO q6h for 30 days. **Penicillin-allergic** patients may be treated with double the above-mentioned tetracycline or erythromycin doses if they are also allergic to ampicillin (many are not) or cannot be desensitized to penicillin. **Topical** treatment with steroids and mydriatic-cycloplegics is similar to that for congenital syphilis.

2. **Lyme disease** an infectious and immune-mediated inflammatory disease caused by the spirochete *Borrelia burgdorferi,* has numerous ocular, neuroophthalmic, and systemic manifestations. There are three defined stages of disease.

   a. **Stage 1.** Within 1 month of an infected deer tick bite, a characteristic macular rash of varying severity and often with a clear center usually appears at the area of the bite. There may be associated fever, chills, fatigue, and headache. A malar rash and **conjunctivitis** (11% incidence) may also occur.

   b. **Stage 2.** After several weeks to months, neurologic (meningitis, radiculoneuropathies, severe headache) and cardiac (atrioventricular block, myopericarditis) signs may begin. **Neuroophthalmic** findings include optic neuritis and perineuritis, papilledema, ischemic optic neuropathy, optic nerve atrophy, pseudotumor cerebri, diplopia secondary to third and sixth nerve palsies, Bell's palsy, and multiple sclerosis–like disease. **Other ocular manifestations** include retinal hemorrhages, exudative retinal detachments, iritis followed by panophthalmitis, and bilateral keratitis. The keratitis is characterized by multiple focal, nebular subepithelial opacities at all levels of the stroma, limbus to limbus, and possibly progressing to corneal edema and neovascularization.

   c. **Stage 3.** Up to 2 years after the bite a migratory oligoarthritis may develop initially without joint swelling but later with effusions and degeneration. Extreme fatigue, lymphadenopathy, splenomegaly, sore throat, dry cough, testicular swelling, mild hepatitis, and nephritis are not uncommon. The **ocular manifestations** of Lyme disease may appear at **any stage** but are more common in the later two stages and may occur despite "adequate" treatment. Most resolve spontaneously, waxing and waning.

   d. **Diagnosis.** Either the indirect fluorescent antibody (IFA) method or the enzyme-linked immunosorbant assay (ELISA) is reliable. Lyme titers of 1 : 256 are diagnostic. In chronic Lyme disease, absence of antibodies against the spirochete does not exclude the disease; a specific T-cell blastogenic response to *B. burgdorferi* may make the diagnosis in seronegative patients. There is CSF pleocytosis.

   e. **Systemic treatment** is still controversial, and any manifestation of the disease may recur and require retreatment.

      (1) **Definite neuroophthalmic, ocular, neurologic, or cardiac disease**

         (a) **Adults.** Penicillin G IV, 24 million units/day in 4 divided doses for 14 days, or ceftriaxone IV, 2 mg/day for 14 days.

         (b) **Children.** Penicillin G, 250,000 units/kg/day in 4 divided doses for 14 days, or ceftriaxone, 100 mg/kg/day in 2 divided doses for 14 days.

      (2) **Nonspecific symptoms with positive Lyme titers**

         (a) **Adults.** Doxycycline, 100 mg PO bid, or tetracycline, 500 mg PO qid, or penicillin, 500 mg PO qid, each regimen 4-6 weeks.

         (b) **Children.** Penicillin V potassium PO, 50 mg/kg/day in 4 divided doses, or amoxicillin, 125–250 mg PO tid, or erythromycin, 40 mg/kg/day in 4 divided doses, each regimen 3-4 weeks.

   f. **Topical treatment** is adjunctive to systemic therapy. Vision-debilitating keratitis is responsive to 1% prednisolone qid with taper over several months and reinstitution as needed. Iritis may self-resolve and require only mydriatic-cycloplegic therapy (homatropine 2% or 0.25% scopolamine bid) or be more severe, requiring addition of intensive topical steroids, 0.1% dexamethasone q1-2h initially.

M. **Leprosy (Hansen's disease).** The interstitial keratitis of leprosy *(Mycobacterium leprae)* is a deep infiltration usually extending from the periphery to the center of the cornea, particularly in the upper outer quadrant, and is frequently bilateral. The interstitial keratitis may be associated with a punctate epithelial keratitis, and while corneal nerves are notably thickened and beaded, the interstitial vascularization is not prominent. The keratitis rarely occurs alone but can occur with involvement of the ciliary body or a limbal leukoma or glaucoma. Nodular lepromas are frequently seen in the subconjunctival tissues and iritis is severe. The cornea can be greatly thickened, and the opacity usually does not clear.

Treatment. Systemic sulfone therapy is usually required with topical steroid and atropine needed for control of the local reaction. Tuberculous (neuraesthetic) leprosy is treated with dapsone, 100 mg PO qd and 600 mg of rifampin monthly for 6 months. For lepromatous (granulomatous) leprosy, 50 mg of clofazimine is added to this regimen daily and 300 mg of it is given monthly. Such treatment should be carried out by a physician familiar with lepromatous disease.

N. Fungal keratitis. Fungal infection of the eye poses a threat not only because of the damage that can be caused by the fungus but also because of the limited number of approved antifungal agents available for treatment.

   1. Yeast fungi. *Candida* ulcers commonly occur in eyes with predisposing alterations in host defenses, including chronic use of corticosteroids, exposure keratitis, keratitis sicca, herpes simplex keratitis, and prior keratoplasty. *Candida* is a common offender in the northern and coastal regions of the United States, constituting 32–43% of keratomycoses. It is unwise and often not possible to determine the species of infecting organism by the clinical features, but the clinical appearance may suggest the infecting agent. *Candida* ulcers occasionally have distinct oval outlines with a plaquelike surface or can produce a relatively indolent stromal infiltration with smaller satellite lesions.

   2. Filamentous fungi. *Fusarium, Cephalosporium,* and *Aspergillus* are the most common filamentous fungi in the United States, with *Fusarium* causing 45–61% of filamentous keratitis cases. These organisms usually infect normal eyes following mild abrasive corneal trauma, especially after injury from vegetable matter. The organisms are ubiquitous and can be isolated readily from soil, air, and organic waste. These organisms are particularly responsible for keratitis in the southern United States. The clinical appearance can be characteristic, with a gray or dirty-white dry, rough, textured surface that often has an elevated margin. There may be feathery extensions beneath epithelium into the adjacent stroma. Satellite lesions separated from the central infectious area may occur and correspond to microabscesses in the surrounding tissue. Occasionally, **ring abscesses** have been described. If the infection is deep there can be endothelial plaque formation. Anterior chamber reaction and hypopyon can occur with large or deep infections. In **contact lens wearers,** filamentous fungi are more associated wtih cosmetic or aphakic lens wear and yeasts with therapeutic lenses.

   3. Diagnosis. Probably the most important step in early diagnosis is prompt and rigorous laboratory investigation. Scraping and inoculation of media should be performed (see sec. **III.C**), but several points deserve emphasis. It is important to scrape multiple sites in the ulcer crater, particularly at the margins, to enhance recovery of organisms. Since the organisms tend to be deep within the stroma, superficial keratectomy (corneal biopsy) may be necessary to obtain diagnostic material. Since the organism is often not seen on the scraping, it is important to inoculate each culture medium with multiple scrapings. Although Gram stain may identify some fungal forms, particularly the yeast forms of *Candida,* Giemsa stain is more likely to define the structure of filamentous fungi. Though not generally available, the Grocott modification of Gomori methamine silver stain often provides greater definition of fungal cytology. Sabouraud's broth and agar and a blood agar plate kept at room temperature, as well as brain heart infusion broth, are essential. More specialized media (such as Nickerson's media for identification of *Candida* organisms) may be used but are not essential.

4. **Treatment** is initially medical and potentially surgical since fungal infection can be rapidly destructive to the integrity of the eye, with ulceration of the cornea to the point of perforation with involvement of the iris and posterior chamber by synechiae and secondary glaucoma.

   a. **Medical therapy** is limited by the number of approved **antifungal drugs** and by the poor penetration of the available agents. Table 5-8 summarizes the most commonly used drugs, dosages, and indicated organisms. Prior to identification of the infectious agent, therapy should begin with as broad a spectrum as possible. Natamycin (Natacyn, pimaricin) 5% suspension or amphotericin B 0.075-0.3% is readily available and active against yeast and filamentous fungi. Substitution of a specific antifungal agent according to the clinical response or in vitro sensitivities is then indicated. Cultures may take from 3-14 days to become positive. When fungal elements are confirmed on direct smears, culture, or from histologic biopsy examination, therapy should be oriented toward the type of organism and extent of disease. **Filamentous** cases are usually responsive to the topical polyenes, natamycin, or amphotericin B, but refractory cases may be successfully treated with the addition of topical and subconjunctival miconazole. Ketoconazole PO is usually used as an adjunct therapy for patients unresponsive to purely topical medication. *Candida* or other yeasts usually respond to the **synergistic** combination of topical amphotericin B and oral flucytosine or to topical and subconjunctival miconazole with or without adjunctive oral ketoconazole (see Table 5-8 for doses and indicated organisms). Daily **epithelial debridement** by the physician (if the surface heals over) is useful in aiding drug penetration for at least the first several days of therapy. **Systemic amphotericin B** is indicated if the infection spreads to sclera or perforation threatens or occurs (see Table 8-7).

   Cycloplegics such as atropine or scopolamine should be used liberally to prevent posterior synechiae and to help reduce uveal inflammation. Secondary glaucoma may require oral carbonic anhydrase inhibitors or hyperosmotic agents. During early therapy of a fungal ulcer, **corticosteroids** are **contraindicated** due to the documented enhancement of fungal growth. If there is evidence that an effective antifungal agent is being used and that the clinical infection is well under control, corticosteroids can be used cautiously late in the treatment to reduce stromal or anterior segment inflammation.

   b. **Surgical therapy** may be required not only for complications of the acute infectious processes but also should medical management fail. Debridement and superficial keratectomy, although mostly of diagnostic benefit, may enhance the effectiveness of medical treatment. Conjunctival flaps have been advocated for nonhealing ulcers and are often effective, although fungal organisms have been found to persist under a conjunctival flap. Lamellar keratoplasty is usually ineffective in treating fungal keratitis because of the inability to remove completely the infectious agent, and it is probably contraindicated. If the area of infection can be completely encompassed by a penetrating graft and if there has been inadequate response to medical treatment, the corneal graft may provide an effective cure. Lens extraction should be avoided if the posterior segment is not involved.

O. **Nontrue fungi of the family Actinomycetaceae and Nocardiaceae.** Two organisms that superficially resemble fungi but are related to the true bacteria cause disease in humans.

   1. *Actinomyces* can infect the lacrimal system, particularly the canaliculi, producing a chronic conjunctivitis and canaliculitis. Rarely, a nodular keratitis may be produced. The gram-positive, non-acid-fast, nonmotile filamentous organism microscopically shows branching filaments when gran-

Table 5-8. Antifungal therapeutic regimen used in fungal keratitis[a, b]

Drug	Efficacious against
Amphotericin B (Fungizone) *Topical:* 0.075–0.3% drop q1h; taper over several weeks *Subconjunctival:* 100–300 mg q48h for 1–2 doses	*Candida, Aspergillus, Cryptococcus, Coccidioides, Sporothrix, Blastomyces, Histoplasma, Paracoccidioides, Mucor*
Clotrimazole[c] *Topical:* 1% drop q1h; taper as above	See Miconazole
Fluconazole (Diflucan) *Oral:* 200–400 mg PO initial dose; 100–200 mg/day PO for 3 wk *(Candida)* and for 10–12 wk *(Cryptococcus)*	*Candida, Cryptococcus*
Flucytosine (5-FC, Ancobon) *Topical:* 10 mg/ml drop q1h; taper as above *Oral:* 150 mg/kg/day	*Candida, Aspergillus, Cryptococcus, Cladosporium*
Ketoconazole (Nizoral) *Oral:* 400 mg–1.0 gm/day PO in single dose	Dermal mycoses; see Miconazole
Miconazole (Monistat) *Topical:* 10 mg/ml drop q1h; taper as above *Subconjunctival:* 10 mg q48h for 2–3 doses	*Candida, Fusarium, Penicillium, Aspergillus, Alternaria, Rhodotorula, Histoplasma, Cladosporium, Coccidioides, Mucor, Paracoccidioides, Phialophora, Actinomyces*
Natamycin (Pimaricin) *Topical:* 5% drop q1h; taper as above	*Candida, Fusarium, Cephalosporium, Aspergillus*

[a] For systemic doses in addition to ketoconazole, see Table 8-6.
[b] Only Pimaricin is FDA-approved for ocular use.
[c] Under FDA-IND, Compassionate Plea. Schering Plough Corp. (301) 443-4310.
Source: Adapted from D. Pavan-Langston and E. Dunkel, Antifungal Agents. *The Handbook of Ocular Drug Therapy and Ocular Side Effects of Systemic Drugs.* Boston: Little, Brown, 1991.

ules expressed or curetted from the canaliculi are smeared. The organism grows on blood agar or in chopped meat infusion, usually anaerobically. **Treatment** of the canaliculitis usually requires surgical removal or expression of the granules, but the organism is sensitive to **penicillin** and **sulfa** drugs (see Appendix B). Irrigation of the expressed canaliculus with a penicillin solution is often effective.

2. **_Nocardia asteroides_** is a gram-positive filamentous organism and may stain acid-fast. The organism grows aerobically very slowly on many simple media. It can produce a chronic corneal ulcer with a gray sloughing base and undermined overhanging edges. *Nocardia* can rarely produce endophthalmitis. **Sulfonamides** are the drugs of choice (see Appendix B).

P. **Amoeba.** Corneal ulceration and keratitis due to **_Acanthamoeba_** species is rare in the United States but must be considered in a nonhealing, culture-negative infection. Typically, it has been noted in patients who wore contact lenses (even disposables) or who had exposure to hot tubs, communal baths, or just plain tap water.

1. **Diagnosis.** About 65% are initially diagnosed as herpetic keratitis, and 30% of patients are not definitely diagnosed for 4–7 months after onset. **Inordinate pain** is one of the cardinal signs. The lesions are often multicentric,

but a ring-shaped lesion with stromal infiltrate is characteristic. Amoeba can be cultured from scrapings or biopsy on confluent layers of coliform bacteria or in *Enterobacter* suspensions. Calcofluor white stain of scrapings is positive in 70% of cases.

2. **Therapy** is still controversial and unsatisfactory; many medical cures have now been reported, but penetrating keratoplasty in combination with medical treatment may still be required. The organism exists in the cornea in both trophozoite and encysted states, thus requiring extremely prolonged therapy. Currently used regimens are 1% propamidine isethionate (Brolene, Bausch and Lomb, Tampa, Fla.—under FDA-IND study; OTC in Great Britain), 1 drop followed 5 minutes later by 1 drop of neomycin–polymyxin B–gramicidin (Neotricin, AK-spore) every 15 minutes to 1 hour, 18 hours per day, or dibromopropamidine (Brolene ointment; OTC in Great Britain) and neomycin–polymyxin B–bacitracin q2h for 1 week. Frequency is then tapered, e.g., q2h by day, q4h by night to 1 drop of each medication bid–qd for a year. In severe infections, oral ketoconazole and 2% clotrimazole may be added to the above regimen. Oral itraconazole, 150 mg PO every morning coupled with 0.1% miconazole q1h for 20 days with gradual tapering of both medications and discontinuation after just 2 months of therapy, has been reported as successful. Mild topical steroids will reduce inflammation and possibly scarring, but their use is not established.

V. **Noninfectious keratitis, keratoconjunctivitis, and keratopathies**

A. **Exposure keratopathy.** Any loss of the normal protective mechanisms of corneal sensation or lid blinking function can lead to exposure keratopathy.

1. **Causes** are Bell's palsy, traumatic facial palsy, or exophthalmus and incomplete lid closure.

2. **Clinically,** there is corneal desiccation, most notable in the inferior interpalpebral area of the conjunctiva and cornea, which can lead to a frank epithelial defect and a noninfiltrated ulceration. Superinfection is a constant threat.

3. **Treatment**

a. **Mild exposure.** Frequent instillation of artificial tears during the day and lubricant ointment at night with taping of the lid closed is usually sufficient. Frequent observation is needed.

b. **Moderate exposure.** Application of a soft contact lens with frequent instillation of lubricant may suffice. Usually lid surgery (intermarginal lid adhesions, cerclage, or spring implant) is required.

c. **Severe exposure.** Usually associated with marked exophthalmus often of endocrine etiology, severe exposure requires emergency treatment with high-dose systemic steroids, e.g., prednisone, 80–100 mg/day for a few days, to control the acute infiltrative ophthalmopathy or orbital decompression, most commonly into the maxillary and ethmoid sinuses (Ogura technique). Antibiotic prophylaxis and lubrication should be instituted.

B. **Thygeson's superficial punctate keratitis.** The clinical entity of a coarse punctate ("snowflake") epithelial keratitis running a chronic course with exacerbations and remissions, and associated with foreign body sensation, photophobia, and tearing is usually bilateral but can be asymmetric. These circular to oval epithelial lesions usually occur centrally and are slightly elevated with central fluorescein staining and a cluster of heterogeneous, granular gray dots. The disease is epithelial and not associated with inflammation elsewhere in the eye. It usually self-resolves in 6 years or less.

Treatment. The lesions and associated symptoms usually respond quickly to application of topical corticosteroids. The steroids can usually be tapered rapidly, but recurrence of the keratitis is common. One drop of prednisolone 0.12% weekly or even less may keep a patient asymptomatic. It is not necessary to treat to the level where all lesions are gone but only to the point of comfort. Application of a therapeutic soft contact lens will often relieve symptoms if the use of steroids is not possible or advisable. **Antiviral drugs are not** advised, as they may induce scarring beneath the lesions.

C. **Filamentary keratopathy.** A variety of conditions can produce filamentary keratopathy, which is probably best considered as a form of aberrant epithelial healing. Consequently, any condition that leads to focal epithelial erosions may produce filamentary keratopathy.

1. The **following conditions** are probably most commonly associated with this entity.

   a. **Keratitis sicca.** Filaments frequently occur in corneas that are subject to the epitheliopathy of keratitis sicca. These filaments can be distributed diffusely and are often associated with areas that stain with fluorescein on the corneal surface. Excess mucous production in this syndrome probably aggravates filament formation.

   b. **Superior limbic keratoconjunctivitis.** This condition, initially described as mild inflammation and vascular injection of the superior conjunctiva associated with rose bengal staining of the superior bulbar conjunctiva, often is associated with filaments distributed over the superior portion of the cornea.

   c. **Prolonged patching** following cataract or other ocular surgery.

   d. **Epitheliopathy** due to aerosol or **radiation** keratitis.

   e. **Following epithelial defects** of herpes or Thygeson's superficial punctate keratitis.

   f. **Systemic disorders,** including diabetes, psoriasis, and ectodermal dysplasias.

2. **Treatment.** The specific etiology of the filamentary keratopathy should be identified, and specific treatment for this should be given.

   a. **Debridement.** If only a few filaments exist, they may be removed at their base with a pair of jeweler's forceps following topical anesthetization of the cornea.

   b. **Medication.** In the dry eye or in the eye with unstable tear film, lubricants in the form of drops q2h or ointments q4h may be tried. Lid hygiene should be encouraged.

   c. **Therapeutic contact lens.** If symptoms are severe or if medication has failed, application of a high-water-content (70%) soft contact lens (Permalens, Sauflon) will provide relief and usually allow adequate epithelial healing without filament formation. Antibiotic drops bid (sulfacetamide, Polytrim) should be used for the first few weeks of wear. Lenses should be discarded for new ones q4–6 months until the disease resolves.

D. **Superior limbic keratoconjunctivitis** presents as bilateral ocular irritation with dilatated conjunctival vessels over the superior bulbar conjunctiva. It is often associated with superior corneal filaments. Rose bengal reveals prominent staining in the superior bulbar conjunctiva. The superior conjunctival cells are often keratinized. No organisms have ever been associated conclusively with superior limbic keratoconjunctivitis, and the role of the tarsal conjunctiva in provoking the reaction is speculative.

Treatment. Topical lubricants and low-dose topical steroids may alleviate the symptoms but usually do not completely reverse the conjunctival changes. Some success has been achieved with topical application of silver nitrate solution 1.0% to the involved area. The silver nitrate application frequently has to be repeated. Silver nitrate cautery sticks should **not** be used for this purpose as severe conjunctival burn and necrosis can occur. Various surgical procedures have been advised. Acceptable results can be achieved after application of faint diathermy in a checkerboard pattern across the superior bulbar conjunctiva. Recession or resection of a perilimbal strip of conjunctiva from the superior limbus is usually effective if other measures fail. Long-term wear of therapeutic soft contact lenses may be required (see sec. **C.2.c**). Superior limbic keratoconjunctivitis has been reported to occur with greater frequency in patients with hyperthyroidism.

E. Neuroparalytic keratitis

1. **Bell's palsy.** Idiopathic palsy of the facial nerve results in paralysis of the obicularis muscle and lagophthalmos, with incomplete closure of the lids and incomplete lubrication of the ocular surface, with resultant desiccation and epithelial breakdown. Particularly if Bell's phenomenon is weak or absent, frank ulceration of the corneal surface can occur. Emergency treatment of acute palsy is prednisone, 40 mg PO bid for 7–10 days, or aspirin, 650 mg q4h around the clock for 10 days.

2. **Herpes zoster ophthalmicus.** Involvement of the eye by herpes zoster ophthalmicus can result in severe corneal epithelial defect during the acute episode but also in diminished corneal sensitivity in the recovery stage. Loss of the protective corneal innervation results in a surface that breaks down readily and is very prone to desiccation with minimum exposure. The predisposition of the eye to inflammation makes treatment with contact lenses or surgery hazardous.

3. **Status posttrigeminal section for tic douloureux.** Neurosurgical procedures to interrupt the sensory root of the trigeminal nerve often result in corneal anesthesia. These corneas are also very sensitive to desiccation and exposure, with subsequent epithelial breakdown.

4. **Postradiation keratopathy.** After radiotherapy to lesions of the head and neck, trophic changes can occur in the eye, with corneal epithelial breakdown.

5. **Syphilitic (luetic) neuropathy.** Hypesthesia of the corneal nerves from luetic involvement also predisposes to epithelial breakdown.

6. **Neuroparalytic keratitis treatment**
   a. **Lubricants.** The mainstay of treatment of exposure keratopathy, particularly in the mild stages, is topical lubricants consisting of artificial tears (the more viscous bases being more effective) instilled q1–2h during the day with lubricant ointment or antibiotic ointment at night. In many cases this treatment will be sufficient.
   b. **Mechanical.** If significant lid dysfunction or lagophthalmos is present, it needs to be treated. Taping the lid shut at night is often efficacious, and patching, although inconvenient, can be used intermittently during the day. Application of an aqueous-impermeable shield or plastic coating to form a moist chamber may help. Side shields for glasses worn during the day are also somewhat effective. For more severe cases, lateral tarsorrhaphy can be performed with good effect.
   c. **Soft contact lens.** Application of a therapeutic, high-water-content soft contact lens (Permalens, Sauflon) in conjunction with supplemental tears can provide a reservoir to prevent desiccation. It must be remembered, however, that eyes with impaired sensation do not tolerate soft contact lenses as well as those with normal sensation, and the patient requires close follow-up to detect any signs of neovascularization, infiltration, or anterior chamber reaction. Antibiotics such as chloramphenicol or sulfur should be instilled to minimize the chance of infection. If any question of intolerance develops, lubricants or partial lid adhesion should be considered. Lid taping may be used in short-term treatment.

F. A **pterygium** is a fleshy triangular band of fibrovascular tissue with a broad base on the nasal or temporal epibulbar area, a blunt apex or head on the cornea, and a gray zone, or cap, which just precedes the apex. It is most common in the 20- to 30-year age group, in males, in tropical climates, and in people exposed to the elements and ultraviolet light. The episcleral portion usually develops rapidly over 2–3 months, but corneal growth takes many years. Signs and symptoms include congestion, photophobia, tearing, foreign body sensation, progressive astigmatism, diplopia, and restriction of extraocular movement. Often pterygia will spontaneously become inactive before any vision-threatening lesions occur. There is absence of periodic congestion, loss of punctate staining over the body and shrinkage of the cap. Involution usually occurs, leaving a flat inconspicuous scar. Because of a strong tendency to **aggressive recurrence** after surgical excision, and the good chance for involution, great care must be taken to **document** progressive, vision-threatening, or disturbing corneal or episcleral **growth** with recorded sequential size measurements and, if possible, photography before any **surgical** therapy is performed. The key to prevention of pterygium if surgery is performed is prevention of new vessel formation in the bared episcleral surface by cauterization of existing vessels and **beta irradiation** (2000 rep) with a strontium 90 applicator at the time of surgery. As topical **steroids** and rapid epithelization also help to prevent growth of granulation tissue, **conjunctival autograft** to cover all exposed episclera followed by frequent topical antibiotic and steroid has been very successful in lieu of irradiation or in excision of recurrent pterygia. The excision itself should leave a pterygium-free bed in the cornea and be episcleral outside the limbus, leaving a 0.75-mm margin around the periphery. For deep corneal lesions a lamellar corneal graft may be required. At the first sign of recurrence (brushlike vessels) if bare episclera is present, the new vessels should be scraped, cauterized under local anesthesia, or closed with argon laser and an additional 1000 rep of beta irradiation or 1ary 2000 rep given. Recently **mitomycin C**, 0.02–0.04 mg/ml drop bid for 5–10 days, has proved effective in preventing recurrence of these aggressive lesions, but this drug is available only in major medical centers at this time.

G. **Marginal degenerations and ulcerations**
1. **Terrien's marginal degeneration** is an uncommon, nonulcerative thinning of the marginal cornea. Usually occurring bilaterally, the condition predominantly affects males in the late teens or older. Usually involving the superior peripheral cornea, the process begins with opacification and progresses over many years with thinning and superficial vascularization and, in younger patients, may be inflammatory. Lipid deposits may be seen at the leading edge. Symptoms of mild irritation may occur and respond to lubricants or, in the inflammatory cases, to intermittent mild steroid qd-bid (0.1% FML). The most bothersome problem can be progressive astigmatism with some diminution of vision. Rigid toric contact lenses or piggyback hard or soft lenses often correct this. Spontaneous perforation is rare, but trauma can rupture the thin cornea. **Treatment** is nonspecific. Surgical reinforcement with corneal patch grafting may occasionally be required if severe thinning occurs.
2. **Furrow degeneration** is a thinning of the peripheral cornea occurring in older patients in the area of an arcus senilis. There is no ulceration or epithelial defect, no vascularization, and no tendency to perforate. **Treatment** is usually not necessary.
3. **Furrow degeneration associated with rheumatoid arthritis** can occur as an inflammatory thinning of the cornea with epithelial defect and progressive ulceration of the stroma. The **ulcer may perforate,** particularly when it is treated with topical steroids. Systemic treatment of the basic disease with nonsteroidal anti-inflammatory drugs (NSAIDS), steroids, immunosuppressives, gold, or penicillamine is essential (see Chap. 8, sec. **VIII.D**). Local ocular therapy is lubrication, soft contact lenses, and tissue adhesive (Nexacryl [FDA-IND]) if perforation threatens or occurs.
4. **Inflammatory ulceration associated with rheumatoid arthritis** may occur in marginal and central cornea and is seen with greater infiltration than furrow degeneration. Progressive melting to perforation is common. Systemic steroids may slow the disease but are limited for long-term use. Immunosuppressive agents such as cyclophosphamide and azathioprine or methotrexate appear to control both the ocular inflammation and may prolong survival by controlling other vasculitis. Such therapy for rheumatoid or collagen-vascular disease should be undertaken in consultation with a rheumatologist or oncologist familiar with immunosuppression (see Chap.

8, sec. **VIII.D**). Local ocular therapy is as outlined under sec. **3**. Topical mild steroids are useful in sclerosing or acute stromal keratitis but should be avoided in furrowing or keratolysis.

5. **Mooren's ulcer** is a severe inflammatory ulcerating disease of the marginal cornea running a **painful** and progressive course. The characteristic clinical picture is that of an overhanging advancing edge of an epithelial defect with vascularization of the ulcer base. The condition has been described in two forms, the first a more benign unilateral affliction of older males and the second a bilateral ulceration of relentless progression in younger patients. Advancement of the inflammatory ulceration is both centrally and peripherally around the limbus and may extend into the sclera in severe cases. Spontaneous perforation is uncommon but certainly can occur. Vascularization can advance to cover the cornea (autoconjunctival flap).

   Treatment is often disappointing. Topical and systemic steroids are of some help, but immunosuppression with cyclosporine A or cytotoxic agents may be quite useful (see Chap. 8, secs. **VI.A, C**, and **D** for use and dosage of these drugs). Conjunctival excision and recession with or without cryotherapy of the recessed edge has been reported successful in some cases but the condition can recur. Soft contact lens therapy may benefit milder cases. Lamellar or full-thickness corneal grafts often melt or vascularize.

6. **Noninfectious systemic vasculitic diseases** associated with **peripheral ulcerative keratitis (PUK)** include Wegener's granulomatosis, relapsing polychondritis, systemic lupus erythematosus, Sjögren's syndrome, polyarteritis nodosa, and giant-cell arteritis. **Other autoimmune** disorders include progressive systemic sclerosis and graft-versus-host reactions. **Hematologic** diseases include porphyria and leukemia, and **dermatologic** diseases are acne rosacea, psoriasis, cicatricial pemphigoid, and Stevens-Johnson syndrome. Many of these are discussed in this chapter, in Chapter 8, and in Tables 14-1, 14-2, and 14-9.

VI. Dry eyes (keratoconjunctivitis sicca)

A. Etiologies. One of the most common causes of chronic low-grade irritations of the eyes, particularly in the elderly population, is lacrimal insufficiency or the dry eye. Although reflex tearing can decrease with advancing age, a variety of diseases can also diminish basal tear secretion. The height of the tear meniscus or marginal strip (less than 0.3 mm), the presence of rose bengal staining, particularly of the inner palpebral conjunctiva and inferior cornea, or a consistently diminished Schirmer strip test is of diagnostic importance.

1. **Idiopathic.** Many patients with chronic low-grade keratoconjunctivitis sicca, usually of a mild degree, will demonstrate no systemic disease or other ocular disease to account for the lacrimal insufficiency. It is important to exclude **drug-induced** tear hyposecretion, as can occur with a variety of drugs, including phenothiazines, antihistamines, and anticholinergics.

2. **Lupus erythematosus.** Both systemic and diskoid lupus erythematosus can result in the complex of keratoconjunctivitis sicca and xerostomia due to infiltration of the lacrimal and salivary glands. Superficial punctate epitheliopathy and corneal erosions accompany the dry eye. Diagnostic features of importance are the butterfly rash of the cheek, nose, and lower lids. Treatment is systemic with NSAIDs, steroids, and cytotoxic agents (see Chap. 8, secs. **VI.A, C**, and **D**). Local ocular therapy is lubrication.

3. **Pemphigoid** (essential shrinkage of the conjunctiva, benign mucous membrane pemphigoid). While chronic low-grade irritation is a common feature of this disease, the more severe dry eye is encountered late in the disease, after significant scarring of the accessory lacrimal glands and ducts has occurred. Keratinization of the surface is further aggravated by distortion of the lid anatomy and trichiasis. Dry eye and keratinization with scarring may be prevented with early systemic therapy. Dapsone orally may arrest the disease, but immunosuppression with cytoxan or chlorambucil may be prequired and should be done in consultation with an oncologist (see Chap. 8, sec. **VI.C**).

4. **Sjögren's syndrome** (Gougerot-Sjögren syndrome) with keratoconjunctivitis sicca, xerostomia, and arthritis has been described as the prototype of this disease state. Seventy-five percent of the patients have associated rheumatoid arthritis. Approximately 15% of patients with rheumatoid arthritis will develop the sicca syndrome.

5. **Erythema multiforme (Stevens-Johnson syndrome).** The postinflammatory mucosal scarring that occurs as a result of an acute episode of erythema multiforme involving the eyes can result in chronic dry eye. Resolution of the acute mucosal necrosis leaves symblepharon and scarring of the accessory lacrimal glands and the ducts of the main lacrimal gland. Keratinization can occur. Immunosuppressive agents (see Chap. 8, sec. **VI.C**) may be useful in therapy of chronic complications and cycloplegia, and mild topical steroids may be needed for chronic iritis. Lubrication is discussed in sec. **B** and acute disease in sec. **VII.F.**

6. **Scleroderma (progressive systemic sclerosis)** in rare instances can produce keratoconjunctivitis sicca.

7. **Periarteritis nodosa.** Keratoconjunctivitis sicca occurs as a late development in some patients with inflammatory ocular involvement from periarteritis.

8. **Sarcoidosis.** In this chronic granulomatous disease, infiltration of the lacrimal gland can result in keratoconjunctivitis sicca and occurs with relative frequency in the older patients afflicted with the disorder.

9. **Status postexcision of the lacrimal gland.** In most patients, excision of the lacrimal gland or obliteration of its ducts by removal of the palpebral portion will not be associated with keratoconjunctivitis sicca, because the basal and mucosal secretors are preserved. In a small number of patients, however, a frank keratoconjunctivitis sicca can be provoked by such extirpation of the lacrimal gland.

10. **Mikulicz's syndrome** can result from a variety of causes, including infiltrative disease from tuberculosis, leukemia, Hodgkin's disease, or sarcoidosis. Characterized by symmetric enlargement of the lacrimal glands and salivary (parotid) glands, the condition can result in keratoconjunctivitis sicca.

B. **Treatment.** The following sequence of therapy is indicated.

1. **Tear replacement.** Hypotonic solutions have been recommended but are not always helpful. More viscous vehicles, such as methylcellulose or polyvinyl alcohol, provide a longer contact time. The many different brands confirm the variable effectiveness of these solutions (see Appendix A).

2. **Ocular inserts.** Hydroxypropyl methylcellulose slow-dissolving polymers are occasionally effective. Patient tolerance and acceptance are variable.

3. **Soft contact lens therapy.** Hydrophilic bandage lenses often provide a tear reservoir but must be used in conjunction with replacement tears. These patients are prone to contact lens intolerance and superinfection and should be followed carefully. Forniceal scarring may dislodge the lenses.

4. **Punctal occlusion.** Temporary punctal occlusion can be achieved by insertion of 0.2–0.4 mm collagen plugs (Eagle Vision, Inc., Memphis) or miniature teflon plugs. Permanent occlusion of the puncta is achieved by electrocautery after local anesthesia. Temporary occlusion may be used to predict those patients who would suffer from epiphora if permanent occlusion were performed. Application of a hot platinum spatula to the puncta after pylocaine anesthesia also provides temporary closure to establish the risk of epiphora.

5. **Lateral tarsorrhaphy** will decrease tear evaporation.

6. **Other methods.** Moist chambers achieved by an occlusive plastic shield across the eye have helped in some cases. Close-fitting glasses with side shields often achieve the same effect. Parotid duct transplants and mechanized pumps with implanted tubes to the conjunctival sac have been used with limited effectiveness.

7. Associated conditions. Interference with the normal lubrication and cleansing function of the tears as well as the association of decreased lysozyme content place these patients at risk for chronic low-grade infections. Such infections of the eyelid margin can aggravate the underlying tear deficiency and should be treated with adequate lid hygiene and antibiotic therapy when necessary.

VII. Allergy and hypersensitivity

A. Atopic keratoconjunctivitis

1. Conjunctivitis is an acute or chronic inflammatory reaction of the conjunctiva manifested by chemosis, conjunctival vascular engorgement, and papillary conjunctival reaction. This condition is usually provoked by a specific allergen, which may include the pollens, inhalants, and other vegetable substances, as well as animal danders and dusts. There can be a mild punctate keratopathy, but pannus formation is rare. Epithelial scrapings reveal eosinophils. Differentiation from acute viral infections can be made by lack of adenopathy, but differentiation from contact or toxic exposure often relies on the history.

2. Treatment. The most effective treatment is removal of the offending allergen, although its identity is often difficult to establish. Palliative treatment with topical decongestants or antihistamines or both may be effective, although severe reactions require topical steroids. Patients with a history of atopy, hay fever, eczema, or other systemic allergy often respond well to **4% cromolyn** (disodium chromoglycate, Optichrome) 4–6 times daily. This **mast cell stabilizer** must be used as directed to be effective. It may be used alone or in combination with other ocular allergy drugs, topical and systemic antihistamines and decongestants (antazoline, naphazoline, phenylephrine). Desensitization should be reserved for more severe cases in which a specific allergen can be unequivocally identified.

B. Atopic eczema may rarely cause keratoconjunctivitis. Acute exacerbations of atopic eczema with scaly dermatitis affecting especially the face, neck, popliteal, and antecubital areas can be associated with keratoconjunctivitis that is characterized by thickening and hyperemia of the conjunctiva with superficial opacification and vascularization of the cornea. Multiple other allergies, including hay fever, rhinitis, asthma, and urticaria, are often concurrently present. All may cause allergic keratoconjunctivitis. A higher occurrence of keratoconus than in the normal population has been reported with this condition.

Treatment. Acute episodes usually require topical steroids but considerable residual scarring may occur. Cromolyn 4%, 4–6 times a day may relieve symptoms.

C. Vernal conjunctivitis. This seasonally recurrent bilateral inflammation of the conjunctiva, producing itching, tearing, photophobia, and foreign body sensation, occurs in two forms.

1. The palpebral form is distinguished by **cobblestone** papillae on the tarsal conjunctiva and may be associated with shield ulcers of the superior cornea.

2. The limbal form occurs with papillary hypertrophy on the limbal conjunctiva associated with white, chalky concretions known as **Trantas' dots** near the limbus.

3. Diagnosis. One of the main diagnostic features is the conjunctival scraping showing prominent eosinophils, many of which will be fractured, releasing their granules. A seasonal predilection is for the spring and early summer as well as for the fall. In addition to the clinical appearance of the papillary changes, a thick, ropy mucous discharge is a hallmark of the disease. The condition usually occurs in young people and tends to run a course of from 4–10 years before remission occurs.

4. Treatment. The mainstay of treatment in the past has been topical steroids (1%–⅛% prednisolone bid–qid), but the frequent and often long-term use of steroids has been complicated by development of cataracts or elevation of the intraocular pressure (IOP). These must both be monitored. Recent attempts at treatment with **4% cromolyn** solution topically 4–6 times a day often results in control of symptoms, although little change in the papillae is noted. **Aspirin** may markedly relieve symptoms if initiated as 600 mg 5 times daily for a week, with subsequent taper of 600 mg/week until a minimum maintenance level necessary to control symptoms is reached.

Occurrence of shield ulcers requires adequate antibiotic prophylaxis and occasionally soft contact lens therapy in the form of a hydrophilic bandage lens. Some relief can be seen on a change of locale or environmental exposure, but extensive allergy workup and hyposensitization are usually unsuccessful.

D. **Phlyctenular keratoconjunctivitis.** This nodular inflammatory response of the conjunctiva or cornea appears to be an allergic reaction to an antigen. The clinical evolution of the phlyctenule is usually that of a small vesicle that forms a nodule that subsequently breaks down, with subsequent spontaneous healing. A local leash of vessels is common and may be most prominent when the phlyctenule moves onto the corneal surface. Formerly associated with tuberculosis in a debilitated patient, it is now most commonly secondary to staphylococcal blepharoconjunctivitis. Symptoms of irritation, tearing, and redness tend to be more severe when corneal involvement occurs. The condition must be distinguished from an inflamed pinguecula, small pterygium, or from limbal corneal involvement by acne rosacea or limbal herpes simplex keratitis.

1. **Treatment.** Topical steroids are the treatment of choice. Treatment may require prednisolone 1% or dexamethasone 0.1% q2-4h for several days. If photophobia is severe, cycloplegics will provide comfort. An epithelial breakdown should be treated with prophylactic antibiotics.

E. **Ligneous conjunctivitis** is a rare, chronic disorder of the conjunctiva and other mucous membranes characterized by multiple inflamed (lymphocytes, plasma cells, eosinophils) granulomatous lesions. Treatment with excision followed by steroids, cromolyn, fibrinolysin, and silver nitrate usually fails with rapid recurrence. Recent success using excision followed by topical cyclosporine, 20 mg/ml q2-6h over several weeks, has been reported (not FDA approved). Prophylactic topical antibiotics should be used under this treatment.

F. **Erythema multiforme (Stevens-Johnson syndrome).** Usually occurring before the age of 30 and primarily a **cutaneous eruption** of sharply defined erythematous vesicular and bulbous patches scattered about the hands, forearms, face, and neck, this condition can affect mucous membranes, resulting in severe stomatitis and conjunctivitis. It occurs as an idiopathic entity or secondary to infections (herpes, mumps, Coxsackie virus, echovirus, mycoplasma, psittacosis, scarlet fever) or drug reaction (sulfonamides, sulfones, penicillin, barbiturates). Ocular complications are common. The **conjunctivitis** usually occurs in one of three forms: (1) catarrhal—circumscribed raised patches of edema that may lead to frank bullae formation that resolves with disappearance of the eruption, (2) purulent—usually severe and associated with extreme chemosis and corneal involvement (epithelial keratitis, ulceration) or exudative iridocyclitis, or (3) pseudomembranous—most common and associated with extensive discharge and pseudomembrane formation with subsequent symblepharon and scarring. Optic neuritis may develop in either. Corneal involvement is most likely to occur with the pseudomembranous form and can result in frank ulceration and perforation. Iritis or panophthalmitis may occur. Severe keratoconjunctivitis sicca is a sequela. **Systemic treatment** of acute disease is high-dose systemic steroids (prednisone, 60-100 mg/day or equivalent initially) and systemic antibiotic to combat potential secondary infection (tetracycline or erythromycin, 250 mg PO qid). Ocular therapy in acute disease is topical antibiotic particularly for staphylococcal infection, which is common. Bacitracin, erythromycin, gentamycin, or tobramycin drops or ointment is given q2-4h up to 48 hours after the eyes heal. Topical corticosteroids will help to control inflammation—1% prednisolone qid initially with monitoring for corneal ulceration with thinning, in which case they should be reduced or stopped. Use of steroids, topical or systemic, is under dabate. The fornices should be gently swept qd-bid with a glass rod after topical anesthetic to break fresh adhesions. Late management is that of keratoconjunctivitis sicca and iritis (see sec. **VI**). Immunosuppressives may be therapeutically effective.

G. **Acne rosacea** is primarily a disease of the sebaceous glands of the skin, predominately involving the malar and nasal areas of the face. There can be a **chronic blepharoconjunctivitis** present in up to 30% of cases. Of those showing ocular involvement, approximately 7% will develop **corneal ulceration.**

1. **Facial eruption.** The rash is often present as a butterfly configuration across the malar area and consists of small macular, slightly scaling lesions on an erythematous base. Although the lesions may be slightly elevated, they can be very faint and subtle. Numerous small telangiectasia may be present. The chronic form with hyperplasia of sebaceous glands and periglandular fibrosis presents as rhinophyma, particularly in males. The patient often gives a history of prominent blushing and facial erythema, particularly after ingestion of alcohol or coffee.

2. **Ocular findings**

   a. **Blepharitis.** Probably the most common manifestation of ocular rosacea, this nonulcerative condition of the lid margins is usually bilateral and can be associated with prominent plugging and inspissation of meibomian gland secretion, which can be expressed on pressure to the lid. Staphylococcal superinfection may be present.

   b. **Conjunctivitis.** A low-grade conjunctivitis that fluctuates in severity is frequently associated with the blepharitis.

   c. **Keratitis** may present as marginal infiltrate with a fascicle of vessels from the limbus or as a frank ulceration that progressively advances across the cornea. Rarely do these ulcers perforate unless intensive steroids are used in treatment. Chronic scarring at the site of the ulcer usually results.

   d. **Cutaneous** and **ocular** lesions of rosacea need not coincide in severity. Skin lesions should be sought in any patient with chronic blepharitis or vascularized keratitis.

3. **Treatment**

   a. **Local measures.** Lid hygiene should be emphasized with daily massage, hot compresses, and removal of crusts from the lid margins. Mild topical antibiotics such as erythromycin or bacitracin ointments may be used to control any superinfection. Instability of the tear film or surface irregularities often necessitate lubricant tears.

   b. **Systemic treatment.** The most effective treatment for the ocular manifestations of acne rosacea is **systemic tetracycline.** Treatment is begun with 250 mg of tetracycline 1–2 times a day on an **empty stomach** for a period of 10 days and then tapered to bid, or qd dosage, to be maintained for 3–6 months. The effect of the tetracycline is apparently independent of its antibiotic effectiveness and may relate to anti-inflammatory effect and meibomian lipid composition. **Alternative drugs** are erythromycin, 250 mg PO qd, or doxycycline (a tetracycline), 100 mg PO qd with meals. The usual precautions with use of tetracycline should be observed, and it should not be used in women who are pregnant or breast-feeding. Relapse of the condition after discontinuation of tetracycline may occur.

   c. **Steroids.** The inflammatory and vascular aspects of the keratitis are extremely sensitive to low doses of topical steroid. Steroids must be used with caution, however, as there is a tendency for ulceration to perforate. It is probably best to **limit steroid treatment** to no more than prednisolone 1.0%, or its equivalent, twice a day; and 0.12% prednisolone is probably safer.

H. **Cicatricial pemphigoid (ocular pemphigoid)** is a relatively rare chronic inflammatory systemic disease of the mucous membranes probably due to anti-basement membrane antibody reaction. In the eye there is conjunctival subepithelial fibrosis with foreshortening of the fornices, symblepharon formation, entropion, trichiasis, and ultimately dry eye with corneal ulceration, neovascularization, and keratinization.

Treatment is primarily systemic, and the earlier started the better. Initial treatment for mild, nonprogressive early ocular disease is suppression with **steroids**, e.g., prednisone, 40–60 mg PO qd, tapering to alternate–day therapy ranging from 2.5–60.0 mg/day. Steroids do not stop progressive pemphigoid but the **sulfone, dapsone,** is effective for mild to moderately progressive oral and ocular lesions. The starting dosage is 50 mg PO qd for 1–2 weeks, then, if tolerated, increasing to 50 mg PO bid but monitoring for the expected side effect of hemolytic anemia and adjusting dosage up and down as needed. Successful maintenance doses range from 50–150 mg PO qd for years. **Glucose-6-dehydrogenase–deficient patients** should **not** receive this drug or hemolysis will be severe. Rapidly progressive pemphigoid is usually responsive to combined **cyclophosphamide**, 1–2 mg/kg PO qd, and **prednisone**, 1 mg/kg PO qd, for 1 month. If disease activity is still significant, cyclophosphamide is increased in 25-mg amounts monthly and prednisone tapered to 40 mg PO qd. Once disease is controlled, therapy is usually continued for 12–18 months total. **Lid hygiene,** topical **lubricants,** and **blepharitis therapy** should be maintained indefinitely. Oculoplastic surgery may be required for more advanced cases. Unfortunately, these advanced disease states do not respond well to systemic or topical treatment.

VIII. **Dystrophies.** Corneal dystrophy describes primary, inherited, bilateral changes of the cornea that occur unaccompanied by systemic disease. Characteristic corneal changes are also encountered in certain inherited metabolic and skin disorders.

A. **Meesman's epithelial dystrophy.** This dominantly inherited dystrophy presents in the fully developed form a corneal epithelium diffusely studded with minute flecklike opacities of variable density and distribution that, on retroillumination with the slit lamp, appear to be minute collections of debris in an otherwise clear, spherical microvesicle. These spherical microcysts may elevate the corneal surface sufficiently to disturb the tear film. Superficial corneal scarring is rare. The epithelial changes have been demonstrated as early as 7 months and tend to increase with age. Although usually asymptomatic, some pedigrees have shown mild ocular discomfort and slight decrease in visual acuity to the 20/40 range. This condition must be differentiated from bilateral microcystic epithelial changes that may also be seen with corneal edema, with vernal conjunctivitis, or in association with disturbed tear function. Pathologically, the small round intraepithelial cysts appear to represent degenerate epithelial cells and contain periodic acid Schiff (PAS)–positive cellular debris. Pathologic changes are usually confined to the epithelium. **Hereditary epithelial dystrophy** (Stocker-Holt, Schneider) occurs as a dominantly inherited dystrophy presenting with minute epithelial droplets that are transparent and have predilection for the center of the cornea. There can be fluorescein staining but pathologic changes are confined to the epithelium. This condition may be a variant of the Meesman's corneal dystrophy. **Treatment** is usually not necessary. If the discomfort is severe, soft contact lenses can be considered. If visual impairment is unusually severe, lamellar keratoplasty may be indicated.

B. **Anterior membrane dystrophy.** There is an increasing tendency to lump together and label some of the epithelial basement membrane disorders as anterior membrane dystrophies.

1. **Cogan's microcystic epithelial dystrophy.** This epithelial disorder, with no obvious hereditary tendency, appears in females as bilateral, gray-white, round or comma-shaped deposits in the corneal epithelium ("putty marks"). Mild foreign body sensation is often a complaint but visual acuity and corneal sensation are unaffected. Histologically, the deposits represent intraepithelial cysts containing cellular debris. PAS-positive nodular substance on the anterior surface of an irregular basement membrane is also seen.

2. **Fingerprint dystrophy.** Bilateral curvilinear lucent opacities, seen best on retroillumination at the slit lamp, at the level of Bowman's layer and var-

iously described as "fingerprint" or "mare's hair" lines are the characteristic of this condition in which no consistent hereditary pattern is described.

3. **Map-dot-fingerprint (MDF) dystrophy.** Polymorphic epithelial and anterior Bowman's layer opacities described as map-dot pattern or a fingerprint-like wrinkling of the basement membrane (seen best by slit-lamp retroillumination) have been observed in bilateral distribution, again not associated with visual symptoms but often associated with recurrent epithelial erosions.

4. **Recurrent epithelial erosion.** The three preceding changes can be accompanied by recurrent epithelial erosions. Often a fourth category of dystrophic recurrent erosion is described with similar epithelial changes but occurring in a dominantly inherited fashion. All are probably associated with an abnormality of basement membrane adhesion that accounts for the recurrent erosive episodes, giving the eyes discomfort and foreign body sensation.

5. **Treatment** of these disorders is essentially that of treatment of recurrent erosion and includes patching with an antibiotic during the acute phase and an attempt at aborting recurrences by use of hypertonic (5%) sodium chloride ointment nightly. For frequent or more severe erosions, a high-water-content **therapeutic soft contact lens** (Permalens, Sauflon) should be fitted and left in place for 2–3 months. Antibiotic drops bid and lubrication should also be used. Abnormalities of the lids, including chronic low-grade blepharomeibomitis, can aggravate the epithelial changes and predispose to recurrent erosion. Meticulous lid hygiene and control of the blepharitis are often necessary to prevent repeated attacks of erosion. **Superficial debridement** or **anterior stromal puncture** are advocated in persistent cases. The puncture technique is done under topical anesthesia at the slit lamp. A 20- to 30-gauge bent needle tip is used to place 20 to 40 micropunctures directly over and surrounding the erosion. Depth is through epithelium to its underlying basement membrane with the purpose of creating microfibrotic adhesions that will hold the epithelium in place. After treatment, antibiotic ointment is instilled and a 24-hour pressure patch applied. Lubricants are used regularly starting 1 day postoperatively. Occasionally the erosion will recur in the same area or adjacent to it, requiring retreatment with anterior stromal puncture or, if due to local edema, treatment with ointment only.

C. **Reis-Buckler's dystrophy** is an autosomal dominant condition of the cornea characterized by a network of ringlike opacities occurring at the level of Bowman's layer and protruding irregularly into the epithelium, with subsequent distortion of the anterior corneal surface. The disorder may present at about 5 years of age and shows a progressive course, with increasing frequency of attacks of recurrent erosions that usually result in a diffuse anterior scarring corresponding to a fall in visual acuity and a decrease in corneal sensation. Histopathologic studies show widespread destruction of Bowman's layer, with replacement by irregular scar tissue interspersed with aggregates of microfilamentous material. Absence of hemidesmosomal attachments accounts for the faulty adherence of epithelium. Early **therapy** with soft contact lenses or corneal scraping has been recommended but in severe cases lamellar keratoplasty may be indicated.

D. The **anterior dystrophy** described by **Grayson** and **Wilbrandt** is similar to Reis-Buckler's dystrophy, with variable effects on vision and preservation of corneal sensation.

E. **Vortex dystrophy** was the diagnosis once applied to the pigment lines occurring in a whorl-like fashion over the surface of the cornea and located in the area of Bowman's layer and adjacent stroma. This appears to be the same corneal lesion seen in Fabry's disease and is thought to be a manifestation of the asymptomatic carrier state of females with X-linked **Fabry's disease.** In general, it must be distinguished from the corneal deposits seen in **phenothi-**

Table 5-9. Histologic staining characteristics of stromal dystrophies

Dystrophy	Masson's trichrome	PAS	Congo red	Birefringence
Granular	Bright red	Negative	Negative	Negative
Macular	Negative	Pink	Negative	Negative
Lattice	Red	Pink-red	Red	Positive

PAS = periodic acid Schiff (reaction).

azine keratopathy, amiodarone, chloroquine indomethacin or **tamoxifen toxicity,** and occasionally the pattern of **fingerprint lines.** The appearance of drug-induced vortex keratopathy is **not** an indication to stop the drug. The condition is reversible if the medication is stopped, however.

F. **Granular dystrophy (Groenouw type I)** is an autosomal dominant dystrophy characterized by stromal opacities of dense, milky granular-appearing deposits occurring in the axial portion of the cornea, more prominently in the anterior stroma. Intervening stroma is clear. The lesions may be manifest in the first decade of life, but visual acuity is usually not affected until late in the disease. The histochemical characteristics are listed in Table 5-9. The deposits are thought to be principally **noncollagenous protein.** Occasionally, when visual acuity is severely impaired, penetrating keratoplasty is indicated.

G. **Macular dystrophy (Groenouw type II),** an autosomal recessive dystrophy, appears as a diffuse clouding in the central cornea between the ages of 5 and 9. Gradual increase in the density of the opacity with development of gray-white nodular deposits of varying size within the corneal stroma is accompanied by progressive diminution of vision and episodic irritation and photophobia. The severe decrease in visual acuity often necessitates penetrating keratoplasty. Histologically and histochemically, the deposits in and around the keratocytes appear as accumulation of **mucopolysaccharide** as a result of a local enzyme deficiency.

H. **Lattice dystrophy (Biber-Haab-Dimmer)** is an autosomal dominant dystrophy characterized by the appearance in the corneal stroma of relucent branching filaments interlacing and overlapping at different levels and forming an irregular latticework with dichotomous branching. Fine dots, flakes, and stellate opacities may appear between the filaments. Although appearing as early as 2 years of age, the occurrence of recurrent erosive episodes and progressive clouding of the central cornea is apparent by the age of 20 and is associated with decreased visual acuity such that penetrating keratoplasty is often indicated in the forties. Histopathologically, the stromal deposits appear as hyaline fusiform deposits of amyloid. The histochemistry and fibrillary ultrastructure are that of **amyloid.**

I. **Fleck dystrophy (central speckled dystrophy)** is an autosomal dominant condition involving all layers of the cornea with oval to round gray-white opacities. The lesions are well circumscribed and separated from each other by clear cornea. Corneal sensation and visual acuity are usually not affected. Treatment is usually not necessary.

J. **Central cloudy and parenchymatous dystrophy** is an apparently autosomal dominant condition that involves particularly the deep stroma but sometimes extends to Bowman's layer. The condition is quite variable and usually does not result in visual impairment. Treatment is usually not indicated.

K. **Schnyder's crystalline dystrophy,** an autosomal dominant condition, is characterized by a round ring-shaped central corneal opacity consisting of white-to-yellow or polychromatic crystals in the stroma. Peripheral deposits separated from the limbus by a clear line also appear. The lesions may be apparent as early as 18 months and may progress but usually are not destructive to visual acuity. Corneal sensation is usually normal. Pathologically, the needlelike crystals are found to contain **cholesterol**. Occasionally, the visual acuity is depressed to the point where penetrating keratoplasty is indicated. Some patients with this dystrophy may exhibit abnormally elevated blood lipids, xanthelasma, and corneal arcus.

L. **Congenital hereditary endothelial dystrophy (CHED)** is characterized by diffuse milky or ground-glass opacification of the stroma associated with a thickening of the cornea up to 4 times normal. It has been described as both a dominantly and a recessively inherited disorder. Despite the gross stromal edema, the epithelium has only a mild roughening associated with fine microbullae. Visual acuity varies according to the degree of corneal clouding. Corneal sensation is normal and vascularization is rare. Histopathologically, there are **rare to absent endothelial cells** and an overall **increase in thickness of Descemet's membrane**, in contrast to Fuchs's dystrophy. The **prognosis** for penetrating keratoplasty in these patients is **poor**. Examination of asymptomatic relatives of patients with congenital hereditary endothelial dystrophy may reveal clear vacuolar lesions with surrounding white haze and an irregular endothelial mosaic despite normal corneal thickness and visual acuity. The high risk of producing offspring with congenital hereditary endothelial dystrophy makes examination of relatives important.

M. **Fuchs's epithelial-endothelial dystrophy** is a condition seen most often in females in the fifth to sixth decades of life and can be transmitted in a dominant fashion. It tends to be progressive, with increasing corneal thickness due to edema that culminates in epithelial edema and bullous keratopathy. It is impossible to predict progression or the ultimate degree of visual impairment, but if the endothelial function fails and epithelial edema ensues, painful epithelial breakdown can occur. Chronic edema can sometimes be associated with peripheral vascularization. Frequently, the condition is associated with cataractous changes in the lens nucleus, and a higher incidence than normal of chronic open-angle glaucoma has been reported. Histopathologically, there is a paucity of endothelial cells most notable on specular microscopy. Initial palliative **therapy** includes the use of hypertonic sodium chloride ointments at night and drops during the day. If painful bullous keratopathy ensues, a soft contact lens will often provide relief although it rarely improves visual acuity. Penetrating keratoplasty is the mainstay of therapy for both visual rehabilitation and relief of pain.

N. **Posterior polymorphous dystrophy,** a dominantly inherited dystrophy of the endothelium and Descemet's membrane, presents clinically with a variable number of round, elliptical, or irregular lesions, often with vesicular appearance, bulging into the stroma or projecting into the anterior chamber. While generally benign and nonprogressive, it can be associated with corneal edema, requiring penetrating keratoplasty for restoration of vision. Abnormal iris processes and peripheral anterior synechiae have been described. Histopathologically, a **thickening** of the posterior lamellae of **Descemet's membrane** and the presence of **atypical cells** on the posterior corneal surface suggestive of metaplasia to a fibroblastic cell suggest that it may represent a form of the anterior cleavage syndrome.

O. **Keratoconus (ectatic corneal dystrophy)** is a disorder characterized by conical ectasia (bulging) of the central cornea, with thinning and scarring resulting in a painless, progressive loss of vision due to an increasingly severe irregular myopic astigmatism. Familial occurrence has been noted, although the majority of cases show no definitive inheritance pattern. In the early stages, distortion of the retinoscopic reflex, keratoscopic figures, and keratometric mires are apparent. As the condition advances, vertical striae may be seen in the posterior stroma along with axial thinning and an increase in the axial corneal curvature. Reticular scarring of Bowman's membrane can occur, and the appearance of a Fleischer ring is often noted. Stromal corneal nerves tend to be more visible and fine fibrillary lines may be seen along the internal edge of the

Fleischer ring. Occasionally a break in the endothelium and Descemet's membrane results in gross stromal edema (corneal hydrops) accompanied by pain and a rapid decrease in vision. **Treatment** is correction of the refractive error by spectacles or contact lenses or, in advanced cases, penetrating keratoplasty, which gives a good prognosis for this condition. Patients should **not be dilated postoperatively,** as permanent mydriasis may ensue even if the drops are given years later. Preoperative dilation should be done with mild mydriatics only, e.g., 2.5% phenylephrine. Keratoconus has been described in association with various **ocular anomalies** such as blue sclera, ectopia lentis, cataract, aniridia, retinitis pigmentosa, and optic atrophy. It has been **associated with** Down's syndrome, Ehlers-Danlos syndrome, Marfan's syndrome, Addison's disease, neurofibromatosis, Apert's anomaly, and allergic disease, including vernal conjunctivitis and atopic eczema. Association with chronic rubbing of the eyes and eyelids has been suggested.

IX. **Corneal edema.** Corneal deturgescence is achieved when pump function of the corneal endothelium balances the fluid-accumulating effect of intraocular hydrostatic pressure and corneal swelling pressure. Disturbance of this balance or disruption of the limiting membranes of the cornea (epithelium and endothelium) results in corneal edema. Stromal edema may minimally decrease visual acuity; epithelial edema, however, results in significant visual impairment and painful surface breakdown.

A. **Causes of corneal edema**
1. **Elevated IOP**
   a. **Acute angle-closure glaucoma** results in marked and often rapidly increased IOP. Corneal stroma thickness may not be increased despite prominent epithelial edema, but in some cases the pressure will aggravate prior endothelial dysfunction or produce temporary dysfunction resulting in stromal edema. Epithelial edema is a classic sign of acute glaucoma with resultant decreased vision. While both epithelial and stromal edema usually clear with control of the IOP, there occasionally can be residual stromal haze, which does not greatly affect vision.
   b. **Congenital glaucoma** can produce corneal haze that is usually most marked centrally but that can involve the entire cornea. Edema involves stroma and epithelium. Normalization of the pressure may permit clearing of the cornea, although residual endothelial damage as manifested by horizontal (Haab) striae of Descemet's membrane may predispose to future corneal decompensation and edema late in life.
2. **Endothelial damage**
   a. **Trauma**
      (1) **Birth trauma** (forceps injury) results in relucent double-contoured striae of Descemet's membrane that signal endothelial damage. The cornea is often clear during youth but can become edematous after an interval of several decades, with both stromal and epithelial edema.
      (2) **Nonsurgical contusion injury** can cause focal endothelial dysfunction, with typical annular or diskiform areas of endothelial and stromal edema. Often transient and resolving over a few days, these focal areas of edema usually cause little long-term visual disability.
      (3) **Penetration of a foreign body** into the anterior chamber can result in a retained foreign body in the inferior anterior chamber angle, with resultant focal (wedge-shaped) inferior corneal edema. Removal of the foreign body can be curative.
      (4) **Surgical trauma** from cataract extraction, intraocular lens (IOL) implantation, and prolonged or profuse anterior chamber irrigation can damage endothelial cells to produce corneal edema. The edema can occur following vitrectomy or retinal detachment surgery and is more prone to occur in diabetics. Extensive extraocular muscle detachment procedures can also result in corneal decompensation if anterior segment necrosis occurs. Vitreous adherent to the cornea

following cataract extraction may produce focal edema. Chronic touch can stimulate metaplasia of the endothelium with resultant persistent edema.

  b. Dystrophy

    (1) Fuchs's dystrophy, first described as stromal and epithelial edema, subsequently was found to be caused by dystrophic endothelium characterized clinically by a beaten metal appearance of the posterior corneal surface associated with excrescences of Descemet's membrane and occasionally endothelial pigment deposits (see sec. **VIII.M).**

    (2) Congenital hereditary endothelial dystrophy, present at birth, produces modest epithelial edema and a markedly thickened and edematous corneal stroma usually involving both eyes (see sec. **VIII.L).**

    (3) Posterior polymorphous dystrophy, while often not causing significant visual deterioration, can, if progressive, produce corneal edema (see sec. **VIII.N).**

    (4) While usually not considered as a cause of corneal edema, the **anterior membrane dystrophies** are characterized by corneal changes that can be accompanied by epithelial edema in very discrete distribution, especially if recurrent breakdowns have occurred.

    (5) An acute and painful cause of corneal edema occurs in some cases of **keratoconus (acute hydrops).** This seems to occur more commonly in patients affected with trisomy 21 (Down's syndrome). Ruptures in Descemet's membrane occasionally result in scarring that flattens or alters the conical contour. Moderate pressure patching of the lid relieves discomfort in most cases.

  c. Endothelial dysfunction secondary to inflammation

    (1) Uveitis or intraocular inflammation can temporarily depress endothelial function to produce edema. Control of inflammation often restores endothelial integrity and reversal of edema. Herpetic uveitis is a common offender and should be suspected in patients with unilateral corneal edema and uveitis.

    (2) Focal keratitis (bacterial, fungal, viral) can provoke edema both by local inflammatory response and by compromising endothelial function. The infectious nature of the disease process is often suggested by the clinical features of focal infiltration of inflammatory cells that accompany the edema.

    (3) Corneal graft rejection in patients who have undergone penetrating keratoplasty is a classic example of endothelial damage. The clinician should be alert to any inflammation or the earliest sign of edema in a corneal graft no matter how distant the surgery.

3. Epithelial damage resulting from **mechanical, chemical,** or **radiation** injury disrupts the barrier effect of the epithelium, allowing passage of fluid into the anterior corneal stroma. Metabolic disturbance of the cornea, such as hypoxia of contact lens overwear or toxic effects of medications and anesthetics, can also provoke intra- and intercellular epithelial edema.

B. Treatment is first to restore the normal physiologic balance of corneal hydration. Should that be impossible, attempts should then be made to compensate for the fluid accumulation. Although visual acuity may be improved, the treatment often must strive for comfort and protection of the cornea.

1. Lower IOP. If IOP is pathologically elevated, attempts should be made medically or surgically to lower that pressure. In patients with borderline endothelial function and early corneal edema, reduction of the pressure from high normal to low normal levels will often relieve the edema.

2. Control of inflammation may improve corneal edema if dysfunction is due to that inflammation. Topical steroids often are sufficient to achieve this.

3. Hypertonic agents such as sodium chloride 5% (drops or ointment), colloidal osmotic solutions, or anhydrous glycerine may provide sufficient dehydrating effect. Discomfort from such applied solutions can be significant, especially with glycerine, and limits their acceptance. Other mechanical measures for encouraging evaporation of tears, such as dehumidification of the environment or use of hot forced air from a hair dryer, may be used with some success.

4. **Graft (penetrating keratoplasty) rejection** requires urgent therapy with **topical steroids,** e.g., 0.1% dexamethasone q1h by day and q2h by night for several days followed by taper down to qid by about 3-4 weeks and to qd by 2-3 months. Rejections with edema delimited by an endothelial lymphocyte (KP) line respond far better than total diffuse edema of the entire graft. If there is no response to therapy within 1-2 weeks, the graft has probably failed due to permanent endothelial damage and will need to be replaced. Herpetic graft rejections should be treated with steroids as above plus trifluridine drops 6 times a day or vidarabine ointment tid because of the high incidence of dendritic keratitis in the face of rejection. **Topical cyclosporine,** a selective T-cell immunosuppressant, has been used successfully as prophylaxis against rejection in high-risk patients (previous rejection and graft failure, deep stromal neovascularization, severe alkali burn). Topical 2% cyclosporine is formulated by the pharmacy using the oral preparation diluted in olive oil. Dosage is 1 drop q2h by day for 2 days preoperatively and for 4 days postoperatively, then qid with topical steroid for 3 months. Both drugs are decreased to tid by 3-6 months and bid thereafter. Cyclosporine A is not FDA approved for this purpose.

5. For those cases of corneal edema unresponsive to more conservative measures, **penetrating keratoplasty** offers the most effective method of restoring vision. Obviously, the prognosis for successful keratoplasty depends on the etiology of the corneal edema, with inflammatory conditions being less sure than dystrophic causes.

6. If **visual rehabilitation is not essential,** several procedures may be used to assure comfort and protection of the edematous cornea.
   a. **Soft contact lens therapy,** particularly the use of the ultrathin hydrophilic contact lens, will often ensure comfort but at the risk of stimulating vascularization or infection of the cornea (see sec. **XI.A**).
   b. **Conjunctival flap** surgery after epithelial debridement is often helpful. This surgery does not preclude subsequent keratoplasty.
   c. **Electrocautery** or **corneal micropuncture** (see sec. **VII.B**) of the corneal surface will produce scarification of the surface to prevent recurrent bullous keratopathy.
   d. **Implanted fluid barriers ("artificial endothelium")** may be of benefit in limited cases but pose technical surgical problems. **Prosthokeratoplasty** also has been advocated but should probably be reserved for those patients with severe vascularization or prior keratoplasty failures.

X. **Congenital anomalies of the cornea.** Congenital lesions of the cornea may be inherited as developmental defects or errors of metabolism or may be due to intrauterine infection or injury.
   A. **Anomalies of size, shape, and contour**
      1. **Megalocornea** is an enlargement of the cornea beyond 13 mm in diameter. The cornea is usually clear with normal vision, but there may be astigmatic refractive errors. The condition is usually not progressive and requires no treatment. The developmental condition must be distinguished, however, from corneal enlargement due to congenital glaucoma. The buphthalmic cornea often has central or peripheral clouding and Haab striae or Descemet's tears. IOP is elevated in buphthalmus but normal in megalocornea.
      2. **Microcornea** is a cornea with a diameter less than 11 mm. Occurring as a developmental defect, the cornea is often steeper than normal, producing myopia. Microcornea can occur as part of other congenital abnormalities, including the rubella syndrome. If there is no corneal opacification, **treatment** is often not necessary except for correction of the refractive error.

3. **Cornea plana** is a rare flattening of the anterior contour of the cornea. The cornea may be small in addition to its markedly flattened shape. Marked astigmatism can occur.
4. **Keratoglobus** is a rare bilateral enlargement of the cornea in which it assumes a globular shape. Myopic and astigmatic refractive errors often occur.
B. **Congenital corneal opacities**
1. **Edema** can occur as a result of congenital hereditary endothelial dystrophy or congenital glaucoma. Edema can also occur with Descemet's ruptures due to forceps injury or birth trauma.
2. **Congenital malformations.** A rather confusing array of congenital corneal opacities associated with abnormalities of the anterior chamber angle have been described as part of the anterior chamber cleavage syndrome. A recent classification helps to categorize the appearance of central or peripheral opacification with or without corneal-iris or corneal-lenticular touch (Fig. 5-2).
3. **Epibulbar and limbal dermoid tumors** also can occur as congenital lesions. Treatment for these congenital malformations can be difficult and usually requires penetrating keratoplasty or anterior segment reconstruction with or without lensectomy. Since the surgical technique can be difficult and graft rejection is not uncommon, it is probably best to perform surgery on the worse eye only. Developmental abnormalities of the posterior segment may be present and further interfere with visual function.
4. **Inborn errors of metabolism** (see also Chap. 10)
   a. **Mucopolysaccharidoses** occurring as autosomal recessive traits can present with corneal hazy opacification, particularly in the Hurler, Scheie, Morquio, and Maroteaux-Lamy syndromes.
   b. **Corneal opacification** can also be noted in cystinosis, mucolipidosis, gangliosidosis, Lowe's syndrome, Riley-Day syndrome, and von Gierke's disease.
5. **Chromosomal defects** can be associated with corneal opacification, especially with trisomy 21, trisomy 13–15, and trisomy 18.
6. **Postinflammatory opacities** of the cornea can be present with the rubella syndrome, luetic interstitial keratitis, or congenital herpes simplex infection.
XI. **Contact lenses**
A. **Therapeutic soft contact lenses.** The expanding array of hydrophilic soft contact lenses offers a valuable method of treatment for a variety of corneal abnormalities. The most frequent use for soft contact lenses is as a protective bandage for a diseased epithelial surface (epithelial defect, corneal edema), but the hydrophilic lens can also provide a reservoir for tears or medications and can be used for cosmetic or therapeutic occlusion. **Specific indications and precautions** are as follows:
1. **Alkali burns.** After immediate removal of the offending chemical and appropriate irrigation, the ocular surface is often left deepithelialized or populated by a markedly abnormal epithelium. A soft contact lens applied to the alkali-burned eye when conjunctival edema has subsided will aid in the reepithelialization and provide protection to the fragile and easily dislodged epithelial layer. Encouragement of reepithelialization of the ocular surface is necessary to avoid the progressive ulceration that can occur in response to local collagenase production in the second to third week following the injury. Topical antibiotics are used to prevent infection.
2. **Bullous keratopathy.** Epithelial edema of aphakic bullous keratopathy or Fuch's combined dystrophy that does not respond to topical hyperosmotic agents can result in bullous epithelial lesions that are painful on breakdown. Therapeutic soft contact lenses can protect against recurrent epithelial breakdown and will provide comfort in many patients. Visual acuity is rarely improved but comfort is attained. Prolonged epithelial edema, particularly with the use of a large contact lens, can lead to vascularization that can interfere with future corneal surgery.

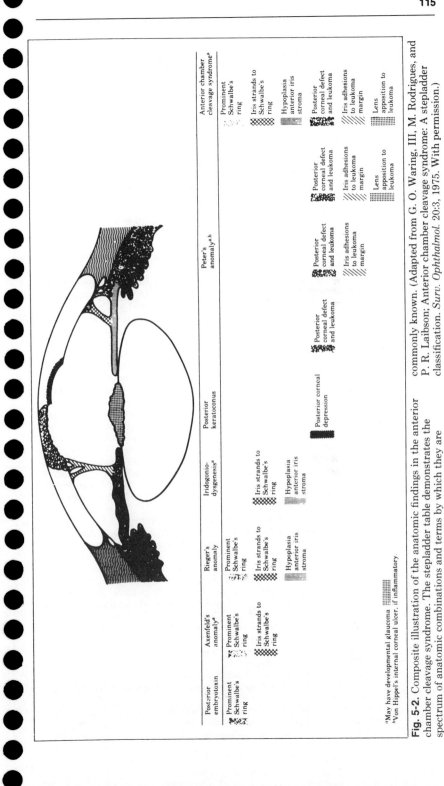

Fig. 5-2. Composite illustration of the anatomic findings in the anterior chamber cleavage syndrome. The stepladder table demonstrates the spectrum of anatomic combinations and terms by which they are commonly known. (Adapted from G. O. Waring, III, M. Rodrigues, and P. R. Laibson; Anterior chamber cleavage syndrome: A stepladder classification. *Surv. Ophthalmol.* 20:3, 1975. With permission.)

Posterior embryotoxin	Axenfeld's anomaly[a]	Rieger's anomaly	Iridogonio-dysgenesis[a]	Posterior keratoconus	Peter's anomaly[a,b]	Anterior chamber cleavage syndrome[a]
Prominent Schwalbe's ring	Prominent Schwalbe's ring	Prominent Schwalbe's ring				Prominent Schwalbe's ring
	Iris strands to Schwalbe's ring	Iris strands to Schwalbe's ring	Iris strands to Schwalbe's ring			Iris strands to Schwalbe's ring
		Hypoplasia anterior iris stroma	Hypoplasia anterior iris stroma			Hypoplasia anterior iris stroma
				Posterior corneal depression		
					Posterior corneal defect and leukoma	Posterior corneal defect and leukoma
					Iris adhesions to leukoma margin	Iris adhesions to leukoma margin
					Lens apposition to leukoma	Lens apposition to leukoma

[a]May have developmental glaucoma

[b]Von Hippel's internal corneal ulcer, if inflammatory.

3. **Corneal perforations.** Pinpoint perforations or flap lacerations that are otherwise in good apposition can often be splinted with a soft contact lens until wound healing occurs. Frank perforations that can be sealed with cyanoacrylate tissue adhesive are best managed by application of a soft contact lens to improve patient comfort and prevent the mechanical dislodgment of the adhesive by the action of the lids.

4. **Corneal transplants.** In cornea with diseased epithelium (chemical burns, herpes simplex keratitis), delay in epithelialization of the corneal donor or secondary breakdown of that epithelial layer frequently responds to soft contact lens treatment. Pinpoint leaks at the wound margin or slight anterior shifting of the wound edge that is not sufficient to require positioning of new sutures can often be splinted and sealed with the use of a soft contact lens. Soft contact lens therapy also provides comfort in those patients with epithelial defects; it is often best to use a firm soft lens to vault the corneal defect.

5. **Dry eye syndrome.** Patients with lacrimal insufficiency that does not respond to replacement lubricants can sometimes be benefited by a soft contact lens that provides a tear reservoir. These eyes are often less tolerant of a soft contact lens, due to desiccation of the hydrophilic polymer, and there is great risk of infection.

6. **Epithelial erosions.** Epithelial defects occurring in a cornea prone to epithelial breakdown (diabetes mellitus, anterior membrane dystrophy, lattice corneal dystrophy) are often effectively managed with a soft contact lens. This condition usually requires a very thin (0.02 μ central thickness) lens. Treatment is usually required for several weeks to months for complete reformation of the basement membrane adhesions.

7. **Filamentary keratitis.** This abnormality of the epithelial surface, probably due to aberrant healing of multiple small erosions, usually responds well to a soft contact lens. Relief of the irritative symptoms and loss of the filaments is usually rapid. In a dry eye, the tear reservoir effect of the lens is also of some benefit.

8. **Irregular astigmatism.** Whereas a soft contact lens usually is not effective in relieving high degrees of astigmatism, a mildly irregular anterior corneal surface can be smoothed to better optical clarity with a soft contact lens, and any tendency to dellen formation can be minimized.

9. **Keratoconus.** Soft contact lenses alone are inadequate to treat most cases of keratoconus. It is possible, however, in patients who are intolerant of hard contact lenses to provide a better surface for a hard contact lens by application of a soft contact lens. The "piggyback" technique can provide tolerance of an optically efficient lens system.

10. **Neuroparalytic keratopathy.** Patients with neurotrophic breakdown of the corneal epithelial surface (herpes zoster ophthalmicus, status posttrigeminal rhizotomy) often will have epitheliopathy and recurrent epithelial breakdown. These patients can be treated with a bandage soft contact lens but great care is required, as the protective mechanisms of sensation are diminished and a greater incidence of intolerance with corneal infiltration and vascularization as well as superinfection is possible. If intolerance develops, partial tarsorrhaphy should be considered instead, adjunctively or prophylactically.

11. **Trichiasis.** Scarring of the lids or inturning of the lashes from any etiology will result in chronic irritation of the epithelium, which can be minimized by wearing a soft contact lens as a protective barrier. Posttraumatic or cicatricial entropion are especially well treated this way, particularly if lid surgery is difficult or inadvisable. Patients with benign mucous membrane pemphigoid are more difficult to fit, due to the frequent shortening of the cul-de-sac.

12. **Postherpetic or postinfectious (trophic) defects.** Following an infectious epithelial defect, when the primary infection has been adequately controlled, a soft contact lens may be of value in encouraging reepithe-

lialization. It is essential that the underlying infectious element be controlled before such lens insertion.

13. Descemetocele. In an eye that has sustained a thinning of the stroma to the point of descemetocele formation, a soft contact lens may be applied as reinforcement until such time as definitive therapy of tissue adhesive, lid adhesion, or keratoplasty may be necessary.

14. Medications. Although a soft contact lens can serve as a barrier to penetration of some medications, it is also possible by saturation of the lens to provide a higher and more uniform concentration of delivery to the anterior corneal surface. Instillation of drops into the eye with a soft contact lens will also provide a mild reservoir effect. Epinephrine-containing compounds can become entrapped in the soft contact lens and oxidize to the adrenochrome pigments, producing a black tint to the lens. Fluorescein is a well-known stain that can be absorbed by the hydrophilic material, but with time will usually leach free. Collagen shields are discussed in sec. **IV.B.6.**

B. Care of the soft contact lens. The flexibility of the soft contact lens sometimes poses problems on insertion and removal. The tendency of the lens to desiccate and deform its contour is also at times a problem. The lens should be kept hydrated at all times in a saline solution without preservatives. It should be cleaned and sterilized prior to insertion. Care should be taken not to apply any sharp object to the lens, as this may tear it. In many cases where there are organic abnormalities of the cornea, it is advisable to use prophylactic antibiotics, usually in the form of sulfacetamide or Polytrim ophthalmic drops. Antiviral ointment may be used, but there is a greater chance of dislodging the lens. Due to the large diameter of the lens, scleral compression and peripheral vascular engorgement may occur.

C. Complications of soft contact lens therapy (see also Chap. 13, sec. **VIII** for cosmetic hard, gas-permeable, and daily and extended wear lenses).

a. Foreign body sensation and irritation of the eye are felt by some patients.

b. Loss of lens. The flexibility of the lens and an irregular contour of the diseased cornea can result in repeated loss of the lens.

c. Damage to lens. Tears or fractures in the lens can cause discomfort and irritation.

d. Infiltrates can be infectious or noninfectious. The noninfectious infiltrates tend to appear peripherally but can be central and are usually epithelial or immediately subepithelial. They disappear with removal of the lens.

e. Infection. The soft contact lens has been associated with the most serious complication, that of infection. Although this is usually bacterial, fungal infection can also occur. It is therefore essential that the lens be periodically sterilized and that a prophylactic topical antibiotic be used. Frequent follow-up is essential (see secs. **E** and **F**).

f. Anterior chamber reaction. The inflammatory reaction that can be provoked by a contact lens can include flare and cell or frank hypopyon. This reaction is usually sterile and resolves after removal of the lens.

g. Vascularization. Peripheral vascularization can occur, particularly in a patient with chronic epithelial edema or postinfectious ulcer. Since stromal vascularization can interfere with the success of future surgery, the lens should be removed.

h. Giant papillary conjunctivitis. A cobblestone hypertrophy of papillae on the upper tarsal conjunctiva has been associated with the wear of soft contact lens and can lead to chronic irritation. The reaction usually subsides after removal of the lens.

D. Hard contact lenses are most effective in optically correcting high degrees of ametropia or corneal astigmatism such as in keratoconus or post-thinning distortion.

E. Studies on the **microbiology of contact lens–related keratitis** indicate that cosmetic contact lenses were worn in about 45% of cases, with extended-wear soft contact lens incidence 2.5 times that of daily-wear soft contact lenses and daily-wear hard lenses in only 3%. Aphakic contact lenses were worn in about 32% of cases, with aphakic extended-wear soft contact lenses accounting for about 90% of this group. Therapeutic soft contact lenses were worn in about 25% of cases. Of organisms cultured, 52% were gram-positive, 36% gram-negative, and fungi and *Acanthamoeba* 4% each. *Pseudomonas* was highly associated with cosmetic soft lens use. Other studies on contact lens–related fungal keratitis indicate 4% incidence in cosmetic or aphakic hard or soft contact lenses and 27% incidence in therapeutic soft lenses. *Fusarium* and *Cephalosporium* predominated in cosmetic lenses and *Candida* in therapeutic lenses. Disposable extended-wear soft contact lenses have also been associated with bacterial keratitis even with proper lens care.

F. **Contact lens disinfection** studies indicate that while available hard lens regimens and soft lens cold hydrogen peroxide or heat disinfection effectively eliminate **bacteria** from the lenses, bacterial contamination was found in the contact lens cases or solutions: 75% in chemical disinfection, 50% in peroxide disinfection, and 28% in heat procedure. **Acanthamoeba** was effectively eliminated from lenses by not less than 2-hour exposure to 3% hydrogen peroxide followed by enzyme catalyst. Also effective in eliminating the trophozoite and cysts from solutions and lens cases was 4-hour exposure to thimerosol 0.001–0.004% or benzalkonium chloride 0.005%, both with edetate or 1-hour exposure to chlorhexidine 0.005% with edetate. Other commercial preparations were not effective or effective only with prolonged exposure (12–24 hours). The safest and best proven method of *Acanthamoeba* disinfection is still **heat sterilization. AIDS virus** and the **herpesviruses** are also all effectively killed by heat and the above disinfecting systems. Cold cleaning/disinfection effective against these viruses includes Boston cleaner and Boston conditioner for hard contact lenses and Pliagel, Miraflow, or Softmate for soft contact lenses.

XII. **Radial keratotomy** is the use of surgical incisions (bicycle spoke with clear optical center zone, tangential, or both) for correction of myopia and astigmatism by altering corneal curvature. Surgical variables affecting outcome are diameter of the clear central zone (3–5 mm) and the number (4–16) and depth of the incisions. Greatest flattening occurs with smaller central zones, four to eight cuts, and deeper incisions. Patient variables affecting outcome are greater effect with higher myopia and more advanced age, making **outcome only relatively predictable.** Multiple other variables exist (sex, IOP, corneal thickness), but their effect is not yet established. Current results indicate that 85% of patients undergoing radial keratotomy see 20/40 or better uncorrected compared to only 1% preoperatively. Radial keratotomy on the second eye has a 66% chance of being within 1 d correction of the first eye and 98% within 3 d. On the negative side, 20% of patients are undercorrected, there is a 5%/year trend toward progressive hyperopia of yet to be determined duration, endothelial cell loss may be enhanced, and soft contact lenses should not be fitted for at least 3 months postoperatively because of increased tendency to neovascularization. Glare and daily fluctuation in vision are common and decrease markedly over the first year, although some may persist for years. Rare complications are surgical perforation, cataract, infectious keratitis, and traumatic corneal rupture. In general up to 71% of patients are very satisfied and only about 10% dissatisfied with this procedure.

XIII. **Sclera and episclera**

A. **Anatomy and physiology**

1. **The sclera** constitutes five-sixths of the anterior tunic of the globe as an almost spherical segment 22 mm in diameter. It is continuous with the cornea at the limbus anteriorly and with the optic nerve posteriorly at the scleral fibers of the lamina cribrosa.

a. The **thickness** of the sclera varies from a maximum of 1 mm near the optic nerve to 0.5 mm at the equator and 0.8 mm anteriorly. The thinnest portion (0.3 mm) is found just behind the insertions of the recti muscles.

b. **The stroma** is composed of collagen bundles varying in size from 10–15 μ in thickness and 100–150 μ in length, interlacing in an irregular crisscross pattern roughly parallel to the surface of the globe. When compared to cornea, the scleral fibers have greater birefringence, absence of fixed spacing, and greater variation in fiber diameter. All these anatomic features contribute to the opaque character of the sclera.

c. The **avascular** sclera transmits blood vessels but retains scant supply for its own use, obtaining nutrition from the underlying choroid and the overlying episclera. The long posterior ciliary vessels course anteriorly in the horizontal meridian of the sclera, while six to seven oblique channels posteriorly transmit the vortex veins.

d. **Innervation** of the sclera is from the long and short posterior ciliary nerves and is especially prominent in the anterior portion where stimulation of the nerve endings by inflammation or distention can produce marked pain.

2. **The episclera** provides much of the nutritional support of the sclera, which itself is permeable to water, glucose, and proteins. The episclera also serves as a synovial lining for the collagen and elastic sclera and reacts vigorously to scleral inflammation. The fibroelastic episclera has a visceral layer closely opposed to the sclera and a parietal layer that fuses with the muscle sheath and the conjunctiva near the limbus. These two layers are connected and bridged by delicate connective tissue lamellae. The posterior episcleral plexus of **vessels** comes from the short posterior ciliary vessels. The anterior episcleral circulation is more complex, with communications among a conjunctival plexus, superficial episcleral plexus, and deep episcleral plexus that anastomose at the limbus with the superficial and deep intrascleral venous plexus. This interconnection of intrascleral and episcleral venous systems drains the anterior portion of the ciliary body. The conjunctival and episcleral vessels can be blanched with 1 : 1000 adrenalin or 10% phenylephrine while the deep vessels are little changed, thus providing a useful method **of differentiating superficial from deep** inflammatory congestion.

3. **The function of the sclera** is to provide a protective shell for the intraocular contents that will prevent distortion of the globe in order to maintain optical integrity yet allow for variation in IOP. The viscoelastic ocular coat provides mobility without deformation by the attached muscles. Primarily supportive, the metabolic activity of the sclera is low and easily satisfied by the adjacent vascularity of episclera and choroid. The high hydration of the sclera contributes to the opaque nature of the tissue, which can become translucent if the water content is reduced to about 40%, as is seen clinically in scleral dellen. The collagenous nature of the sclera and its encasement by an episclera that acts much like a synovium have suggested the comparison of the eye to an exposed and modified ball-and-socket joint. This comparison has some merit since diseases that affect articular structures often can involve the scleral-episcleral coat.

B. **Diseases of the sclera and episclera: inflammation.** The most important clinical afflictions of the sclera and episclera are inflammatory. Although congenital, metabolic, degenerative, and neoplastic disease can also affect the sclera and episclera, the most common, diagnostically perplexing, and therapeutically difficult conditions are inflammatory.

1. **Classification**

   a. **Episcleritis**—simple and nodular.

   b. **Anterior scleritis**—diffuse, nodular, or necrotizing with or without inflammation (scleromalacia perforans).

   c. **Posterior scleritis**

2. **Clinical differentiation** of these types of inflammations is of diagnostic and therapeutic importance. Episcleritis is often a benign condition requiring

modest treatment; scleritis, however, can signal destructive disease involving collagen tissues in general and can require potent therapy.

C. **Episcleritis**

1. **Simple episcleritis** is a usually benign, often bilateral, inflammatory reaction occurring in young adults, with a tendency for spontaneous regression in 7–10 days and then recurrence. There is discomfort localized to the eye, accompanied by variable degrees of lacrimation and photophobia. Segmental or diffuse vascular engorgement and edema of the episclera are usually present. Women are more often affected than men, and the peak age incidence is the fourth decade.

2. **Nodular episcleritis** is similar in its incidence and pattern but may run a more protracted course. The incidence of episcleritis is difficult to determine since many patients undoubtedly do not seek treatment. About three-fourths of the cases are simple and the remainder nodular in character. About 30% of cases of nodular episcleritis can be associated with general medical problems: 5% occurring with collagen vascular disease (rheumatoid arthritis), 7% with prior herpes zoster ophthalmicus, and 3% with gout. Extensive laboratory workup is not rewarding with most episcleritis cases, but clinical examination for evidence of rheumatoid arthritis, herpes zoster ophthalmicus, or gout can be supplemented by **serologic tests for rheumatoid arthritis** and serum **uric acid.** Most cases of episcleritis resolve within 3–6 weeks without complication, although there can be an associated uveitis (7%), and intraocular inflammation should be excluded.

3. **Corneal complications** of episcleritis occur in approximately 15% of cases but are usually not severe or permanent. Elevation of the limbal area due to episcleral edema or nodule can result in **corneal dellen.** This local desiccation phenomenon may respond to patching, lubrication, or resolution of the limbal swelling. With significant inflammation, there can be superficial and midstromal infiltration and edema of the cornea that rarely provoke vascularization.

4. **Treatment** is often not required, and symptoms can sometimes be relieved by topical decongestants. More symptomatic cases usually respond to modest topical steroid treatment (prednisolone 1% tid or qid). Recalcitrant cases may be treated with systemic NSAIDS: oxyphenbutazone (Tandearil, Oxalid), 100 mg qid, or indomethacin (Indocin), 25 mg bid, gradually increased to 50 mg bid. Also of use are naproxen (Naprosyn), 250 mg q12h, or diflunisal (Dolobid), 500 mg q12h, with a meal.

D. **Scleritis.** Inflammation of the sclera can result in severe destructive disease that causes pain and threatens vision. Occurring more commonly in females than in males, with a peak incidence in the fourth to sixth decades, the condition is bilateral in approximately 50% of cases. Pain can be severe and is often described as a deep boring ache. There is often associated photophobia and lacrimation as well as chronic systemic inflammatory disease.

1. **Anterior scleritis.** Ninety-five percent of cases of scleritis are in the anterior portion of the sclera.

   a. **Diffuse anterior scleritis** occurs approximately 40% of the time, and **nodular anterior scleritis** approximately 45% of the time. **Necrotizing scleritis,** occurring 14% of the time, is usually more severe and is twice as frequent with inflammation as without. The specific pattern of scleritis is usually not distinctive enough to prove an etiology, although the clinical course and prognosis are often predictable on the basis of the pattern of inflammation. The diffuse anterior variety is most benign; the nodular anterior form is more painful. The necrotizing form is the most severe and unremitting.

   b. **Diseases** associated with the various types of scleritis vary.

      (1) The **diffuse anterior** pattern can be associated with rheumatoid arthritis (24% of cases), prior herpes zoster ophthalmicus, and gout.

      (2) The **nodular anterior** variety has been associated most frequently with prior episodes of herpes zoster ophthalmicus.

(3) The **necrotizing** variety is the most ominous and can be associated with ocular or systemic complications in 60% of patients. Forty percent may show decreased visual acuity. Twenty-nine percent of patients with necrotizing scleritis may be dead within 5 years. The necrotizing variety must be distinguished on the basis of focal areas of avascular scleral dropout. In those cases of **necrotizing scleritis without inflammation (scleromalacia perforans),** most patients have long-standing rheumatoid arthritis involving multiple joints. More than half of the time the condition is bilateral in patients with rheumatoid arthritis. Clinically, large areas of avascular sclera may appear as a sequestrum with adjacent exposure of the uveal pigment through a markedly thin sclera. Anterior chamber reaction can occur with this type of scleritis and is an ominous sign. Perforation is not common but can occur.

2. **Posterior scleritis** is difficult to diagnose and often overlooked. One histopathologic series of enucleated eyes documented posterior involvement in 43% of eyes diagnosed with anterior scleritis. Certainly, posterior scleritis can occur alone but is then more difficult to diagnose. **Symptoms** suggesting posterior scleritis are pain and reduced visual acuity. Physical **signs** suggesting posterior scleritis include fundus changes, particularly exudative retinal detachment, annular choroidal folds or detachments, subretinal mass, patchy chorioretinal changes, vitritis optic nerve edema, or macular edema. Severe posterior inflammation can result in shallowing of the anterior chamber, proptosis, limited extraocular movement, and lower lid retraction. Posterior scleritis can be associated with rheumatoid arthritis or systemic vasculitis. **Ultrasound** or **CT scan** will reveal diagnostic scleral thickening.

3. **Complications of scleritis**
   a. Corneal changes occur in approximately 37% of cases of **anterior diffuse and nodular scleritis.** There are four characteristic patterns of corneal involvement.
      (1) Diffuse stromal: midstromal opacities occurring with immune ring patterns and keratic precipitates.
      (2) Sclerosing stromal keratitis: edema and infiltration of the stroma with vascularization and scarring resulting in subsequent crystalline formation.
      (3) Deep keratitis: white, opaque sheets of infiltration at the level of Descemet's membrane.
      (4) Limbal guttering: a limbal gutter progressing to ectasia and characterized by lipid deposits with or without vascularization.
   b. The **necrotizing** forms of scleritis can produce more significant corneal changes, occurring primarily in three forms.
      (1) Acute stromal keratitis: edema and dense white infiltration associated with ring infiltrates and keratic precipitates.
      (2) Corneal guttering: marginal thinning with prominent inflammation indicative of a vasculitis that must be differentiated from Mooren's ulcer.
      (3) Keratolysis: diffuse areas of corneal infiltration that will suddenly thin by stromal melting to result in descemetocele surrounded by irregularly scarred and vascularized tissue.
   c. **Other ocular complications** of scleritis include uveitis in approximately 35% of cases and scleral thinning in 27%. There can also be both open-angle and narrow-angle glaucoma (13.5%), as well as cataract, retinal detachment, and optic nerve swelling.

4. Because of the high incidence of associated systemic or collagen disease, it is often wise to obtain ancillary **laboratory investigations** as a diagnostic routine.
   a. **Hematology studies**
      (1) Complete blood count and erythrocyte sedimentation rate.
      (2) Plasma protein and immunoglobulin level.

      (3) Antinuclear and rheumatoid factors.

      (4) Serum uric acid.

      (5) Serologic tests for syphilis.

  b. X rays: chest, hands and feet, lumbosacral spine.

  c. Fluorescein angiography, anterior or posterior segment, for evidence of vasculitis.

  d. Unfortunately, **laboratory investigations** are often not helpful in the earliest stages of scleritis; particularly, x rays may be normal. It is obvious that these tests have limited specific diagnostic value, as they can be positive in a variety of systemic conditions. Results of the tests need interpretation in light of the history, associated physical findings, and the pattern of positive results (see Chap. 8, sec. **V**).

5. Treatment of scleritis

  a. Medical therapy is the first line of defense.

    (1) Although **topical steroids** frequently increase comfort and occasionally maintain a remission, the topical preparations may not be sufficient to induce a remission and will exacerbate keratolysis.

    (2) If topical steroids are ineffective, systemic treatment with **NSAIDS** is possible. Such treatment (oxyphenbutazone, 100 mg qid, or indomethacin, 25 mg bid, increasing to 25 mg tid) may suppress the inflammation in diffuse and nodular varieties but is not likely to control the necrotizing form. Naproxen, 250–375 mg q12h, and diflunisal, 500 mg q12h, also have proved effective in nonnecrotizing scleritis.

    (3) For unresponsive cases, scleromalacia perforans, or severe necrotizing inflammation, the mainstay of treatment is **systemic steroids** in a dosage of 80–120 mg prednisolone/day for the first week with rapid tapering to 20 mg daily, within 2–3 weeks, and then tapered slowly by 2.5-mg steps. Topical steroids may be used to sustain a remission. Subconjunctival steroids are to be discouraged because the scleral thinning per se and sustained local suppression of wound healing by subconjunctival route can be hazardous.

    (4) Severe or unremitting cases may require treatment with penicillamine or **immunosuppressive drugs.** The drug of choice is cyclophosphamide (Cytoxan), starting at 100 mg PO qd and increasing the dosage to 150–200 mg PO qd over 2 weeks. Patients should be warned of the potential serious side effects (see Chap. 8, sec. **VI.C**). An internist or other physician familiar with the use of these drugs should be consulted before and during the course of treatment.

    (5) If fluorescein angiography reveals a vasculitis or blood tests indicate immune complex disease, both life-threatening processes, and/or the presence of a progressive destructive ocular lesion, inflamed or not inflamed, cyclophosphamide, 100 mg PO qd or less, with prednisolone, 15 mg PO qd, may control the process. If there is little response, pulsed IV methylprednisolone over 1–2 hours should be given with 500 mg of cyclophosphamide IV over several hours and washed through with IV 5% D/W or saline over 24 hours to decrease the incidence of hemorrhagic cystitis. This pulsed therapy is not without hazard and may be repeated if necessary under desperate circumstances to save not only vision but life itself. Once the disease process is under control using systemic therapy, **mild topical steroids** should be used qd–tid to maintain suppression and systemic treatment stopped. **Subconjunctival steroids** should **never** be given, as scleral or keratolysis may result.

    (6) Adverse effects. It is important to recognize the potential serious adverse reactions to systemically administered anti-inflammatory agents. The serious adverse effects of steroid therapy with adrenal suppression can be avoided with short-term therapy, but gastrointestinal disturbance, aggravation of hyperglycemia, fluid retention, and acute psychoses may occur. Long-term systemic or local steroid therapy obviously can produce cataracts and elevate IOP. Oxyphenbutazone may cause gastrointestinal ulceration and occasionally hematologic suppression. Indomethacin also has gastrointestinal toxicity. (See Chap. 8, sec. **VI.D**).

  b. **Surgical treatment**
    (1) Extreme scleral thinning or **perforation** requires reinforcement. Whatever material is used must be covered with conjunctiva to maintain its integrity. Donor sclera or cornea may be used but usually swells with edema and softens. Fascia lata or periosteum is somewhat more resistant to the melting process. All grafts should be completely covered by sliding conjunctiva or using donor conjunctiva from the same or opposite eye.
    (2) Extreme corneal marginal ulceration or keratolysis may require corneal grafting, usually as a lamellar patch graft.

The Crystalline Lens and Cataract

Deborah Pavan-Langston

I. **Basic anatomy, biochemistry, and physiology.** The crystalline lens is suspended by thin filamentous zonules from the ciliary processes between the iris anteriorly and the vitreous humor posteriorly. It is an encapsulated, multicellular organ with an anterior layer of cuboidal epithelium covering concentric layers of fibers (Fig. 6-1). The epithelial cells contain nuclei, mitochondria, endoplasmic reticulum, and other cytoplasmic organelles; metabolic activity is both aerobic and anaerobic. At the equator, epithelial cells differentiate into lens fibers; all cells are gradually incorporated into the lens, and no cells are lost. Cellular organelles are lost during differentiation from epithelial to fiber cells, and in lens fibers aerobic metabolic activity is absent. The nucleus, the innermost part of the lens, contains the oldest cells, and metabolic activity in this region is virtually nil. Metabolic activity supports active transport of amino acids and cations across the epithelium as well as protein synthesis in the fibers. Cations move actively across the anterior epithelium, but passively across the posterior lens capsule—a so-called pump-leak system. The maintenance of homeostasis is essential to lens clarity. Physiologic stresses may disrupt this homeostasis and lead to opacification of part or all of the lens.

A. **Incidence.** Ninety-five percent of persons over 65 years of age have some degree of lens opacity; many have cataracts sufficiently dense to warrant cataract extraction. Over 1 million cataract extractions are done each year in the United States alone. Cataract accounts for a significant amount of treatable blindness in the world; extraction may lead to complete visual rehabilitation.

B. **Physiologic optics.** In the cataractous lens, fluctuation in the index of refraction creates foci of light scattering and a loss of transparency. In cortical, supranuclear, and subcapsular cataracts, protein-deficient fluid collects between fibers. The index of refraction of this fluid is much less than that of fiber cytoplasm, and light scattering occurs at this interface. Light scattering also occurs from large protein aggregates linked to the cell membrane by disulfide bonds. In nuclear cataract, light is scattered by huge, soluble protein aggregates with molecular weights in excess of 5×10^6 daltons. The mechanisms responsible for these cortical and nuclear changes are slowly being defined, but until we fully understand them, our ability to delay cataract maturation with medical (as contrasted to surgical) means will be severely limited.
The lens and cornea form an optical system that focuses light from a distant object on the retina (emmetropia), anterior to the retina (myopia), and posterior to the retina (hyperopia). Myopic and hyperopic refractive errors are corrected with spectacle or contact lenses. The ability to focus near objects is called "ocular accommodation." Contraction of the ciliary muscle relaxes zonular tension on the lens and allows the intrinsic elasticity of the lens capsule to increase the central convexity of the anterior lens. This change reduces the focal length of the lens and moves the point of clear vision closer to the face (see also Chap. 8, sec. I.B and Chap. 13, sec. V.B).

II. **Aging effects.** Infants possess great powers of accommodation; with age, this power decreases; about the age of 40, much accommodative power has been lost (pres-

Sections I through V in this chapter were written by Leo T. Chylack, Jr., and are taken from the previous edition.

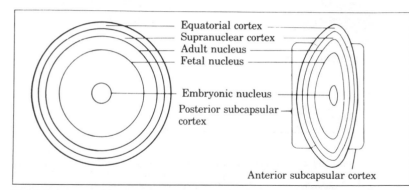

Fig. 6-1. Anatomic layers of the crystalline lens. Between the fetal and adult nuclei lie the lamellae of the infantile and adolescent nuclei.

byopia). At this time, reading glasses are needed for clear near vision. This is one of the earliest age-related lenticular changes. The lens nucleus also becomes increasingly yellow with age (nuclear sclerosis), and in some cataracts the nuclear color may be brown or black. Nuclear sclerosis per se is not associated with any loss of clarity. A change in color perception may result from the superimposition of a yellow filter between the retina and the incident light. **Sclerosis** is to some degree a misnomer; the water content of the adult nucleus is the same as that of the young lens. This implies that there is no significant increase in density or hardness. The older nucleus is harder or more sclerotic, however, if judged by its resistance to ultrasonic disintegration (in phacoemulsification) or aspiration.

III. **Definition of cataract.** When the transparency of the crystalline lens decreases enough to disturb vision, a clinically significant cataract exists. Such a decrease is usually due to foci of light scattering or absorption in the axial part of the lens; however, similar changes in the peripheral parts of the lens may exist without any loss of vision. *Although these changes are strictly cataractous in nature, they usually are not labeled as such, as long as vision is normal.* It is necessary to understand this distinction so that patients with lens opacities, but no visual symptoms, are not worried unnecessarily by a premature diagnosis of cataract.

A cataract is characterized by the zones of the lens involved in the opacity: anterior and posterior subcapsular, anterior and posterior cortical, equatorial cortical, supranuclear and nuclear. In certain congenital cataracts, the nuclear zone is further subdivided into adult, adolescent, infantile, fetal, and embryonic zones (Fig. 6-1).

IV. **Detection of significant lens opacification**
  A. **Symptoms of cataract formation**
    1. **Glare.** One of the symptomatic manifestations of light scattering is glare. When a patient looks at a point source of light, the diffusion of bright white and colored light around it drastically reduces visual acuity. The effect is akin to looking at automobile headlights at night through a dirty windshield. Posterior subcapsular opacification is responsible for much of the glare.
    2. **Image blur.** An image blur occurs when the lens loses its ability to differentiate (resolve) separate and distinct object points. When this occurs, near-visual tasks, such as reading and sewing, become more difficult. Many older patients may tolerate considerable glare if their night driving is minimal, but they may not be as tolerant of a blur that interferes with their indoor activities.
    3. **Distortion.** Cataracts may make straight edges appear wavy or curved. They may even lead to image duplication (monocular diplopia). If a patient complains of double vision, it is essential to determine if the diplopia is binocular or monocular. If monocular, the examiner is usually dealing with corneal, lens, or macular disease.

4. **Altered color perception.** The yellowing of the lens nucleus steadily increases with age. Artists with significant nuclear sclerosis may render objects browner or yellower than they are.
5. **Unilateral cataract.** A cataract may occur in only one eye or may mature more rapidly in one eye than in the other. Unless the patient is in the habit of checking the acuity of each eye, he or she may not be aware of the presence of a dense cataract in one eye. It is not uncommon for a patient to claim that the vision in the cataractous eye was lost precipitously. Since cataracts rarely mature precipitously, it is more likely that the slowly evolving lens opacity was unrecognized until the patient happened to test his or her monocular acuity.
6. **Behavioral changes**
   a. **Children.** Children with congenital, traumatic, or metabolic cataracts may not verbalize their visual handicap. Behavioral changes indicative of a loss of acuity or binocular vision may alert the parents or teachers to the presence of a visual problem. Inability to see the blackboard or read with one eye may be one such symptom; loss of accurate depth perception, e.g., the inability to catch or hit a ball or to pour water from a pitcher into a glass, may be another.
   b. **Prepresbyopic adults.** Difficulty with night driving is frequently an early sign of cataract.
   c. **Presbyopic adults.** Frequently, maturation of nuclear cataracts is associated with a return of clear near vision due to increasing myopia secondary to the higher refractive power of the rounder, harder nuclear sclerotic lens. Reading glasses or bifocals are no longer needed. This change is called "second sight." Unfortunately, the improvement in near vision is only temporary as the nuclear zone becomes more opaque.
B. **Signs of cataract formation**
   1. **Leukocoria.** The "white pupil" is seen in mature cataracts; in certain immature cataracts, whitish, gray, or yellow patches are seen in the pupillary zone. These are due to foci of light scattering located in the anterior subcapsular or cortical zone.
   2. **More subtle signs.** Examination of the red reflex with the direct ophthalmoscope set on +4 (black) diopters at approximately 20 cm from the patient frequently will reveal a black lens opacity against the reddish-orange hue of the reflex. This is an extremely sensitive method of detecting cataractous change. If, on upgaze, the opacity appears to move down, the opacity is in the posterior half of the lens; if the opacity moves up with upgaze, it is in the anterior half of the lens.
   3. **Reduced visual acuity.** Although it is not part of the usual physical examination, the measurement of visual acuity will alert the examiner to the presence of cataract as well as other ocular disorders. The examiner should always inquire about monocular acuity when conducting a review of systems.
C. **Diagnostic tests and glasses correction for cataract**
   1. **Visual acuity.** Distant and near acuity with the appropriate glasses should be tested.
   2. **Flashlight examination of lens and pupil.** The direct and consensual pupillary responses are not affected by lens opacities if a bright light is used; if a dim flashlight is used, the responses may be less pronounced when illuminating the eye with a dense cataract. A flashlight may also render anterior lens opacities more visible to the examiner if pupil size is not reduced excessively. The flashlight may also reduce the patient's acuity as a result of miosis and glare.
   3. **Direct ophthalmoscopy.** Nuclear cataracts often appear as a "lens within a lens" when viewed against the red reflex (with a +4 to +6 lens).
   4. **Slit-lamp biomicroscopy** allows the most detailed examination of the an-

terior part of the eye. The extent, density, type, and location of the cataract can be easily determined.

5. **Refraction and retinoscopy.** Nuclear myopia occurring in the early stages of nuclear cataract formation can be detected by routine refraction. Patients may be well corrected for months or even years with a stronger myopic distance lens and little or no reading add. Retinoscopy will reveal the abnormal reflexes associated with lenticonus, a condition in which the anterior or posterior surfaces of the lens (or both) are excessively convex or conical.

6. **A-scan and B-scan ultrasonography** are techniques for measuring the thickness and location of a cataract. They are particularly useful in evaluating partial or total dislocation of the lens. They also provide a means of detecting abnormalities in the posterior half of the eye with a very dense cataract. Some secondary cataracts form in response to posterior segment tumors or inflammation, thereby necessitating ultrasonography to ascertain the anatomic state of the eye behind the lens (see Chap. 1, sec. III.E).

V. **Abnormalities of the lens**

A. **Congenital abnormalities: ectopia lentis (dislocated lens)** (see also Chap. 10, **VII.E** and **F**)

1. **Homocystinuria.** This autosomal recessive condition is associated with a deficiency of cystathionine synthetase, an enzyme responsible for condensing homocystine and serine to cystathionine. Bilateral lens dislocation occurs in this disease; if the lens dislocates into the anterior chamber, acute glaucoma may develop. Cataractous changes do not usually occur. Systemic manifestations include malar flush, mental retardation, osteoporosis, pectus excavatum, decreased joint mobility, and eczema. Abnormal physical findings are usually apparent by age 10, but may be delayed until the third decade. Surgical removal of dislocated lenses is fraught with complications, including vitreous loss, iris prolapse, and retinal detachment. **General anesthesia is to be avoided,** if possible, because of the increased risk of vascular thrombosis. Defective cross-linking of collagen has been detected in the skin of these patients.

2. **Marfan's syndrome.** Inheritance of this disorder is autosomal dominant. In contrast to homocystinuria, in which lens dislocation is usually inferior, in Marfan's syndrome dislocation is superior and only occasionally into the anterior chamber. Acute secondary glaucoma may result from lens dislocation into the anterior chamber. Surgical extraction of these lenses is complicated by many of the same problems encountered in homocystinuria. The systemic manifestations of this disease are tall and thin body habitus, scoliosis, arachnodactyly, elastic skin, hyperextensible joints, aortic insufficiency, and aneurysm. The biochemical basis is unknown. The diagnosis is usually established by the physical examination and the characteristic patient habitus. If the urinary cyanide-nitroprusside reaction is normal, the physician can exclude the diagnosis of homocystinuria and be more confident of the diagnosis of Marfan's syndrome.

3. **Weill-Marchesani syndrome** is inherited as an autosomal recessive trait. Patients are short with broad hands and fingers. There may be joint stiffness, prominence, and decreased mobility. Carpal tunnel syndrome may result from fibrous tissue hyperplasia. Lenses are small, spherical, and frequently dislocate anteriorly, precipitating acute glaucoma. Patients are easily distinguished from those with Marfan's syndrome or homocystinuria by their characteristic body habitus.

B. **Congenital abnormalities: cataract** (see also Chap. 10, sec. **XIV**)

1. **Galactosemia** is due to an inborn error of galactose metabolism, a deficiency of galactose-1-phosphate uridyltransferase, the enzyme that converts galactose-1-phosphate to uridine diphosphogalactose. In the presence of milk sugar (lactose), this deficiency leads to the accumulation of galactose-1-phosphate and galactose. Galactose is converted by the enzyme aldose reductase to the sugar alcohol, galactitol. The accumulation of this

sugar alcohol within lens cells creates a hypertonic intracellular milieu that is neutralized by the influx of water. The entry of water leads to swelling, membrane disruption, and opacification of the lens. Cataracts are not apparent at birth but usually develop within the first few months of life. A central nuclear opacity resembling a drop of oil appears within the lens. This opacity may progress to opacification of the fetal nucleus. The disease is manifest in **patients fed milk products** that contain the disaccharide lactose (glucose plus galactose). In addition to the cataracts that appear in these patients, there is frequently mental retardation, growth inhibition, and hepatic dysfunction. The diagnosis can be made with an assay for uridyltransferase in peripheral red cells.

2. **Galactokinase deficiency.** The enzyme galactokinase converts galactose to galactose-1-phosphate. Lack of this enzyme leads to the accumulation of galactose, which is then converted to galactitol. The same osmotic events as in galactosemia occur and lead to cataract formation. In these patients, however, hepatomegaly, mental retardation, and other systemic manifestations of galactosemia are absent. Except for cataracts, these patients usually enjoy normal health. Treatment is dietary restriction of galactose-containing foods.

3. **Hypoglycemia.** Neonatal hypoglycemia occurs in approximately 20% of newborn infants. The incidence is significantly increased in premature infants. Blood sugars of 20 mg/dl or less may cause repeated episodes of somnolence, diaphoresis, unconsciousness, and convulsions. Repeated hypoglycemic episodes may lead to a characteristic lamellar cataract in which layers of cortical opacity are separated from a deeper zonular cataract by clear cortex. The cataract does not usually appear until the child is at least 2–3 years old; in many patients, no visual disability is encountered. Experimental evidence obtained by incubating rabbit and rat lenses in glucose-deficient media suggests that this cataract may be due to an inactivation of type II hexokinase. Treatment of this condition is aimed at the restoration and maintenance of normal glucose levels in the blood.

4. **Lowe's syndrome (oculocerebral renal syndrome).** Bilateral nuclear cataracts and microphakia are frequently found in this disorder. Aspiration of these cataracts is associated with a poor prognosis for full visual recovery. Other ocular abnormalities include glaucoma and malformation of the anterior chamber angle and iris. Most striking is the **blue sclera,** a manifestation of scleral thinning. Frequently, there is associated mental retardation, failure to thrive, absence of eyebrows, and vitamin D–resistant rickets. Vomiting, glucosuria, proteinuria, renal caliculi, and convulsions are not unusual.

5. **Myotonic dystrophy** is inherited as an autosomal dominant trait. Early cataracts are characteristic and consist of fine scattered dustlike opacities in the cortex and subcapsular region. Multicolored, refractile bodies are scattered among these finer dustlike opacities. The nucleus is completely clear. Later on in the disease, a granular, posterior subcapsular cataract develops. Cataract extraction usually is performed in adulthood, and the visual prognosis is good if there is no serious posterior segment involvement, such as optic atrophy or retinal degeneration. Associated systemic findings include dystrophic changes in muscles, including impaired contraction and relaxation, gonadal atrophy, and frontal baldness. Unfortunately, the characteristic features of this cataract are best appreciated by slit-lamp biomicroscopy and cannot be seen with direct ophthalmoscopy or flashlight examination.

6. **Congenital ichthyosis.** Morphology of cataracts in this disorder is varied. The dermatologic abnormalities usually make the diagnosis quite straightforward.

7. **Rothmund-Thomson syndrome.** Rapidly progressive bilateral cataracts occur in approximately 15% of individuals with this disorder. Morphology is varied and not characteristic. The presence of hypogonadism, poikilod-

erma, atrophy, and sclerosis of the skin, with dystrophic changes in hair and nails, makes the diagnosis reasonably easy. Inheritance is not fully understood but is believed to be autosomal recessive.

8. **Rubella cataract** results from fetal infection with rubella virus prior to the ninth week of gestation. This virus is known to inhibit mitosis and cell division in many fetal tissues. Involvement of the lens vesicle at the time of elongation of the posterior epithelial cells leads to the abnormal lens development. The cataract has a characteristic morphology: a slightly eccentric dense white core opacity and lesser opacification of the surrounding cortex. The anterior suture may be visible. Other ocular manifestations of this disease are microophthalmus, pigmentary retinopathy, and iritis. Due to the involvement of dilator fibers, pupillary dilation is frequently incomplete. Early referral to an ophthalmologist will optimize chances for successful cataract extraction. Surgery is frequently difficult due to poor pupillary dilation, shallow anterior chamber depth, and the small size of the eye. The newest techniques, however, with phacoemulsification and other forms of cataract aspiration give this procedure a better prognosis.

Rubella prevention, through vaccination, probably offers the safest and most effective method of reducing the incidence of this disease.

9. **Other congenital abnormalities** in which cataracts are found are Werner's syndrome and Hallermann-Streiff-François syndrome (see Chap. 10, sec. **X.A**).

C. Adult cataract

1. **Diabetic: osmotic cataract.** In the preinsulin era, the acute onset of a mature cataract in an untreated or brittle diabetic was not uncommon. Since blood sugar control is now relatively easy with insulin, this form of acute osmotic cataract is extremely rare. It is possible to precipitate this cataract, however, by abruptly lowering a markedly elevated blood sugar with insulin. The intracellular hypertonicity, due to the accumulation of sorbitol and glucose, remains after the serum osmolarity drops precipitously with the blood sugar. A rapid influx of water leads to acute swelling and opacification of the lens.

   a. **Poorly controlled diabetics** frequently experience changes in their refractive status. Increasing blood sugar is associated with myopic change; decreasing blood sugar is associated with hyperopic change. These changes are most noticeable during periods of poor control. Restoration of control eliminates these refractive error fluctuations.

   b. The **reversible appearance and disappearance of a posterior subcapsular cataract** has been documented in adult diabetics. This is believed to be a somewhat lesser response to the same osmotic stress that opacifies the entire lens of the uncontrolled juvenile diabetic.

   c. **Incidence.** In a population of adult diabetics, cataract extraction is done more frequently and at an earlier age when compared with the general population. It is not clear whether this is due to the increased incidence and more rapid maturation of cataract in diabetics or whether it is a manifestation of the increased detection of cataracts in a population already under medical supervision. Abundant experimental evidence suggests that diabetes is a significant cataractogenic stress that, added to other age-related stresses, may lead to earlier maturation of cataracts. The development of aldose reductase inhibitors to block the conversion of glucose to sorbitol may provide a means of eliminating this cataractogenic stress. The morphology of the adult diabetic cataract is indistinguishable from that of the nondiabetic senile cataract.

2. **Hypocalcemic (tetanic cataract).** The morphology of the cataract associated with hypocalcemia varies with the age at which hypocalcemia occurs. In the infant, depression of serum calcium produces a zonular cataract with a thin opacified lamella deep in the infantile cortex. In the adult, acquired or surgical hypoparathyroidism is associated with punctate, red, green, and highly refractile opacities occurring in the subcapsular area. In **pseudo-**

hypoparathyroidism, lamellar opacities are found in the nucleus of the lens. Ocular involvement may include papilledema, diplopia, photophobia, and strabismus. It is believed that calcium is necessary for the maintenance of membrane integrity and that calcium deficiency leads to membrane disruption and increased permeability.

    3. **Aminoaciduria** (see **V.A** and **B;** Chap. 10, sec. **VII.E**).

D. **Senile cataract.** The term *senile* was previously used to describe cataracts in older adults with no specificity with regard to morphology or etiology. With the emergence, however, of surgical procedures specifically suited to certain forms of cataract extractions and with the increased understanding of mechanisms of cataract formation, it has become more important to distinguish one form of cataract from another. In **cortical** and **subcapsular cataracts,** light scattering is believed to occur as a result of the interfibrillar accumulation of protein-deficient lakes of fluid. Wide discrepancies in the index of refraction of the intra- and extracellular spaces lead to light scattering. In contrast, in the **nuclear cataract,** the presence of high-molecular-weight protein aggregates (with molecular weights $> 50 \times 10^6$ daltons) leads to light scattering.

E. **Toxic cataract**

    1. **Corticosteroids.** The use of topical and systemic corticosteroids is associated with the appearance of axial posterior subcapsular cataracts. These cataracts frequently assume a diskoid morphology and, by virtue of their position in the visual axis near the nodal point of the eye, cause a great deal of visual disability. The higher the dose of corticosteroid and the longer the course of treatment, the more likely the patient is to develop cataract. By reducing the dose and duration of treatment, the cataractogenic process can be slowed or stopped. All patients with diseases requiring prolonged corticosteroid therapy should be evaluated by an ophthalmologist with particular attention to the crystalline lens.

    2. **Miotics (anticholinesterase drugs including echothiophate, diisopropyl fluorophosphate, and demecarium bromide)** are used in the treatment of glaucoma and some forms of strabismus in children. Prolonged use is associated with the appearance of anterior subcapsular vacuoles and granular opacities in this same region. Removal of the drug reduces the risk of progression and may even be associated with reversal of cataract.

    3. **Infrared radiation** (glassblower's and glassworker's cataract). Prolonged exposure (over several years) to infrared radiation leads to exfoliation of the anterior lens capsule. In contrast to the pseudoexfoliation seen in elderly patients, in true exfoliation large pieces of the lens capsule flake off and may curl back on themselves in the pupillary zone of the lens. Although this is not a true cataract, prolonged exposure may lead to the appearance of a diskoid posterior subcapsular opacity with many highly refractile spots. This cataract is rarely seen now but was common in the nineteenth century.

    4. **X-ray radiation.** Ionizing radiation is capable of producing a characteristic posterior subcapsular opacity. The degree of cataract formation is a function of the dose of radiation. As little as 300–400 rad, as a single dose, may lead to cataract formation. These opacities do not necessarily progress. With higher doses, the cataract may progress to involve the entire posterior subcapsular zone; in the case of extreme exposure to radiation, cataract formation may involve the entire lens. There is usually a latent period between the exposure and the onset of cataract that may be as brief as 6 months (after intensive exposures such as atomic bomb injury) or as long as several years. Neutron and alpha beams produce the greatest ionization and pose the greatest risk of cataract formation. The most frequently used radiation in medicine is gamma and x rays; therefore, these forms are most frequently associated with cataract formation. Appropriate shielding of the lens is necessary when tumors around the eye are being treated.

    5. **Microwave radiation.** Although it is possible to produce cataracts in animals exposed to high doses of microwave radiation, it is believed that microwave exposure in humans has not been associated with cataract for-

mation. Surveys of armed service personnel exposed to microwave radiation at radar installations have not revealed an increased incidence of cataracts. This remains, however, a potential cataractogenic factor.

6. **Ultraviolet (UV) radiation.** Exposure to UV radiation has been linked to human cataracts in many studies. This radiation is divided into three wavelength bands: UV-A (400–320 nm), UV-B (320–290 nm), and UV-C (290–100 nm). UV-A induces suntanning, UV-B blistering and skin cancer, and UV-C does not normally reach the earth's surface. Depletion of the ozone layer, however, is allowing more UV-B and potentially UV-C to penetrate our atmosphere. The cornea absorbs some of the UV-B (snow blindness is UV-B keratitis), but all wavelengths longer than 300 nm are transmitted into the eye. While the lens tends, in turn, to transmit UV-A, it absorbs almost all intraocular UV-B, the wavelength shown experimentally and clinically to be most damaging to the lens, particularly in formation of cortical and nuclear cataracts. Only the retina is susceptible to damaging effects from visible light. Ocular exposure to UV-B may be reduced by 50% by just wearing a hat with a brim, 95% by wearing ordinary glasses with plastic lenses, and 100% by using UV coat or UV screener incorporated into glasses lenses. Such UV screener may protect against cataract formation.

The ability of the natural lens to absorb UV light may have a protective effect on the retina. UV irradiation can cause macular degeneration in patients whose natural lenses have been removed because of cataracts. Because of this, manufacturers of intraocular lenses (IOLs) are incorporating filters in their lenses that block transmission of wavelengths below 400 nm. In 1989, 89% of all IOLs implanted had UV-absorbing chromophores bonded to polymethyl methacrylate (PMMA) of the optic. Similar filters are being used in spectacles. The patient benefits from both the filtered spectacles and the implants by experiencing less glare in bright light and perhaps greater macular longevity. Darkly tinted glasses block transmission of visible light but not of UV radiation. The patient must have UV screener to be fully protected.

7. **Electrical cataract.** Electrocution injury can be associated with cataract formation. The cataracts may involve both the anterior and the posterior subcapsular and cortical regions and are usually more extensive on the side with the greater electrical burn. The morphology of these cataracts varies but may include punctate dustlike vacuoles as well as linear and cortical spokes. Nuclear opacification is unusual.

8. **Copper (chalcosis) and iron (siderosis) cataracts.** Intraocular foreign bodies containing copper and iron may lead to cataract formation.

   a. **Copper** is extremely toxic to the eye and produces a sunflower cataract with small yellowish-brown dots in the pupillary zone in the subcapsular cortex. The petals of the sunflower may extend toward the equator. This cataract is frequently seen with a flashlight examination and should be looked for in any person with a history of an intraocular copper foreign body.

   b. Intralenticular **iron** may produce a brownish anterior subcapsular opacity without characteristic morphology. The brown color may involve other parts of the eye such as the iris or the cornea.

   c. Both copper and iron may lead to significant loss of vision.

9. **Syn- and cocataractogenic factors.** Many investigators have advocated the concept of cataractogenesis as the result of multiple subthreshold cataractogenic stresses. Each stress acting alone is insufficient to cause cataract; however, when these stresses act in concert, a cataract may form. It is possible that age is one of these cataractogenic stresses, and that the superimposition of other toxic stresses on an aging lens may accelerate the rate of cataract formation. Conversely, the elimination of one or more subcataractogenic stresses may delay or entirely prevent cataract formation.

F. **Other forms of secondary cataract**

1. **Traumatic cataract.** Lens opacification may occur in response to blunt and penetrating trauma.
2. **Cataract secondary to ocular inflammation.** Chronic keratitis, iritis, and posterior uveitis may all lead to cataract formation. The exact mechanism of lens opacification is poorly understood, but treatment of this cataract is addressed primarily to the control of the ocular inflammation and the minimization of the dose of corticosteroid used to treat the inflammation.
3. **Neoplasia.** Anterior and posterior segment tumors such as ocular melanoma and retinoblastoma may lead to cataract formation. Metastatic tumors involving the choroid or anterior segment may also cause cataract.

G. **Miscellaneous lenticular abnormalities**
   1. **Exfoliation or pseudoexfoliation.** Exfoliation is described in sec. **E.3.** Pseudoexfoliation is the deposition of a dandruff-like material on the anterior lens capsule, posterior iris, and ciliary processes and is associated with a form of open-angle glaucoma. The material does not derive from the lens capsule and is therefore called "pseudoexfoliation." It is of visual significance as it indicates a coexisting, potentially severe **glaucoma** and **weak lens capsule zonules,** which may make use of an **anterior chamber lens implant** advisable at the time of cataract surgery despite a successful extracapsular procedure.
   2. **Lens-induced inflammation.** A hypermature cataract may leak lens protein into the anterior chamber. These proteins may act as antigens and induce antigen-antibody formation, complement fixation, and inflammation. The lens proteins per se are not toxic or inflammatory, and suppression of the immune response will temporarily relieve the inflammation; however, permanent relief of this condition is obtained only by cataract extraction.
   3. **Lens-induced glaucoma.** In a similar manner, the leakage of lens protein into the anterior chamber may elicit a macrophage response. Macrophages engorged with lens protein obstruct the trabecular meshwork outflow tract, and aqueous humor produced within the eye cannot exit freely. An acute glaucoma called **phacolytic glaucoma** may arise. Treatment is by immediate cataract extraction.
   4. **Pupillary block glaucoma.** As a mature lens swells and becomes hypermature, the disintegration of protein molecules into smaller molecules results in intralenticular hypertonicity, and swelling may obstruct the iridolenticular interface. This leads to iris bombé and an acute form of **angle-closure glaucoma.** Peripheral iridectomy is inadequate treatment. The lens must be extracted to relieve the pupillary block. In other forms of pupillary block glaucoma, in which an intumescent lens is not involved, peripheral iridectomy is sufficient treatment.

VI. **Medical treatment of cataract**
   A. **Mydriatics.** The patient with a small axial cataract frequently may benefit from pupillary dilation (mydriasis); this allows the clear, paraxial lens to participate in light transmissions, image formation, and focusing. Mydriatic drugs may completely eliminate the glare and blur from these small central cataracts. Phenylephrine 2.5%, 1 drop bid in the affected eye, may clarify vision. In the hypertensive patient, the use of a short-acting, mydriatic-cycloplegic drug such as tropicamide 1% or cyclopentolate 1% will obviate the chance of aggravating the hypertension; i.e., these drugs are safer than phenylephrine.
   B. **Diabetes**
   1. **Senile cataracts** are widely believed to occur more frequently and mature more rapidly in diabetics. Although data on these points are inconclusive, it is clear that diabetic patients have their cataracts extracted earlier and in greater numbers than similar nondiabetic patients. Just as careful control of blood sugar levels can minimize the troublesome changes in refractive error that occur in patients with poorly controlled diabetes, some cataracts can be reversed through diabetic control. Advanced cataracts are not benefited by better diabetic control.

2. **Aldose reductase inhibitors** have been used successfully in animals to prevent "sugar cataract" (diabetic and galactosemic) formation. This finding has led to widespread optimism that such drugs will be beneficial in human diabetics. Blocking the conversion of glucose to sorbitol by aldose reductase might delay or prevent the adverse osmotic stress resulting from the intracellular accumulation of sorbitol, a sugar alcohol. These drugs are now under clinical evaluation.

C. **Removing cataractogenic agents. Irradiation** (infrared and x-ray radiation) as well as **drugs** (corticosteroids, phenothiazines, cholinesterase inhibitors, and others) can cause cataracts. Conversely, their removal may delay or prevent further progression of the cataract. Any drug or agent with known cataractogenic properties should be used as briefly or at as low a dose as possible (or both). Ophthalmologic evaluation before and during treatment can alert the physician to signs of further cataract formation.

VII. **Surgical treatment of cataract**

A. **When to operate**

1. **Visual considerations.** The mere presence of a cataract is insufficient reason for its removal. If the cataract is uniocular, surgery may be delayed until the cataract is mature, as long as the vision in the fellow eye is sufficient for the patient's needs and the patient does not need stereoscopic vision. If bilateral cataracts are present, extraction of the cataract from the eye with the lower visual acuity may be done when the patient regards the visual handicap as a significant deterrent to the maintenance of his or her usual life-style.

2. **Anesthesia options.** Cataract extraction can be done under local or general anesthesia. Local anesthesia minimizes the risk of wound rupture, a complication frequently associated with coughing during extubation and postoperative nausea and vomiting. The use of 1 : 4 mixed 2% xylocaine and 0.75% bupivacaine in facial and peribulbar or retrobulbar blocks achieves rapid anesthesia, akinesia, and postoperative analgesia for the first 8–10 hours. Plain (no epinephrine) anesthetics are much less painful and have less risk of cardiac effect. Care to avoid intravascular injections of anesthetic is essential, since refractory cardiorespiratory arrest may result from an inadvertent IV or intraarterial injection. Patients who are extremely apprehensive, deaf, mentally retarded, or unstable are frequently more suitable for general anesthesia. Many patients express an inappropriate dread of the facial and retrobulbar injections; although these injections are somewhat uncomfortable, proper preoperative sedation, e.g., IV versed, and good rapport with the surgeon make them quite tolerable.

3. **Preparation of a patient for surgery** should include a full explanation of the potential risks and benefits of proposed surgery and anesthesia as well as the technique for administering eye drops and ointments and other postoperative care. A model consent form to be signed by the physician and patient is now available from the American Academy of Ophthalmology, or doctors may elect to design their own. **Preoperative topical antibiotics** such as tobramycin qid for 3 days just before surgery is advisable prophylaxis against endophthalmitis. Studies indicate a reduction in incidence from 0.71–3.05% to 0.05–0.11% when preoperative antibiotics are given. Any blepharitis or dacryocystitis should be treated and resolved before intraocular surgery.

4. **Both outpatient and inpatient surgical facilities** are used for cataract surgery, with the latter reserved for patients at risk for medical complications. Well-designed, certified outpatient surgical facilities offer the patient the briefest possible surgical experience and reduce to a minimum the disruption of the patient's normal living routine. Such facilities offer the surgeon an opportunity to deliver state-of-the-art surgical care without tying up a hospital bed for 2 or 3 days; in addition, the patient is not exposed to nosologic infections. The cost of outpatient surgical care is also much less

than inpatient care. Of paramount importance in outpatient cataract surgery is proper preoperative and follow-up care.

B. Types of surgical techniques
   1. Intracapsular cataract extraction. Removal of the entire lens (with capsule intact) is performed with a forceps or cryophake. Usually the supporting zonules are dissolved with the enzyme alpha-chymotrypsin. This procedure was the most widely employed surgical technique of cataract extraction for nearly 50 years but has almost entirely been replaced by planned extracapsular technique in the past decade.
   2. Planned extracapsular extraction (Fig. 6-2). The vast majority of patients benefit from this technique that is designed to remove the opaque portion of the lens without disturbing the integrity of the posterior capsule and anterior vitreous face. This procedure is the procedure of choice in the great majority of cases due to the lower incidence of postoperative cystoid macular edema and retinal detachment, improved prognosis of subsequent glaucoma filtering surgery or corneal transplantation, reduced incidence of vitreocorneal touch and bullous keratopathy, and reduced secondary rubeosis in diabetics (especially compared with intracapsular cataract extraction). In this technique, the anterior capsule is opened, the nucleus expressed through a 9- to 10-mm incision, and the residual equatorial cortex aspirated, either manually or mechanically using an irrigation-aspiration (I-A) machine (e.g., Kelman, Site) or a hand-held device (e.g., Simcoe, McIntyre). The posterior capsule may be polished but is otherwise undisturbed, and serves as the resting site for posterior chamber lens implants and to stabilize the vitreous gel, thus minimizing cystoid macular edema. Some posterior capsules may opacify within a few months or years of surgery. These are easily opened on an outpatient basis using the neodymium YAG (yttrium, aluminum, garnet) laser (see sec. **VII.C.9**).
   3. Phacoemulsification and aspiration (Fig. 6-3).
      a. Technique. A titanium needle vibrating at ultrasonic frequencies (40,000 cps) can disrupt even hard adult nuclei. The resulting emulsion is then easily aspirated. Irrigating fluid enters the eye through a concentric sleeve around the titanium needle. This technique requires only a 3.5-mm incision in the wall of the eye **if no IOL is to be inserted** (unless foldable; see below) and allows the patient to resume normal activities (exclusive of contact sports) postoperatively. Contact lens fitting can be done after 3 weeks, compared with 2–3 months after planned extracapsular cataract extraction (PECCE) or intracapsular cataract extraction (ICCE). If a currently standard IOL is inserted, the wound is opened to 7.0–7.5 mm after phacoemulsification.
      b. Risks. The difficulty of emulsifying sclerotic brunescent cataracts deterred ophthalmic surgeons from offering phacoemulsification to patients with this type of cataract. Despite new designs of the titanium needle (thin-walled, oval, 15-, 30-, and 45-degree tip angles) and more powerful sonicators, which facilitate emulsification of brunescent nuclei, many surgeons feel that too much vibration and power release occur in the eye to be safe. Emulsification of the nucleus in the posterior chamber (behind the iris plane) has reduced the risk of damage to the corneal endothelium and, in certain patients, has reduced the importance of corneal endothelial dystrophy as a contraindication to phacoemulsification. There is a higher risk of capsular rupture, however. With the development of synthetic hyaluronic acid and chondroitin sulfate, both clear viscoelastic substances, and topical nonsteroidal anti-inflammatories (flurbiprofen), it has become possible in many cases to deal with shallow chambers and poorly dilating pupils—two conditions that dissuaded surgeons from considering this operation. In spite of the decreasing number of contraindications to phacoemulsification, the number of surgeons using this technique remains small because of the technical difficulty of the procedure and potential for rapidly occurring

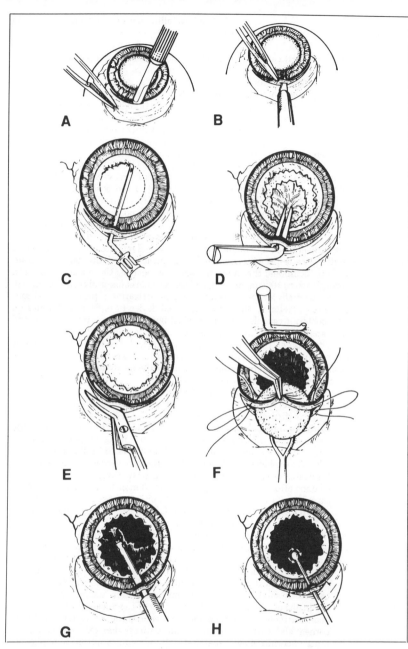

Fig. 6-2. Planned extracapsular cataract extraction by irrigation-aspiration technique.
A. Posterior limbal groove, 10–11 mm, 2/3 scleral depth. **B.** 3.5-mm entry into anterior
chamber (AC) with microsurgical blade, then placement of viscoelastic substance in
AC. **C.** 360-degree round cystotome opening of anterior capsule. **D.** Removal of anterior
capsule. **E.** Corneal scissors angled at 45 degrees extend wound to 10 mm. **F.** 10-0 nylon
or 7-0 Vicryl sutures 7 mm apart displaced from wound and nucleus expressed by
gentle pressure at 6 o'clock (muscle hook) and 12 o'clock (lens loop). Assistant lifts
cornea and rotates and "teases" nucleus out with 19-gauge needle. **G.** Irrigate AC, tie
sutures and place third suture at 12 o'clock before irrigation-aspiration of residual lens

Fig. 6-3. Planned extracapsular cataract extraction by phacoemulsification technique.
A. 7.0-mm groove (as in Fig. 6-2) if standard IOL to be placed and 3.2-mm keratome opening made into AC. **B.** Open anterior capsule as in Fig. 6-2. Perform phacoemulsification, sculpting nucleus from superior to inferior direction to create bowl shape, always keeping ultrasound port in view. **C.** Displace nucleus inferiorly with cyclodialysis spatula through paracentesis, irrigate, allow nucleus to rise, and slip phako tip behind superior lens equator (viscoelastic injection may aid in creating cleavage plane). **D.** Stabilize lens with spatula and complete phacoemulsification using aspiration mode (footswitch position 2), alternating with bursts of ultrasound (footswitch position 3) to emulsify, staying near center of pupil near iris plane. Eye is then ready for I-A and IOL as in Fig. 6-2. (Adapted from P. Hersh, *Ophthalmic Surgical Procedures.* Boston: Little, Brown, 1988. Pp., 103–105. With permission).

Fig. 6-2 (*continued*).
cortex. **H.** Gently clean posterior capsule (if necessary) with polisher, remove 12 o'clock suture, put viscoelastic in AC, and eye is ready for IOL (close pupil with intraocular carbachol or acetylcholine if AC IOL to be placed). Create peripheral iridectomy after IOL placement. (Adapted from P. Hersh, *Ophthalmic Surgical Procedures.* Boston: Little, Brown, 1988. Pp. 91–93. With permission).

intraoperative complications. Most surgeons elect to deliver the nucleus intact through a 10.5-mm corneoscleral incision, rather than to emulsify it through a 3.5-mm incision and then open the wound to 7 mm to place an IOL.

c. With the **advent of viscoelastic gels, better equipment, and foldable IOLs** (thus smaller wound openings) on the horizon, however, some surgeons are gradually turning to phacoemulsification (see sec. **C**), especially under the pressure of lay publicity. Recent data indicate that while there is an earlier visual recovery and return to full activity with smaller incisions of phacoemulsification, by 1–2 months postoperatively there is no significant difference in the visual outcome among patients who had 3.5-, 7.0-, or 10.0-mm incisions and uncomplicated I-A versus phacoemulsification. This must be balanced against the not widely publicized higher intraoperative phacoemulsification complication rate, which occurs in even the best surgeons' first few hundred cases (e.g., vitreous loss, nucleus loss into the vitreous), and the continued higher rate among surgeons who do not perform several hundred cataract extractions annually. There is no compelling evidence at this time to suggest that phacoemulsification is superior to standard I-A techniques or that the visual end results differ between the two procedures.

4. **Pars plana lensectomy and phacofragmentation.** Cataracts frequently obscure the vitreous pathology; to deal surgically with such pathology, the cataract may have to be removed. This is accomplished with an ultrasonic needle introduced through the sclera and pars plana. The emulsified lens is aspirated through the same needle; irrigation fluid enters the eye through a separate portal. This technique is not used for cataract extraction alone.

C. **Intraocular lenses (intraocular implants, IOLs).** In the past decade, the replacement of a cataractous crystalline lens with a clear lens of PMMA has become an integral part of almost every cataract procedure; more than 1 million IOLs were implanted in 1989. Of these lenses, 93% were the posterior chamber type (PC IOL), and 7% were anterior chamber type (AC IOL). Of the PC IOLs, 89% were UV absorbing, 26% had a laser ridge to hold the posterior capsule away from the optic (allowing more room for laser capsulotomy), and 0.6% were soft (hydrogel or silicone). Iris-fixation and iridocapsular IOLs are no longer used because of a higher complication rate. The rapid rise in number of IOLs implanted from 1983–1989 has now plateaued as the backlog of cataract patients who would benefit from this procedure have already undergone it. The number of implants largely reflects new cases of visually significant cataracts. The rapid rise in IOL implants and their popularity are a function of many factors such as increasing acceptance by doctors and patients alike, a growing appreciation of the improved visual rehabilitation and quality of vision compared to aphakia corrected by spectacles or the lesser convenience of contact lenses, the lowered postoperative complication rate of cystoid macular edema and retinal detachment with the extracapsular technique, improved instrumentation, better lens design, and the advent of viscoelastic substances.

1. **Anterior chamber intraocular lenses (AC IOLs)** are relatively easy to insert after ICCE or PECCE, and most are easy to remove if so indicated (Fig. 6–4A; Table 6-1). The first AC IOLs to gain acceptance were either rigid, vaulted, four-footed lenses or rigid, closed loop lenses, some of which had rough edges that induced the **UGH syndrome** of **uveitis, glaucoma,** and **hyphema** (blood in the anterior chamber) and had a higher incidence of corneal endothelial decompensation and cystoid macular edema than the newer flexible, open lenses. While the former IOLs are no longer available, there are an estimated 100,000 (of the more than 200,000 implanted) in patients with well-functioning eyes still in the population.

To reduce the postoperative complications and to avoid sizing problems that resulted from rigid, too large lenses eroding into and painfully inflaming the intraocular AC structures or too small lenses "propellering" in the AC, manufactures developed AC IOLs with flexible supporting loops that

Anterior Chamber Lenses

Fig 4. Full C-loop.

Fig 8. Spanflex type.

Fig 15. Modified C-loop with eyelets.

Fig 16. Kelman omnifit.

Fig 17. Choice Mark IV.

Fig 18. Choice Mark IX.

Fig 19. Four legs.

A

Posterior Chamber Lenses: J-Loop and Modified J-Loop Design

Fig 1. J-loop.

Fig 2. Modified J-loop.

Fig 3. Oval optic.

Posterior Chamber Lenses: C-Loop and Modified C-Loop Design

Fig 4. Full C-loop

Fig 5. Modified C-loop.

Fig 6. Extra long C-loops

Posterior Chamber Lenses: Other Lens Types

Fig 7. Two narrow, closed loops.

Fig 8. Spanflex type.

Fig 9. One closed, one open loop

Fig 10. Single loop design.

Fig 11. Two closed loops, Annis type.

Fig 12. Two small loops.

Fig 13. Dubroff type.

Fig 14. Silicone

B

Fig. 6-4. Currently available anterior **(A)** and posterior **(B)** chamber IOL styles, either FDA approved, under premarket approval, or investigational new drug (IND). See Tables 6-1 and 6-2 for specific data on various styles. (Adapted from A. Colenbrander, L. Woods, and R. Stamper, Intraocular lens data. *Ophthalmology* 96 [Suppl.]: 20, 1989. With permission).

Table 6-1. Anterior chamber intraocular lenses

Fig. no.[a]	Optics[b] Size (mm)	Powers (d)	Positioning holes[c]	Haptic size	Loop material	UV absorption[d]	Manufacturer[e]
4	5.5	10–27	0, 4	12.50/14	PMMA	0	1
8	5.0, 5.5, 6.0	4–30	0, 1, 4	12.25, 13.00, 13.50, 14.00	PMMA	0, +	2–8
15	5.5, 6.0	4–32	0/2		PCQ	0, +	1, 3, 7
16	5.5, 6.0	11–24	0/1	11.50, 13.20, 13.50, 14.20	PMMA	0	1, 9
17	6.0	5–30	0	11.50/13.50	PMMA	0	3
18	5.0	14–23	2	11.00/14.00	PMMA	+	7
19	6.0	6–28	0	12.50/13.50	PMMA	+	6

Key: PMMA = polymethyl methacrylate; PCQ = Perspex-CQ.
[a] Shown in Fig. 6-4A.
[b] All optics are made of polymethyl methacrylate.
[c] Positioning holes may be in or outside of optic, depending on lens design.
[d] UV + or 0 = lens with (+) or without (0) UV screener.
[e] Manufacturer:
1 = Allergan Medical Optics (800-348-6554).
2 = Alcon Surgical (800-862-5266).
3 = Cooper Vision CILCO (800-426-8903).
4 = Intraoptics (800-843-1137).
5 = IOPTEX Research (800-423-6557).
6 = Optical Radiation Corp. (800-423-1887).
7 = Storz Ophthalmics (800-237-5906).
8 = Surgidev Corp. (800-235-5781).
9 = IOLAB Corp. (800-423-1871).

rested gently against the angle structures. It has been shown that all closed-looped and open broad-loop AC IOLs have varying angle contact during flexion of the globe. This results in chronic irritation, secondary angle synechiae, endothelial cell loss, and/or cystoid macular edema. Current evidence indicates that the optimal IOLs are the three- and four-footed flexible open design (Kelman style), which maintain a small but constant area of angle contact with external ocular pressure. Flexible AC IOLs are available with or without UV screener, with a 6-mm optic with or without positioning holes, in size range 12-, 13-, and 14-mm diameter with a 0.75-mm range of flexion in the angle-to-angle diameter. In general, visual results are excellent, complications are low, and surgical outcome comparable with PC IOLs. Even with flexible loops, rarely a patient may have ocular tenderness upon touching the eye postoperatively. This is not an indication for removal of the IOL but that the patient stop rubbing the eye.

  2. Secondary IOL. For those patients who did not have an IOL implanted at the primary cataract extraction, a **secondary IOL** may be put in at a later time, thus avoiding need for cataract lenses and their inconvenience or aphakic spectacle correction with its distortion of vision, and giving the superior, more normal vision of the IOL. Preoperative evaluation for suitability should include specular microscopy (endothelial cell count should be greater than 1200 mm^2), no active intraocular inflammation, an intact posterior capsule (for PC IOLs), and a sufficiently intact iris for the AC IOL feet to rest upon with stability.

  3. Posterior chamber implants (PC IOLs) are by far the IOLs most commonly inserted after PECCE by I-A or phacoemulsification with the posterior capsule relatively intact (a small hole may still allow use of a PC IOL) (Figs. 6-4B and 6-5; Table 6-2). The loops fit either within the capsular "bag" of the lens or in the ciliary sulcus, a ridge just anterior to the ciliary processes. The loops prevent the lens from moving by becoming enmeshed in a fibrous cuff. The optic rests against the zonules and the posterior capsule. In certain patients with no intact capsule, a few surgeons are successfully suturing PC IOLs just behind the iris plane using iris or scleral fixation and 10-0 prolene sutures. Any advantage of this technique over AC IOLs has not yet been demonstrated.

   a. Design modifications. The first PC IOLs had simple J-loop prolene haptics and PMMA optics all in one plane. Since then, modification in designs in Fig. 6-4B include

     (1) A gentler J-curve or broadening the haptic all the way to a C-curve to increase the fixation contact.

     (2) Anterior angulation of the loops to minimize iris capture.

     (3) Reduction or elimination of fixation holes that might cause glare in an inordinately large pupil.

     (4) Varied optic sizes from 6.0 to 6.5 or 7.0 mm.

     (5) Incorporation of UV chromophores to screen out harmful UV-B rays.

     (6) Use of PMMA for both haptic and optic construction to reduce potential inflammatory reaction to prolene degradable haptics.

     (7) Use of single-piece construction.

     (8) Biconvex optics to decrease posterior capsule hazing.

     (9) Laser ridges.

     (10) Introduction of multifocal and soft foldable IOLs (see secs. **5** and **6**).

       All of the above are generally aimed at various levels of IOL improvement, but each lens design must be selected on the basis of its suitability for a given patient situation, and not all modifications invariably achieve the desired end point.

   b. Disadvantage. Although the reduced incidence of cystoid macular edema and retinal detachment following extracapsular cataract extraction with PC IOL implantation is well documented, the technical difficulty of

Fig. 6-5. Insertion of PC IOL. **A.** After AC deepening with viscoelastic, place inferior haptic into capsular bag or ciliary sulcus, depending on type of IOL fixation desired. **B.** Secure superior haptic with forceps and advance lens into eye. **C.** Push haptic into anterior chamber, pronate hand to flex knee of haptic behind iris, and release haptic into desired position. **D and E.** Use Sinsky hook to center optic and rotate lens to horizontal orientation, using positioning holes if present. **F.** Remove viscoelastic with irrigation-aspiration on minimum, close pupil with intraocular carbachol or acetylcholine, and perform peripheral iridectomy. **G.** Close wound with 10-0 nylon (90% depth) and replace any Vicryl sutures. Retract beyond posterior limbus and, if possible, bury knots. Finish by standard techniques. (Adapted from P. Hersh, *Ophthalmic Surgical Procedures.* Boston: Little, Brown, 1988. P. 95. With permission.)

Table 6-2. Posterior chamber intraocular lenses

Fig. no.[a]	Optics[b] Size (mm)	Optics[b] Powers (d)	Positioning holes[c]	Haptic size (mm)	Loop material	Haptic angle (degrees)	UV absorption[d]	Manufacturer[e]
1	6.0	4–32	0, 2	13, 14	PMMA, Prol	0/10	0, +	1–4
2	6.0, 6.5, 7.0	4–35	0, 4	12, 13 13.5, 14, 14.5	Polyprop PMMA, Prol	0/10	0, +	1–3, 5–14
3	5.0, 6.0	4–32	0, 2	13.5, 14	Prol	0/10	+	6
4	6.0, 6.5 7.0	4–35	0, 4, 6	13.2, 13.5 13.8, 14.0	Prol, PMMA Polyprop	0/8 9/10	0, +	1–8, 10–13
5	6.0, 6.5 7.0	4–35	0, 2, 4	11.0, 13.50 13.80, 14.00	Prol PMMA	0/3/6 7/10	0, +	1–13, 15
6	5.8, 6.0 6.5, 7.0	4–32	0, 2	11.00, 12.00 13.50, 14.00	PMMA	0/6 7.5/10	0, +	1–3, 6, 9–11, 13, 15
7	6.0	8–28	0	12.50	PMMA	0/3	0, +	11, 14
8	6.0	8–30	0, 4	12.00, 13.50, 14.00	PMMA	—	0, +	3, 13
9	6.0	5–30	0, 1	12.50, 13.25	Prol, PPMA	0	0, +	2, 3, 6
10	6.0	14–27	2	12.00	PMMA	0	+	13
11	6.0	4–32	2	10.50	Prol, PMMA	0	0, +	2, 3, 6
12	6.5	4–32	0, 1	10, 11.35	PMMA	0	+	6, 13
13	6.0	10–28	3	14.00	PMMA	0	+	3
14	6.0	4–32	0, 2	10.5, 11.00, 11.50	Silicone	0	0	6, 12

Key: PMMA = polymethyl methacrylate; Prol = prolene;
Polyprop = polypropylene.
[a] Shown in Fig. 6–4B.
[b] All optics are made of polymethyl methacrylate except for #14 (silicone).
[c] Positioning holes may be in or outside of optic, depending on lens design.
[d] UV + or 0 = lens with (+) or without (0) UV screener.

[e] Manufacturer:
1 = Alcon Surgical (800-862-5266).
2 = Optical Radiation Corp. (800-423-1887).
3 = Pharmacia Intermedics Ophthalmicus (800-423-4866).
4 = Surgidev Corp. (800-235-5781).
5 = Allergan Medical Optics (800-348-6554).
6 = Cooper Vision CILCO (800-426-6903).
7 = Eye Technology (800-722-3985).
8 = International Ophthalmics (800-284-IOLS).
9 = Intraoptics (800-843-1137).
10 = IOLAB Corp. (800-423-1871).
11 = IOPTEX Research (800-423-6557).
12 = Staar Surgical Corp. (800-352-7842).
13 = Storz Ophthalmics (800-237-5906).
14 = 3M Vision Care (800-322-6981).
15 = Domilens (800-426-5968).

removing a PC IOL remains a major potential disadvantage of this type of implant. Fortunately, the need for removal of PC IOLs has been far less than for all other styles of implants, and it is the hope of all ophthalmologists that this risk will remain a potential one.

4. **Complications of AC and PC IOLs** are rare, often self-resolving or resolved with medical therapy, and usually less than 1 or 2%. In order of approximate decreasing frequency the most common are macular edema, secondary glaucoma, hyphema, iritis, corneal edema, pupillary block, retinal detachment, vitritis, endophthalmitis, and cyclitic membrane.

5. **Foldable PC IOLs** made of hydrogel or silicone are now under study in a few centers under an FDA Investigational New Drug (IND) status.
   a. The proposed **advantages** of such lenses are
      (1) Insertion through a small incision: 6 mm for standard designs; 4.5 mm for expansile hydrogel lenses, which increase in size by 30% after insertion; and although not a true soft IOL, 3 mm for the PMMA Phakofit lens with foldable lateral wings, which spring open behind the iris after insertion.
      (2) Good to excellent tolerance and flexibility.
      (3) Hydrophilic properties that reduce endothelial damage through low interfacial energy.
      (4) Autoclavability.
      (5) Reduced astigmatism and faster rehabilitation due to smaller incisions.
      (6) Thicker lens (silicone), which fills and distends the posterior capsular bag more fully, possibly decreasing incidence of capsular haze [however, see sec. **b.(2)**].
      (7) Development of **capsulorhexis** (round continuous tear anterior capsulotomy), which may enhance ease of "in the bag" lens placement. This procedure is difficult to learn.
   b. The **disadvantages** of the current generation of foldable PC IOLs occasionally reported are
      (1) A tendency to decenter.
      (2) Increased capsular opacification, zonular, or capsular fibrosis.
      (3) Imperfect surface finishing especially with silicone lenses (possible potential for UGH syndrome).
      (4) Severe iris chafing.
      (5) Weak tensile strength with lens tears and increased susceptibility to damage.
      (6) Groove marks from insertion instruments.
      (7) Tissue damage when lens released from folding instrument.
      (8) Visual acuity possibly not as good.
      (9) Suboptimal insertion instruments and difficulty inserting lens without tissue damage.
      (10) Pitting during YAG capsulotomy.
   c. As with phacoemulsification, neither surgeon nor patient should be pressured by peers or publicity into having a procedure that is not yet fully developed or shown to be superior to current standard PECCE with PMMA IOLs.

6. **Multifocal PC IOLs** are also being studied under an FDA-IND status. These lenses focus both near and far objects, placing images on the macula simultaneously. The brain decides which image to concentrate on via selective vision. Success will be determined by whether the patient can distinguish between the two objects. For the best-case patients in the current FDA study, 82% had near vision of J-1 to J-3 with distance correction only. Clinical trials of two multifocals, a diffractive style lens and a modification of this, are now under way, and preliminary results are encouraging. A third style, an aspheric lens, is awaiting IND status, and a fourth style with five optical zones is awaiting clinical trials as well. More than 5000 diffractive

lenses have been implanted worldwide, but follow-up of at least 1–2 years is needed to begin to have reliable safety and efficacy data.

7. **Contraindications to IOL implantation** include active, uncontrollable uveitis (see sec. **VII.E**), proliferative diabetic retinopathy, glaucoma with progressive visual field loss (although with PC IOLs this may be a relative contraindication), and youth. The lower limit of age at which it is safe to implant a lens is not known. Ophthalmologists in only a few centers are implanting lenses in children, and they are doing so according to carefully designed and monitored clinical research protocols. Most centers regard 30–40 years of age as the limit below which patients may be too young for IOL implantation. There is considerable difference of opinion regarding this lower limit however, some surgeons believing it to be too low, others too high. Other contraindications include aniridia and a history of IOL intolerance in a fellow eye unless judged due to suboptimal lens style or intraoperative complication. Over the years, the list of contraindications has decreased in size as surgical techniques and implant quality have improved.

8. **Results of IOL implantation** have been generally excellent with final visual acuity of 20/40 or better in greater than 90% of AC and PC IOLs. PC IOLs may give slightly better results regardless of age by currently available studies (94% versus 90%). There is evidence, however, that PECCE surgery coupled with an AC IOL may give equally good results and should be considered in certain patients, e.g., pseudoexfoliation with weak zonules.

9. **YAG capsulotomy.** In patients over 65 years of age, the posterior capsule usually remains clear behind the optic. In younger patients, and in some older patients, the capsule often opacifies and must be opened. Prior to the advent of the YAG laser, the posterior capsulotomy with a PC IOL in place was a formidable surgical challenge. The YAG laser has simplified this procedure, however, and in fact has prompted lens manufacturers to place small ridges on the posterior surfaces of the optic to keep the capsule away from the surface of the optic and avoid inadvertent damage to the optic when the laser light is used to cut the posterior capsule (see sec. **B.2**). If the lens dislocates sideways during normal postoperative fibrosis, however, otherwise clear vision may be blocked by the ridge. It is possible to fracture or pit the optic with the YAG laser beam, but fortunately these small imperfections are usually insignificant. Whether these ridges are useful will be seen. Photodisruptive powers used range from 0.6 mJoules for thin capsules to 3.5 mJoules for dense fibrous bands (usually posttraumatic).

D. **Postoperative care**
   1. **Wound healing** occurs slowly over a 6- to 8-week period, but refractive changes due to further healing of the incision occur up to 9 months postoperatively. As corneal anesthesia decreases, contact lenses can be fitted if the patient did not receive an IOL. Nonabsorbable sutures may be cut or removed if protruding or inducing astigmatism usually between 6 and 8 weeks; some are not removed. Topical corticosteroids, used to control postoperative inflammation, may retard healing slightly, but patients with nonphysically-straining jobs are often back to work in 3–5 days.
   2. **Postoperative medications.** Patients often receive subconjunctival tobramycin (40 mg), gentamicin (40 mg), or cefazolin (100 mg) and a steroid such as methylprednisolone (50 mg), 1–4% pilocarpine drop, and antibiotic ointment at the end of the procedure, with regular topical medicine deferred until the next day. If elevated pressure is anticipated, a carbonic anhydrase inhibitor may be given immediately postoperatively and for taking at home. Common postoperative regimen includes antibiotic-steroid combinations, e.g., Pred-G or Tobradex bid-qid for 2–3 weeks and then a mild steroid (FML) qd for 3–4 weeks. Pilocarpine 1% bid for 7 days is useful for pressure control and to prevent pupillary capture of the optic in the immediate postoperative period.

3. **Dressings.** An eye patch is used for only a few days postoperatively; a protective shield is worn at night to avoid injury to the eye during sleep for 6 weeks.

4. **Activities and limitations.** Due to the advances in the manufacture and use of suture materials, the postoperative wound strength is sufficient to allow resumption of normal daily activities with little risk of wound rupture. It is still prudent, however, to avoid contact sports, vigorous exertion, excessive bending from the waist, and heavy lifting for approximately 6 weeks postoperatively.

5. **General medical considerations.** Constipation, coughing, and wheezing should be avoided. Any stressful diagnostic procedure, such as sigmoidoscopy, barium enema, pulmonary function studies, and exercise tolerance tests, should be delayed, if possible, for 6 weeks. Anticoagulant therapy should be delayed for at least a few weeks. Most topical medications used postoperatively (topical steroid drops and antibiotics) have minimum and easily recognizable systemic side effects. Carbonic anhydrase inhibitors used to treat postoperative glaucoma may lead to potassium depletion and cardiac arrhythmias. The control of diabetes mellitus is usually easily reestablished, but ocular complications of cataract surgery may interfere with this.

E. **Cataract surgery in uveitis patients.** Posterior subcapsular cataracts are common complications of uveitis, particularly cyclitis. It is possible, however, to control the uveitis and place an **IOL** successfully in many of these patients through judicious uses of perioperative anti-inflammatory therapy.

Drug management in cataract surgery in the uveitic eye includes the following: Inflammation should be suppressed to 0-2 leukocytes/0.2 mm high slit beam in the aqueous or anterior vitreous for at least 3 months preoperatively. This may be done through the previously discussed use of topical, periocular injected, and systemic corticosteroids, NSAIDS, and, where indicated, immunosuppressive agents. For the 3 days prior to surgery, each patient is treated with 1 mg/kg/day of oral prednisone with breakfast, diflusinal, 500 mg PO bid, and topical 1% prednisolone or 0.1% dexamethasone qid along with continuation of any immunosuppressive therapy on which the patient may have been placed. If an IOL is to be placed, a posterior chamber lens is recommended to minimize uveal tissue contact. At the end of the surgical procedure, 80 mg of subconjunctival methylprednisolone is injected and usually an antibiotic such as 40 mg of tobramycin or gentamycin or 100 mg of cefazolin. Postoperatively, topical 1% prednisolone or 0.1% dexamethasone is used 4–8 times daily, depending on the anterior chamber inflammation, and systemic prednisone is tapered and discontinued after the inflammation has cleared (unless the patient is maintained on this drug for systemic disease). Diflusinal is continued for 2 months postoperatively along with any immunosuppressives indicated for the primary disease.

F. **Cystoid macular edema therapy with nonsteroidal anti-inflammatory drugs.** A leading cause of visual loss after cataract extraction, about 3–5%, is aphakic or pseudophakic cystoid macular edema. Although the majority of affected eyes will ultimately regain good vision, cystoid macular edema prolongs the postoperative recovery period and causes concern for physician and patient alike.

1. **Etiology.** Cystoid macular edema is a nonspecific response, which may result from a variety of ocular conditions, leading to a disruption of a blood-ocular barrier as well as clinical and histologic evidence of inflammation, particularly following cataract surgery. These factors include excessive or prolonged postoperative uveal inflammation, intraoperative vitreous loss, intracapsular cataract extraction, and extracapsular cataract extraction with primary capsulotomy.

Prostaglandins are unsaturated fatty acid derivatives formed from arachidonic acid. Their effects on the eye include disruption of the blood-ocular barriers, dilatation of iris vessels, miosis, and alteration of the intraocular pressure. They are found in increased concentrations in the aqueous during cataract extraction and are hypothesized an etiologic factor in the development of aphakic cystoid macular edema.

2. **Aphakic cystoid macular edema** frequently undergoes transient periods of relapse and recovery and, while not entirely benign, is generally considered self-limited regardless of treatment regimen.

3. **Pseudophakic cystoid macular edema** is more persistent and often requires therapeutic intervention.

4. **Medical therapy** of cystoid macular edema (CME) is still a controversial topic, as there are no well-controlled studies. Nonetheless, NSAIDs are prostaglandin inhibitors and are currently favored for management of macular edema, although guidelines for specific indications of use are not well defined. Current recommendations for use of NSAIDs in cystoid macular edema are when topical steroids cannot be used, as in the occurrence of ocular hypertensive response to steroid therapy or a history of preexisting ocular hypertension or glaucoma, or as primary therapy. One regimen that has been successful in numerous patients is flurbiprofen 0.03% drop to the affected eye q2h for 1 week followed by 1 drop q4h for 2 weeks. If improved, patients are then continued on flurbiprofen 3–6 times daily for 1–3 months, then bid for 8–12 months or for at least 2 months after fluorescein angiogram has shown resolution of CME. Systemic NSAIDs, e.g., naprosyn or indocin PO tid, are also often effective.

G. **Visual rehabilitation**

1. **Temporary cataract glasses** are dispensed to patients who have not received an IOL immediately postoperatively if the vision in the unoperated eye is poor. Although vision with these glasses is not perfectly clear, acuity is usually sufficiently good so that patients accept them. Aphakic spectacles contain thick convex lenses; unavoidable optical aberrations with these lenses are (1) 30–35% magnification of objects in the field of view, (2) a dramatic restriction of the width of the visual field, (3) a circular zone around the central field in which the patient sees nothing, and (4) the annoying "jack-in-the-box" phenomenon, an apt term describing the manner in which objects in the blind circular paracentral field suddenly pop into view. If the patient's unoperated eye has good vision, usually he or she will not willingly wear temporary or permanent cataract glasses for ambulation and driving due to these optical problems. *It is not possible to use an aphakic lens over only the operated eye, since this would lead to intolerable diplopia based on image size discrepancy.* It would also lead to tilting of the glasses, since the weight of the cataract lens is greater than the phakic lens. To many patients, monocular aphakia is a visual handicap far greater than the blurred but otherwise normal vision before cataract surgery. It is therefore advisable to defer cataract extraction of a unilateral cataract unless the patient has a mature lens, a lens-induced complication, or a willingness to use contact lenses or IOLs.

2. **Tinted lenses** are very helpful postoperatively (see sec. **V.E.6**).

3. **Contact lenses** (soft, hard, gas permeable). Without going into the specific advantages and disadvantages of each form of contact lens, it is important to understand that contact lenses offer the postoperative cataract patient many advantages. Image magnification is usually less than 7% and does not lead to image size diplopia. Binocular fusion is possible, so depth perception is normal. Visual field size is unrestricted, and there are none of the other optical disadvantages of aphakic spectacles. Contact lenses may be more difficult to insert and remove, however, and the rate of contact lens failure increases with age. **Continuous-wear lenses** are available as hard, semisoft, and soft lenses. They may be worn continuously, being removed for cleaning only every 6 months in the ideally fitted patient. It is difficult, however, to predict for an individual patient the likelihood of a successful fit. The success rate decreases with increasing age, climate (patients in dry dusty areas do poorly), and intercurrent illness (e.g., keratitis sicca, arthri-

tis, senility, seborrheic blepharitis). Approximately 70% of all patients are successful with continuous-wear aphakic lenses (see Chaps. 5 and 13).

4. **IOLs** spare patients the challenge of insertion and removal that they experience with contact lenses. Image magnification is usually less than 3%, and visual field size is unrestricted. It is necessary, however, to measure corneal curvature and axial length of the eye accurately in order to select an IOL based on A-scan ultrasound calculations that will yield a refractive error postoperatively that is similar to the unoperated eye. It is not advisable to insert an "average" IOL, because many patients will have significant inequality of refractive errors postoperatively.

VIII. Referral criteria for internists, pediatricians, and primary care physicians

  A. Congenital cataracts. Of utmost importance in the restoration of vision in an infant with congenital cataracts is detection of the cataracts in the first few months of life. Prompt referral to a pediatric ophthalmologist is indicated. The prognosis for visual improvement surprisingly is better for children with bilateral rather than unilateral congenital cataracts.

  B. Strabismus. An imbalance of eye movement or an abnormality of eye position may be due to cataract. A lens examination is done as part of any strabismus evaluation. Once again, prompt referral of children with strabismus is most important.

Retina and Vitreous

Mohandas M. Kini

I. **Normal anatomy and physiology** (see frontispiece)

A. **The retina** is the innermost layer of the eye and is derived from neuroectoderm. It is composed of two layers, the outer retinal pigment epithelium (RPE) and the inner neural retina, with a potential space between the two layers. The RPE, a single layer of hexagonal cells, is continuous with the pigment epithelium of the ciliary body at the **ora serrata**. The inner sensory retina is a delicate sheet of transparent tissue varying in thickness from 0.4 mm near the optic nerve to approximately 0.15 mm anteriorly at the ora serrata. The center of the **macula** contains the thin sloping **fovea** that lies 3 mm temporal to the temporal margin of the optic nerve. The macula is close to the insertion of the inferior oblique muscle and is made almost entirely of cones. It is the site of detailed fine central vision (20/20 normal). Visual acuity drops off rapidly in the paramacular areas and is only 20/400 at a distance of 2 or 3 mm from the fovea. The ora serrata is located 6 mm posterior to the corneoscleral limbus nasally and 7 mm temporally. The scleral insertions of the medial rectus and the lateral rectus serve as landmarks for the location of the ora serrata nasally and temporally.

Nutritional support for the sensory retina comes largely from the Müller cell, which spans almost the entire thickness of the retina. The retina is nourished by the retinal vessels posteriorly to the level of the outer plexiform layer. The photoreceptors and the RPE are nourished by the choriocapillaris of the choroid.

B. **Histology.** The retina consists of 10 parts, proceeding from outward in.
   1. Retinal pigment epithelium.
   2. Photoreceptor cells (rods and cones).
   3. External limiting membrane.
   4. Outer nuclear layer.
   5. Outer plexiform layer.
   6. Inner nuclear layer.
   7. Inner plexiform layer.
   8. Ganglion cell layer.
   9. Nerve fiber layer.
   10. Inner limiting membrane.

C. **Physiology.** The neuronal component of the retina consists of rods and cones that transduce light signals into electric impulses, which are amplified and integrated through circuitry involving bipolar, horizontal, amacrine, and ganglion cells, and transmitted through the nerve fiber layer to the optic nerve.

D. **Vitreous.** The vitreous body, which makes up the largest volume of the eye, provides support for the delicate inner structures of the eye. It is limited by the lens anteriorly and by the ciliary body and the retina posteriorly. The vitreous is a clear jellylike substance consisting of a delicate framework of **collagen** interspersed with a hydrophilic mucopolysaccharide, **hyaluronic acid.** Delicate collagen fibrils attach the vitreous to the internal limiting membrane of the retina, the attachment being strongest at the ora serrata, optic disk, and the foveal area.

II. **Test of retinal function** (see Chap. 1, secs. **II.A, C, G, I** and **III.A–E**; Chap. 12, sec. **I.**)

 A. **Visual function** is classified under the terms *light sense, form sense,* and *color sense.* Scientifically, these characteristics of incident light striking the eye are analyzed in terms of spatial, luminous, spectral, and temporal functions.

  1. **Visual acuity.** In clinical practice, form sense is assessed by use of such tests as the Snellen chart test (see Chap. 1, sec. **II.A**). This test is primarily of macular function. It is subjective and depends on patient cooperation. Objective tests are of value in assessing visual acuity of infants, mentally disturbed patients, and malingerers. The amplitude of the visual evoked response (VER) or the optokinetic nystagmus response can be correlated with visual acuity. Thus, it is estimated that the visual acuity at birth is approximately 20/600, improving by the age of 5 months to 20/60 and to adult levels by the age of 2 years.

  2. **Perimetry.** Light sense is assessed by visual field examination, which reflects any damage to the visual pathway from the retina to the visual cortex. The conventional method of testing the visual field is called **kinetic perimetry** and consists of moving a target to identify points of equal retinal sensitivity. The normal visual field extends at least 90 degrees on the temporal side, 70 degrees nasally and inferiorly, and 60 degrees superiorly. **Static perimetry** involves the determination of the differential light threshold in chosen areas of the retina. This method is more sensitive and reproducible than kinetic perimetry.

  3. **Color vision.** The retinal cones mediate color vision. Many abnormalities of visual function are characterized by defects in color vision. The simplest and best known method of testing color vision is by the use of **Ishihara** pseudoisochromatic plates. The Ishihara plates can only identify defects in red-green discrimination, whereas the American Optical *Hardy-Rand-Rittler* (HRR) plates are useful in detecting red-green and blue-yellow defects. The Farnsworth-Munsell *100 Hue* test and anomaloscopes are more sophisticated devices used in clinical research on color vision testing.

  4. **Dark adaptation.** This test depends on the increase in visual sensitivity occurring in the eye when it goes from the light-adapted state to the dark-adapted state. The Goldmann-Weekers machine is used to plot the dark adaptation curve. The eye to be tested is exposed to a bright light for 10 minutes and then all lights are extinguished. At intervals of 30 seconds a measurement of light threshold is made in one area of the visual field by presenting a gradually increasing light stimulus until it is barely visible to the patient. The graph of decreasing retinal threshold against time shows an initial steep slope denoting cone adaptation and a subsequent gradual slope due to dark adaptation. Depression of the dark adaptation curve occurs in conditions affecting the outer retina and RPE, such as retinitis pigmentosa.

  5. **Fluorescein angiography** is the study of retinal and choroidal vasculature using fluorescein (see Chap. 1, sec. **III.A**).

   a. **Technique.** Fluorescence is a physical property of certain substances that, on exposure to light of short wavelength, emit light of longer wavelength in a characteristic spectral range. Sodium fluorescein, a yellow-red substance, absorbs light between 485 and 500 nm in aqueous solution and exhibits a maximum emission between 525 and 530 nm. A 5-ml bolus of dye is rapidly injected via the antecubital vein, and rapid retinal photographs are taken with a fundus camera containing an excitatory filter with maximum transmission between 485 and 500 nm and a barrier filter peaking close to the maximum of the fluorescein emission curve (between 525 and 530 nm). The value of fluorescein angiography is based on the fact that fluorescein dye leaks freely from the normal choriocapillaris but does not penetrate healthy RPE and normal retinal capillaries because of the tight endothelial junction present in the latter. Under optimum conditions, the smallest retinal capillaries (5–10 μ in diameter) can be seen with this technique, a feat impossible by ophthalmoscopy or by color photography.

b. **Use in retinal disease.** Fluorescein angiography is of particular value in elucidating small vessel disease such as diabetic retinopathy, outlining clearly such changes as microaneurysms, shunt vessels, and early sites of neovascularization. New retinal vessels, both on the surface of the retina and those proliferating into the vitreous, characteristically leak fluorescein because of the absence of tight endothelial junctions. Angiography provides a valuable means of identifying such vessels in diabetes, sickle cell disease, and retinal vein obstruction, and of assessing the efficacy of treatment, particularly photocoagulation, in eliminating these vessels.

c. **Use in choroidal disease.** Fluorescein angiography is useful in assessing **choroidal circulation,** particularly in identifying foci of choroidal neovascularization as seen in conditions such as senile macular degeneration and ocular histoplasmosis.

d. **Use in RPE and optic nerve evaluation.** Although angiography does not provide any clue regarding the function of RPE, it anatomically delineates the true extent of atrophy of RPE in diseases affecting RPE, such as rubella, retinitis pigmentosa, drusen, and fundus flavimaculatus. Angiography is also helpful in distinguishing early papilledema, in which both the superficial and deep vascular networks become dilated and leak fluorescein. Papillitis shows many of the fluorescein characteristics of early papilledema. In optic atrophy there is a loss of vessels in both the superficial and the deep networks.

6. **Electrophysiology.** There are three major electrophysiologic tests used in the investigation of the visual system (see also Chap. 1, sec. III.C and D).

a. **Electrooculography (EOG)** measures slow changes in the resting retinal potential. Electrodes are attached to the skin over the orbital margin opposite the medial and lateral canthi, and the potential difference between the electrodes is amplified and recorded, after both light and dark adaptation. The maximum height of the potential in light divided by the minimum height of the potential in dark is multiplied by 100 to give the **Arden** ratio. Since the EOG reflects the presynaptic function of the retina, any disease that interferes with the functional interplay between the RPE and the photoreceptors will produce an abnormal or absent light rise in the EOG. Thus, the EOG is affected in diseases such as **retinitis pigmentosa, choroideremia, vitamin A deficiency, toxic retinopathies, and retinal detachment.**

b. **Electroretinography (ERG)** reflects the chain of graded electric responses from each layer of the retina. The human response, for clinically useful purposes, is a biphasic wave, an early negative *a* wave, generated by the rods and cones, followed by a larger positive *b* wave, generated at the bipolar cells. The recording is done with a corneal contact lens electrode and a reference electrode on the forehead. Both scotopic and photopic responses can be elicited in the ERG. In addition, rod-mediated and cone-mediated responses can be differentiated because of the fact that cones are sensitive to longer wavelengths (red) and rods are sensitive to shorter wavelengths (blue). In addition, the ERG can distinguish the differences in response between the rods and cones to flickering flash, since the cones have a much higher temporal resolution than the rods. The ERG is very useful in evaluating early retinal function loss before ophthalmoscopic changes are evident. The ERG is normal in diseases involving only the ganglion cells and the higher visual pathway, such as optic atrophy.

c. **VER.** The VER is the response of the electroencephalogram (EEG) recorded at the occipital pole and is a macula-dominated response, due to the disproportionately large projection of the macular retina in the occipital cortex. The VER can be recorded using an intense flash stimulation or a pattern stimulation. The VER is the only clinically objective technique available to assess the functional state of the visual system beyond the retinal ganglion cells. The flash VER can assess **retinocortical function in infants and demented or aphasic patients,** and it can distinguish patients with psychological blindness from those who have an organic basis for poor vision.

III. Retinal vascular disease

A. Retinal vascular anomalies cause loss of visual function primarily through incompetence of the endothelial lining of the anomalous vessels, permitting escape of exudate and, less often, blood into the retinal tissues and the subretinal space. The serous component of the exudate is resorbed, resulting in a massive ring-shaped deposit, often in the macular area. The presence of such a deposit in a young person should lead to the search of the peripheral retina for a vascular anomaly. The only effective method of treatment of these lesions is **photocoagulation** for lesions less than 2.5 disk diameter (dd) and located posterior to the equator, and **cryotherapy** with repeated freeze and slow thawing for lesions larger than 2.5 dd or located anterior to the equator. Photocoagulation and cryotherapy have largely replaced diathermy and irradiation as therapeutic modalities for these conditions. Photocoagulation or cryotherapy is hardly effective once serous detachment of the retina has occurred. Retinal vascular anomalies may be classified as follows.

1. Retinal telangiectasia or Coats's disease. The basic lesion in Coats's disease is a congenital anomaly of the vasculature of the retina and optic nerve, manifested ophthalmoscopically as telangiectasia. Fluorescein angiography shows an abnormally coarse net of dilatated capillaries, often with irregular aneurysmal dilations and leakage of fluorescein. The telangiectasis may involve either superficial or deep retinal vessels or both. Hemorrhage may occur from the deep telangiectasia, producing subretinal mounds of exudate. Even advanced cases may regress spontaneously. Retinal telangiectasia is often bilateral. Patients with loss of central vision from subretinal or intraretinal exudation are ideal candidates for photocoagulation. There is a high incidence of recurrence after treatment; therefore, these patients should be followed indefinitely.

2. Retinal angiomatosis or von Hippel-Lindau disease. The basic lesion in von Hippel-Lindau disease is a vascular hamartoma consisting of capillaries with proliferating endothelial cells, a feeding artery, and draining veins. Partly through abnormal hemodynamics and partly through hypertrophy and hyperplasia of the constituent elements, these lesions may enlarge over a period of time. However remote the lesion may be, abnormal permeability results in changes at the macular region, including development of hard exudates, retinal edema, serous detachment of the retina, and intraretinal deposits such as cholesterol. Photocoagulation of selected parts of the tumor may temporarily reduce the amount of exudation, but treatment of angiomas on or near the temporal margin of the optic nerve head is difficult without destroying central vision.

3. Retinal cavernous hemangioma may arise in the retina or optic nerve head. The lesion is composed of clusters of saccular aneurysms filled with dark venous blood. Fluorescein angiography shows that these lesions do not leak and that they have a sluggish blood flow. Dermal vascular lesions and intracranial lesions may be associated with this condition. Photocoagulation may be used when spontaneous hemorrhage occurs.

4. Arteriovenous (AV) aneurysms, a rare condition, have been called "racemose" or "cirsoid" aneurysms. Small-caliber aneurysms are well compensated and stationary and usually do not require any treatment. Large-caliber AV aneurysms often have a breakdown of the blood-retinal barrier, with development of macular edema and a reduction of vision. Photocoagulation may be of benefit in these cases. Severe cases of widespread AV aneurysms, often with intracranial associations, are not amenable to therapy because of widespread retinal disorganization.

5. **Retinal macroaneurysms** occur in the retinal arteries of arteriosclerotic and often hypertensive elderly patients. The aneurysms present as a large local retinal hemorrhage, but they tend to become thrombosed and resolve. The artery beyond the aneurysm is often sclerosed and occluded. If macular edema or exudate formation is present, photocoagulation may be of help.

B. **Vascular retinopathies** affect the retina by means of two basic mechanisms: (1) abnormal vascular permeability, resulting in changes seen in retinal vascular anomalies such as Coats's disease, and (2) **retinal ischemia.** The ischemic response of the retina results in the following changes:

1. Acute intracellular edema.
2. Neovascularization.
3. Vitreous hemorrhage and fibrosis.
4. Retinal traction with detachment.
5. **Management** of the vascular retinopathies consists of treatment of the underlying medical condition. **Photocoagulation** is of benefit in treating the retinal complications of the ischemic response. Newer surgical techniques such as pars plana vitrectomy are useful in managing vitreous hemorrhages and traction retinal detachments.
6. **Hypertensive retinopathy.** The retinal changes in hypertension are essentially the same as in the retinopathies seen in the collagen diseases and are secondary to local ischemia. At least 15 million Americans suffer from hypertension with its effects on the arteries of the heart, brain, kidneys, and the retina.

   a. **Pathology.** Essential hypertension is associated with thickening of the arteriolar wall caused by hypertrophy of muscle fibers in the media and by increase of fibrous tissue in the intima. Sustained elevations of blood pressure cause necrosis of vascular smooth muscle and seepage of plasma into the unsupported wall through a damaged endothelium. Angiography at this stage will demonstrate a focal leak of fluorescein. Progressive plasma insudation into the vessel wall with further muscle necrosis results in secondary occlusion and the typical picture of advanced **fibrinoid necrosis.**

   b. **Grading of hypertensive** retinal changes is done by the **Keith-Wagener-Barker** classification into four grades because of the significance of the individual changes.

      (1) **Group I** shows moderate arteriolar attenuation, often combined with focal constriction and a brightened copper-wire or silver-wire arteriolar reflex. These patients have essential benign hypertension with adequate cardiac and renal function.

      (2) **Group II** demonstrates pronounced arteriolar attenuation with focal and diffuse constriction and AV crossing phenomena, with partial concealment of the venous blood column and alteration of the angle of crossing. Hard shiny deposits and tiny hemorrhages may develop. These patients have a continuously higher blood pressure but are still in good health.

      (3) **Group III** includes patients with retinal edema, hemorrhages, and cotton-wool spots. Retinal hemorrhages are usually linear and flame shaped and lie in the nerve fiber layer. They are usually located near the optic disk and may be associated with a branch retinal vein occlusion (BRVO). The soft exudate, or **cotton-wool spot,** is the hallmark of malignant or accelerated phase of hypertension. It consists of gray-white patches about 0.5 dd in size, located in areas around the disk, and due to focal ischemia in the nerve fiber layer. Cotton-wool spots in the retina can occur in a number of other conditions, such as **anemia, leukemias, collagenases, dysproteinemias, infective endocarditis, diabetic retinopathy and AIDS.**

      (4) **Group IV** consists of patients with all signs of group III along with disk edema. These patients have the most adverse prognosis, since they have severe nervous system, renal, and other organ disturb-

ances. A protracted hypertensive state often results in the development of a **macular star** of **hard exudates.** These shiny exudates consist of collections of macrophages filled with lipid material. They are located in the outer plexiform layer of the macula.

c. **Prognosis.** Serious impairment of vision does not usually occur as a direct result of the hypertensive process unless there is local arterial or venous occlusion. The Keith-Wagener-Barker classification helps in assessing the hypertensive damage to the heart, the brain, and the kidneys. Patients with group IV changes with papilledema, hemorrhages, and exudates have a mean life expectancy of 10.5 months from diagnosis; group III patients without papilledema have a mean life expectancy of 27.6 months.

7. **Venous retinopathy.** Retinal vein occlusion can manifest itself either as a **central retinal vein occlusion** (CRVO), in which the site of occlusion is behind the cribriform plate, or as a **branch retinal vein occlusion** (BRVO), in which the occlusion is anterior to the cribriform plate. Obstruction of outflow occurs in retinal vein occlusion, resulting in a rise of intravascular pressure and stagnation of flow. The rise in intravascular pressure is responsible for the **edema, abnormal leakage, and hemorrhage** leading to the formation of **collaterals** over several weeks. Stagnation of flow is manifest by delayed perfusion, leading to ischemia of endothelial cells and the surrounding retina, resulting in capillary nonperfusion. The development of large areas of capillary closure stimulates the growth of new vessels that may revascularize nonperfused areas but also become preretinal new vessels leading to often to vitreous hemorrhage.

a. **BRVO**

   (1) There are four **sites of occlusion** in BRVO:

      (a) At the edge of the optic disk, causing hemisphere occlusion.

      (b) At AV crossings, causing classic quadrantic or small macular occlusions.

      (c) Peripherally, as a result of systemic disease such as sickle cell disease.

      (d) Along main veins, as in diabetes.

   (2) The most common **cause** of BRVO is systemic **hypertension.** The clinical picture consists of superficial and deep intraretinal hemorrhages with many cotton-wool spots indicating areas of focal retinal infarction. Subhyaloid and vitreous hemorrhages also occur.

   (3) The **natural history** of BRVO varies from complete resolution with no long-term visual difficulties to a progressive situation with complications leading to permanent visual loss. Most patients with BRVO maintain good central vision without treatment. In those who do not, the most common causes are **macular edema** and **preretinal neovascularization.** Macular edema occurs in 57% of cases with temporal branch occlusion. Treatment is controversial. **Photocoagulation** may be considered in those patients who have been followed for at least 6 months and who demonstrate objective and fluorescein angiographic evidence of deterioration.

b. **CRVO**

   (1) Clinical course. CRVO presents a wide spectrum of clinical appearances. The variation depends on the severity of obstruction of venous outflow. In the mildest cases, minimum dilation of veins and hemorrhages are present with little macular edema and little decrease in vision. In the severe cases, vision may deteriorate to hand motions, with extensive deep and superficial hemorrhages with stagnant blood columns in grossly dilated veins and numerous cotton-wool spots. As in BRVO, the principal vascular response in CRVO consists of dilation of retinal capillaries, abnormal vascular permeability, and retinal capillary closure. **Macular edema** is often present in the **nonischemic** CRVO with dilated, leaking capillaries.

Macular vision often improves if the perifoveal capillary arcade is not damaged in the acute process. **Ischemic** CRVO is characterized by capillary closure. Serious neovascular complications are extremely common, leading to **retinal neovascularization, rubeosis iridis, and neovascular glaucoma.** Rubeosis iridis is usually visible by 1 month and neovascular glaucoma within 3 months of the occlusion. The incidence of the latter complication is about 10–15%.

(2) **Differential diagnosis.** There are four conditions from which CRVO must be differentiated:

(a) **Hypertension.** Hypertension often coexists with CRVO. Hypertensive retinopathy (groups III and IV of Keith-Wagener-Barker classification), however, is usually bilateral and often symmetric with superficial hemorrhages, with a macular star of hard exudates present. Retinal hemorrhages do not extend to the periphery as in CRVO. Severe macular edema and visual loss are rare in hypertensive retinopathy.

(b) **Hyperviscosity syndromes** such as macroglobulinemia, leukemias, polycythemias, and some hyperlipemias show a clinical picture similar to CRVO. These conditions are usually bilateral with few hemorrhages and little macular edema.

(c) **Diabetic retinopathy** is usually bilateral. Beading and reduplication of the vein is rare in CRVO.

(d) **Venous state retinopathy** has been described in patients with internal carotid occlusion. Unlike CRVO, venous stasis retinopathy is characterized by the presence of only mild hemorrhages, arterial dilation, and the absence of disk hyperemia.

(3) **Treatment.** There is no medical treatment, such as anticoagulants or steroids, that will guarantee improvement or even maintenance of vision in patients with CRVO. Fluorescein angiography is of help in delineating large areas of retinal ischemia. Early **panretinal photocoagulation** in eyes with an ischemic CRVO pattern virtually eliminates the dreaded complications of neovascular glaucoma.

8. **Diabetic Retinopathy** is the leading cause of new cases of blindness in the United States in patients between the ages of 20 and 74. In the developing Western countries, at least 12% of all blindness is due to diabetes. In the United States, a diabetic patient has over a 20-fold chance of becoming blind compared to a nondiabetic counterpart.

a. **Risk factors.** The duration of diabetes is the main factor in the appearance of diabetic retinopathy, with two-thirds of those with diabetes for 15 years or more having retinopathy. The relationship of metabolic control of diabetes to the frequency of severe retinopathy is unsettled. Studies show an association between high blood sugar levels and the prevalence of severe retinopathy. When diabetes is diagnosed before age 30, the risk of developing retinopathy is about 2%/year if the disease has lasted for a similar length of time.

b. **Types of diabetes.**

(1) **Type I (juvenile onset)** diabetes cases are autoimmune (pancreatic destruction) and have a high risk for developing severe proliferative retinopathy.

(2) **Type II (adult onset)** have normal to high insulin production but insulin-resistant receptor cells. There are more type II patients with blinding sequelae because of the greater number of type II diabetic patients.

c. **Medical evaluation.** Every diabetic patient deserves the benefit of a comprehensive eye evaluation, which should check for symptoms of diabetic retinopathy such as decreased vision, distortion of vision, loss of color vision, and the presence of floaters. The duration of diabetes and the method of control of diabetes should be assessed. The presence of associated systemic disease should be noted. Hypertension is present in 20% of insulin-dependent diabetics and in 58% of non-insulin-dependent diabetics. Optimal medical control is key to minimizing ocular and systemic complications.

   d. Clinical appearance. Diabetic retinopathy is classified into three groups:

   (1) Background retinopathy (nonproliferative retinopathy). The diabetic lesions of background retinopathy are

   (a) Microaneurysms.
   (b) Hemorrhages.
   (c) Soft exudates (cotton-wool spots).
   (d) Hard exudates.

   (2) Preproliferative diabetic retinopathy represents the most severe stage of background retinopathy (nonproliferative retinopathy). Preproliferative retinopathy is categorized by the presence of intraretinal microvascular abnormalities such as shunt vessels, multiple cotton-wool spots, and venous beading. Severe macular edema is present in these patients. Approximately 10–40% of patients with preproliferative retinopathy develop proliferative retinopathy within a year.

   (3) Proliferative diabetic retinopathy occurs in 5% of patients with diabetic retinopathy. Vascular abnormalities appear on the surface of the retina or within the vitreous cavity. Visual loss can be severe. New blood vessels grow on the surface of the retina and the optic nerve and are usually attached to the posterior hyaloid surface of the vitreous body. Contraction of the vitreous body causes traction on the optic disk or retinal neovascularization resulting in vitreous hemorrhage. Fibrous bands subsequently form to the vitreous organization, causing traction detachment of the retina.

e. Pathology. Histology of eyes with diabetic retinopathy shows loss of intramural pericytes and extensive capillary closure in trypsin-digest flat preparations of the retina. The greatest amount of pathology is temporal to the macula, as is seen in vivo by fluorescein angiography. The most widely accepted working hypothesis for the pathogenesis of proliferative retinopathies such as diabetes, retinopathy of prematurity (ROP), and sickle cell retinopathy is that retina rendered ischemic by widespread capillary closure elaborates a vasoproliferative factor that stimulates retinal neovascularization in order to establish blood supply to poorly perfused tissue. Retinal neovascularization invariably develops at the interface between well-perfused and poorly perfused retina.

f. Management

Fluorescein angiography and color fundus photography are ancillary tests that are used in the management of diabetic patients. The retinal periphery must be examined, as approximately 27% of retinal abnormalities are found outside the central 45-degree area. Diabetic patients are best examined using binocular indirect ophthalmoscopy or Goldmann contact lens with maximal pupillary dilatation.

   (1) Three major clinical trials over the past 10 years have been carried out by the National Eye Institute to elucidate the retinal history of nonproliferative and proliferative diabetic retinopathy, as well as guidelines for the value of treatment. The three major clinical trials are:

   1. Diabetic Retinopathy Study (DRS)
   2. Early Treatment Diabetic Retinopathy Study (ETDRS)
   3. Diabetic Retinopathy Vitrectomy Study (DRVS)

   Argon laser photocoagulation is the recommended preferred treatment of diabetic retinopathy in patients with high-risk proliferative disease and in patients with clinically significant macular edema. The DRS, ETDRS, and DRVS demonstrated the value of an early vitrectomy in these patients and in some patients with very severe proliferative diabetic retinopathy.

(2) The management guidelines for diabetic retinopathy as recommended by the American Academy of Ophthalmology are as follows:

Patients with minimal non-proliferative diabetic retinopathy are usually followed at yearly intervals as are also patients with non-proliferative diabetic retinopathy without macular edema. Patients with macular edema that is not clinically significant are examined at six month intervals.

(3) Clinically significant **macular edema** includes any of the following features:
  (a) Thickening of the retina at or within 500 μ of the center of the macula.
  (b) Hard exudates at or within 500 μ of the center of the macula.
  (c) Zones of retinal thickening one disk area or larger, any part of which is within 1 dd of the center of the macula.
  Appropriate argon laser photocoagulation reduces the risk of visual loss substantially.

(4) Preproliferative diabetic retinopathy represents the most severe stage of nonproliferative diabetic retinopathy. In patients with bilateral preproliferative retinopathy, one eye should deserve the benefit of panretinal photocoagulation.
  The **characteristics of high risk for proliferative retinopathy** are as follows:
  (a) Neovascularization of the disk greater than one-quarter to one-third of the disk area.
  (b) Vitreous or preretinal hemorrhage associated with less extensive NVD, or neovascularization elsewhere in the retina (NVE) one-half disk area or more in size.

(5) Laser applications in different patient categories. The risk of severe visual loss in patients with these high-risk characteristics is substantially reduced by means of **panretinal laser photocoagulation** done either with the argon laser or the Xenon arc photocoagulator. The laser burns are applied to the disk on the nasal side and to within 2 dd of the temporal side of the macula. At least 500 Xenon arc burns of 4.5-μ spot size for a 0.5-second duration or 2000 argon laser burns of 500 μ for a 0.2-second duration are applied. In addition, focal lesions are also treated. In those patients with proliferative diabetic retinopathy who do not have the above high-risk characteristics, treatment of one eye is recommended when bilateral disease is present. In addition, focal argon laser photocoagulation is preferred for **macular edema** in the non-high-risk proliferative diabetic retinopathy patients. These patients need to be followed at 3-month intervals. When severe vitreous or preretinal **hemorrhage** is present, laser photocoagulation is impossible. In some cases, proliferative diabetic retinopathy may continue to be active in spite of panretinal laser photocoagulation. Panretinal cryoablation is useful in selected patients. Early pars plana vitrectomy is beneficial in type I diabetics with severe hemorrhage. Intraoperative laser photocoagulation is often performed when these patients undergo pars plana vitrectomy when dense vitreous hemorrhage is present. B-scan ultrasonography should be used to rule out underlying traction retinal detachment.
  When traction **macular detachment** or a combination traction and rhegmatogenous **retinal detachment** is present, vitreous surgery is indicated. Vitrectomy surgery should be undertaken with careful consideration of potential risks and benefits for the patient.

9. **Sickle cell retinopathy.** About 100,000 blacks in the United States are at risk of developing sickle cell retinopathy, which often occurs in the most productive years of life. Proliferative retinopathy is most common in sickle cell disease but can occur in several other hemoglobinopathies.
   a. **The five progressive stages** of sickle cell retinopathy are
      (1) Peripheral arteriolar occlusion.
      (2) Peripheral arteriovenous anastomosis.
      (3) Sea fan (retinal arterial) neovascularization, which is most frequent at about the equatorial plane superotemporally. Fluorescein angiography is valuable in detecting early sea fans.
      (4) Vitreous hemorrhage.
      (5) Retinal detachment, which usually begins in areas affected by fibrovascular proliferation and local vitreous traction.
   b. **Treatment** consists of photocoagulation in obliterating neovascular fronds. An alternative treatment involves obliteration of areas of capillary nonperfusion using scatter laser photocoagulation. This treatment involves low energies, thereby potentially reducing complications. Peripheral **cryotherapy,** causing mild retinal whitening of the nonperfused areas, is an alternative mode of therapy. Pars plana vitrectomy is useful in treating patients with prolonged vitreous hemorrhage. Special precautions should be taken if retinal detachment surgery is undertaken. Since these eyes are prone to develop **anterior segment ischemia,** special measures to prevent this should include partial exchange blood transfusion, local anesthesia omitting the use of vasoconstrictors such as epinephrine, and reduced intraocular pressure (IOP). Cryotherapy is preferable to diathermy to create chorioretinal adhesion. Subretinal fluid is drained where technically possible. A segmental scleral buckle is preferable to one with an encircling band.
10. **Retinopathy of prematurity (retrolental fibroplasia).** See Chap. 10, sec. XII.
11. **Ischemic Retinopathies**
    a. **Cotton-wool spots** are seen in the early stages of ischemic retinopathies. Although diabetes, AIDS, and hypertension are the most frequent systemic diseases associated with cotton-wool spots on the retina, they may also occur in collagen vascular diseases such as dermatomyositis, systemic lupus erythematosus, polyarteritis nodosa, and giant-cell arteritis.
    b. **Systemic etiology** should be searched for in any patients with cotton-wool spots. Other conditions where cotton-wool spots are found include cardiac valvular disease, radiation retinopathy, carotid occlusive disease, pulseless disease, syphilis, radiation retinopathy, leukemia, trauma, AIDS, metastatic carcinoma, intravenous drug abuse, and partial retinal artery obstruction. With severe ischemia, development of optic disk and retinal neovascularization occurs.
    c. **Treatment.** In addition to treating the underlying systemic condition, photocoagulation may be used when the ischemic condition is well established, the guidelines being the same as in the management of proliferative diabetic retinopathy. Lupus anticoagulant, an acquired serum immune globulin, should be considered in all patients with collagen vascular diseases, retinal artery occlusion, ischemic optic neuropathy, or transient visual loss or diplopia. It is important to recognize lupus anticoagulant in young and middle-aged patients not otherwise at high risk for stroke. Lupus anticoagulant and other vascular occlusive disease (see Chap. 8, sec. **V.C.9**) may be screened for using anticardiolipin antibodies.
12. **Retinal arterial occlusion**
    a. **Clinical appearance.** Retinal arterial occlusion results in **infarction** of the inner two-thirds of the retina, reflex constriction of the whole retinal arterial tree, and stasis in retinal capillaries. The infarct is is-

chemic; therefore, unlike retinal vein occlusion, hemorrhage is minimal. The retina at the posterior pole becomes milky white and swollen, and the choroid is seen through the fovea as a **cherry-red spot.** Usually the patient has either painless, total loss of vision or bare light perception temporal to fixation (unless the patient has a cilioretinal artery supplying the papillomacular nerve fibers). Although some circulation is reestablished, it is small in volume so that the retinal arteries remain narrow and ultimately are reduced to white threads.

   b. **Histology.** The retinal cells undergo necrosis, disintegrate, and are phagocytosed by macrophages. These macrophages appear foamy because of the high lipid content of the retina. In time the edema and necrotic tissue are resorbed, leaving a thin retina with loss of bipolar cells, ganglion cells, and nerve fibers. Gliosis is minimal because glial cells are destroyed along with the nerve cells. Extensive hyalinization of the retinal vessels is seen in late stages.

   c. **Etiology.** The most common cause of retinal arterial occlusion is **embolization** of the retinal vascular tree due to emboli arising from the major arteries supplying the head or from the left side of the heart. The emboli may be fatty material from **atheromas,** calcium deposits from diseased heart valves, septic and nonseptic fibrin, and platelet thrombi. In the absence of visible emboli, other causes include **giant-cell (temporal) arteritis, collagen vascular diseases,** and increased orbital pressure in conditions such as **retrobulbar hemorrhage** and **endocrine exophthalmus.** Rare causes include **sickle cell disease** and **syphilis.**

   d. **Treatment.** Retinal arterial occlusion is an ophthalmic emergency, and prompt treatment is essential. An anoxic retina is irreversibly damaged in about one hour. Specific factors should be carried out as indicated, e.g., orbital decompression for acute retrobulbar hemorrhage, and ocular hypotension for acute glaucoma. Nonspecific methods to increase blood flow, to dilate the retinal vessels, and to dislodge emboli include inhalation of a 95% oxygen–5% carbon dioxide mixture, digital massage, 500 mg IV acetazolamide and 100 mg IV methylprednisolone (for possible arteritis). Additional measures include paracentesis of aqueous humor. Improvement can be determined by visual acuity and visual field testing, and by ophthalmoscopic examination. Patients with **transient blurring of vision (amaurosis fugax)** should have a thorough evaluation of the carotid artery. Amaurosis fugax demands urgent attention because it is a warning sign of an impending stroke.

13. **Retinal vasculitis** is a complex group of conditions in which there is evidence of retinal vascular disease along with signs of inflammation such as cells in the aqueous or vitreous. Fluorescein angiography shows staining of the vessel walls with leakage, macular edema, and all the other signs associated with ischemic response of the retina. Retinal vasculitis is seen in a number of conditions such as **sarcoidosis** and **Behçet's disease. Eales's disease** is considered to be retinal vasculitis and is responsible for idiopathic vitreous hemorrhage, especially in young males. The etiology of Eales's disease is obscure. Photocoagulation is of benefit if an ischemic response has been established with retinal and disk neovascularization.

14. **Acquired immunodeficiency syndrome (AIDS).** See Chap. 8, sec. **X.E.**

IV. **Degenerative diseases of the macula.** Macular degenerations form the most common cause of patients being reported to the Registry of the Blind. Their treatment presents a formidable clinical challenge. Fluorescein angiography and photocoagulation in selected cases represent major advances in the classification and therapy of these conditions. The basic pathology in these conditions appears to be confined to the choriocapillaris, Bruch's membrane, and the RPE. The sensory retina is affected secondarily, in contrast to retinal vascular disease, in which the sensory retina is affected primarily. The choroid and the RPE may be affected by inflammation or degeneration that can be the result of a variety of factors, such as vascular, metabolic, or toxic influences. The response of the macula can be either a serous (or hemorrhagic) detachment of the retina or a primary atrophic or degenerative response.

A. Serous detachment of the macula

  1. Central serous retinochoroidopathy

  a. Clinical characteristics. Central serous retinochoroidopathy occurs usually in young adult males and has an unknown etiology. The usual symptoms are decreased visual acuity, distortion, generalized darkening of the visual field, increased hypermetropia, and a decreased recovery from glare. Patients can be symptomatic even if their vision is 20/20. Ophthalmoscopy shows shallow detachment of the sensory macular retina, but the detachment may occur anywhere in the posterior pole. Fluorescein angiography demonstrates one or more point stains of hyperfluorescence appearing in the AV phase, demonstrating the site of origin of leakthrough of the RPE into the subretinal space. The leaking point may lie anywhere within the serous detachment.

  b. Differential diagnosis. Serous detachment of the macula can occur in association with a **congenital pit of the optic disk.** Secondary retinal changes are often seen in chronic detachments associated with an optic pit.

  c. Treatment. The disease usually lasts 3–6 months and a majority of the patients recover gross visual acuity. The condition is not inflammatory in nature, and systemic steroids are not indicated. The duration of the disease, the initial visual acuity, and the age of the patient do not appear to have any effect on the final visual outcome. Almost all patients show some disturbance of the RPE even after complete visual recovery. The role of **photocoagulation** in management of this condition is unsettled. Duration of the disease for longer than 4–6 months and detectable morphologic changes in the retina, such as cystic edema and lipid deposition on the outer retinal surface, are frequently accepted as indications for treatment.

  2. Diskiform degeneration of the macula. In this condition, the retina and RPE are detached from the underlying structures by serous fluid, and the subpigment epithelial space is occupied by blood vessels derived from the choroid, the so-called **choroidal neovascular membrane (CNM).** The CNM may cause subpigment epithelial hemorrhages, and the subsequent organization of these hemorrhages gives rise to a typical subretinal fibrovascular **diskiform scar,** most often located in the macular region.

  a. The predisposing cause of diskiform degeneration is **drusen** in the posterior fundus. Drusen are colloid bodies and occur between the inner collagenous layer of Bruch's membrane and the basement membrane of RPE. They are considered to be the accumulation of discharged contents of pigment epithelial phagosomes. Drusen occur in the following conditions:

    (1) During aging, the drusen become larger and more numerous. Ten percent of these eyes eventually develop CNM. Occasionally they are seen in young eyes.

    (2) During retinal and choroidal degeneration in disease states, especially if the disease phenomenon involves a vascular, inflammatory, or neoplastic condition. Thus, they can be seen overlying choroidal **malignant melanomas** and in **phthisic eyes.**

    (3) As a **primary dystrophy** in which they appear to be transmitted as an **autosomal dominant.** Drusen can also be seen in dystrophies such as **fundus flavimaculatus.**

  b. Clinically, drusen appear as small, bright, sharply defined, circular points lying beneath the retinal vessels and mostly confined to the posterior pole. These bright yellow-to-white masses may coalesce to form larger rounded masses, often with some pigmentation around their edges. Central vision is rarely affected unless there is a concomitant degenerative change in the function of the RPE and choriocapillaris. Minimum metamorphopsia may be present in patients with drusen.

  c. The **causes of CNM** are as follows:

    (1) Age-related maculopathy (ARM), often associated with drusen.

    (2) Maculopathy of presumed histoplasmosis (see Chap. 8, sec. **XI.E**).

    (3) High myopia.

    (4) Angioid streaks. These are dark lines radiating from the region of the disk and represent breaks in Bruch's membrane. Angioid streaks occur bilaterally and may superficially resemble retinal vessels in their appearance and course. They are associated with **pseudoxanthoma elasticum, Paget's disease of the bone** (osteitis deformans), and **sickle cell disease.**

    (5) Traumatic choroidal ruptures.

    (6) Drusen of the optic nerve.

    (7) Retinal dystrophies such as Best's vitelliform dystrophy.

  d. Treatment consists of obliteration of the CNM by **photocoagulation.** The CNM is identified and delineated by **fluorescein angiography.** During the initial transit of dye, a lacy meshwork or a bicycle-wheel pattern of the CNM can be identified before there is a progressive leakage of dye from the capillaries into the subretinal space. Since CNM and its complications may be responsible for up to 90% of severe visual loss (visual acuity of 20/200 or less) in ARM and since ARM is responsible for 14% of all new cases of blindness in the United States in persons over the age of 65 years, the National Eye Institute initiated in 1979 a collaborative clinical trial of laser photocoagulation in the treatment of CNM in SMD. This study demonstrated that argon laser photocoagulation is effective in reducing the risk of visual loss in extrafoveal CNM (between 200 and 2500 μ from the focal center). Treatment, which should be done as soon as possible after identification of the CNM by fluorescein angiography, consists of high-energy contiguous laser burns. After the initial treatment, patients should be followed at close intervals with repeat fluorescein angiography and, if necessary, retreated if residual or recurrent CNM is still present.

  The conventional **argon laser photocoagulator** has blue and green wavelengths. The blue wavelength is absorbed significantly by the macular xanthophyll and can result in foveal damage. The blue light is also phototoxic to the sensory retina. The green wavelength is absorbed by the hemoglobin and may dispose the eye to retinal vascular damage. The **krypton red photocoagulator,** because of its ability to spare the inner retina by its virtual lack of absorption by hemoglobin, is useful in the treatment of CNM closer than 200 μ but not under the fovea.

3. Pigment epithelial detachments. A local detachment of the RPE may occur in the macular region and may involve a much greater area than that seen in central serous retinochoroidopathy, although the symptoms are the same. Fluorescein angiography shows that the entire dome of the pigment epithelial detachment lights up early in the angiogram, unlike the lacy or bicycle-wheel pattern seen in a CNM. In older patients, these detachments occur with **drusen,** and there may be a **diskiform lesion** in the fellow eye. Spontaneous resolution of the detachment can occur, but there may be minor disturbances in visual function associated with disturbance of the RPE. Guidelines for the use of photocoagulation in this condition are not well established, although it has been shown that these detachments can be flattened by a grid of photocoagulation marks covering the entire lesion but avoiding the fovea. Photocoagulation may provoke the development of a CNM.

B. Atrophic macular degeneration is characterized by a bilateral progressive atrophy of the RPE and the choriocapillaris. It arises either from ischemic changes, from exposure to toxic substances that have a predisposition to the macula, or as a result of genetically transmitted diseases. Since the condition is primarily atrophic, **treatment** is symptomatic and consists of rehabilitation with **low vision aids.**

1. **"Dry" ARM** is due to arteriosclerotic changes at the macula, with chronic choroidal ischemia giving rise to degenerative changes in the RPE, Bruch's membrane, and the choroid. Drusen may be seen in this form of degeneration, just as in early diskiform (pre-CNM) disease. Varying stages of retinochoroidal atrophy may be seen, with minor atrophy of the RPE to large punched out areas of complete loss of the choroid and the overlying RPE and sensory retina. These changes can be demonstrated by the extent of RPE changes.

2. **Toxic maculopathies.** Certain drugs have a toxic effect on the macula by producing degeneration of RPE and loss of vision. It is important to detect these changes at an early stage, by either fluorescein angiography or electrophysiologic diagnostic tests.

   a. **Chloroquine.** This aminoquinoline along with hydroxychloroquine is used in the long-term treatment of rheumatoid arthritis and lupus erythematosus. A total dose of 100–300 gm or more of chloroquine leads to a toxic effect on the macula characterized by a horizontally oval area of RPE atrophy, giving rise to a bull's eye appearance of the macula. Hydroxychloroquine is tolerated in large cumulative doses (1000 to nearly 5000 gm) as long as the daily dose does not exceed 400 mg/day or 6.5 mg/kg body weight/day. **Bull's eye maculopathy** can be detected at its earliest stages by **fluorescein angiography.** The earliest functional changes are a relative or absolute scotoma to red, red-green defect on the Ishihara color test, an abnormal EOG, and elevation of threshold on static perimetry.

   b. **Thioridazine** also has toxic effects on the RPE. Patients receiving high doses (> 1 gm/day) may develop pigmentary retinopathy of the macula with central or ring scotomas and diminished photopic and scotopic responses of the ERG.

   c. **Chlorpromazine,** when taken in large doses (> 2 gm/day for a year) may cause mild pigmentary changes of the retina with no significant functional deficits.

3. **Hereditary macular dystrophies.** A number of genetically transmitted conditions such as Stargardt's disease, Best's vitelliform dystrophy, and cone dystrophy show a marked similarity in appearance to the toxic maculopathies (see sec. 2).

C. **Vitreoretinal macular diseases.** Disturbances at the vitreoretinal interface are common causes of reduced central vision in elderly patients.

1. **Idiopathic preretinal macular fibrosis.** These patients, who present themselves with blurry vision and metamorphopsia (distorted vision), show a glinting reflex, traction lines, and mild, gray preretinal fibrosis in the macula. These characteristics may arise spontaneously or may be related to vitreous detachment, or they may be secondary to local vascular or inflammatory changes. Preretinal macular membranes may also arise after photocoagulation or after retinal detachment surgery. Pars plana vitrectomy with peeling of the epimacular membrane is done if there is significant visual loss due to epimacular membranes.

2. **Senile macular holes.** Idiopathic macular hole is a common cause of reduced central vision in otherwise healthy patients, usually women, in the sixth and seventh decades. These holes may be "lamellar" or true full-thickness macular holes. Bilaterality is often seen. These holes rarely give rise to retinal detachment. The cause of this condition is unknown but may represent an ischemic change combined with traction forces from a vitreous detachment. No treatment is indicated unless a retinal detachment occurs.

V. **Retinal inflammatory diseases.** A variety of diseases cause inflammation primarily of the sensory retina, the RPE, or both the choroid and the retina. These diseases cause loss of central vision either by direct involvement of the macula or from secondary retinal edema or detachment from a paramacular lesion. Cells in the vitreous are always present.

A. Retinitis. A variety of bacterial and fungal agents can be carried to the retina as septic emboli. If the agent can be identified by blood cultures, culture of aqueous humor, or vitreous aspirates, and appropriate therapy instituted immediately, many of these eyes can be saved with maintenance of varying degrees of visual function. **Pars plana vitrectomy** to remove the infected vitreous gel is a major advance in the treatment of endophthalmitis. At the conclusion of vitrectomy for identifying the offending bacterial organism, 400 μg of gentamicin and 1 mg of vancomycin is injected in the midvitreous (see Chap. 8, sec. **XV**).

   1. Bacterial retinitis. A variety of bacterial emboli may be carried from focal areas of infection elsewhere to the retina. If the nature of the bacteria is established promptly and appropriate antibiotic therapy, both intravenous and subconjunctival, instituted, useful visual function may be preserved.

   2. Fungal retinitis. Candidal retinitis is the most important fungal retinitis and occurs in patients receiving prolonged IV antibiotic therapy by a catheter. Candidal retinal abscesses also occur in severely debilitated patients such as those receiving immunosuppressant therapy. Candidal retinitis appears as focal retinal abscesses. Antifungal therapy with amphotericin B and 5-fluorocytosine is effective in treating this condition. Pars plana vitrectomy is effective in removing the infected vitreous gel and in permitting the easy diffusion of the antifungal agent. Amphotericin, 5–10 μg, is injected in the midvitreous cavity after vitrectomy (see Chap. 8, sec. **XV**).

B. Infectious disease of the retinal pigment epithelium. Certain viral diseases appear to primarily involve the RPE.

   1. Rubella retinitis. Children born of mothers who contracted rubella in the first trimester of pregnancy show a high incidence of salt-and-pepper mottling of the RPE. Multiple other ocular and other organ involvement may be present. In the absence of other ocular problems, such as cataracts or glaucoma, these children may have normal visual function. Fluorescein angiography shows mottled hyperfluorescence due to extensive and irregular loss of pigment.

   2. Acute posterior multifocal placoid pigment epitheliopathy (APMPPE), along with the related condition of focal retinal pigment epithelitis **(Krill's disease),** appears to involve the RPE, particularly in the macular region, causing visual loss with subsequent spontaneous resolution and residual pigmentation. The affected patients are young (average age 25 years) and have a history of viral illness preceding the onset of visual symptoms. Bilateral involvement is present. One or more flat, gray-white, subretinal lesions are present in the posterior pole. These lesions block out background choroidal fluorescence during the early stages of fluorescein angiography. The late stages of APMPPE may show extensive pigmentary changes and appear similar to atrophic macular degenerations or widespread retinal dystrophies. Unlike the latter conditions, patients with APMPPE retain good visual acuity and good electrophysiologic function.

C. Retinochoroiditis (see Chap. 8 and Chap. 10, sec. **II**). Focal or diffuse retinitis may be associated with a number of conditions involving the uvea, such as toxoplasmosis, cytomegalic inclusion disease, peripheral uveitis, sarcoidosis, and rare diseases such as Behçet's disease and subacute sclerosing panencephalitis.

VI. Retinal dystrophies are genetically transmitted diseases of the retina that lead to premature cell changes and cell death (see Chap. 10, sec. **XVII**). These conditions must be differentiated from congenital stationary retinal disorders such as stationary night blindness or achromatopsia (autosomal recessive). Electrophysiologic tests are important in diagnosing these disorders, especially in young children, the main tests being **ERG** and **EOG**. An abnormality of the RPE photoreceptor complex plays a primary role in these diseases, with probable secondary abnormality of the choriocapillaris. In three conditions—retinitis pigmentosa, choroideremia, and sex-linked retinoschisis—the female carrier may show ocular signs. In most instances the female carrier is asymptomatic and has normal test findings. Although a metabolic abnormality—hyperornithinemia—has been shown to be associated with gyrate atrophy of the choroid and retina, most retinal dystrophies do not appear to have any systemic or metabolic associations. Within the past decade advances in molecular genetics using DNA probes have identified the genetic defect in dominant retinitis pigmentosa and choroideremia.

A. Primary retinal dystrophies

1. **Retinitis pigmentosa** is the most common retinal dystrophy. The most common symptom is **night blindness.** Ophthalmoscopy demonstrates attenuation of the retinal vessels, retinal pigmentary changes consisting of bone-corpuscular clumping of pigment clustering around retinal vessels in the midperiphery of the fundus, and waxy pallor of the optic disk. The visual fields show annular scotomas. The EOG and scotopic ERG are primarily affected; the photopic ERG is relatively spared. The autosomal recessive is the most severe form of the disease; the autosomal dominant is the most benign form. There is no treatment beyond the provision of low vision aids and genetic counseling.

2. **Cone dystrophy.** Unlike retinitis pigmentosa, in which the rod system is primarily affected, in cone dystrophy the cone system is initially affected, with changes in the rod system later in the course of the disease. The patient complains of poor visual acuity, poor color vision, and photophobia. Ophthalmoscopy may show a bull's-eye macula with a ringlike depigmentation around the macula. The end stage of cone dystrophy has the same appearance as retinitis pigmentosa.

3. **Differential diagnosis of retinitis pigmentosa.** A number of diseases and syndromes are associated with retinitis pigmentosa.

   a. **Acanthocytosis (Bassen-Kornzweig syndrome)** is an autosomal recessive disorder characterized by crenated red cells, serum abetalipoproteinemia, and spinocerebellar degeneration. In its early stages the pigmentary retinopathy can be reversed by large doses of vitamin A.

   b. **Alström's syndrome** is a rare autosomal recessive disease whose clinical features include profound childhood blindness, obesity, diabetes mellitus, and neurosensory deafness. Chronic renal disease is seen in later stages.

   c. **Bardet-Biedl syndrome** is an autosomal recessive disorder characterized by polydactyly, obesity, mental retardation, and hypogonadism.

   d. **Cockayne's syndrome** is a rare, autosomally inherited condition. Afflicted patients have a prematurely senile appearance, mental retardation, deafness, peripheral neuropathy, and photosensitive dermatitis.

   e. **Friedreich's syndrome** is a recessively inherited spinocerebellar ataxia with deafness and mental deficiency.

   f. **Kearns-Sayre syndrome.** The symptoms of this disease, which begins in childhood, include progressive external ophthalmoplegia and cardiac conduction defects. Early recognition and the use of a cardiac pacemaker may avert a fatal cardiac arrest.

   g. **Leber's congenital amaurosis** is an autosomal recessively inherited disease and is associated with profound visual loss at birth or in the first year of life. The ERG is nondetectable and provides an important means of differentiating retinal disease from "cortical blindness."

   h. **Mucopolysaccharidosis.** There are two types of mucopolysaccharidoses associated with pigmentary retinopathy. In **Hunter's disease** (type II) the clinical features are gargoylism, mental retardation, hepatosplenomegaly, and early death. **Sanfilippo's disease** (type III) is characterized by mental retardation, seizures, and deafness.

   i. **Refsum's disease** is a recessively inherited condition characterized by peripheral neuropathy, deafness, and cerebellar ataxia. There is an increase of **phytanic acid** in the blood. Early dietary control consisting of withholding phytol, a precursor of phytanic acid, may retard neurologic and retinal changes.

j. Syphilis. Both acquired and congenital syphilis show extensive signs of pigmentary retinopathy.

k. Usher's syndrome is an autosomal recessively inherited condition responsible for 3–6% of severe childhood deafness and 50% of deaf-blindness. Both the cochlear and vestibular systems are involved.

l. Pseudoretinitis pigmentosa. Certain retinal degenerations and inflammations may culminate in a clinical and electrophysiologic picture similar to that seen in retinitis pigmentosa. This condition is encountered with detachment of the retina and following injury, especially concussive ocular injuries occurring early in life.

B. Primary macular dystrophies. Most macular dystrophies show ophthalmoscopic and retinal functional changes outside the macular area; however, their early manifestations are first seen in the macular area.

1. **Vitelliform dystrophy (Best's disease)** is an autosomal dominant disorder that begins in childhood and is characterized by an egg-yolk-like lesion in the macular region bilaterally. It is compatible with near-normal visual acuity. The EOG is specifically afflicted; the ERG is normal. The yolklike material eventually absorbs, resulting in extensive pigmentary degeneration of the macula.

2. **Stargardt's disease.** This well-known macular dystrophy occurs between the ages of 6 and 20 and is inherited as an autosomal recessive condition. Unlike vitelliform dystrophy, Stargardt's disease begins with rapid loss of vision without ophthalmoscopic changes. Subsequently, the macula shows pigmentary disturbance with a peau d'orange appearance. Many yellowish flecks surround this central area of beaten bronze atrophy. Central vision is ultimately lost, but the visual fields remain intact. The ERG is normal. *Fundus flavimaculatus* is reserved for cases without macular involvement, whereas Stargardt's disease denotes atrophic macular dystrophy with fundus flavimaculatus.

C. Primary choroidal dystrophies (see Chap. 8, sec. **XIX**). The best known disorders in this group are the sex-linked choroideremia, the autosomal recessive gyrate atrophy of the choroid and retina, and the autosomal dominant central areolar choroidal dystrophy.

D. Primary vitreoretinal dystrophies primarily affect the superficial retina and the vitreous body and include juvenile retinoschisis, Goldmann-Favre dystrophy, Wagner's disease, and clefting syndromes with palatoschisis and maxillary hypoplasia (see Chap. 10, sec. **XVII.C**). These clefting syndromes are closely related to the **Pierre Robin syndrome** of glossoptosis, micrognathia, and cleft palate. **Retinal detachment** is frequently associated with clefting syndromes.

VII. Retinal detachment. In retinal detachment, fluid collects in the potential space between the sensory retina and the RPE that remains attached to Bruch's membrane. Fluid may accumulate by three major mechanisms. It may escape from the vitreous cavity into the subretinal space through a retinal hole or tear (break) in the retina. This tear is called a **rhegmatogenous retinal detachment.** Extravasation from the choroid or the retina may result in retinal detachment, the so-called **secondary retinal detachment.** Lastly, the retina can be detached from its normal position by fibrous bands in the vitreous, resulting in a **traction retinal detachment.**

A. Rhegmatogenous retinal detachment occurs in patients over the age of 45. It is more common in males, frequently bilateral, and more common in myopic than hyperopic eyes. It occurs in 2% of patients who have undergone cataract surgery.

1. **Signs and symptoms.** The patient initially experiences flashing lights (photopsia), vitreous floaters, or both. These symptoms are often associated with acute **posterior vitreous detachment** (PVD), a condition perhaps indicative of more serious vitreoretinal pathology. The complications of acute PVD include retinal break formation. Collection of subretinal fluid

causes retinal separation, resulting in a field loss corresponding to the area of detachment. Ophthalmoscopy shows that the retina has lost its pink color and appears gray and opaque. If the collection of subretinal fluid is large, the retina shows a ballooning detachment with numerous folds. Binocular indirect ophthalmoscopy with scleral depression is valuable in locating the retinal breaks in order to repair the retinal detachment. Surgical reattachment should be performed as soon as possible as the macular undergoes cystic changes, with progressive degeneration of rods and cones, since the photoreceptors are separated from the choriocapillaris, their normal source of nourishment.

2. The following conditions **predispose** to retinal break formation:
   a. **Peripheral cystoid degeneration** is generally found in eyes after age 20. These microcysts are considered to be a normal aging change and are located from the ora serrata extending backward into the retina.
   b. **Senile retinoschisis.** Microcystoid degeneration may lead to extensive splitting of the retina, particularly in the inferotemporal periphery. This condition is often bilateral and is seen in older persons. Retinoschisis produces an absolute field defect. Retinal detachment develops only if there are holes in the inner and outer walls of the schisis. The risk of a retinal detachment from double layer holes in retinoschisis is about 1.4%.
   c. **Peripheral chorioretinal degeneration.** These lesions develop after the age of 40. They are often located inferiorly near the ora serrata and are bilateral. Vitreous traction over these thinned areas may lead to retinal hole formation.
   d. **Lattice degeneration** of the retina is characterized by patches of white lines that intersect each other in the peripheral retina and are concentric with the ora serrata. The retina becomes atrophic in these areas, with hole formation and pigmentary disturbance. Vitreous traction can cause large horseshoe breaks at the posterior margin of lattice degeneration. Lattice degeneration is present in 6–12% eyes. The risk of developing retinal detachment in eyes with lattice degeneration is 0.3%.
   e. **Dialysis** or disinsertion of the retina from its attachment to the ora serrata can occur spontaneously or as a result of trauma. Most dialyses occur in the inferotemporal retina, although superonasal dialyses can be seen after ocular contusion. A **giant retinal break** is when the tear extends 90 degrees or more along the circumference of the globe. It is often due to a traumatic dialysis.

3. **Treatment.** Rhegmatogenous retinal detachment is treated with a **scleral buckling** procedure. All retinal breaks are localized and a chorioretinal adhesion is initiated around the break with diathermy or the cryoprobe. The subretinal fluid is drained surgically, and the detached retina is indented toward the vitreous cavity by a scleral implant or explant. The buckled sclera and choroid close the retinal break, pushing the retina toward the vitreous cavity, and release vitreous traction at the site of the retinal break.

B. **Secondary retinal detachments** can occur with systemic or retinovascular diseases or as a response to inflammation of the retina or choroid.
   1. **These conditions** include
      a. Severe hypertension, especially toxemia of pregnancy.
      b. Chronic glomerulonephritis.
      c. Retinal venous occlusive disease.
      d. Retinal angiomatosis.
      e. Papilledema.
      f. Choroidal detachment, especially after intraocular surgery.
      g. Primary or metastatic choroidal tumor.
      h. Vogt-Koyanagi-Harada disease.
      i. Retinal vasculitis.

2. Treatment is directed toward correcting the underlying condition. Secondary retinal detachments are not amenable to standard scleral buckling surgery.

C. Traction retinal detachments are due to fibrous bands in the vitreous arising from the organization of inflammatory exudates and of hemorrhages in the vitreous, the most common cause being **diabetic retinopathy.** Other causes include retained **intraocular foreign body, perforating ocular injury,** and **vitreous loss** after cataract surgery. In eyes in which scleral buckling surgery is repeatedly unsuccessful, a preretinal membrane develops, leading to **massive preretinal retraction** and a funnel-shaped retinal detachment. **Treatment** of these traction retinal detachments is difficult. **Pars plana vitrectomy** with vitreous membrane cutting and pealing appears to be the only way of treating these detachments.

VIII. Vitreous. The vitreous undergoes significant physical and biochemical changes with **aging.** The most striking changes are liquefaction (**syneresis**) and **PVD** (posterior vitreous detachment). Complications of PVD include retinal break, vitreous and retinal hemorrhage, and cystoid maculopathy. Syneresis and PVD occur an average of 20 years earlier in myopes than in emmetropes. Aphakic eyes have a much higher prevalence of PVD. Forward movement of the vitreous may be a reason for the higher prevalence of retinal detachment in aphakic eyes and also for development of **pupillary block glaucoma** and **malignant glaucoma.**

A. Developmental abnormalities (see Chap. 10, sec. **XVII**). Persistent hyperplastic primary vitreous (PHPV) and the various vitreoretinal dystrophies belong to this group. Eyes with PHPV, which are microophthalmic, develop cataract, pupillary block, and secondary glaucoma. Early intervention with a vitrectomy instrument to remove the cataract and retrolental tissue, either via the anterior or pars plana approach, is advisable. Visual results are naturally poor because of the associated amblyopia.

B. Vitreous opacities

1. Blood. Vitreous hemorrhage usually comes from the retina and may be preretinal or diffusely dispersed in the vitreous cavity. Massive hemorrhages may reduce vision severely. The blood in a long-standing vitreous hemorrhage often becomes converted to a white opaque mass resembling an inflammatory exudate, endophthalmitis, or an intraocular tumor. A detailed history along with a complete ocular examination combined with **ultrasonography** usually establishes the diagnosis. The components of blood such as platelets and leukocytes probably contribute to the development of pathologic vitreous membranes.

Vitreous hemorrhage and membrane formation are seen in a number of ocular conditions. **Diabetic retinopathy** is the most important cause, followed by **retinal tear.** Other conditions include PVD, retinal vein occlusion, sickle cell retinopathy, congenital retinal vascular anomalies, trauma, diskiform macular lesions, choroidal malignant melanoma, and subarachnoid hemorrhage.

2. Asteroid hyalitis, also known as **Benson's disease,** is characterized by minute white or yellow solid bodies suspended in an essentially normal vitreous. This condition probably represents a dystrophy with fairly weak penetrance. Calcium palmitate and stearate are present in these vitreous deposits.

3. Cholesterolosis bulbi (synchysis scintillans) is typified by freely floating, highly refractile crystals in liquefied vitreous and is seen in eyes with severe intraocular disease.

4. Other conditions. Vitreous opacification can be seen in **primary amyloidosis** and **reticulum cell sarcoma.** In **retinoblastoma,** tumor cells may be seen freely floating in the vitreous.

C. Inflammation. The response of the vitreous is characterized by liquefaction, opacification, and shrinkage whenever it is exposed to inflammatory insult. The vitreous is an excellent culture medium for the growth of bacteria, leading to **endophthalmitis.** The presence of white blood cells results in the laying down of fibrous connective tissue and varying degrees of capillary proliferation. Organization of these membranes may lead to a **cyclitic membrane,** formed by the cells from the ciliary body and the adjacent retina and located along the plane of the anterior hyaloid surface. Cyclitic membranes often lead to total retinal detachment. In addition to bacteria and fungi, vitreous abscesses with intense eosinophilia may be seen with **parasitic infections,** such as *Taenia,* microfilaria, and nematode infections due to *Toxocara canis* and *Toxocara cati* (see Chap. 10, sec. **III.B**).

D. **Vitrectomy** is the most significant advance in the surgical management of vitreous disease. The technique is used to clear vitreous opacities and relieve or prevent vitreoretinal traction. Vitrectomy through the pars plana approach is the best established procedure. A variety of vitrectomy units is currently available. All instruments perform vitreous cutting and aspiration, the procedure being performed under microscopic control with the aid of fiberoptic illumination. The following are indications for pars plana vitrectomy:

1. Nonresolving vitreous opacities (e.g., diabetic hemorrhage).
2. Certain retinal detachments:
   a. Traction detachments.
   b. Giant retinal tears with rolled posterior edges.
   c. Rhegmatogenous detachment and vitreous hemorrhage or severe vitreous traction.
   d. Massive preretinal retraction.
3. Trauma:
   a. Certain penetrating injuries of the posterior segment.
   b. Selected magnetic and nonmagnetic intraocular foreign bodies.
4. Vitreous biopsy (amyloidosis, reticulum cell sarcoma).
5. Anterior segment reconstruction (pupillary membranectomy).
6. Vitreous complications in the anterior segment:
   a. Vitreous "touch" with corneal edema.
   b. Aphakic pupillary block glaucoma.
7. Secondary open-angle glaucoma:
   a. Hemolytic glaucoma.
   b. Phacolytic glaucoma.
8. Endophthalmitis.
9. Proliferative diabetic retinopathy.

   The ophthalmologist who does not perform pars plana vitrectomy must consider this procedure in patients with ocular pathology other than vitreous hemorrhage. With further refinement of instrumentation and techniques, this procedure should become even more useful in the future.

IX. **Trauma** (see Chap. 2; Chap. 8, sec. **XVII**). Ocular injuries often cause vitreoretinal and choroidal changes. Vitreoretinal trauma can be considered under the following headings.

A. **Contusion injuries** are caused either by a direct blow applied to the eye or from indirect force, as in head injuries or explosions. The force distorts the globe and alters pressure relations in the retinal and uveal vessels. The following are the sequelae of contusion.

1. **Commotio retinae** is due to vasoparalysis of the small retinal blood vessels and results in widespread marked retinal edema with scattered hemorrhages. Commotio retinae usually resolves without permanent damage. No treatment is indicated.
2. **Purtscher's retinopathy,** also known as traumatic retinal angiopathy, occurs after crushing injuries of the chest or long bones. The condition is usually bilateral. The characteristic appearance is of multiple patches of superficial white exudates and hemorrhages surrounding the optic disk. These exudates and hemorrhages disappear with some loss of vision. The condition appears to be due to acute capillary ischemia.
3. **Macular hole.** Sometimes retinal edema after contusion is confined to the macular area. This edema subsides in 3–4 weeks, and there is often some residual loss of central vision. A **macular cyst** may form due to the coa-

lescence of edema fluid. An early intraocular gas-fluid procedure may prevent progression. Rupture of the cyst results in a macular hole.

4. **Retinal tears** or dialysis of the retina along with retinal detachment occurs after trauma. There is a high incidence of retinal dialysis after blunt trauma. This is a major cause of retinal detachments in children and young adults. Retinal dialysis appears to occur at the time of ocular contusion. If it is not recognized initially, it may go undetected until symptoms develop. Patients who have had blunt trauma should be examined periodically, especially if vitreous hemorrhage obscures part of the retinal periphery.

5. **Retinal hemorrhages.** The effects of retinal hemorrhages vary considerably according to their sizes and locations. Small retinal hemorrhages absorb completely without any significant visual defects. Hemorrhages rupturing into the vitreous may provoke a fibrovascular reaction (**retinitis proliferans).** Peripheral retinal hemorrhages may organize on the anterior vitreous surface, resulting in a **cyclitic** membrane and later a traction retinal detachment. Large vitreous hemorrhages may cause **erythroclastic glaucoma** or they may organize, causing traction retinal detachment.

6. **Massive gliosis.** Elevated glial masses found in the posterior pole in infants and children are ascribed to organization of traumatic **hemorrhage in the newborn,** due to obstetric trauma. This picture may be also seen in adults after severe inflammation due to endophthalmitis.

B. **Perforating injuries** through the posterior sclera are less common than perforating wounds of the anterior segment. An eye that has sustained a penetrating or lacerating injury may develop persistent vitreous hemorrhage or fibrovascular proliferation in the vitreous, leading to traction retinal detachments that are inoperable by standard scleral buckling surgery. Infection directly introduced into the vitreous will result in endophthalmitis and loss of the eye unless it is rapidly and adequately controlled. Pars plana vitrectomy gives good results in such a severely traumatized eye.

C. **Intraocular foreign bodies.** The presence of intraocular foreign bodies is frequently overlooked, and radiologic studies are often neglected. A high index of suspicion should be maintained whenever there is a laceration or penetrating ocular injury. This is commonplace in industrial accidents involving the eye. Most of the intraocular foreign bodies involve vitreoretinal trauma. The adjacent choroid and sclera are also affected. Foreign bodies entering the posterior segment of the eye are usually metallic splinters traveling at high speed. Although most of these high-velocity foreign bodies are sterile, all foreign bodies must be assumed to be contaminated and prophylactic antibiotic therapy must be instituted. Retinal foreign bodies may ricochet off the retina once or twice before coming to rest, resulting in **retinal tears** and subsequent fibrovascular proliferation into the vitreous. Contraction of these bands of tissue results in **traction retinal detachment.**

Intraocular foreign bodies may be divided into two types, based on the ocular reaction they elicit (see Chap. 2).

1. **Inert substances** such as gold, silver, glass, and plastics cause no specific reaction in the eye based on their composition. Apart from traumatic infection and hemorrhage, these substances cause slow liquefaction and opacification of the vitreous and fibroglial proliferation from the local retina.

2. **Irritant metals.** Iron and copper have serious effects on the eye.

   a. **Iron foreign bodies. Siderosis** is the complication of intraocular iron foreign bodies. The degree depends on the size, number of ferrous particles, and location in the eye. Retained iron, especially soft iron, undergoes electrolytic decomposition, combines with tissue cells, and causes eventual cell death. Siderosis affecting the retina results in diminution and ultimate extinction of the ERG. Iron can be demonstrated in tissues by **Perls's stain,** a specific histochemical test. Late effects of siderosis include **heterochromia,** cataract, and secondary glaucoma.

   Treatment consists of removal of the foreign body by a magnet either through the pars plana or transclerally if the foreign body is lying directly on the retina. Of course, the retinal tear should be treated and late complications, such as fibrovascular proliferation into the vitreous, should be watched for. High-grade steel alloys are poorly magnetic and cannot be removed by a magnet. Removal, if indicated by the clinical course, is done using a vitreous forceps under direct ophthalmoscopic control combined, when necessary, with pars plana vitrectomy.

b. Copper foreign bodies cause profuse suppuration in the eye. Copper is oxidized as readily as iron. Intraocular foreign bodies with less than 85% of copper cause **chalcosis,** signs of which include a greenish-blue peripheral ring in Descemet's membrane in the cornea, a greenish-red iridescent sunflower cataract, and retinal atrophy. **Management** consists of pars plana vitrectomy and removal of the foreign body using vitreous forceps.

D. Radiant energy. Ocular lesions can be produced by radiant energy of almost any wavelength. Vitreoretinal pathology is seen in the following conditions.

1. Solar retinopathy (foveomacular retinitis) refers to a specific foveolar lesion occurring in patients who gaze directly at a solar eclipse, sunbathers, and people gazing at the sun while under the influence of a hallucinogenic agent. Soon after exposure, these patients complain of metamorphopsia and a central scotoma. Vision is reduced to between 20/40 and 20/200, but almost complete recovery is seen over the ensuing months. During the period immediately after the exposure, a small gray zone develops around the foveolar area due to photochemical injury to the sensory retina and the RPE. This zone is slowly replaced by a sharply circumscribed lamellar hole.

2. Radiation retinopathy describes alterations in the retinal vasculature in patients several months or years after receiving roentgen radiation to the skull and orbital region. An ischemic ocular response may be established as is seen in diabetic retinopathy. Macular function may be affected with decrease in central vision. Photocoagulation may be of value in controlling these complications.

3. Retinal phototoxicity. Wavelengths between 400 and 1400 nm are transmitted by the mammalian ocular media to the retina, causing mechanical, thermal, and photochemical damage. Melanin granules in the RPE play a key role in mediating all three types of damage. Absorption of energy by the RPE and choroid causes elevation of temperature above the ambient temperature present in the neural retina, with thermal denaturation of sensitive macromolecules such as proteins. Photochemical damage results from extended exposure of the retina by shorter wavelengths in the visible spectrum (450–550 nm). The lens absorbs wavelengths below 450 nm, with the result that fewer photons in the blue and near-ultraviolet region reach the retina.

The physician, especially the ophthalmologist, should be aware of retinal irradiance levels for all ophthalmologic instruments such as ophthalmoscopes, intraocular fiberoptic light sources, surgical microscopes, and overhead surgical lamps. Infrared radiation should preferably be filtered from these sources because it causes actinic damage and does not contribute to visibility. Aging or diseased retinas may be more susceptible to actinic damage as compared to normal retinas.

X. Lasers have been a major therapeutic modality in the management of the retinochoroidal and vitreal disorders. Lasers have been variously used to perform **photocoagulation, photodisruption, photovaporization,** and **photoradiation.**

A. Photocoagulation is the most commonly used modality. The incident light energy is absorbed and converted into heat by the pigment in the target tissues such as RPE. The threshold temperature rise for retinal photocoagulation is approximately 10°C. Excessive temperature rise can cause vaporization and hemorrhage in target tissues. The wavelength of the incident light contributes to the efficiency of the photocoagulation process. The white light from a xenon arc lamp was used in the early photocoagulators and was followed by the **ruby laser,** which produced monochromatic light of 695 nm. The ruby laser was highly effective in producing an adhesive chorioretinitis but was not useful in the treatment of vascular diseases.

B. Photoradiation therapy (PRT) is a new technique currently under investigation for the treatment of a variety of solid malignant tumors such as malignant choroidal melanoma. Malignant tumors selectively absorb systemically administered **hematoporphyrin derivative** (HpD), a photosensitizing compound. Photoactivation of the tumor by a red laser (630 nm) results in the formation of highly reactive singlet oxygen and also superoxide, which causes tumor death. Tumor vasculature appears to be particularly sensitive to PRT damage.

C. Laser types (see also Chap. 9, sec. **VI**).

1. The **argon** laser has been a major advance in the treatment of major blinding conditions such as diabetic retinopathy, SMD, severe open-angle glaucoma, and angle-closure glaucoma. This laser has both blue (488 nm) and green (514 nm) wavelengths. The advantage of the argon laser is that it is well absorbed by hemoglobin and also by melanin in the RPE. The delivery system is precise with wide range of power densities possible, thereby affording a large coagulation range. The argon laser is minimally absorbed by the ocular media. It can be delivered through fiberoptic systems so that laser photocoagulation can be done intraoperatively such as during vitreous surgery for diabetic traction detachments and hemorrhages. Its major disadvantage is that the argon laser cannot be applied close to the fovea because of the absorption of the laser energy by the xanthophyll pigment in the macula.

2. The **krypton** laser with the red wavelength (657 nm) is an excellent alternative when CNM is present in the parafoveolar area, since this wavelength is minimally absorbed by the macular xanthophyll. The red krypton laser produces a good adhesive chorioretinitis and is useful in the treatment of hemorrhagic retinopathies.

3. The short-pulse **neodymium yttrium-aluminum-garnet (Nd-YAG)** laser is an example of a **photodisruptor.** This laser delivers a very high-power density in the pico- to nanosecond range (10^{-11} to 10^{-9} seconds), thereby ionizing tissue in a small volume of space at the laser beam focus, creating a **"plasma."** The clinical Nd-YAG laser delivers energy in the near infrared (1064 nm) and is coupled with a helium-neon laser to provide a visible, red focusing beam that identifies the focal point of the invisible Nd-YAG laser beam. This modality is primarily used to disrupt relatively transparent targets in the anterior segment such as lens capsular membranes and anterior vitreous bands.

4. **Dye lasers,** with intermediate wavelengths between green and red, are used for photocoagulation in the macular region. Laser technology has improved so that small, solid-state diode lasers are currently available for retinal photocoagulation.

5. **Excimer lasers** are currently being tested to alter the refraction of the cornea and may be soon used to treat myopia.

6. The **carbon dioxide** (CO_2) laser is a laser of great power with an emission located in the far infrared (10,600 nm). It is not clinically used in the management of vitreoretinal diseases, although its **photovaporization** characteristics have been used occasionally to seal fibrovascular fronds at the time of vitrectomy.

Uveal Tract: Iris, Ciliary Body, and Choroid

Deborah Pavan-Langston

I. **Normal anatomy and physiology.** The middle vascular layer of the eye, the uveal tract, is composed of three portions: **iris, ciliary body,** and **choroid.** The primary function of this tract is to supply nourishment to the ocular structures (see frontispiece).

   A. **The iris** is the anterior extension of the ciliary body dividing the aqueous compartments into anterior and posterior chambers. The anterior surface of the iris consists of loosely structured stromal tissue of mesodermal origin lined posteriorly by a pigmented layer that extends from the pupillary margin of the iris back to the ciliary body. The pupil is the central iris aperture that changes in size to control the amount of light entering the eye. The pupillary sphincter muscle is supplied by the parasympathetic fibers of the third nerve, and the dilator pupillary muscle is supplied by the sympathetic nervous system (see Chap. 12, sec. III).

   B. **The ciliary body** is the posterior extension of the iris and contains the ciliary muscle, which functions in accommodation. The epithelium extending posteriorly from the iris becomes two distinct layers. The outer pigmented epithelial layer is continuous posteriorly with the retinal pigment epithelium (RPE). The inner nonpigmented epithelial layer of the ciliary body produces aqueous humor and extends posteriorly to become the sensory retina.

      1. **The aqueous humor** from the ciliary body epithelium contributes to the maintenance of intraocular pressure (IOP) and supports the metabolism of the avascular lens and cornea. The composition of aqueous is approximately that of blood plasma with nearly all protein removed. Once secreted, the aqueous concentration is modified by water and chloride in the posterior chamber and by accumulation of lactic acid from the lens. The pressure of the eye depends on the rate of secretion of aqueous humor, which is approximately 1.0–2.0 µl/minute, and on the ease with which the aqueous passes through the trabecular meshwork to the canal of Schlemm and then into the aqueous veins.

      2. **Accommodation,** or focusing of the lens, is a function of both the inner radial muscle lying posterior to the iris root and the outer longitudinal muscle running between scleral spur and choroid. Between these muscles run the oblique muscles of the ciliary body. Contraction of the round muscle shortens the diameter between the ciliary processes, allowing relaxation of tension on the lens capsule. The lens, by virtue of its own elasticity, tends to assume a more spherical shape, thus increasing its refractive power to focus on an object closer to the eye. Contraction of the longitudinal and oblique muscles has a similar effect. Conversely, relaxation of these three muscle bundles increases tension on the zonular fibers, thereby increasing tension on the elastic lens capsule to flatten the lens, causing the eye to become focused on a more distant object.

   C. **The choroid** makes up the major portion of the uveal tract. It runs between retina and sclera from the ora serrata to the optic nerve. This vascular layer supplies nutrition to the external half of the retina and is composed primarily of an inner layer of capillaries known as *choriocapillaris* and externally by succeedingly larger collecting veins (medium vessels—Sattler's layer; outer large vessels—Haller's layer). The choroid is thickest posteriorly (0.25 mm) and thin near the ora serrata, where it is 0.1 mm. The anterior uveal tract is fed primarily by long posterior ciliary arteries; the posterior uveal tract is fed primarily by short ciliary arteries, although there is free anastomosis between vessels. Bruch's membrane is part of the choroid and lies between the choriocapillaris and the retinal rods and cones. Uveal melanocytes are scattered throughout the choroid, and their numbers account for variation in degree of choroidal pigmentation. The nerve supply to the choroid is from both short posterior and long anterior ciliary nerves.

II. Uveitis

A. Definition. *Uveitis* is a general term referring to inflammation of the uveal tract. It may be divided into iritis, cyclitis (ciliary body inflammation), iridocyclitis, and choroiditis, according to specific areas of the uveal tract involved. Although the term *uveitis* refers primarily to inflammation of this vascular structure, adjacent structures such as retina, vitreous, sclera, and cornea are also frequently involved secondarily in the inflammatory process.

B. Incidence. In a population of 100,000 people, over a period of 1 year, 15 individuals will develop uveitis. Of these patients, about 75% will have anterior uveitis (iritis, iridocyclitis), 8% intermediate uveitis (pars planitis), and 17% posterior or panuveitis.

C. Demography

1. **Age.** Patients most commonly afflicted are 20–50 years of age. There is a marked decrease in incidence in individuals over 70 years of age. In the elderly patient, the most common forms of uveitis are toxoplasmosis, herpes zoster, and aphakic uveitis. In the young, congenital toxoplasmosis, toxocariasis, and peripheral uveitis are found.

2. **Sex.** Forms of uveitis more common in men are sympathetic ophthalmia, due to a greater incidence of penetrating injury, and acute anterior nongranulomatous uveitis secondary to systemic ankylosing spondylitis and Reiter's syndrome. In women there is a greater incidence of chronic anterior uveitis of unknown etiology, toxoplasmosis, and pauciarticular juvenile rheumatoid arthritis.

3. **Race.** In the United States toxoplasmosis and histoplasmosis are less common in blacks than in whites. Sarcoid is more common in blacks and Behçet's disease in Japanese (not Americans of Japanese extraction).

4. **Geographic location.** Sympathetic ophthalmia is almost unheard of in the Southwest Pacific. Histoplasmosis is found almost exclusively in the midwestern United States. Sarcoidosis is most common in Sweden and the South Atlantic and Gulf regions of the United States. Leprosy is found almost entirely in the subtropics. Onchocerciasis is found in tropical Africa and Central America; Behçet's disease is found in the Mediterranean and Japan. Vogt-Koyanagi-Harada (VKH) syndrome is several hundred times more common in Japan than in the United States.

5. **Social factors.** Fungal endophthalmitis and AIDS are seen more frequently in IV drug users and AIDS and syphilitic ocular disease in promiscuous heterosexuals, homosexual males, and their sexual contacts. Other contributing factors are low social economic status and psychological depression in the 2-month period prior to the onset of an attack of uveitis.

6. **Immunologic factors.** The histocompatibility leukocyte antigen (HLA) system in humans influences immunologic homeostatic functions and cellular and humoral immune responses, as well as coding for histocompatibility antigens on cell surfaces. The uveitis syndromes for which there is a strong HLA-disease association may be due to inherited genetic factors that control the expression of HLA antigens, immune responses, and possibly responses to endogenous inflammatory mediators (see sec. **V.C.5**).

7. **Endocrine factors.** There is a correlation between hypothyroidism and uveitis and a tendency for reactivation of chorioretinitis during pregnancy. The mechanism of either is unknown.

Table 8-1. Anatomic locations potentially involved in major types of uveitis

Anterior only	Both segments	Posterior only
AIDS	AIDS	AIDS
Ankylosing spondylitis	APMPPE	APMPPE
Behçet's disease	Behçet's disease	Aspergillosis
Herpes simplex	Brucellosis	Behçet's disease
Herpes zoster	Coxsackie virus	Birdshot
Heterochromic iridocyclitis	Epstein-Barr virus	retinopathy
Idiopathic	Herpes simplex and	Candidiasis
Reiter's disease	zoster virus	Cryptococcosis
Sarcoidosis	Intermediate uveitis	Cysticercosis
Tuberculosis	Rubella	Cytomegalovirus
	Rubeola	Geographic
	Sarcoidosis	choroiditis
	Sympathetic	Histoplasmosis
	ophthalmia	Lyme disease
	Syphilis	Malignancy
	Toxoplasmosis	Nocardiosis
	Tuberculosis	Onchoceriasis
	Vogt-Koyanagi-	Periarteritis nodosa
	Harada syndrome	Sarcoidosis
		Syphilis
		Toxocariasis
		Toxoplasmosis
		Tuberculosis

AIDS = acquired immunodeficiency syndrome; APMPPE = acute multifocal placoid pigment epithe-liopathy.

III. **Signs and symptoms of uveitis** may be unilateral or bilateral, isolated attacks or repeated episodes. Autoimmune disease tends to be bilateral, while unilateral disease is often infectious or of unknown origin. Table 8-1 lists systemic infections and diseases of possible significance in uveitis.
   A. **Granulomatous versus nongranulomatous uveitis.** Although morphologic description is still of some value, the rigid division of uveitis into these two categories has become largely anachronistic. By the original definition, *nongranulomatous uveitis* was typically acute or chronic, located in the iris and ciliary body, and characterized by a cellular infiltrate of lymphocytes and plasma cells that tended to form hypopyon and fine precipitates on the corneal endothelium known as **keratic precipitates (KPs).** The etiology was thought to be noninfectious. *Granulomatous uveitis* was thought to be chronic and to involve any portion of the uveal tract but with a predilection for the posterior area. It was typically characterized by nodular collections of epithelioid cells and giant cells surrounded by lymphocytes. The KPs were larger than those seen in nongranulomatous disease, greasy in appearance (mutton fat), and composed primarily of epithelioid cells and pigment. The etiology was thought to be infectious and due to such organisms as tuberculosis, toxoplasmosis, and spirochetes; however, granulomatous uveitis was also seen in noninfectious disease such as sarcoidosis and sympathetic ophthalmia. It is now known that **transitional forms** of uveitis are not uncommon and that the basic pathology

lies somewhere between the rigidly defined granulomatous and nongranulomatous uveitides. Nonetheless, the classification is often useful in orienting the physician toward workup and therapy.

B. Acute anterior uveitis is usually sudden in onset (a few days) and lasts from 2–6 weeks. The typical clinical findings in acute nongranulomatous uveitis are an acute onset with ocular pain, hyperemia, photophobia, and blurred vision. There is perilimbal flush caused by dilation of the radial vessels and frequently fine white KPs on the posterior corneal and trabecular meshwork. The pupil is miotic, and cells and flare are found in the anterior chamber with or without fibrin exudation. Posterior synechia formation between iris and lens may be present, but **iris nodules** (pupillary Koeppe and anterior iris Busacca) and vitreous haze are typically absent. The course of disease is acute and the prognosis relatively good, although recurrence is not uncommon. More than 50% of cases are associated with HLA-B27 or HLA-B8.

C. Chronic anterior uveitis is often insidious in onset and lasts longer than 3 months. Chronic iridocyclitis may be either nongranulomatous or granulomatous in character and usually is not associated with much hyperemia. In fact, in several forms the eyes may be white (juvenile rheumatoid arthritis [JRA], white iritis in young girls, and Fuchs's heterochromic iridocyclitis). Common diagnoses of chronic iridocyclitis are sarcoidosis, tuberculosis, and Fuchs's heterochromic iridocyclitis.

D. Intermediate uveitis (pars planitis) is usually bilateral with patients presenting with blurred vision (macular edema) and/or floaters and little or no pain, photophobia, or anterior segment inflammation. The ora serrata is the site of vitritis and exudates that may progress to "snowbank" appearance, especially inferiorly. Twenty percent of children with uveitis have pars planitis.

E. Posterior uveitis. In disease limited entirely to the posterior segment of the eye, granulomatous disease is more commonly seen. Onset may be acute but is often more insidious with little or no pain, minimum photophobia and blurring of vision (unless the macular area is involved), and no perilimbal flush. Choroidal lesions may be diffuse but tend to be focal patchy yellow-white areas of infiltrate with overlying vitritis. Because of the anatomic relationship between choroid and retina, a retinitis is also usually present, and resolution of the process results in a chorioretinal scar with a corresponding visual field scotoma. If the macula is not involved, central visual acuity may return to normal. Examples of diseases involving predominantly the choroid are sympathetic ophthalmia and VKH (often with retinal detachment). Toxoplasmosis is a necrotizing retinitis with secondary inflammation in the choroid, as are the viral infections cytomegalovirus, herpes simplex and zoster, rubella, and rubeola. Behçet's disease, however, is a retinitis with retinal vasculitis and only rarely has choroidal involvement. It is not, then, truly a uveitis, although it is almost always included in this ocular disease category.

F. Panuveitis may involve the entire uveal tract in any inflammatory type. Onset may be acute or insidious and the course variable, depending on etiology. The KPs, if present, tend to be large and greasy (mutton fat), and the pupils small and occasionally scarred down to the lens by posterior synechiae. In the anterior chamber, cells and flare are sometimes present, but not to the extent commonly seen with acute anterior uveitis. Iris nodules and vitreous haze are occasionally present. The course tends to be chronic with a fair to poor prognosis, and recurrence occasionally is seen despite an apparent cure.

Certain types of uveitides may be ruled out on the basis of location alone. Table 8–1 lists potential anatomic location of several uveitis types.

IV. Differential diagnosis of uveitis. It is first necessary to determine whether a lesion is an inflammation, a tumor, a vascular process, or a degeneration. Although flare and cells in the anterior chamber are a hallmark of uveitis, they themselves are not diagnostic. Necrotic or metastatic tumors may produce an inflammatory response. Vitreous cellular debris may result from degenerative conditions such as retinitis pigmentosa or retinal detachment. Study of cells from the aqueous or vitreous or both may be diagnostic (see Chap. 1, **III.G**).

A. **Conjunctivitis** is an inflammatory condition of the mucous membrane overlying the sclera. Hyperemia is usually diffuse or may be confined to just the lateral and medial angles but is not primarily confined to the perilimbal area as in iritis. In conjunctivitis, vision is generally not blurred and pupillary responses are normal. A watery or purulent discharge may be present. There is no notable photophobia or deep pain. Moderate irritation and itching may also be present.

B. **Anterior scleritis,** while not a disease of the retinal vasculature, may have a sufficiently intense inflammatory reaction to induce an anterior or intermediate uveitis in about 40% of patients (see chapter 5). **Posterior scleritis** is also not a uveitis but may cause ocular pain, boggy conjunctiva, vitritis, and chorioretinal edema. Ultrasound will reveal the posterior scleral inflammatory process indicating need for systemic steroid therapy.

C. In **acute angle-closure glaucoma** the vision is markedly reduced, and pain may be so severe that the patient presents with nausea and vomiting. Attention may be incorrectly misdirected to the gastrointestinal tract and the red eye ignored as the source of this disturbance.

The pupil is fixed in mid-dilation at about 4–5 mm and nonreactive. The cornea is diffusely hazy. Occasionally, it may be difficult to differentiate angle-closure glaucoma from glaucoma secondary to uveitis. Gonioscopy of an eye with angle closure will reveal obstruction of the trabecular meshwork by iris, whereas an eye with acute glaucoma secondary to uveitis will have a normal open angle unless there has been extensive peripheral anterior synechia formation to the posterior cornea. In this latter case the scarring will be self-evident (see Chap. 9, sec. **IX**).

D. **Retinoblastoma** is seen in young children and is characterized by pseudohypopyon with nodules in the iris as well as free-floating cells in the aqueous humor. The fundus should be carefully searched for retinal lesions. An x ray of the globe revealing calcification scattered throughout the retinoblastic tumor is helpful in differentiating the disorder. **Anterior chamber aspiration** should be performed only if there is serious doubt concerning diagnosis (see Chap. 1, sec. **III.G**; Chap. 10, sec. **XI.A**).

E. **Juvenile xanthogranuloma of the iris (nevoxanthoendothelioma)** is characteristically associated with recurrent hyphema (blood in the anterior chamber), elevated IOP, and yellowish, poorly defined tumors. Therapy varies and includes local systemic corticosteroids, local irradiation, and excision. This disease is most commonly seen in the first year of life, but it may occur in adults. The physician should look for yellow tumors in the skin.

F. **Malignant lymphoma** such as lymphatic leukemia involving the anterior chamber is diagnosed primarily by the absence of KPs and by cell type on aqueous aspiration.

G. **Neurofibromas** of the iris appear as brownish pinhead-sized tumors level with the iris stroma or projected in a mushroom from the stroma. They may be congenital or develop after birth, puberty, pregnancy, or menopause. Pigmentation may appear and disappear spontaneously.

H. **Pigment "cells"** in the anterior chamber may be confused with iritis. The anterior chamber should be graded for flare and cells before dilating drops, especially phenylephrine hydrochloride, are used, because the process of dilation may release cells into the aqueous that are actually benign pigment granules. This is most common in patients over the age of 40 and in myopes. These cells are one-tenth the size of white cells and brownish in color. This benign pigment dust may also appear on the back of the cornea and is finer in appearance and more diffuse than that seen with leukocytic KPs.

I. **Pseudoexfoliation of the lens** presents as blue, white, or gray dandrufflike flecks on the pupillary margins, anterior surface of the lens, trabecular meshwork in the angle, lens zonules, or ciliary body. Diagnosis is confirmed by the presence of a dandruff ring, the central edge of which is lifted and curled, on the anterior lens capsule.

J. **Primary familial amyloidosis** may present as globules that are slightly larger than inflammatory cells suspended in the anterior vitreous or as dense veil-like opacities of wavy contour resembling glass wool. Protein electrophoresis and biopsy are indicated.

K. **Reactive lymphoid hyperplasia** frequently presents as an iridocyclitis. This condition may also simulate malignant melanoma. These pseudotumors respond to topical or systemic corticosteroids.

L. **Reticulum cell sarcoma** involving the eye frequently presents as a uveitis. Occasionally, the diagnosis may be made by aqueous or vitreous tap, with the better yield being from vitrectomy. Malignancy should be suspected in individuals over 40 years of age, particularly those with neurologic manifestations.

V. **Diagnostic tests in uveitis.** The three stages of diagnosis are (1) integrate information, (2) name the uveitis, and (3) order indicated tests. After a careful history and physical (Table 8-2), **name** the uveitis, e.g., a nongranulomatous iridocyclitis with band keratopathy in both eyes of a 4-year-old girl with arthritis in one knee. These characteristics suggest JRA, so the main test would be an antinuclear antibody (ANA), which is positive in 80% of patients with iridocyclitis in JRA. Other tests that should be considered are as follows (Table 8-3):

A. **Skin testing** is a frequently used useful diagnostic tool, although the risks of severe local reaction or reactivation of quiescent ocular lesions, e.g., macular histoplasmosis, must be borne in mind.

1. The **tuberculin** and **histoplasmin** tests are among the most important skin tests in uveitis. Even a very small area of reactive induration may be significant. The intermediate-strength PPD should be used routinely, and a positive test is regarded as an indication of tuberculous disease unless the patient was vaccinated with BCG previously. A positive PPD does not, however, rule out other etiologic factors, as it may be a coincidental finding.

2. The **Kveim test** for sarcoid varies with the antigen batch used, and a negative test may merely reflect the anergy seen in many sarcoid patients.

3. The **Behçetin** skin test for pathergy is rarely used now, as it appears to be effective primarily in Behçet's disease patients from the Middle East but not in the United States.

4. Other skin tests such as for cat hair, coccidioidin, lens antigen, and uveal pigment are of little or no value.

5. **Anergy** or hyporeactivity to skin testing may be of diagnostic value, as it is a phenomenon seen in sarcoidosis, lepromatous leprosy, pars planitis, and possibly herpes zoster or other immunocompromised patients.

6. **Hyperreactivity** to skin tests is seen in presumed ocular histoplasmosis and Behçet's disease. Mumps and trichophyton skin tests are used to test for the degree of reactivity.

7. **Systemic steroids** taken every other day will not suppress skin test reactions. If, however, corticosteroids are in daily use the physician must not require much of a reaction for a positive response; the response may be drug suppressed altogether or, rarely, anergy may be reversed by these drugs. Systemic **cyclosporine** may also suppress a positive skin test.

B. **Skin snips** are biopsy specimens used in making a diagnosis of onchocerciasis. The snip should be taken from one or two of the skin nodules.

C. **Blood tests** used in diagnosis of uveitis are numerous; the shotgun approach is rarely rewarding and very expensive. The tests should, therefore, be based on a high index of suspicion based on clinical findings. Some of these are obvious in their objective, e.g., VDRL or fluorescent treponemal antibody (FTA) test for syphilis. Others warrant the following discussion, and all are listed in Table 8-3.

1. A **complete blood count** (CBC) with differential showing eosinophilia indicates parasitic infestation.

2. An **elevated erythrocyte sedimentation rate** (ESR) is a nonspecific indication of systemic disease that may or may not be related to the ocular disease.

3. **Antibody titers against infectious organisms.** A *Toxoplasma* fluorescent

Table 8-2. Signs and symptoms of possible diagnostic significance in uveitis

Sign or Symptom	Possible Clinical Disease
Alopecia	VKH
Arthritis	Behçet's, colitis, JRA, RA, Reiter's, sarcoid
Cerebrospinal fluid pleocytosis	APMPPE, Behçet's, sarcoid, VKH
Cough, shortness of breath	Sarcoid, tuberculosis, malignancy
Diarrhea	Colitis, Whipple's disease
Erythema nodosum	Behçet's, sarcoid
Genital ulcers	Behçet's, Reiter's
Headaches	Sarcoid, VKH
Immunosuppression	CMV, HSV, VZV, AIDS, fungal (especially *Candida*), parasitic (pneumocystitis, *Toxoplasma*), chorioretinitis, other opportunistic infections
Lymphoid swelling	AIDS, sarcoid
Neurosensory deafness	Sarcoid, VKH
Oral ulcers	Behçet's, colitis
Paresthesia, weakness	Behçet's, multiple sclerosis
Psychosis	VKH
Salivary or lacrimal gland swelling	Sarcoid
Sacroiliitis	Ankylosing spondylitis, colitis, Reiter's
Skin nodules	Onchocerciasis, sarcoid
Skin rash	Behçet's, HSV, psoriasis, RNA viral exanthem (mumps, measles, rubella), sarcoid, syphilis, VZV
Systemic vasculitis	Behçet's, polychondritis, sarcoid
Tracheal, nasal, or ear lobe pain	Polychondritis
Vitiligo, poliosis	VKH

AIDS = acquired immunodeficiency syndrome; APMPPE = acute posterior multifocal placoid pigment epitheliopathy; CMV = Cytomegalovirus; HSV = herpes simplex virus; JRA = juvenile rheumatoid arthritis; RA = rheumatoid arthritis; VKH = Vogt-Koyanagi-Harada syndrome; VZV = varicella-zoster virus.
Source: Adapted from R. Nussenblatt and A. Palestine, *Uveitis.* Chicago: Year Book, 1988. P. 58. With permission.

antibody or hemagglutination titer is considered positive at any level, even 1 : 1. Antiviral titers (herpes simplex, varicella, zoster, cytomegalovirus, Epstein-Barr and others listed in Tables 8-1 and 8-2) are, with the exception of HIV titers (AIDS), meaningful only when drawn as acute and convalescent sera about 1 month apart and demonstrating at least a two- to fourfold rise in titer. A single "positive" test for virus does not indicate whether a viral infection took place recently or not.

4. **Angiotensin converting enzyme (ACE)** is often routinely drawn in cases of suspected sarcoid, yet it is not specific for this disease, normal values in children are not known, and the predictive value is not established in the absence of other signs of sarcoid.

5. **HLA (histocompatibility leukocyte antigen)** testing is of significance when positive in a patient exhibiting signs of disease compatible with the appro-

Table 8-3. Diagnostic aids for uveitis by anatomic classification

Anterior uveitis	Intermediate uveitis	Posterior uveitis
Anergy workup	Anergy workup	Anergy workup
Angiotensin converting enzyme	Angiotensin converting enzyme	Angiotensin converting enzyme
Anterior chamber paracentesis	Behçetin skin test	Anticardiolipin antibody
Antiviral antibodies	CT scan	Antifungal antibody
Behçetin skin test	Chest x-ray study	Antitoxoplasma antibody
Chest x-ray study	Conjunctival biopsy	Antitoxocara antibody
Chlamydial complement-fixation test	Fluorescein angiography	Antiviral antibody
Conjunctival biopsy	Gallium scan	Behçetin skin test
Fluorescein angiography	Hand x-ray studies	Cell-mediated responses to antigen(s)
Gallium scan	Laser interferometry	Chest x-ray study
Hand x-ray studies	Lacrimal gland biopsy	Chorioretinal biopsy
Heterophile	Liver function tests	Electrooculogram
HLA typing	Lumbar puncture	Electroretinogram
Immune complexes	Potential acuity meter	Fluorescein angiography
Lacrimal gland biopsy	PPD	Gallium scan
Laser interferometry	Stool evaluation	Histoplasmin skin test
PPD	Vitreal biopsy (cytology, subsets)	HIV testing
Sacroiliac x-rays		HLA typing
Skin snips		Immune complexes
Stool evaluation		Laser interferometry
VDRL/FTA-ABS		Liver function tests
		Lumbar puncture
		Potential acuity meter
		Pathergy
		PPD
		Skull x-rays
		Stool evaluation
		T-cell subsets
		Ultrasound
		Viral cultures
		Visual evoked response

Source: Adapted from R. Nussenblatt and A. Palestine, *Uveitis: Fundamentals and Clinical Practice.* Chicago: Year Book, 1988. P. 81. With permission.

priate known HLA immunogenetic test. HLA tests associated with specific ocular inflammatory states include
  a. Acute anterior uveitis: HLA-B27, HLA-B8.
  b. Ankylosing spondylitis: HLA-B27, HLA-B7.
  c. Behçet's disease: HLA-B51.
  d. Birdshot retinopathy: HLA-A29.
  e. Ocular pemphigoid: HLA-B12.
  f. Presumed ocular histoplasmosis: HLA-B27.
  g. Reiter's syndrome: HLA-B27.
  h. Rheumatoid arthritis: HLA-DR4.

   i. Sympathetic ophthalmia: HLA-A11.
   j. Vogt-Koyanagi-Harada disease: MT-3.
HLA typing is now considered an important diagnostic test in determining the etiology of certain uveitides. The HLA system is the main human leukocyte isoantigen system. Human leukocyte antigens are present on most nucleated cells and comprise the major histocompatibility systems in humans. In practice, the blood lymphocyte is tested by cytotoxicity methods by incubation with antiserum complement. The genetic loci belonging to the system are designated by the loci A, B, C, and D. These alleles are designated by numbers. In practice, it is seen that HLA-B27 is commonly associated with iridocyclitis in ankylosing spondylitis. A patient with a positive HLA-B27 has a 35% chance of developing acute iritis, compared with a 7% chance for those with a negative HLA-B27. The VKH syndrome has an increased frequency of HLA-BW22J, a unique Japanese antigen. HLA-B7 appears to predispose a patient to the development of histoplasmic maculopathy. This testing is generally done in university hospital centers.

  6. **Circulating immune complexes** present in ocular inflammatory disease may be a secondary or protective reaction rather than a destructive primary cause of disease. A positive ANA is of diagnostic significance in juvenile rheumatoid arthritis and lupus erythematosus, however.

  7. **Serum globulin** and **calcium** are elevated in sarcoidosis as is **urine calcium.**

  8. The **lymphocyte transformation test** may demonstrate T-cell or cellular hypersensitivity to many antigens in the laboratory. These highly specialized tests may or may not aid in diagnosis and are still being refined.

  9. **Anticardiolipin antibodies** should be drawn in cases of retinal vascular occlusive disease especially suspected lupus with vasculitis (see Chap. 7, sec. **III.B.11**).

  10. **Antineutrophil cytoplasmic antibodies** (ANCA) for diagnosis of Wegener's granulomatosis and efficacy of cyclophosphamide or trimethoprim sulfisoxasole DS tablets daily, using sequential ANCA titers.

D. **Radiographic analyses** of diagnostic significance are

  1. **Skull films** for calcification indicative of toxoplasmosis.

  2. **Gallium scans** of the lungs, salivary, or lacrimal glands for sarcoidosis.

  3. **Chest x ray** for sarcoid, tuberculosis, or malignancy.

  4. **Sinus films** for periocular inflammatory disease are now of controversial value in diagnosing intraocular inflammatory disease.

  5. **Sacroiliac and spinal x rays** for evidence of ankylosing spondylitis.

  6. **Hand, wrist, foot, and knee x rays** for arthritic changes of rheumatoid disease or Reiter's syndrome.

E. **Anterior chamber aspiration.** Cytologic examination and antibody titers of the aqueous humor after keratocentesis may be of diagnostic assistance (see Chap. 1, sec. **III.G**).

  1. **Cytology** may vary depending on etiology. A small drop of **aqueous** is placed on a slide from the aspirating needle, fixed in absolute methanol for 10 minutes, and allowed to air-dry. The slide is stained with Giemsa solution for 1 hour and then rinsed with 95% ethanol and allowed to dry. Acute uveitis involving binding of complement to immune complexes (Behçet's syndrome) may have an abundance of neutrophils. Lens-induced uveitis produces many macrophages as well as some neutrophils. In parasitic infections numerous eosinophils are present. Bacterial uveitis may reveal both organisms and multiple neutrophils. Gram staining should be performed on another single-drop slide preparation of aqueous to confirm the type of bacteria seen.

  2. **Local production of antibody** resulting in higher intraocular than serum titers may be indicative of an active intraocular lesion such as toxoplasmosis, herpes simplex virus, or varicella-zoster virus. A normal antibody coefficient is 1.0. A range of 2–7 is suggestive and over 8 diagnostic. These tests are done only in major medical centers.

F. Fluorescein angiography may be of use in diagnosis and clinical follow-up of chorioretinitis secondary to toxoplasmosis, toxocariasis, and histoplasmosis and as an invaluable aid in following the clinical course of the many changes seen in a variety of uveitis patients.

1. The most common **fluorescein angiographic changes** found in uveitis include
   a. Cystoid macular edema.
   b. Disk leakage.
   c. Late staining of the retinal vasculature.
   d. Retinal pigment epithelial disturbances.
   e. Retinal capillary dropout, ischemia, and neovascularization.
   f. Subretinal neovascular membranes.
2. **Visual acuity impairment** is correlated directly with increased macular thickening but not with late-phase leakage as determined by angiography.

G. Other ophthalmic tests of use in uveitis are as follows:

1. The **electroretinogram (ERG;** local retinal damage) and the **electrooculogram (EOG;** retinal pigment epithelial status assessed by corneal retinal potentials) will indicate the extent of widespread damage to the eye but are not diagnostically specific.
2. **Laser interferometry** is a useful predictor of which patients will do well with immunosuppressive therapy. Visual acuity measured by laser interferometry is often better than that measured by standard eye charts. The difference probably indicates potentially reversible macular disease. Thus, if a patient reads two lines better with laser testing than on the eye chart, one may predict about a two-line potential improvement with therapy with better than 80% accuracy.
3. **Stool samples** are of diagnostic value if parasitic disease is the suspected etiologic agent.
4. **Conjunctival biopsy** is useful in sarcoidosis only if there is an obvious lesion. Even if shown to be a granulomatous reaction, it may be hard to prove it is not an old chalazion.
5. **Lumbar puncture for CSF cytology** is indicated in cases of suspected VKH syndrome or intraocular neoplasm.

VI. Nonspecific treatment of uveitis. Since the etiology of a uveitis is often unknown or no specific treatment is available despite specific diagnosis, nonspecific measures are frequently employed. These measures include corticosteroids, mydriatic-cycloplegics, immunosuppressive drugs, nonsteroidal anti-inflammatory agents, and photocoagulation.

A. Corticosteroids are very effective, not too difficult to administer, not too expensive, and therefore are the most common agents used. These drugs reduce inflammation by (1) reduction of leukocytic and plasma exudation, (2) maintenance of cellular membrane integrity with inhibition of tissue swelling, (3) inhibition of lysozyme release from granulocytes and of phagocytosis, (4) increased stabilization of intracellular lysosomal membranes, and (5) suppression of circulating lymphocytes. Corticosteroids should be used with caution in uveitis secondary to an infectious process, particularly that of herpes simplex or bacterial etiology. Relative drug potency for conversion of doses is listed in Table 8-4.

1. **Topical preparations.** The strongest ophthalmic corticosteroid drop preparations are dexamethasone phosphate 0.1%, dexamethasone alcohol 0.1%, prednisolone acetate 1.0%, and prednisolone phosphate 1.0%. Of lesser strength and of great use in tapering or treating less severe anterior segment inflammation are the prednisolone 0.20% and 0.12% preparations. Fluorometholone (FML) is useful in patients with a tendency to IOP rise secondary to corticosteroids. It is one-third as effective, however, as the stronger corticosteroids mentioned. Corticosteroid ointments, although readily available, are significantly less effective than drops.

Table 8-4. Relative dose potency of commonly used corticosteroids

Drug	Equivalent anti-inflammatory dose (mg	Relative anti-inflammatory potency
Cortisone	25.0	0.8
Hydrocortisone	20.0	1.0
Prednisolone	5.0	4.0
Prednisone	5.0	4.0
Methylprednisolone	4.0	5.0
Tramcinolone	4.0	5.0
Dexamethasone	0.75	26.0
Betamethasone	0.60	33.0

2. **Topical corticosteroid administration.** If the uveitis is posterior to the lens iris diaphragm, drops or ointments will not be adequate. For an anterior iridocyclitis, however, the frequency of corticosteroid drops is dependent on the severity of the reaction and varies from 1 drop q2-4h around the clock for the first few days to 1 drop every other day. Titration should be slow over many days to weeks and generally reduced by 50% at each step as the disease improves. The starting point is dependent on how severe the reaction is. In general, the presence of a fibrinous hypopyon uveitis would indicate high-dose therapy starting at q2-4h; the presence of a mild to moderate cell and flare reaction would indicate therapy starting at a level of strong corticosteroids 2-4 times daily with taper within several days to the weaker steroid preparations. Corticosteroids should not be used topically more than 2 or 3 times daily without concomitant antibiotic ointment or drops administered once or twice daily.

3. **Systemic corticosteroids** are of use in intractable anterior uveitis not responding satisfactorily to topical drops alone and for posterior uveitis or panuveitis where the deeper uveal structures can be reached only by systemic administration of drug or by periocular injection (see sec. **4**). With the exception of concurrent systemic disease that demands systemic therapy or severe vision-threatening disease, children should be treated only with topical and/or periocular injection, as immunosuppressive agents have lifelong effects on growth and development. **Systemic steroids should never be used in children without consultation with or the concomitant care of a pediatrician.** Table 8-4 lists the relative dose potencies of commonly used corticosteroids for dose conversion from one drug to another.

   a. **Daily therapy** for marked inflammatory activity, in which an immediate high dosage is necessary over a period of several days for maintenance of the integrity of critical visual structures such as the macula or optic nerve, is necessary for up to 2 weeks before switching to alternate-day therapy. Common dosage is 60-100 mg of prednisone each morning for 7-14 days, followed by 100 mg every other breakfast (to reduce adrenal suppression) and later by a reduction of the milligrams to minimum maintenance.

   b. **Alternate-day therapy.** The advantages of alternate-day steroid dosage include avoidance of adrenal suppression, preservation of intact neutrophil and macrophage function, and decrease in systemic side effects. It is important in using this approach to use short-acting preparations that will not carry over through the nonsteroid day. Table 8-4 lists steroid preparations according to the duration of their effects. In the absence of acute disease, alternate-day therapy may begin immediately with prednisone, and the usual dosage ranges from 50-100 mg every other breakfast, with subsequent reduction as noted under daily therapy (see sec. **3.a**).

4. **Periocular injection.** Because of the danger of intraocular injection, such medication should be given only by an ophthalmologist. Periocular injections are indicated to supplement systemic therapy in patients who cannot be trusted to take their medications, at eye surgery in an eye with uveitis, and when topical and systemic steroids are not sufficiently effective. Children must be placed under general anesthesia and **never maintained on injected steroid without monitoring by a pediatrician** for adrenal suppression and other adverse side effects.

   a. **Medication.** Although depot medication remains in the periocular tissues for 6 weeks, its major effect is during the first week. (Depomethylprednisolone, 40-80 mg subconjunctivally, subtenon, or retrobulbar, is commonly used). These injections are ordinarily given once every 2 weeks for 4-5 times, although some patients may require such an injection only once every 6 months. Soluble, short-acting steroids may be used for acute cases, in patients who have to take injections every week, or in patients in whom the physician is concerned about a rise in IOP from corticosteroids. Aqueous methylprednisolone, 40-80 mg, or decadron, 4-24 mg/ml, may be given daily, every other day, or as needed to control inflammation.

   b. The **injection** is most safely made above the temporal subtenon area over the pars plana, over the peripheral retina, or back near the macular region depending on the disease target. Topical anesthetics are necessary, but mixing injectable anesthetic with steroid increases volume and initial pain. Preinjection oral analgesics should be given for the lingering discomfort. Such injections may be used at the end of an intraocular surgical procedure, in unilateral uveitis, in cystoid macular edema, and in children. All are situations where systemic effects of steroids are minimized, yet good therapeutic doses are delivered to the target site.

5. **Complications of corticosteroid therapy**

   a. **Topical therapy.** Potential side effects of topical therapy include temporary partial lid ptosis, pupillary mydriasis of 0.6-2.0 mm, increased IOP in approximately 30% of patients treated for 3 weeks or more, posterior subcapsular cataract formation that will not progress if corticosteroids are discontinued, bacterial or fungal superinfection secondary to suppression of cellular defense systems, and decreased wound healing.

   b. **Systemic and repeated periocular therapy.** Complications of systemic or repeated periocular therapy are all the above plus extraocular muscle fibrosis (periocular injection), Cushing's syndrome, peptic ulcers, systemic hypertension, sodium retention, hyperglycemia in diabetics, psychosis, failure of growth, amenorrhea, and Addison's disease.

B. **Mydriatic-cycloplegics** are used to give comfort by relieving iris sphincter and ciliary muscle spasm and to prevent scarring between the pupillary border and anterior lens capsule (posterior synechiae). Atropine, the strongest mydriatic-cycloplegic, is used in strengths of 1-4%. It should be reserved for moderately severe to severe anterior uveitis and should be used 1-4 times daily. As uveitis lessens, the atropine dosage may be reduced or the patient placed on homatropine 5% at bedtime. For mild to moderate anterior uveitis, homatropine 5% qd-bid will suffice to move the pupil. Bedtime use is beneficial only in milder cases, since the pupil is mobilized primarily during sleep and iatrogenic presbyopia is not present during the day. Pupils that fail to dilate on atropine should have additional help of bandages on the eye between applications to increase the effect of the atropine. Phenylephrine 2.5% bid-tid (in the absence of significant cardiovascular disease) and cocaine 4% drops q30min tid only are also useful in mobilizing the otherwise scarred-down pupil. **Phenylephrine 10% should not be used at home because of its cardiotoxic**

effects. Additionally, it has no therapeutic effect on inflammation and does loosen pigment into the anterior chamber, thereby complicating the grading of the inflammation and possibly contributing to pigmentary glaucoma. Atropine may also complicate or precipitate urinary retention in patients with prostatism. Scopolamine 0.5% has almost the same cycloplegic strength as atropine and may be substituted for it in patients with urinary retention problems. Scopolamine itself, however, in very frequent doses may also aggravate this condition. **Cyclopentolate may aggravate iritis** because of its neutrophilic chemotactic effect.

C. **Immunosuppressive agents.** Immunosuppressive drugs should usually not be prescribed by an ophthalmologist alone but in concert with an oncologist or hematologist who is familiar with them and confident in their management. In making a decision as to which patient should receive immunosuppressive therapy, the physician must remember that the use of these drugs for nonneoplastic and non-life-threatening illness is a great clinical responsibility. To date there appear to have been very few severe complications from the combined regimen of corticosteroids and immunosuppressive agents, probably because of the lower dosages used and the better general health of the ophthalmic patients receiving them. Patients should be fully informed as to potential risks and benefits. A signed consent form or chart note to that effect is advisable.

1. **Selection of patients** involves choosing those who
   a. Failed to respond to conventional corticosteroid therapy or have an unacceptable side effect from them.
   b. Have progressive, usually bilateral vision-threatening disease.
   c. Have adequate follow-up.
   d. Are reliable about following instructions.
   e. Are willing to undergo therapy with full knowledge of the possible deleterious side effects.
   f. May potentially benefit from the use of the drugs.
   g. Have no unequivocal contraindication such as active tuberculosis, toxoplasmosis or other infectious process.

2. **Three classes of immunosuppressive agents** are used in ocular inflammatory disease: alkylating agents, antimetabolites, and antibiotics.
   a. **The alkylating agents cyclophosphamide and chlorambucil** work by suppression of lymphocyte T-cell (cell-mediated immunity) and, to a lesser extent, B-cell (antibodies) function.
      (1) **Clinical indications** are not fully established but are most commonly Behçet's disease, sympathetic ophthalmia, Wegener's granulomatosis, rheumatoid arthritis, polyarteritis nodosa, relapsing polychondritis, bullous pemphigoid, and malignancy.
      (2) **Cyclophosphamide dosage** in adult patients starts at 150–200 mg/day (2 mg/kg/day) taken on an empty stomach. A white blood count is taken at day 1 and every 2–3 days until it begins to drop at about 7 days. At this point, dosage is reduced by 25–50 mg to stabilize the white cell count at about 3000 cells/µl. The white cell count and differential are then followed weekly.
      (3) **Chlorambucil dosage** is begun at 2 mg/day and increased every 3–4 days to total dosage of 6–12 mg/day if there is no idiosyncratic reaction. The white cell count and differential are followed as for cyclophosphamide.
      (4) **Adverse side effects** of alkylating agents are uncontrolled leukopenia, thrombocytopenia, anemia, opportunistic infections, gastrointestinal disturbances, alopecia, jaundice, pulmonary interstitial fibrosis, renal toxicity, and testicular atrophy. Hemorrhagic cystitis is an indication for discontinuing the medication. There is an increased incidence of myeloproliferative and lymphoproliferative malignancy in patients on these drugs.
   b. **The antimetabolite azathioprine** interferes with purine metabolism

and **methotrexate** interferes with folate action, both functions essential to nucleic acid synthesis.

(1) **Clinical indications** are in therapy of rheumatoid arthritis, pemphigoid, and regional ileitis. Azathioprine has also been used successfully in some cases of sympathetic ophthalmia, VKH syndrome, pars planitis, and Behçet's disease. Methotrexate has been effective in certain recalcitrant cases of intermediate uveitis and sympathetic ophthalmia but ineffective in Behçet's disease and iridocyclitis.

(2) **Azathioprine dosage** starts at 1 mg/kg/day, working up to 2.5 mg/kg/day. The usual dose range is 50–100 mg/day in one or divided doses.

(3) **Adverse side effects of azathioprine** are uncontrolled leukopenia, thrombocytopenia, hyperuricemia, and gastrointestinal disturbances.

(4) **Methotrexate dosage** is variable due to high drug toxicity. Generally a weekly oral or intramuscular injection dose of 2.5–7.5 mg is given until a therapeutic response is noted and then maintained per hematologic (weekly) and renal and hepatic (monthly) monitoring.

(5) **Adverse side effects of methotrexate** include leukopenia, thrombocytopenia, hepatic and renal toxicity, gastrointestinal disturbances, interstitial pneumonitis, CNS toxicity, and sterility.

(6) **Hematologic monitoring** for both antimetabolites is similar to that of cyclophosphamide (alkylating agents).

c. **The antibiotic cyclosporine A** probably interferes with T-cell lymphocyte activation and **dapsone** works by an, as yet, unknown mechanism.

(1) **The clinical indications** for **cyclosporine** are Behçet's disease (for which corticosteroids are contraindicated by some Japanese investigators) and sympathetic ophthalmia. Relative indications are all noninfectious cases of uveitis unresponsive to maximum tolerated steroid therapy, Eales's disease, retinal vasculitis (noninfectious), and serpiginous choroiditis. Anterior segment disease responsive to this drug includes pamphigoid, Mooren's ulcer, and corneal transplant rejection.

(2) **Cyclosporine A dosage** is 5 mg/kg/day given orally in an olive oil–ethanol solution with milk or juice. Maximum dosage is 7 mg/kg/day.

(3) **Adverse side effects** of the given **cyclosporine A** dosage are systemic hypertension, partially reversible renal toxicity, opportunistic infection, gastrointestinal disturbances, breast tenderness, hyperuricemia, and hepatotoxicity. Monthly and, if warranted, weekly blood tests should monitor these effects.

(4) **Dapsone** is discussed in Chap. 5, sec. **IV.M.**

d. **Combination steroid and cyclosporine A therapy.** These drugs augment each other such that addition of prednisone (10–20 mg/day or short-term 1mg/kg/day) may allow a lowering of the cyclosporine A dosage (2–4 mg/kg/day) with no loss of therapeutic efficacy.

D. **Nonsteroidal anti-inflammatory drugs (NSAIDs)** appear to act by blocking local mediators of the inflammatory response such as the polypeptides of the kinin system, lysosomal enzymes, lymphokines, and the prostaglandins. The prostaglandins are one of the many chemical mediators involved in the pathogenesis of uveitis; they are synthesized by the enzyme prostaglandin synthetase and found in all tissues of the eye. Prostaglandins cause a marked increase in protein content of the aqueous humor and mild smooth muscle contraction (pupillary miosis). Certain prostaglandins lower IOP, and others (E_1 and E_2) may raise it. The increased permeability of the ciliary epithelium may be a critical factor in inducing increased IOP secondary to prostaglandin release. All should be **taken with meals.**

1. **Salicylates** are effective in reducing inflammatory response and protein rise in the anterior chamber after keratocentesis. Aspirin must be used in the range of 4–5 gm or more per day to be effective and may be given in several divided doses.

2. **Phenylbutazone** is of use in ankylosing spondylitis and is used in 3 or 4 divided doses not totaling more than 600 mg/day and not for longer than 1 week. Oxyphenbutazone, 100 mg PO qid, is useful in management of anterior uveitis.

3. **Antiprostaglandin drugs** such as naproxen and diflunisal have been of use in patients in whom aqueous flare is a prominent finding, but treatment of flare alone is not necessary and is inconsequential (see sec. **VII.D**).

4. There is no evidence that any NSAID is effective when used as the **primary agent** in therapy of intraocular inflammation. They are, however, useful in long-term therapy of **recurrent anterior uveitis** initially controlled by steroid therapy. Diflusinal (Dolobid), 500 mg PO bid, naproxen (Naprosyn), 250 or 375 mg PO bid, or indomethacin (Indocin SR), 75 mg PO bid, may allow a patient to reduce or even discontinue steroid therapy without reactivation of disease.

E. **Photocoagulation** in toxoplasmic chorioretinitis has not been confirmed as valuable therapy either in the acute or atrophic stage. It is, however, the treatment of choice in ocular histoplasmosis where a neovascular net has developed under the retina. Such a net tends to leak and produce detachment of the sensory retina. Coagulation of the net usually leads to obliteration of capillaries and some recovery of vision. See Chap. 7, secs. **III** and **IX**.

VII. **Complications of uveitis**

A. **Corneal band-shaped keratopathy** usually indicates that the individual had uveitis as a child. The calcified opacity at the level of Bowman's membrane and the palpebral fissure is separated from the limbus by a clear zone and has disk-shaped holes corresponding to nerve channels. This band may be **removed for visual or cosmetic reasons** by the use of chelating agents such as 0.5–1.0% sodium edate (EDTA). The corneal epithelium is gently removed with cocaine 4% on a sterile cotton-tipped applicator and mild scraping with the edge of a Bard Parker blade if necessary. A Weck-cell sponge cut to the shape of the band is soaked in the chelating agent and applied over the area of the band for 5–10 minutes. It is then removed and the band wiped again with a sterile cotton-tipped applicator or blade. The Weck-cell may need to be reapplied to complete removal of the calcium. EDTA may also be dropped onto the cornea but will produce a significant chemical conjunctivitis postoperatively. Antibiotic ointment and a short-acting cycloplegic should be instilled and mild pressure patching applied for 24–48 hours postoperatively.

B. **Cataracts.** See Chap. 6, sec. **VII.E**.

C. **Macular surface wrinkling** is an increased shagreen or reflection and crinkled cellophane-like appearance that has given rise to the term *cellophane maculopathy*. Various types of cells growing on the internal limiting membrane may produce this wrinkling. No specific therapy is available, although retrobulbar depot steroids may retard progression of macular traction. Occasionally surgical peeling of membranes may be successful.

D. **Edema of the disk and macula** may be seen in the more severe posterior uveitides and panuveitides. Edema of the disk does not result in much visual impairment, but macular edema is a major cause of reduced vision. Whenever vision is reduced in uveitic patients, this entity should be suspected and is probably best established diagnostically (in decreasing order) by the photo-stress test, by fluorescein angiography, by slit-lamp microscopy of the macula using a Hruby lens, and least well by direct ophthalmoscopy. Systemic and posterior periocular **steroid** therapy or, if necessary, **immunosuppressive** therapy may be of significant use in reversing or limiting macular damage in appropriately selected cases. **Antiprostaglandin drugs** such as PO naproxen, 250–375 mg bid, or diflunisal, 500 mg qd–bid, may be of use in limiting macular edema in certain cases and may be used with greater safety than steroids for prolonged therapy or after a course of steroid. **Topical indocin** (1 tablet/5 ml saline), **flurbiprofen** 0.03%, or **suprofen** qid is often effective.

E. **Corneal edema** is proportionate to the degree of damaged corneal endothelium and to the height of IOP. Topical steroids should be used q2–6h as needed to quiet inflammation in the vicinity of the endothelium, and measures should be taken to reduce IOP. Ethoxzolamide, 50 mg PO tid, or other carbonic anhydrase inhibitors with or without topical β blockers or epinephrine, are effective.

F. **Secondary glaucoma**
   1. **Etiology.**
      a. **Debris blockage** is probably the most common cause of secondary glaucoma, the uveal meshwork being blocked by inflammatory material. The IOP may not rise until the ciliary body is recovering function and secreting normal amounts of aqueous again.
      b. **Anterior synechiae** result from inflammatory adhesions between cornea and iris, usually due to nodules or infiltration of the trabeculum, thereby closing the angle.
      c. In **rubeosis iridis** a fibrovascular membrane in the angle contracts like a zipper, causing angle-closure glaucoma. Rubeosis signifies an ischemic retina and conveys a poor prognosis.
      d. **Corticosteroids** themselves frequently result in an increase in IOP and may aggravate primary glaucoma. If the patient is a steroid responder, and the pressure cannot be controlled below 25 mm Hg or there is progressive cupping or field loss despite acetazolamide or methazolamide pills and beta blocker or epinephrine drops (or both), the physician may reduce the level of steroid to increase the degree of uveitis and effect a lowered pressure. If the problem is posterior, e.g., toxoplasmic chorioretinitis, prednisone tablets rather than depot injections or corticosteroid drops should be used.
      e. If the iris becomes bound to the lens all around the pupil, **iris bombé** may develop, preventing flow of aqueous in the ciliary body into the anterior chamber and trabecular area. If pressure becomes too high, YAG or argon **laser iridotomy** or, if these fail because of iris edema and inflammation, surgery to produce a peripheral iridectomy opening is necessary.
      f. **Sclerosis** of the trabecular meshwork may follow chronic uveitis.
      g. A **hyaline membrane** may form over the trabeculum, blocking out flow.
      h. **Swelling** of the trabeculum from inflammation (trabeculitis) may reduce its porosity.
   2. **Treatment contraindications**
      a. **Miotics are avoided in secondary glaucoma due to uveitis** because they increase the discomfort from the sphincter pupillae and increase inflammation.
      b. **Laser trabeculoplasty is not useful** and not indicated in uveitis glaucoma (see Chap. 9).

G. **Retinal detachment** may be exudative, as in VKH syndrome. Uveitis may also give rise to detachment by producing shrinkage in the vitreous, with resultant traction and tears in the retina. In patients without uveitis, such a tear in the retina often gives rise to anterior segment changes that simulate uveitis.

VIII. **Endogenous anterior uveitis (iridocyclitis)**
   A. **Idiopathic anterior uveitis** is the most common form of anterior segment inflammation with about 50% of patients having ocular findings only, about 30% iridocyclitis plus a positive HLA-B27 test, and the remainder having associated systemic disease such as Reiter's syndrome, ankylosing spondylitis, or JRA.
      1. **Clinical findings** may involve both eyes but usually only one eye at any given time. These include any or all of the following: pain, photophobia, diffuse redness with predominant circumlimbal flush, tearing, blurred vision,

a nongranulomatous anterior chamber cell and flare reaction, and occasional aqueous fibrin, miosis, posterior synechiae, and secondary glaucoma.

2. **Diagnostic tests** are usually not done for a single attack unless there are systemic symptoms such as backache (see Table 8-2).

3. **Therapy** is topical steroids sufficient to control the attack, e.g., 0.1% dexamethasone 2-6 times/day in combination with cycloplegia such as homatropine 1-3 times/day. Drops are tapered over several weeks and the patient hopefully weaned off between attacks. If **macular edema** develops, a short course of systemic steroid or periocular steroid injection may be needed.

B. **Ankylosing spondylitis** has a 25% incidence of anterior uveitis. Of these patients, 80% will have both eyes involved but usually at different times.

1. **Clinical findings** are the same as in idiopathic anterior uveitis. Recurrences may occur monthly or less than annually.

2. **Diagnostic tests** are listed in Table 8-3, the most important being lumbosacral spine x rays for sacroiliitis and spinal fusion. Many patients are HLA-B27 positive, and some have family histories of ankylosing spondylitis.

3. **Therapy** is similar to that for idiopathic iridocyclitis except that topical steroids may need to be used q1h initially to control the inflammation. NSAIDs such as diflusinal, 500 mg PO bid, or naproxen, 375 mg PO bid, will alleviate joint symptoms but have no apparent effect on the ocular disease.

C. **Reiter's syndrome** is rare in the United States, being seen most often in men and rarely in children. There is a nongonococcal triad of **arthritis, urethritis,** and **conjunctivitis.** Among organisms suspected of having a possible etiologic role are *Chlamydia (Bedsonia)* and *Ureaplasma.* It is been suggested that Reiter's syndrome is caused by one of these organisms by means of an unusual host response. The postvenereal form occurs exclusively in men, but a gramnegative postdysenteric form has been observed in families.

1. **Clinical findings** include the above triad plus nebulous keratitis, an acute frequently recurring nongranulomatous iridocyclitis in up to 12% of patients, a scaling skin eruption (keratoderma blennorrhagicum), balanitis, and aphthous stomatitis. Arthritis will develop in 95% of patients at some point and may involve joints of the hands, wrists, feet, knees, or sacroiliac area. Urethritis occurs in about 75% and conjunctivitis in 30-60% of patients. A multifocal punctate subepithelial and anterior stromal infiltrative keratitis with or without pannus, pupillary synechiae, and cystoid macular edema (CME) may develop. Glaucoma or cataracts almost never develop.

2. **Diagnostic tests** of key importance are HLA-B27 and joint x rays. Rheumatoid factor and autoantibody tests are usually negative. (See Table 8-3.)

3. **Therapy** of the ocular disease is topical steroids. Systemic tetracycline, 250 mg PO qid, or doxycycline, 100 mg PO bid, for 3 weeks should be given if *Chlamydia* is suspected. The disease usually resolves completely between episodes.

D. **Juvenile rheumatoid arthritis (JRA)** has a 20% incidence of anterior uveitis. Patients at highest risk of ocular disease (14%) are young (4 years-teens) female JRA patients with fewer than four joints involved, no wrist involvement, and positive ANA testing. Another high-risk group (75%) for developing ocular disease are teenage males with pauciarticular disease and positive HLA-B27 testing. Arthritis usually precedes ocular inflammation by several years, but occasionally the situation may be reversed.

1. **Clinical findings** in the eye may be similar to those of idiopathic anterior uveitis (acute and symptomatic), especially in males. More dangerous is the insidious chronic smouldering iritis seen in more than 50% of the predominantly female HLA-B27-negative, ANA-positive group who develop iritis. This "silent" anterior uveitis is characterized by a white and quiet, initially asymptomatic eye with 1-2+ cells and flare. The ocular disease tends to progress despite therapy even after the joint disease has become quiescent as the patients mature. Long-term complications include band keratopathy,

posterior synechiae, cataract, secondary glaucoma, hypotony, and occasionally vitritis and macular edema.

2. **Diagnostic tests.** The joint distribution, positive ANA, primarily anterior nongranulomatous uveitis, and normal serum and urine calcium help to differentiate JRA from ocular **sarcoidosis** in children. Positive HLA-B27 and frequently negative rheumatoid factor also support a diagnosis of JRA anterior uveitis.

3. **Therapy.** Mydriatic drops to prevent posterior synechia formation and topical steroids just sufficient to minimize (no need to eliminate totally) the aqueous cells and flare will often carry patients successfully for long periods of time. Steroids should be used as little as possible because of drug cataractogenesis, but in some patients repeated periocular deposteroid injections may be needed to control chronic, active inflammation. Except in the most severe cases, long-term use of oral corticosteroids should be avoided. Children especially suffer adverse effects on growth and bone formation. Alternate-day therapy should be used if possible. **Any child on periocular steroid injection or systemic steroid therapy should be co-monitored by a pediatrician or rheumatologist for adverse drug effect.** Older JRA patients (late teens and on) with systemic as well as ocular inflammatory disease should be considered for immunosuppressive therapy with azathioprine or methotrexate (see sec. **VI.C**).

E. **Miscellaneous endogenous anterior uveitides**

1. **Anticholinesterase agents** include glaucoma drops such as echothiophate iodide and eserine and may produce the rare complications of fibrinous iritis. The miotics, especially the stronger ones, appear to predispose to an increased postoperative iritis and should be discontinued several days prior to surgery. In addition, they should not ordinarily be used in the glaucoma found with uveitis, since they may aggravate the inflammation and lead to synechiae and a small pupil. Mydriatic cycloplegia with **cyclopentolate** may also aggravate iritis due to its neutrophil chemoattractant effect.

2. **Glaucomatocyclitic crisis (Posner-Schlossman syndrome)** is of unknown etiology. The crisis is unilateral, recurrent, and typified by a dilated pupil instead of the constricted pupil that is normally seen in iritis. The mild symptoms are those of blurred vision from corneal edema. Attacks last from a few hours to, rarely, over 2 weeks. Although posterior synechiae do not form, small KPs usually appear with each attack, especially on the trabecular meshwork, and heterochromia may be present. Cells in the vitreous are usually not seen. **Treatment** consists of mild cycloplegics (homatropine 2% hs), topical steroids, epinephrine (1% tid), and systemic carbonic anhydrase inhibitors (ethoxzolamide, 50 mg PO tid, or acetazolamide, 250 mg PO tid–qid).

3. **Fuchs's heterochromic iridocyclitis** is found in about 2% of uveitis patients. The major complaint is blurred vision, which results from the development of a posterior subcapsular cataract or vitreous veils. The affected iris stroma looks less dense, and the pigment layer often has a moth-eaten appearance at the pupil margin. Posterior synechiae never develop. The KPs are most distinctive, being round or star-shaped and usually of medium size. Their most striking feature is that they are not confined to the lower part of the cornea but cover the entire back of the cornea. They do not conglomerate nor become pigmented, and filaments are often seen between the precipitates. White dots are adherent to the framework of the vitreous. The cataract is the typical complicated posterior subcapsular type. Unless the condition is bilateral, there is heterochromia, with a brown eye becoming less brown and a blue eye becoming a more saturated blue. The prognosis for cataract extraction is good, although there is an increased likelihood of progressive recalcitrant glaucoma. In the past, Fuchs's iridocyclitis was considered a degenerative process, but it is now thought to be inflammatory because of the presence of plasma cells on histologic sections. **Treat-**

ment is short-term topical steroids to reduce inflammation. Treatment does not alter the long-term visual prognosis or development of glaucoma.

4. **Ischemic ocular syndrome.** Many patients with ischemic ocular syndrome are over 55 years of age and have familial or medical histories of generalized vascular disease. They may have **fadeouts of vision** on arising or post-prandially. Vision may be poor. The corneas may have mild edema and striate keratopathy. There is a moderate flare in the anterior chamber with some cells. The iris is usually abnormal, with matted stroma, and the pupil irregularly oval. The fundus may have dilated congested veins and mild retinal edema. The retinal artery frequently pulsates with the slightest pressure on the globe. Frequently no carotid pulse is palpable. These eyes usually develop further iris atrophy and mature cataracts in 2–4 months. The clinician's efforts should be directed toward assessment of the **cardiovascular** system.

5. **Kawasaki disease (mucocutaneous lymph node syndrome)** is a systemic vasculitis of children, two-thirds of whom develop a nongranulomatous anterior uveitis in the first week. Systemic findings include fever, lymphadenopathy, erythematous skin rash, oral mucosal erythema, conjunctivitis, disk edema, vascular engorgement, and cardiac abnormalities. As the uveitis is self-limited, a short course of topical steroid and mydriatic or mydriatic alone usually suffices.

6. **Acute angle-closure glaucoma** is a cause of fibrinous iritis. The greater the fibrinous iritis, the greater the probability of adhesions. If medical treatment is effective, the IOP in the involved eye falls lower than in the uninvolved eye, perhaps because of a reduced capacity of the ciliary body to secrete aqueous. **Corticosteroid** drops are indicated for the fibrinous iritis (see Chap. 9, sec. **IX**).

7. **Ulcerative colitis, granulomatous colitis, and Crohn's disease.** Ocular involvement in these gastrointestinal diseases occurs in less than 5% of patients. In both ulcerative colitis and granulomatous enterocolitis, HLA-B27 and ankylosing spondylitis seem to be associated. The iritis, colitis, and arthritis should be considered manifestations of the same immune process rather than as one resulting from the other. Topical corticosteroids are the **treatment** of choice for the iritis.

8. **Psoriasis,** a skin disease due to epidermal hyperproliferation, is strongly HLA-B27 gene associated. An anterior uveitis similar to that seen in other HLA-B27–positive idiopathic iridocyclitis patients may be seen in these patients with or without arthritis of the hands, feet, and sacroileum. The diagnosis of psoriatic uveitis may be made in that subset of patients capable of mounting multiple immune-mediated processes. **Treatment** is mydriasis and topical steroids.

9. **Lyme disease** caused by the spirochete **Borrelia burgdorfi** may cause iritis or panophthalmitis (see Chap. 5, sec. **IV.L.2**).

IX. **Intermediate uveitis (pars planitis, peripheral uveitis, chronic cyclitis)** is an inflammatory process of the peripheral retina and vitreous.

A. **Clinical findings.** This disease of children and young adults is typically bilateral and accounts for about 8% of all uveitis cases in office practice. Symptoms are blurred vision or floaters without pain or photophobia. Children may have some anterior chamber cells and flare and posterior synechiae, but such anterior inflammation is rare in adults. There may be peripheral corneal edema with KPs. The key findings are peripheral retinitis, perivasculitis, and vitritis, often with white snowbanking or snowballs especially over the inferior peripheral retina. If there is snowbanking, areas of neovascular abnormality should be checked as potential sites of hemorrhage. Most cases smoulder for years but do not suffer a loss of visual acuity even without treatment. There are five reported clinical courses:

1. Benign smouldering and resolution with no loss of visual acuity.
2. Inflammatory choroidal and serous retinal detachments.
3. Vascularized high snowbanks and ultimately cyclitic membranes.

4. Significant vascular obliteration with field loss and optic atrophy.
5. Chronic smouldering inflammation with macular edema.
Any of these groups may be seen in combination as well. Long-term visual disability develops in over one-third of patients, and only 5% remit spontaneously.

B. Diagnostic tests are of use only in ruling out other causes of uveitis that may involve this area: sarcoidosis (chest x ray, gallium scan, systemic symptoms, erythema nodosum, elevated serum and urine calcium), toxocariasis (*Toxocara* serology), and idiopathic iridocyclitis (see Table 8–3 and sec. **VIII**). There is no associated HLA phenotype.

C. Therapy is not necessary in many cases. If vision drops below 20/40 due to vitreous haze or macular edema, however, a 20- to 40-mg periocular depot methylprednisolone injection is recommended and should result in improvement for many months. If the injection is not tolerated or ineffective, one or two rows of single-freeze cryotherapy spots are placed along the areas of snowbanking to eliminate the abnormal vascular permeability in the area. If this fails, oral prednisone, 1 mg/kg/day (or equivalent steroid dose [see Table 8–4]) is begun daily and tapered 5–10 mg/week until the minimum maintenance dose for control of the disease is achieved. Periods of exacerbation may require intermittent increase in dosing. A few patients will develop intractable inflammation or macular edema despite maximum tolerable steroid therapy. These cases are usually responsive to systemic immunosuppression with drugs such as cyclosporine (see **VI.C** for drug dosages).

X. Viral uveitis and chorioretinitis

A. Adenovirus may produce subepithelial corneal infiltrates, and rarely a nongranulomatous iritis appears 7–10 days after the onset of infection. Iritis will improve spontaneously with time, although mild cycloplegia with tropicamide 1.0% bid may be advisable during the acute phases. For particularly severe disease, prednisolone 0.125%, bid or tid topically for 7–10 days, may make the patient more comfortable and resolve the intraocular inflammation more quickly. Corticosteroids may possibly prolong the persistence of the corneal infiltrates, however.

B. Herpes simplex virus (HSV) iridocyclitis is a nongranulomatous anterior uveitis that may occur with or without active herpetic keratitis or evidence of facial blistering. With the AIDS epidemic and increasing numbers of iatrogenically immunosuppressed patients in the population (e.g., organ transplant recipients, blood dyscrasia patients), there is a rapidly increasing incidence of HSV **chorioretinitis,** previously a rare form of posterior inflammation. HSV is also one etiologic agent in **acute retinal necrosis.**

1. Clinically, the **iridocyclitis** presents as a red, photophobic, often painful eye with tearing, blurred vision, miosis, and not infrequently active herpetic keratitis and immune stromal or ulcerative infections. There are cells and flare in the aqueous, often KPs, posterior synechiae, secondary glaucoma, and occasionally hypopyon. The etiology is unclear but thought to be primarily an immune reaction to viral antigen, although live or intact virus has occasionally been isolated from these eyes. The chorioretinitis is a direct invasion of the retina by HSV with a secondary choroiditis and vitritis. There are large white retinal infiltrates, vascular sheathing, and hemorrhages. Healing leaves areas of scarred, atrophic retina.

2. Diagnosis is based on clinical evidence of herpetic disease such as keratitis or skin lesions and, if possible, viral cultures or ELISA testing of scrapings taken from active lesions (see Chap. 5). Serology for HSV antibodies is useful only if taken 3–4 weeks apart and demonstrating a four-fold rise in titer. Therapy cannot be delayed for the results of such tests, however.

3. Therapy of HSV iridocyclitis is mydriasis only, e.g., homatropine bid for mild cell and flare. For more marked disease, the mydriatic-cycloplegic therapy is coupled with topical steroid drops using the lowest dosage necessary to control the inflammation and tapering slowly over several weeks to months, reducing the steroid dosage by no more than 50% at any given time, e.g., 1% prednisolone tid for 1 week, bid for 2 weeks, qd for 3 weeks, and then switching to 1/8% prednisolone qid and tapering even more slowly until minimal maintenance level is achieved or the drops may be stopped altogether. If the patient is on the equivalent of 1% prednisolone qd or higher, it is advisable to cover with prophylactic vidarabine or idoxuridine ointment qhs or trifluridine drops qid unless antiviral drug toxicity supervenes. Antibiotic ointment qd is also advisable. If there is corneal ulceration present at the time steroid therapy is to be started or develops during therapy, topical steroids should be reduced or stopped, specific treatment for the ulcer given (see Chap. 5), and, if necessary, a short course of systemic steroids given, e.g., prednisone, 30–40 mg PO each morning for 10 days. The role of systemic acyclovir is not established or FDA approved. Clinical trials using acyclovir, 200 mg PO 5 times daily, during acute disease are still ongoing.

   4. **Therapy of HSV chorioretinitis** is not established, but current evidence indicates that the disease responds to acyclovir, 200 mg PO 5 times daily for 10 days or, in immunocompromised patients, 5–10 mg/kg or 500 mg/m^2/day IV q8h for 5–7 days. Neither regimen is FDA approved for this use, but there is little else to be offered these patients except to reduce, where possible, factors contributing to the immunosuppression.

C. **Herpes zoster virus (varicella-zoster virus [VZV])** may also cause nongranulomatous **anterior uveitis, panuveitis, and chorioretinitis** and probably is the main cause of **acute retinal necrosis.**

   1. **Clinical findings** are those of zoster ophthalmicus as described in Chap. 5. The uveitis is a vasculitis due to live virus invasion and may result in hypopyon, hyphema, posterior synechiae, glaucoma, iris sector atrophy, heterochromia iridis, sympathetic ophthalmia, chorioretinal exudates, vascular sheathing and hemorrhages, and serous retinal detachment.

   2. **Diagnosis** is based on clinical evidence or history of zoster ophthalmicus. The virus is fastidious in its tissue culture requirements (human cells), and serial serology takes too long to be of use in deciding therapy. It may confirm a clinical diagnosis, however. As zoster is associated with deficiency in cell-mediated immunity, **AIDS** (HIV infection) must be considered an underlying risk factor in the absence of other reasons for immunosuppression such as malignancy or organ transplantation.

   3. **Therapy of VZV acute anterior segment and facial inflammation** is acyclovir, 800 mg PO 5 times daily for 10 days, preferably started within 72 hours of onset of disease. Mydriatic-cycloplegics such as 1–2% atropine or 2–5% homatropine qd-tid should be used until only 0–2 cells/0.2-mm slit-lamp beam are seen and only mild to no flare is present. Topical steroids may be instituted if the iridocyclitis persists despite acyclovir therapy. These are used as described under sec. **B.** Antiviral idoxuridine or vidarabine ointments bid may be used for the first 3 weeks when topical steroids are in use if there is any question that HSV might be mimicking zosteriform disease. Topical antibiotics such as erythromycin or bacitracin should be used if ulcerative keratitis is present. Therapy is controversial with regard to systemic corticosteroids. In general, mild or no pain requires no drug except a mydriatic-cycloplegic such as cyclopentolate or homatropine bid. Nonnarcotic or narcotic analgesics for neuralgia may be used during the first 10 days. If there is no relief or if uveitis or pain is not controlled, after chest x-ray, complete blood count, and an immune status evaluation in concert with an internist, the physician may start in the basically healthy patient prednisone, 20 mg PO tid for 7 days, then 15 mg PO bid for 7 days, and then 15 mg PO qd for 7 days, while continuing mydriatics and topical steroids as needed. Frequent monitoring for dissemination of disease should be carried out.

   4. **Therapy of VZV chorioretinitis and acute retinal necrosis** is not established, but current data indicate that effective treatment is acyclovir, 5–10 mg/kg or 500 mg/m^2 IV q8h for 5–7 days. Intravitreal injection of 10–40

μg/0.1 ml coupled with vitrectomy and scleral buckle has been reported as successful therapy of acute retinal disease. None of this treatment is as yet FDA approved for these indications.

D. Cytomegalic inclusion disease (CID) is a multisystem viral infection caused by cytomegalovirus (CMV). There are three means of acquiring infection: (1) transplacentally in utero, (2) during the birth process from an infected maternal cervix, and (3) at any time in life by oronasal droplet infection, sexual transmission, or transfusion of fresh blood or organ transplant that contains infected white cells. Congenital infection is found in 1% of all live births, but of these only 10% will manifest the disease early in life. Over a period of several years, up to 50% of all patients may manifest sensorineural hearing loss and mental retardation. More than 80% of the adult population over 35 years test positive serologically for CMV.

1. **Clinical findings.** In generalized **congenital** CMV infection, ocular involvement may range from mild, with only a few retinal or choroidal blood vessels involved, to total bilateral retinal necrosis, in which few islands of retinal tissue remain intact. Involvement may be peripheral, central, or all-inclusive. There may be an overlying peripheral vitreous haze resembling peripheral uveitis. With resolution of these lesions, the underlying RPE is clumped and mottled. More commonly, the posterior pole is affected and the lesions seen may be identical to those found with congenital toxoplasmosis. The lesions may include necrotizing chorioretinitis, which may be located just in the macula and resolve to a hyperplastic pigmented macular scar, or multiple focal lesions resolving into many small rounded pigmented chorioretinal scars. Retinal involvement with CMV may occur without signs of generalized CID. **Differential diagnosis** includes congenital toxoplasmosis or nematode infection. In the **acquired adult infection,** the eye is not involved despite presence of virus elsewhere in the body. In **immunosuppressed** patients, however, the physician must suspect CMV with the finding of retinal lesions. Clinically, there may be retinal cotton-wool spots (infarcts), extensive retinal hemorrhage and necrosis associated with vitreous haze, and a major retinal vasculitis. Not infrequently, multiple small, yellowish-white granular lesions are scattered along the course of the retinal vessels or in the peripheral retina. CMV retinitis develops in more than one-third of AIDS patients and frequently is the presenting illness as opportunistic infection.

2. **Diagnosis** is made on clinical findings, throat and urine cultures, and leukocyte culture. Serum antibodies should be drawn at the time disease is suspected and 8 weeks later in an attempt to establish a rise in titer as well as to differentiate from toxoplasmosis.

3. **Therapy** of CMV retinitis is only partially satisfactory in that drug must be maintained indefinitely or until the basic immunosuppression can be resolved, if possible. Therapeutic breakthroughs are not infrequent. Currently recommended, FDA-approved treatment is the antiviral antimetabolite, ganciclovir. The drug is given initially as 2.5 mg/kg IV q8h for 10 days and then changed to a maintenance dosage of 5 mg/kg/day for 5 days weekly. Recurrent breakthrough CMV retinitis is treated by giving the initial therapy again and giving maintenance therapy 7 days/week. **Intravitreal** ganciclovir has been used successfully in a limited number of patients intolerant of systemic ganciclovir. Dosage is 200 μg/0.1 ml, which probably has been repeated up to 58 times over several months in some patients, as drug titers fall below therapeutic levels (10 mg/liter) over 48 hours. There is little discernible toxicity, but the usual frequency of injection is 5–8 over 2–3 weeks. An acute rise in intraocular pressure from the volume of the mid-intravitreal injection may be minimized by performing an anterior chamber paracentesis first. Intravitreal use of ganciclovir is not FDA approved. Foscarnet, 60 mg IV over 1 hour q8h for 14 days followed by 8 weeks of 60 mg IV daily, is meeting with some notable success.

E. Acquired immunodeficiency syndrome (AIDS) is caused by the human immunodeficiency virus-1 (HIV-1). The virus destroys the T-lymphocyte (and probably other) immune cells, thus progressively and severely immunocompromising the patient and enhancing susceptibility to a plethora of viral, fungal, and parasitic infections.

1. **Clinically** the ocular findings in AIDS and ARC (AIDS related complex) include punctate or geographic ulcerative keratitis (which may mimic herpes virus), follicular conjunctivitis, Kaposi's sarcoma, nongranulomatous iritis, secondary glaucoma, retinal cotton-wool spots (white, fluffy nerve fiber layer microinfarctions), retinal vasculitis, intraretinal hemorrhages, microaneurysms, Roth spots, ischemic maculopathy, retinal periphlebitis, and papilledema. The HIV itself appears able to produce all of these diseases itself through direct viral invasion and through deposition of immune complexes that clog the vasculature. The opportunistic infections that may be superimposed include HSV, VZV, CMV, cryptococcus, pneumocystis, *Toxoplasma*, *Candida*, and *Mycobacterium* (choroidal granulomas). Several of these may occur simultaneously, e.g., HSV, CMV, and HIV chorioretinitis.

2. **Diagnosis** is made by serologic testing (ELISA and Western blot) for HIV antibody, assessment of the ratio of T-helper to T-suppressor lymphocytes, and, if available, culture of virus from blood, tears, or other body secretions.

3. **Therapy** is not satisfactory in terms of cure. The currently recommended therapy is initiation, as early as possible, of the antiviral antimetabolite azidothymidine (AZT). The drug inhibits viral replication, prolongs patient survival, and improves the quality of life in AIDS patients. AZT dosage is not established and ranges from 300 to 1200 mg/day in 3 to 4 divided doses. There is a report that a recalcitrant iritis in an AIDS patient with no evidence of other infection responded to AZT therapy. CMV retinitis may also respond to AZT therapy, presumably due to an enhanced patient immunocompetence, as AZT has no antiviral effect on HIV-1. Unfortunately AZT and ganciclovir or AZT and acyclovir may interact adversely when used simultaneously in a patient (neutropenia, severe somnolence).
Foscarnet (phosphonoformate, PFA) is an experimental drug effective in HIV strains resistant to ganciclovir and acyclovir. Dosage is 60 mg/kg body weight IV tid for 2–3 weeks before starting qd maintenance dosage. It is not FDA approved for such use. Therapy of opportunistic infections in AIDS patients is discussed under specific disease headings.

F. **Epstein-Barr virus (EBV)** is a herpesvirus and the cause of infectious mononucleosis and probably Burkitt's African lymphoma, nasopharyngeal carcinoma, and some chronic fatigue syndromes.

1. **Clinical findings** in the eye include follicular conjunctivitis, epithelial punctate or microdendritic keratitis, immune anterior stromal pleomorphic nummular or ring-shaped keratitis, acute or chronic nongranulomatous iritis, panchorioretinitis, optic neuritis, papilledema, convergence insufficiency, and extraocular muscle palsy.

2. **Diagnosis** is by heterophile or Monostat serology for EBV antibodies.

3. **Therapy** is still not established. There is one report of an EBV panuveitis responding to combined acyclovir, 600 mg PO 5 times daily, and 3% acyclovir ointment qid over 5 months after failing to respond to 10 months of steroid therapy.

G. **Embryopathic pigmentary retinopathy** presents as a salt-and-pepper chorioretinitis as seen in patients with **congenital syphilis, congenital rubella, varicella, influenza,** and **radiation during the first trimester.** Rubella retinitis is present in 50% of infants with maternal rubella syndrome. Peppering is usually limited to the posterior pole but may involve any or all sectors. Retinal vessels are always normal, but the optic disk may be pale. Rubella chorioretinopathy does not interfere with visual function unless a neovascular net develops in the macula. Occasionally, it may simulate toxoplasmosis.

H. **Other viral infections** that may produce nongranulomatous iridocyclitis or chorioretinitis that are generally self-limited and usually bilateral are inclusion conjunctivitis (iritis), infectious mononucleosis (iridocyclitis), influenza (iridocyclitis or neuroretinitis), lymphogranuloma venereum (no characteristic pattern), measles (chorioretinopathy), mumps (iridocyclitis and neuroretinitis), and ornithosis and psittacosis (chorioretinitis). **Subacute sclerosing panencephalitis (measels)** produces a chorioretinitis of low-grade inflammation characterized by ground-glass whitening of the retina with occasional cotton-wool spots (infarctions), disturbances of the underlying pigment epithelium, and opalescent swelling of the macula. There is no hemorrhage.

XI. Uveitis of predominantly granulomatous nature

A. Tuberculous uveitis is probably caused by immune reaction to or very rarely by direct ocular invasion by the bacterium *Mycobacterium tuberculosis*. It should be suspected in any case of chronic iritis, especially in the older patient, and in any granulomatous disease of the anterior or posterior segment that is not explained by some other agent. Associated lesions are phlyctenules, conjunctival nodules, scleritis, and optic neuritis.

1. **Clinical types.** Iritis may appear in four forms: (a) acute nongranulomatous uveitis, intense but brief, (b) mild nonspecific uveitis with tendency to chronic recurrence, (c) smoldering low-grade granulomatous inflammation resulting in synechiae formation, cataracts, glaucoma, or phthisis bulbi, and (d) fulminating, granulomatous caseating tubercles. In miliary tuberculosis, choroidal tubercles appear as yellow-white nodules 1/6–1/2 disk diameter (dd) in size with blurred borders. They are similar to the disseminated lesions of histoplasmosis, but their occurrence with fever is of diagnostic importance. A retinal periphlebitis and subretinal neovascularization may be present. The **differential diagnosis** of choroidal lesions includes syphilis, coccidioidomycosis, sarcoidosis, and cryptococcosis. With specific therapy the choroidal lesions quiet down and in many cases disappear completely.

2. **Diagnosis**
   a. **Chest x ray and skin testing.** Diagnosis is made in part by chest x ray and by skin testing using the PPD-T (5TU). If the skin reaction to 5TU is completely negative, the 250TU (PPD 2) should be used. Extremely rarely the skin test may be negative and live bacilli present in the eye. Any reaction (even erythema only) suggests that the uveitis could be due to tuberculosis. If there is enough inflammation in the eye, one proceeds to the isoniazid (INH) therapeutic test. Underlying AIDS should be suspected.
   b. **Isoniazid** may also be used as a therapeutic test in suggesting the diagnosis of tuberculosis. One 300-mg tablet is given qd for 3 weeks, and the ophthalmologist observes the eye at weekly intervals to check for improvement. Other therapy is kept constant. After the diagnosis of tuberculosis is strongly suspected, one of the other antituberculosis agents should be added to the regimen. Weaknesses in this mode of diagnosis are the natural waxing and waning of the disease and the concomitant use of steroids, which also cause improvement in most uveitis cases.

3. **Therapy.** The principle of therapy followed is the concomitant use of two or more drugs to prevent the emergence of bacterial resistance to any of the drugs used, without a break of more than 1 or 2 weeks to protect against relapse, for at least 1 year to prevent relapse of active tuberculosis. The primary drugs (isoniazid and rifampin) are the most effective and have the least toxicity. The tertiary drugs (e.g., ethambutol, streptomycin) are the least effective and the most toxic.
   a. **Isoniazid** is given as one 300-mg tablet/day. Since children tolerate large doses, the dosage does not need to be reduced unless the child's weight is under 27.3 kg (60 lb). Peripheral neuritis may be prevented by administering pyridoxine, 25 mg/day. Intolerance to isoniazid, resulting in hepatitis, increases with age and occurs often. Monthly monitoring of patients for liver toxicity has been recommended by the FDA. Isoniazid should be discontinued at least temporarily in patients whose values exceed 3 times the upper limit of normal.

b. **Rifampin.** After the presumptive diagnosis of tuberculosis uveitis has been made, rifampin is usually used as the second drug. The dosage is two 300-mg tablets a day, 1 or 2 hours before or after a meal.

c. **Ethambutol.** In patients with a danger of hepatitis, ethambutol may be a better choice than rifampin. It is given once a day with food, if desired, in a dosage of 15 mg/kg body weight. Patients with decreased renal function need the dosage reduced as determined by serum levels. Ethambutol may produce an optic neuritis. Each eye should be monitored separately.

B. **Syphilitic uveitis and neurosyphilis** caused by the bacterial spirochete *Treponema pallidum* are becoming more common due to the AIDS epidemic. These conditions may be congenital and quiescent, active at birth or in the teenage years, or, most commonly, may be acquired in adult life.

1. **Clinical manifestations of congenital syphilis** include the salt-and-pepper appearance of the fundus on a yellowish-red background. This salt-and-peppering may be found just at the periphery and is invariably bilateral. It may involve the posterior pole or only isolated quadrants. Vision is usually unimpaired. This form of the disease is nonprogressive.

   a. The **differential diagnosis of salt-and-pepper fundus** includes prenatal rubella or influenza, rubeolla, variola, varicella, mumps, vaccination, poliomyelitis, herpes simplex, panuveitis, Cockayne's disease, cystinosis, choroideremia in males, and Leber's congenital tapetoretinal amaurosis.

   b. **Secondary retinal pigmentary degeneration** is manifested by narrowing and sclerosis of choroidal and retinal vessels. There is optic nerve atrophy characterized by a pale disk with sharp margins. Pigment configurations are round, star shaped, or bone corpuscle formation. Many areas of chorioretinal atrophy differentiate it from retinitis pigmentosa. It is always bilateral and may be either in the posterior pole or in the peripheral retina. Vision may be affected.

2. **Secondary syphilis** may be present as an **acute iritis** or diffuse **chorioretinitis.** Three types of secondary syphilitic iritis are iritis roseata (small nets of capillaries), iritis papulosa (highly vascular papules), and iritis nodosa (large well-defined yellowish-red nodules the size of a pinhead or larger). The chorioretinitis of acquired syphilis is bilateral 50% of the time and presents with intermittent photopsia, metamorphopsia, and occasional visual field defect. Fundic examination reveals fine punctate haze in the vitreous and diffuse gray-yellow areas of exudation. These exudates and subsequent pigmentation accumulate along blood vessels and around the nerve head. The choroiditis is particularly noted in the midzone of the fundus and may have scattered superficial flame-shaped hemorrhages and generalized chorioretinal edema. The midfundal localization of the most intense disease results in a partial or complete ring scotoma.

3. **Tertiary syphilis.** A recent survey of patients diagnosed as having presumptive syphilitic uveitis revealed that two-thirds of these patients had negative Venereal Disease Research Laboratory (VDRL) tests but positive fluorescent treponemal antibody-absorption (FTA-ABS) tests. This finding suggests the possibility that some of these patients may be in the tertiary stage. Although syphilis may mimic most types of uveitis, the most common forms seem to be a diffuse or a disseminated chorioretinitis. In **neuroretinitis** the nerve head and adjacent retina are swollen in late stages posttherapy, appearing as arteriolar narrowing and sheathing with pigment migration and bone corpuscle formation.

4. **Diagnosis** is made by the FTA-ABS, which may detect syphilis earlier than the VDRL and rules out almost all biologic false-positives as well as allowing diagnosis of late latent syphilis. The VDRL test becomes negative in two-thirds of cases of late syphilis and in treated syphilis, but the FTA-ABS never becomes negative. Lumbar puncture for CSF serology and cytology should be performed in patients with signs of late-stage syphilis.

5. **Treatment.** No conclusive data are available regarding the best treatment for ocular syphilis. Some physicians have recommended probenecid, which raises the level of penicillin in the aqueous. Probenecid may be helpful not only by its effect on the kidney, leading to higher blood concentrations, but also by its effect on the ciliary body. Ocular cases should be treated as neurosyphilis. Penicillin G, 600,000 units IM or IV q6h for 14 days, accompanied by probenecid, 500 mg PO q6h, should be given to patients with neuroretinitis but no CSF abnormalities. If the CSF is also positive, 12-24 million units of crystalline penicillin G IV should be given qd for 10-15 days along with the probenecid to raise blood and aqueous drug levels. Such doses will also produce treponemicidal levels in the CSF. See Chap. 5, sec. **IV.L.1.** for further discussion and treatment modalities.

C. **Sympathetic ophthalmia** is a bilateral granulomatous panuveitis that may develop about 4-12 weeks after either an injury or rarely intraocular surgery on one eye. It may occur as early as 9 days and as late as 50 years. The **etiology** is unknown, but it is thought to be that injury to one eye results in programming of the body to produce ocular disease autoimmune in nature and predominantly a T-cell lymphocyte reaction in the injured and the sympathizing other eye. Antiretinal antibodies (photoreceptor and Müller cells) have been found in a few patients.

1. **Clinically,** the external eyes are not inflamed, but both uveal tracts are massively thickened by granulomatous lymphocytic infiltration. The iris may be very edematous, and deep nodules and papillitis are common. Disseminated yellow-white spots may appear in the fundus **(Dalen-Fuchs nodules).** There may also be associated signs of vitiligo, poliosis, and alopecia, but these signs are less common than in the VKH syndrome. Sympathetic ophthalmia is extremely rare and may be similar to or associated with phakoantigenic (lens-induced) uveitis. Differentiation is important because removal of lens material will cure the phakoantigenic uveitis.

2. **Diagnosis** is based on the history of injury or ocular surgery and the clinical findings. Fluorescein angiography, ERGs, and EOGs will indicate severity of disease and guide therapeutic response.

3. **Treatment** of sympathetic ophthalmia involves cycloplegia, periocular injections daily to every 6 weeks depending on severity, and systemic medication of 100-200 mg of prednisone or equivalent every morning with breakfast for 7-10 days. Once disease is controlled, dosage may be reduced to a maintenance level (1.0-1.5 mg/kg/day) for at least 3 months, at which time success of the therapy should be reevaluated. If successful, therapy may be continued with 15-20 mg/day of prednisone. The immunosuppressive drugs—cyclosporine A (which should be the first drug tried after steroids or in combination), 6-mercaptopurine, methotrexate, azathioprine, or chlorambucil—have been of use either when corticosteroids are not effective or when they are contraindicated. **Enucleation of the impaired eye should prevent sympathetic ophthalmia if done within 9 days after injury or surgery. After 9 days, enucleation should be performed if the eye has no potential for recovery, since this eye may aggravate the inflammation in the sympathizing eye.**

D. **Sarcoidosis** accounts for about 2% of uveitis patients, and 25-50% of patients with sarcoidosis will develop ocular problems, usually uveitis. There is a concentration of sarcoidosis in Sweden and in the South Atlantic and Gulf regions of the United States. It is more common in black Africans than in black Africans and 10-15 times as common in black Americans (usually females) as in white Americans. It has occurred concordantly in uniovular twins. It usually occurs in the middle years (age 20-50) and lasts about 2 years. The uveitis develops during the silent stage of systemic sarcoidosis in approximately 80% of patients.

1. **Clinically,** although sarcoidosis is typically assumed to be granulomatous in character, it presents equally often in a nongranulomatous form, so the iris may or may not have nodules similar to those seen in tuberculous uvei-

tis. The following types of posterior involvement have been reported: a characteristic chorioretinitis, periphlebitis retinae (candle wax drippings), large chorioretinal granulomas, nonspecific chorioretinitis, optic nerve involvement, including atrophy, edema, and tumor, vitreous opacities, and preretinal infiltrates. The vitreous may have "snowball" opacities inferiorly. CNS manifestations occur in 10-15% of patients with systemic sarcoidosis, but this figure doubles when the fundus is involved.

2. **Diagnosis** is aided by a chest x ray, which is abnormal (hilar adenopathy) in approximately 80% of cases of ocular sarcoidosis. A gallium scan may show increased uptake in areas of inflammation in the parotid and lacrimal glands. Histologic proof is best obtained by biopsy of the conjunctival or lacrimal gland, granulomas, skin lesions, or enlarged lymph nodes. Biopsy may be performed on the liver or gastrocnemius. There is lack of a positive tuberculin reaction in approximately 50% of patients with sarcoidosis as well as a tendency toward hyporeaction on other skin tests (anergy). Other pertinent tests are serum and urine calcium and angiotensin converting enzyme, all of which are elevated in active sarcoidosis. The serum albumin-globulin ratio, pulmonary function, and liver enzymes are also frequently abnormal. Children may have ocular and joint sarcoidosis but no lung involvement. Hand, knee, and foot films may be useful.

3. **Patients diagnosed and treated early** have a favorable outcome and are left with little residual ocular disability. Topical steroids are not always adequate, and periocular steroid injection of 20-40 mg of depomethylpred-nisolone may be needed to supplement drops for anterior nodular iritis and glaucoma. Systemic corticosteroids in high initial doses are often necessary as well, e.g., prednisone, 40-60 mg PO qd with taper over several weeks. Cycloplegics (atropine, homatropine) are continued throughout the steroid course. Cyclosporine A has been used successfully in recalcitrant cases, but no regimen has been established. Cytotoxic agents such as azathioprine or cyclophosphamide offer no advantage.

E. The **fungal disease histoplasmosis** in its ocular form is almost never associated with symptomatic pulmonary histoplasmosis or exposure to *Histoplasma* spores or bird droppings. Over 99% of histoplasmic infections are benign and asymptomatic, with about 2% of adults in the endemic Midwest having histo spots disseminated in the fundus. These spots begin to appear during late childhood and are important as a nidus for future maculopathy. The syndrome has been found occasionally to occur in Europe and in other areas where histoplasmosis is nonexistent; therefore, the best term is "presumed ocular histoplasmosis syndrome" (POHS). In endemic areas, at least 90% of the cases that are seen are probably the result of interaction between the eye's immune response and the exogenous organism, *Histoplasma capsulatum.*

1. The **clinical findings** include disseminated **choroiditis** producing histo spots. These spots vary in number from 1-70, with a mean of 8 per eye. They are more frequent in the left than in the right eye and are bilateral in two-thirds of patients. The majority are found behind the equator and are slightly irregular, round, deeply pigmented, 0.2-0.7 dd in size, and yellow in color. The **macular lesion** is typified in an active stage by a pigment ring and detachment of the overlying sensory retina. This serous and hemorrhagic maculopathy is the result of histo scars that are granulomas eating a hole in Bruch's membrane, which then allows an ingrowth of capillaries. The maculopathy causes legal blindness in 60% of patients having ocular histoplasmosis syndrome. If blood and elevation of the sensory retina are present, the physician may assume the presence of a **neovascular net,** best demonstrated by fluorescein angiography. Changes around the nerve head are similar to histo scars in the periphery except that they may be confluent. Typically, there is a pigmented line next to the nerve, with a depigmented zone outside this line representing old choroiditis. The clinical course is one of exacerbation and recurrence of preexistent histo spots. If spots are

present in the disk macular area, the chances of a symptomatic attack are approximately 20% over the next 3 years. If none are present, the chances of a visually significant attack are reduced to 2%. Occasionally, however, fresh areas of choroiditis may appear; new lesions arise from the edge of old scars.

2. **Differential diagnosis** is aided by the finding in histoplasmosis syndrome of a **clear vitreous,** which immediately differentiates it from most other types of uveitis. Other causes of granulomatous fundus lesions include tuberculosis, coccidioidomycosis, cryptococcosis, and sarcoid. The maculopathy may be simulated by Fuchs's spot of high myopia, the diskiform degeneration of old age, or maculopathy from angioid streaks. Hemorrhagic circumpapillary histoplasmosis is simulated by drusen of the optic disk with hemorrhage.

3. **Diagnosis** is assisted but not confirmed by complement-fixation testing (negative in over two-thirds of typical cases), calcification on chest x ray (previous histoplasma pneumonitis), a positive histoplasmin skin test, and primarily the clinical findings described. Skin testing should not be done in patients with maculopathy, as the test may reactivate the ocular lesions. There is significant association between presence of maculopathy and positive HLA-B27 testing.

4. **Treatment** is not conclusively established. Antifungals have no effect, and peripheral retinopathy is not treated.

   a. **For acute maculopathy,** the patient should be started on 50–150 mg of **prednisone** every other breakfast with retrobulbar injection of long-acting steroid, e.g., 40 mg of depomethylprednisolone acetate about every 2 weeks for 1–2 doses. Tapering of steroids is done over several weeks proportionate to the improvement in maculopathy. Fluorescein angiography may assist the physician with regard to decisions concerning tapering of medications and use of laser therapy.

   b. **Photocoagulation** in the form of argon or krypton laser is used to coagulate capillaries and to eradicate the exudation from a neovascular net that produces a serous hemorrhagic detachment. The laser is the best therapy but is indicated only if the neovascular net is still outside the fovea. Development of nets is not affected by use or nonuse of steroid therapy.

   c. **To decrease leakage into the maculopathy,** aspirin, coughing, and other Valsalva maneuvers should be avoided. Since hemorrhages may appear in the fundus at high altitudes, it is not recommended that patients with an active maculopathy ascend unpressurized to heights over 800 feet. Riding on commercial air flights has not proved detrimental.

F. **Other fungal uveitides.** Although not as common as histoplasmosis, the other fungal infections reported to infect the eye are aspergillosis, blastomycosis, candidiasis, coccidioidomycosis, cryptococcosis, mucormycosis, nocardiosis, and sporotrichosis. Of these, only aspergillosis and candidiasis are common enough to warrant further discussion here.

1. **Aspergillosis.** Most of the recognized aspergillosis infections have occurred in patients who showed no evidence of fungal infection elsewhere. This uveitis should be suspected in drug addicts who infect themselves with contaminated needles or in immunosuppressed patients.

   a. **Clinically,** there are vitritis with fluff balls and yellow-white fundus lesions similar to *Candida* chorioretinitis, intraretinal hemorrhages, and occasional hypopyon.

   b. **Therapy** is combined systemic amphotericin B (IV, intravitreal after vitrectomy) and oral flucytosine. See sec. **XV,** Table 8-7 for drug dosages.

2. **Candidiasis** is the most common of the other fungal infections. It occurs in immunosuppressed and in hospitalized patients who receive systemic antibiotics, especially patients with indwelling IV catheters. A blood culture is valuable in establishing the diagnosis. The chorioretinitis may begin either

in the choroid or in the retina. In mild cases it appears to remain localized in the choroid.

   a. The **clinical picture** simulates that seen in toxoplasmosis. Lesions are usually fluffy, yellow-white elevations, varying in size from those simulating cotton-wool spots to those measuring several disk diameters in breadth. Unlike those seen in toxoplasmosis, these lesions are often multiple and unassociated with previous scars. They often have an overlying vitreous haze, as do the lesions of toxoplasmosis, but unlike toxoplasmosis the process may actually grow into the vitreous.

   b. **Therapy** is similar to that of *Aspergillus* chorioretinitis. See sec. **XV,** Table 8-7 for drug dosages. Vitrectomy is performed if there is progression of disease despite systemic amphotericin B and flucytosine, if there is breakthrough into the vitreous, or in cases of exogenous fungal **endophthalmitis.** Intravitreal amphotericin B may be given 2–3 times if necessary and systemic.

G. Parasitic disease. The following parasitic diseases have been considered causes of intraocular inflammation: amebiasis, angiostrongyliasis, ascariasis, cestodiasis, filariasis, giardiasis, gnathostomiasis, ophthalmomyiasis, porocephaliasis, schistosomiasis, trematodiasis, and trypanosomiasis, toxoplasmosis, and toxocariasis.

   1. Toxoplasmosis is the most common proven cause of chorioretinitis in the world. It is almost always congenital but may be acquired through inhalation of oocytes in cat waste or ingestion of contaminated lamb, pork, or rarely beef. Systemic toxoplasmosis is a benign disease unless the patient is pregnant or immunosuppressed. If a pregnant female becomes infected with *Toxoplasma gondii,* there is a 40% chance that her infant will be affected. **All women getting married should have a serologic test for toxoplasmosis.** If positive, these women can be assured that they are immune and not able to pass toxoplasmosis to any of their children. If negative, they will need to be cautious during pregnancy to avoid infection of the fetus. The probability of a mother having a child with toxoplasmosis is 1 in 10,000 in the United States.

      a. Congenital systemic toxoplasmosis may or may not be active at the time of birth. The symptoms and signs of congenital toxoplasmosis are convulsions, scattered intracranial calcification, and chorioretinitis. The latter is present in 80% of children with congenital toxoplasmosis and is bilateral in 85% of these, with a predilection for the macular area. In children who have been spared the CNS damage of toxoplasmosis, the retinitis may become apparent to an ophthalmologist either by an esotropia or exotropia from macular scarring or by reduced vision at the time of an initial school vision test.

      b. The **etiology** of the initial disease is the protozoan *Toxoplasma gondii,* but reaction of disease may be due to a number of mechanisms, including local proliferation of free forms following rupture of a retinal cyst, delayed hypersensitivity specific for *Toxoplasma* cyst content, hypersensitivity to retinal proteins from tissue breakdown, recurrent parasitemia, and wandering cells that liberate *Toxoplasma* into ocular tissues, allowing invasion of susceptible cells. A change in immune status due to AIDS or immunosuppression should be considered in these patients. The vitritis is much more severe than that seen with CMV retinitis in these patients.

      c. Clinically, in both the congenital **ocular** form and the acquired ocular disease there is an acute focal chorioretinitis having its active onset of recurrence between ages 11 and 40. Lesions may be single and variable in size and are usually posterior to the equator. There is exudation into the vitreous and flare and cells in the anterior chamber. Vitreous may detach from the retina, with hemispheric collections of cells looking like KPs deposited on the back of the vitreous body and dubbed **vitreous precipitates (VPs).** The active disease often occurs next to an old scar to produce the so-called **satellite lesion.** It is usually 1 dd in size, although it may vary from pinpoint to extremely large. Activity in the lesion persists for about 4 months. It is less frequent in blacks and most frequent in teenage girls. Papillitis and papilledema are not uncommon. A rare type of vitreous reaction with the development of "grapevines" in the vitreous covered with "wet snow" may be seen.

d. The **differential diagnosis** of congenital toxoplasmosis includes macular coloboma, cytomegalic inclusion disease, herpes simplex chorioretinitis, neonatal hemolysis, torulosis, cerebral trauma, and foci of retinoblastoma. In adults, tuberculosis, candidiasis, and histoplasmosis need to be considered as well.

e. **Diagnosis** is based on the clinical picture plus serologic tests. The indirect fluorescein antibody test and the ELISA test are now the two most commonly employed. A single positive test even on undiluted serum is considered diagnostically supportive. The presence of IgM antitoxin titers indicates a recent infection. The chances of this test being positive in the population at large are roughly equal to a patient's age. A 50-year-old person has about a 50% chance of having a positive test; therefore, the test can be false-positive, especially in older individuals. Serology is supportive but not definitive. Acquired toxoplasmosis is characterized by fever, myalgia, and lymphadenopathy. In such rare cases, a rising antibody titer is seen.

f. **Treatment** is a combination of systemic corticosteroids and at least one antitoxoplasmic agent and preferably two or three.

(1) **Corticosteroid therapy** is initiated with prednisone, 50–150 mg PO every other breakfast and/or periocular depomethylprednisolone acetate in the area of the lesion every 1–6 weeks. If relapse occurs, dosage is raised just enough to handle the relapse and then tapered again.

(2) **Antitoxoplasmic agents** include sulfadiazine, pyrimethamine, tetracycline, and clindamycin.

(a) **Sulfadiazine and pyrimethamine** are the first drug treatments of choice. Sulfadiazine (triple sulfa) is given as two 500-mg tablets PO q6h for 4–6 weeks along with pyrimethamine. Pyrimethamine is used at levels of 100 mg PO bid the first day and 25 mg PO bid for 6 weeks or until activity subsides. As pyrimethamine acts only on actively dividing *Toxoplasma*, only active cases are treated with this drug. To avoid toxic depression of the bone marrow, **folinic acid** (leucovorin, 3 mg) once or twice weekly counteracts development of thrombocytopenia without interfering with therapeutics. Leucovorin comes in an ampule that may be given by injection, but the patient may be taught to put it in any liquid except alcohol and take it orally. The patient should **not** take folic acid, which would counteract the effect of sulfadiazine or pyrimethamine. **In pregnancy, pyrimethamine should be avoided because of induced congenital malformation.**

(b) **Clindamycin,** 150–300 mg PO every 6h, combined with **sulfadiazine** is a synergistic therapy of second choice. Patients should be warned that if they have four bowel movements per day more than normal they should stop taking clindamycin. In about 1% of patients, severe pseudomembranous colitis develops. The concomitant use of triple sulfa acts to prevent this colitis. If clostridial colitis develops, it is best treated with oral vancomycin.

(c) **Tetracycline** is used with a loading dose of 1000 mg, followed by 500 mg PO qid for 3–4 weeks. For bowel complications, Lactinex is helpful.

(d) **Platelet count** should be checked once weekly if pyrimethamine is used. If it falls to below 100,000, pyrimethamine should be stopped but steroids not discontinued. Leucovorin, 3 mg IM daily, should be instituted until platelet count returns to normal.

(3) **Cryosurgery** and **photocoagulation** are reserved for patients with persistent recurrences. Activity of a lesion is manifested by its softness and elevation and by the presence of cells in the vitreous over it, although the latter may persist in the vitreous for months. Their presence, therefore, is not an absolute guide.

(4) **Fluorescein angiography** is not of great help in following the progress of toxoplasmic chorioretinitis.

2. **Toxocariasis** is the most common parasitic disease in the United States. It is caused by the ascarid *Toxocara canis,* a frequent infestation of puppies. Although 14 types of ocular toxocariasis have been described, only posterior pole and peripheral granulomas in a quiet eye are common.

a. The **systemic disease** of visceral larvae migrans usually occurs before the age of 3; therefore, by the time the child sees the ophthalmologist, systemic manifestations are no longer present. Prophylaxis includes the avoidance of both dirt eating and the handling of cats and dogs. Puppies, especially, should be dewormed with piperazine.

b. **Differential diagnosis** includes *Toxoplasma* and retinoblastoma, which has been the most common erroneous diagnosis. No intraocular calcification has been observed, in contrast with retinoblastoma, which has an incidence of calcification of 75%. Other possible diagnoses are toxoplasmosis, primary hyperplastic vitreous, Coats' disease, sarcoid and retrolental fibroplasia.

c. **Children with diffuse chronic endophthalmitis** are usually 2–9 years of age. They present with chronic unilateral uveitis with cloudy vitreous. There may be an exudative detachment, posterior synechiae, and cyclitic membrane.

d. **Posterior pole granulomas** are usually seen in children 6–14 years of age. The lesion is usually hemispheric, with a diameter roughly equal to or larger than the disk. It seems to be primarily retinal in location. Tension lines radiate out from the granuloma, and fibrous bands may extend into the vitreous and to the pars plana. These granulomas are usually solitary and unilateral. Those at the posterior pole usually lie at the macula or between the macula and the disk.

e. **Patients with peripheral granulomas** in a quiet eye range in age from approximately 6–40 years. These peripheral hemispheric masses are usually associated with dense connective tissue strands in the vitreous cavities that often connect to the disk. Bilateral cases are rare. Heterotopia of the macula may result from the tug of these peripheral masses. These patients need to be differentiated from those with retrolental fibroplasia, which occurs bilaterally in premature infants.

f. **Diagnosis** is made on the basis of clinical findings and the ELISA blood test. Ultrasound and ocular x rays should be negative for calcium deposits.

g. **Treatment** of choice is periocular depomethylprednisolone (40–60 mg) in the area of greatest involvement. This may be repeated weekly or every other week until the process resolves itself. Short-term systemic prednisone may also be used in severe cases. Most inflammation does not start until the larva dies. If antihelminthic therapy is used, it should always be coupled with steroids. A common combination is thiabendazole, 500 mg PO qid or 20 mg/kg/day in divided doses for 5 days, plus 40 mg of prednisone PO qd for 10 days followed by taper as warranted by resolving intraocular inflammation. Cryocoagulation and photocoagulation also kill the larva effectively but should not be used within the foveal area.

XII. Nongranulomatous choroiditis

A. Acute multifocal placoid pigment epitheliopathy. Since inflammatory signs, such as flare and cells, Koeppe's nodules, and episcleritis, as well as cells in the vitreous have been seen in this entity, it should be classified as an intraocular inflammation. The picture on fluorescein angiography differs in the active and inactive stages. In the active stage there is blockage of dye by swollen opalescent plaques. In the inactive stage there is early transmission of background fluorescence through areas of depigmentation. Vision tends to fall to the region of 20/200 as a result of macular involvement. There is **often a dramatic return of vision** in the first 2 weeks. After 10 weeks the vision has usually improved about as much as it will. The etiology is unknown, but it may be related to an inflammatory obstruction of the feeding artery to a segment of the choriocapillaris. No **treatment** has been demonstrated to be of value.

B. Serpiginous or geographic peripapillary choroiditis is characterized by a cream-colored lesion moving in tonguelike spread from the disk area and lasting up to 18 months. If this tongue involves the macula, the vision is usually irreparably lost. The overlying retinal vessels are normal, and there may be a few cells in the vitreous. IV fluorescein enters the extension very slowly. Once the fluorescein appears it remains in a diffuse pattern for several hours. This entity is difficult to differentiate from a degenerative syndrome known as "areolar sclerosis" or choroidal vascular abiotrophy, which has a similar pathology.

C. Acute retinal pigment epithelitis is a minor macular disease characterized by an acute onset, with fairly rapid resolution in 6–12 weeks. A typical lesion is a deep, fine, dark gray, sometimes black spot that, in the acute stages and sometimes afterward, is surrounded by a pale yellow halo. These lesions usually appear in clusters of two to four in the macula and may be unilateral or bilateral.

XIII. Hypersensitivity uveitis.

Although many experimental immunologic studies have been done, they have little pertinence to clinical allergy. A statistical relationship of contact allergy to uveitis has never been established. Uveitis caused by topical epinephrine, inhalants, ingestants, or contactants appears to be rare, and the case reports are usually unconvincing. Three cases of iritis have been reported due to **cat hair.** Uveitis may appear at the time of **serum sickness,** but serum sickness is now a rare phenomenon. **The lens** in phakogenic and other uveitis forms is discussed further in Chap. 6, secs. **V.G** and **VII.E.** and Chap. 9, sec. **XXII.** This immune-iridocyclitis begins 1–14 days after leakage of lens material into the anterior segment or after the development of Elschnig's pearls. It is also believed the lens may become antigenic as a result of a chronic uveitis in which the original cause was completely different. For this reason, cataract extraction may sometimes ameliorate rather than aggravate a uveitis. Lens-induced uveitis and sympathetic ophthalmia coexist in 23% of patients, lending additional support to the allergic theory for both. In addition to nonspecific topical corticosteroids and cycloplegics, surgical removal of all the lens is indicated.

XIV. Childhood uveitis

is uncommon. Approximately 8% of cases are seen in children under 16 years of age. Although panuveitis may occasionally be seen, the disease can ordinarily be divided into the anterior, peripheral, and posterior portions of the eye.

1. Anterior. As the workup seldom discloses an etiology, it should be undertaken only when there is a history of chronicity, frequent recurrences, or failure to respond. The most commonly associated systemic disease is JRA; less common are ankylosing spondylitis, Behçet's syndrome, and sarcoidosis. In the office practice of ophthalmology, traumatic anterior uveitis is the most common diagnosis. Anterior uveitis is also associated with the exanthemas of childhood, occasionally with infectious disease, and with several of the gastrointestinal disorders such as regional enteritis (see sec. **VIII).**

a. A so-called **white uveitis** may occur in children at any age, but especially in those from 4–16 years of age. White uveitis is found in girls 5 times more frequently than in boys. The triad in these children is band-shaped keratopathy, complicated posterior subcapsular cataract, and extensive posterior synechiae. Since the onset of the disease is so insidious, there may be severe damage before it is recognized. A decrease in vision should not be ascribed to flare and cells and turbidity of the vitreous. The physician should look for cysts in the macula, especially with fluorescein angiography. The workup should also include the tuberculin skin test, preferably the intermediate PPD, FTA-ABS for syphilis, and routine roentgenograms of the chest.

   b. Retinoblastoma and juvenile xanthogranuloma are the major diseases in the **differential diagnosis.**

   c. Although the **treatment** in children is the same as that in adults, it is difficult to give periocular steroid injections to children under 12 years of age without a general anesthetic. When long-term atropine is used, the physician must remember to provide bifocals. Prednisone every other breakfast is well tolerated by children, with fewer side effects than adults have, but the systemic route should only be used in severe vision-threatening disease where topical agents or injections are not sufficiently effective or possible. Daily long-term systemic corticosteroids should be studiously avoided in growing children to prevent serious metabolic side effects. A pediatrician should always be consulted, particularly with very young children, as **death from steroid dependence** has been reported.

2. **Peripheral.** Pars planitis or peripheral uveitis is considered in sec. **IX.** Children are usually diagnosed only after the late complications have become apparent. Only those showing cystoid changes in the macula with fluorescein angiography or those with enough vitreous reaction to make a retinal detachment imminent require treatment.

3. **Posterior.** Toxoplasmosis is the most common presumptive diagnosis, with toxocariasis being second (see sec. **XI.G**). Although floaters and blurred vision in a young child occasionally will bring the patient to the ophthalmologist, motility disorders and screening procedures are more frequent reasons. Retinitis pigmentosa provides the most important differential diagnostic problem. Unilateral retinitis pigmentosa simulates syphilitic retinitis. The FTA-ABS test for syphilis and the electroretinogram, which is extinct in retinitis pigmentosa, help differentiate these two.

XV. **Endophthalmitis** is a devastating clinical entity that may be most easily defined as inflammation of the intraocular tissues in response to insult from infection, trauma, immune reaction, physical or chemical changes, vasculitis, or neoplasm.

   A. **Classification**

   1. The most common endophthalmitis is **acute postoperative endophthalmitis,** which may be **infectious** secondary to bacterial or fungal invasion. This condition is seen most commonly in debilitated patients such as diabetics, patients with immunosuppressive disease, or patients with alcoholism, although it is certainly not confined to these groups. The other form of acute postoperative endophthalmitis is the **sterile** endophthalmitis that can be caused by chemical insult such as the use of irrigating agents, the retention of foreign bodies such as sponges or powder from gloves, or the ever-increasing incidence of manipulation of the vitreous, whether in deliberate open-sky vitrectomy or in correcting inadvertent vitreous loss during cataract surgery.

   2. Another form of endophthalmitis is the **long-term postoperative inflammation.** This is commonly associated with filtering blebs, either intentional or unintentional, that allow access to the external organisms directly into the eye through a very thin and tenuous conjunctival covering. The vitreous wick fistula, which is the result of externalization of the vitreous with no protective covering by conjunctiva, affords direct access to the inside of the eye for any external organisms as well. The fistulas seen with epithelial downgrowth are, of course, notoriously difficult to seal off. They also leave

the eye open to direct invasion from the outside by whatever organism may be in the conjunctival cul-de-sac.

3. Endophthalmitis may be seen after **trauma** to the eye, particularly lacerating injuries. Of all causes of endophthalmitis, traumatic injuries seem to be the least common cause of intraocular infection, possibly because the eye is capable of handling a certain level of infection without the assistance of antibiotic or without loss of control over that infection. It may be that, in the course of a laceration, not enough organisms are introduced to make a difference in the vast majority of cases, and therefore a significant endophthalmitis does not develop.

4. One less common form of endophthalmitis is **metastatic endophthalmitis from extraocular locations.** These are infectious loci elsewhere in the body, the most common causes being dermatitis, meningitis, otitis, septic arthritis, and following surgery, particularly of the abdomen, or associated with endocarditis or chronic obstructive pulmonary disease. Drug addicts who mainline heroin introduce into the vascular system fairly significant doses of both bacteria and fungi. Patients with **AIDS** or on **immunosuppressive drugs** for lymphomatous disease, leukemia, or organ transplant are also susceptible to metastatic endophthalmitis, particularly that due to *Candida albicans.* CMV, herpes and zoster viruses, *Pneumocystis,* and numerous other opportunistic infections are also seen more commonly now and should be suspect in any immunosuppressed patient who has blurring of vision.

B. The **etiologic agents** involved in endophthalmitis in general order of frequency are as follows:
   1. **Bacterial—postoperative**
      a. **Acute**
         (1) *Staphylococcus aureus.*
         (2) Gram-negative species:
            (a) *Pseudomonas.*
            (b) *Proteus.*
            (c) *Streptococcus pneumoniae.*
            (d) Miscellaneous *(Serratia, Klebsiella, Bacillus).*
      b. **Chronic low grade**
         (1) *Staphylococcus epidermidis.*
         (2) *Propionibacterium acnes.*
   2. **Bacterial—metastatic**
      a. *Streptococcus* sp.
      b. Pneumococcus.
      c. *Staphylococcus.*
   3. **Bacterial—posttraumatic:** *Bacillus cereus.*
   4. **Bacterial—post filter bleb**
      a. *Haemophilus influenzae.*
      b. *Streptococcus* sp.
   5. **Fungal—postoperative**
      a. *Volutella.*
      b. *Neurospora.*
      c. *Fusarium.*
      d. *Candida.*
   6. **Fungal—metastatic:** *Candida*—yeast.

   Approximately 50% of postcataract endophthalmitis is due to *S. aureus* and 25% is due to gram-negative species. The third most common cause is *S. epidermidis,* previously considered a nonpathogen.

C. **Clinically,** the earliest sign is an unexpected change or exaggeration of the expected **postoperative inflammation.** Patients often but not always complain of pain. There is obvious increased hyperemia. Conjunctival chemosis may be considerable. Lid edema may be so severe as to shut the eye completely, and there may also be spasm. Decreasing vision is invariably part of the process, and corneal edema may be the very first objective sign of an intraocular process gone wrong. Ultimately and often early in the process there will be considerable anterior chamber and vitreous reaction. *S. epidermidis* and *Propionibacterium acnes* may, however, incite only a low-grade inflammatory reaction lasting for weeks. *P. acnes* is particularly associated with intraocular lenses (IOLs). Metastatic endophthalmitis may be acute or slow in onset.

The clinical manifestations of endophthalmitis may sometimes be used to differentiate bacterial, fungal, and sterile etiologic agents. These manifestations are as follows:

1. **Bacterial**
   a. Sudden onset (1–7 days postoperatively), rapid progression.
   b. Pain, very red, chemosis.
   c. Lid edema and spasm.
   d. Rapid loss of vision and good light perception.
   e. Hypopyon and diffuse glaucoma.
2. **Fungal or low-grade bacterial**
   a. Delayed onset (8–14 days or more).
   b. Some pain and redness.
   c. Transient hypopyon.
   d. Localized anterior vitreous gray-white patch extending over face.
   e. Satellite lesions.
   f. Good light perception.
   g. Rare explosive exudation into anterior chamber.
3. **Sterile**
   a. May mimic bacterial or fungal infection.
   b. Undue surgical trauma.
   c. Incarceration of intraocular contents (lens, vitreous, iris) in wound.
   d. Foreign body (sponge, powder) retention.
   e. Vitrectomy

D. The **differential diagnosis** of **sterile endophthalmitis** is late rupture of the anterior vitreous face. This rupture is frequently associated with nonexposed vitreous in the wound. It should be differentiated from vitreous wick syndrome, in which there is actual exposure to vitreous extraocularly. This late rupture is associated with the onset of redness and decreased vision, with anterior chamber and vitreous reaction several months postoperatively. Another process that may be confused with endophthalmitis is cystoid macular edema, which is a common complication of routine as well as complicated cataract surgery. This entity not infrequently presents with decreased vision and increased vitreous inflammatory reaction, coupled with macular edema and occasionally with blurring of the disk. This syndrome can be differentiated from a true endophthalmitis by fluorescein angiography.

E. **Workup** for endophthalmitis includes hospitalization of the patient, a careful history as to any predisposing events, and a clinical examination for some of the previously mentioned predisposing factors.
1. **Cultures** obviously are of critical importance. Numerous studies have shown that conjunctival cultures are probably of very little use, because there seems to be little relationship between the flora growing outside the eye and that growing inside the eye in endophthalmitis.
2. An **anterior chamber paracentesis** (0.2 ml) and a diagnostic and (in some cases) therapeutic **vitrectomy** should be done in the operating room. Approximately 30% of all anterior chamber paracenteses will be positive for organisms. Results of the paracentesis may be correlated fairly well with the prognosis; i.e., eyes with positive cultures have a poor prognosis, whereas those with negative cultures usually regain useful vision. In **vitreous aspiration,** approximately 40–50% of the cultures are positive. In aphakic eyes the vitreous may be aspirated directly into a tuberculin syringe with a 22-gauge needle passed through the limbal incision made for the aqueous sample and on through the pupil. In phakic eyes a pars plana incision should be made and a 22-gauge needle introduced to aspirate a 0.3 ml. of material. If sufficient vitreous is not obtained, a vitreous cutting instrument may be used.

3. The sample should be used for both **culture** and **smears** for staining.
   a. **Culture.** For **bacterial** culture, sheep blood agar plate, chocolate agar plate, beef heart infusion, and thioglycolate broth should be inoculated. These are stored at 37°C and will usually be positive within 12 hours. **Fungal** cultures should be placed on Sabouraud's medium and blood agar plates, as well as beef heart infusion broth with gentamicin in it, to suppress bacterial growth. These are stored at 30°C or room temperature and will be positive in 36–72 hours as a rule.
   b. The **smears** should be Gram stained; any organisms that are found should be classified as positive, gram-positive, or gram-negative. The Giemsa stain smear, although it does not reveal whether the organism is gram-positive or negative, is superior for determining the actual morphology of any organism.

F. **Therapy of bacterial endophthalmitis. After planting the culture, the physician should immediately start treatment** regardless of whether there have been any results on smear. Broad-spectrum therapy should be maintained until definitive culture reports are obtained. The three main forms of therapy for endophthalmitis involve the use of antibiotics, cycloplegic-mydriatics (such as atropine), corticosteroids, and possibly vitrectomy. Antibiotics are delivered by three to four routes: (1) intravitreal, (2) subtenon or subconjunctival injection, (3) systemic (IV, IM, or occasionally PO), and, if point of entry is anterior, trauma, wound leak or ulcer, and (4) topical. See Table 8-5 for intravitreal doses, Chap. 5, Table 5–7 for topical and subconjunctival doses, and Appendix B for systemic doses.

Table 8-5. Intravitreous antibiotic preparations

Drug	Commercial preparation (IV)	First diluent[a] added to 1.0-ml commercial preparation	Initial solution (ml) plus	Second diluent[a] (ml)	Final drug concentration	Injected dose (0.1 ml)
Amikacin	100 mg/ml	4.0	1.0	9.0	1.0 mg/ml	0.1 mg
Carbenicillin	5 gm/10 ml	1.0	1.0	9.0	25 mg/ml	2.5 mg
Cefamandole	1 g/5 ml	1.0	1.0	4.0	20 mg/ml	2.0 mg
Cefazolin	500 mg/ml	1.0	1.0	9.0	25 mg/ml	2.5 mg
Ceftriaxone	1 gm/5 ml	1.0	1.0	4.0	20 mg/ml	2.0 mg
Clindamycin	150 mg/ml	2.0	1.0	9.0	5 mg/ml	0.5 mg
Gentamicin	80 mg/2 ml	3.0	1.0	9.0	1.0 mg/ml	0.1 mg
Tobramycin	80 mg/2 ml	3.0	1.0	9.0	1.0 mg/ml	0.1 mg
Vancomycin	500 mg/10 ml	—	1.0	4.0	10 mg/ml	1.0 mg
Vancomycin[b]	500 mg/10 ml	—	0.4	0.6	20 mg/ml	2.0 mg

The two "Initial solution mix" and "Final solution mix" are spanning headers above the respective columns.

[a] With the exception of carbenicillin and vancomycin (sterile water for injection only), diluent may be sterile water or saline for injection (USP).
[b] If posterior lens capsule not intact.
Source: Adapted from D. Pavan-Langston and E. Dunkel, *Handbook of Ocular Drug Therapy and Ocular Side Effects of Systemic Drugs.* Boston: Little, Brown, 1990.

1. **Therapy before culture data are known**
   a. **Immediately** following diagnosis of bacterial endophthalmitis and anterior chamber and vitreous aspiration for diagnostic purposes, commence **therapy** as follows in the **operating room.**
      (1) **Intravitreal** 0.1 ml injection of 0.2 mg of tobramycin or gentamicin and 1.0 mg of vancomycin for postoperative endophthalmitis, 1.0 mg of vancomycin plus 0.5 mg of clindamycin or 0.2 mg of tobramycin for posttraumatic cases, and 1.0 mg of vancomycin plus 2.0 mg of cefamandole or 2.0 mg of ceftriaxone for postglaucoma filter bleb infections (see Table 8-5 and Appendix B for dosages, mixtures, and other drugs). All are in 0.1 ml volume and may be repeated in 24–48 hours if necessary. After aspiration of fluid from the vitreous for diagnostic purposes, a 22-gauge needle remains in **midvitreous** while two new tuberculin syringes, each containing antibiotic, are exchanged consecutively and the material slowly injected into midvitreous. The small volume of antibiotic delivered into the vitreous should not remain in the bore of the needle. In phakic eyes, both the diagnostic and therapeutic vitreal aspiration and injections are performed behind the lens through a tract made in the sclera 4.0 mm behind the corneal limbus.
      (2) **Periocular injection** should be either subconjunctival (anterior subtenons) or retrobulbar (posterior subtenons). Injections are made with a disposable tuberculin syringe with a 25-gauge needle.
         (a) Gentamicin or tobramycin 40 mg (1 ml), covers most gram-positive and gram-negative organisms.
         (b) Cefazolin, 100 mg (1.0 ml), or vancomycin, 50 mg/ml, covers pneumococcus and streptococci not covered by the aminoglycosides.
   b. **Systemic.** In the operating room or once back in the **hospital room,** if **topical** antibiotics are to be used, start fortified tobramycin or gentamicin, 14 mg/ml, and cefazolin, 133 mg/ml, 2 drops qlh around the clock. **Systemic** amikacin, 15 mg/kg IV or IM q8h, coupled with cefazolin, 1 gm IV q6h for 10–14 days, is broad initial therapy until organisms are known or if they are never identified. See Appendix B for alternative drugs. Before the systemic treatment is started, a blood urea nitrogen (BUN) and creatinine level should be drawn. These should be monitored every 3 days because of the **nephrotoxicity** of these drugs. If the smears show gram-positive organisms, bacitracin drops at a level of 10,000 units/ml (2 drops q2h) should be added. If the smear shows gram-negative organisms, carbenicillin, 4–6 gm IV, or ticarcillin, 200–300 mg/kg IV q6h, should be added for extra protection against *Pseudomonas* and *Proteus.* **Probenecid,** 0.5 gm PO qid, is given to enhance cefazolin, carbenicillin, or other penicillin or cephalosporin levels.
2. **Once the cultures have returned,** the physician adjusts the topical regimen according to the organism found (see Appendix B for specific therapy).
   a. If the organism is a **gram-positive coccus,** the systemic therapy may be adjusted in that direction by vancomycin IV or cephalexin IM or IV qd for 7–10 days and subconjunctivally qd for 2 injections.
   b. If a **gram-negative rod** is found on the culture, the physician should continue to administer either tobramycin and ticarcillin IM or IV or carbenicillin IV qid for 10–14 days and subconjunctivally qd for 2–3 injections.
3. **Steroids**
   a. **Twenty-four hours after the antibiotic therapy** mentioned in sec. **2** is started, steroids may be initiated:
      (1) Dexamethasone phosphate, 4–12 mg (1 ml), or prednisolone succinate, 25 mg (1 ml) subconjunctivally every other day, 1–2 times.
      (2) Prednisone, 40 mg PO qd with rapid taper after 7–14 days.

Table 8-6. Preparation of intravitreous steroid

Drug	Initial solution	Sterile water for injection (USP)	Final concentration	Injected dose (0.1 ml)
Aqueous dexamethasone for injection, 24 mg/ml	1.0 ml	*plus* 5.0 ml	4 mg/ml	400 μg

   b. The role of corticosteroids in endophthalmitis is aimed at limiting inflammatory damage to the intraocular structures. After 24 hours of appropriate antibiotic therapy and only if **fungus is not suspected,** the physician may safely and justifiably start these drugs. If a sterile endophthalmitis is suspected, the physician should continue the steroids at higher levels for a longer period of time. Intravitreal aqueous dexamethasone, 0.4 mg, may be given at the time of a second antibiotic dose or alone (Table 8-6).
   4. The role of vitrectomy is still controversial. It is technically difficult because of poor visualization in infected eyes, but it has the advantage of removing infectious and inflammatory material from the eye. Initial vitrectomy (plus all the aforementioned therapy) should be used in patients presenting with moderately advanced or advanced disease. For patients presenting with milder disease, intravitreal, periocular injected, systemic, and topical antibiotics are preferred. If there is no improvement in 36–48 hours or if a virulent organism such as *Pseudomonas* or fungus is isolated, vitrectomy is recommended along with more intravitreal antibiotic or antifungal agents and appropriate systemic drug adjustment.
G. Therapy of fungal uveitis and endophthalmitis. The general evaluation procedures followed are similar to those just described in secs. **V.A–F.** The drug of first choice for fungal *endophthalmitis* is still amphotericin B given systemically and intravitreally (Table 8-7). **Synergistic** efficacy is obtained by adding oral flucytosine to systemic and intravitreal amphotericin B and continuing maintenance doses of both for 2–4 weeks before tapering. It should also be noted that ketoconazole is **antagonistic** to amphotericin B and should not be used with it. Topical natamycin q1h or amphotericin B q1-2h should be given in addition to systemic and intravitreal drug if the point of entry is anterior and accessible to topical therapy (see Chap. 5 sec. **IV.N**). The role of subconjunctival drug is not well established but may be useful in poorly cooperative patients for pulsing high doses. Toxic sloughing may occur, however. Vitrectomy is discussed in sec. **F.4** and is generally the rule for fungal endophthalmitis.
H. Prophylaxis
   1. Preoperative antibiotics are useful in decreasing the incidence of postoperative endophthalmitis from 0.71–3.05% to 0.05–0.11%. Additionally, the physician should not perform elective surgery if either the lids or lacrimal sac appear inflamed or infected. Culture should be taken and these areas appropriately treated before any surgery is undertaken. The physician should also take great caution and use plentiful preoperative antibiotics in any patients who have keratoconjunctivitis sicca, acne rosacea, or atopic dermatitis, as all of these patients are more prone than normal to carrying highly infectious organisms in the external ocular tissues.
   2. Meticulous operating room technique should be employed, as well as precautions for preserving a sterile approach to the eye.
   3. If the physician observes inadvertent filtering blebs **postoperatively,** an

Table 8-7. Antifungal systemic and intravitreal therapeutic regimen

Drug	Intravitreal	Systemic	Efficacious against
Amphotericin B (Fungizone)	5–10 μg	1 mg in 500 ml of 5% D/W IV over 2–4 hr test dose; work up by 5–10 mg total dose/day to maintenance of 0.3–0.5 mg/kg (4–6 hr infusion); synergistic with flucytosine PO	*Candida, Aspergillus, Cryptococcus, Coccidiodes, Sporothrix, Blastomyces, Histoplasma, Paracoccioides, Mucor*
Flucytosine (5 FC, Ancobon)		150–200 mg/day PO in 4 divided doses, q6h	*Candida, Aspergillus, Cryptococcus, Cladosporium*
Ketoconazole (Nizoral)		200–400 mg/day PO in single dose	See Miconazole Dermal mycoses
Miconazole (Monistat)	40 μg	0.2–0.6 gm IV, q8h (4–6 hr infusion)	*Candida, Fusarium, Penicillium, Aspergillus, Alternaria, Rhodotorula, Histoplasma, Cladiosporium, Coccidioides, Mucor, Paracoccidioides, Phialophora, Actinomycetes*

Fluconazole (Diflucan) for *Candida* or cryptoccosis. Dose: see flucytosine.

attempt should be made to seal these either with cryotherapy or, if necessary, with a secondary surgical procedure. If it is not possible to seal the bleb or in those patients who have intentional filtering blebs for glaucoma, it is advisable to use some form of chronic antibiotic therapy such as erythromycin ointment daily to protect them from building up high levels of gram-positive organisms in the conjunctival cul-de-sac.

XVI. **Panuveitis of suspected autoimmune origin** includes Behçet's syndrome and the uveoencephalitis syndrome of VKH.

  A. **Behçet's syndrome** (recurrent uveitis of young adults) is typified by attacks of nongranulomatous uveitis with hypopyon, aphthous lesions in the mouth, and genital ulceration. It is especially common in the Far East and Mediterranean basin (8 cases/million people). Loss of visual field occurs from widespread **vasculitis.** Skin lesions include erythema nodosum, acne, cutaneous hypersensitivity, and thrombophlebitis. Other findings may include arthritis, gastrointestinal ulcers, aneurysms, and neuropsychiatric symptoms. The disease characteristically follows a chronic recurrent pattern of intervals of 1 week–3 years with intervals between attacks lengthening so that after 15–20 years there are no further attacks, but the average period from onset to blindness from retinal vasculitis is 3 years. From the ocular standpoint Behçet's disease is one of males, but from the genital standpoint it is usually one of females. Both eyes almost always develop disease, sometimes simultaneously, sometimes separately. Age of onset is usually 17–37 years.

   1. The **differential diagnosis** includes acute idiopathic anterior uveitis, but unlike Behçet's disease these uveitides are usually unilateral in any given attack and often HLA-B27 positive. Sarcoid may simulate the posterior uveitis but differs in that it is far more indolent than the explosive retinal vasculitis of Behçet's disease. The latter is, in fact, difficult to differentiate

from the rapidly progressive viral vasculitic chorioretinitis infections. Other causes of **retinal vasculitis** include Eales's disease, birdshot retinopathy, lupus, multiple sclerosis, postvaccination, Wegener's granulomatosis, Takayasu's and Buerger's diseases, polyarteritis nodosa, polymyositis, Whipple's disease, Crohn's disease, Sjögren's A antigen, and numerous fungal, parasitic, viral, bacterial, and rickettsial diseases.

2. **Diagnosis** is based primarily on the clinical findings of uveitis and oral and genital ulcers with or without the other findings described. Japanese patients (not American born) are HLA-B51 positive nearly 60% of the time and Mediterranean patients are HLA-B5 positive more than 50% of the time. Skin hyperreactivity (pathology) is common in these patient groups but not frequently in Americans. Skin testing with Behçetin is highly variable in its results. In contradistinction to the usual uveitis, cells in the anterior chamber are neutrophils. Fluorescein angiography will reveal the extent of retinal vascular occlusive disease and assist in monitoring therapeutic response.

3. **Therapy** is effective but not fully satisfactory. It is critical that these patients be treated in association with an internist familiar with the drugs and disease. Behçet's disease not only blinds but it may also be fatal. Currently recommended treatment in the United States is high-dose systemic steroids for a first attack of mild bilateral disease, e.g., prednisone, 80–100 mg PO qd for several days until improved and then tapered to maintenance levels that control the disease. Over the long run, steroids will reduce inflammation but not prevent blindness or death. For a moderate to severe first attack or for bilateral recurrent attack, the drug of first choice is cyclosporine A in dosages discussed in section **VI.C** for at least 16 weeks and in many patients indefinitely at maintenance dosages. The Japanese almost never use steroids, as they feel it worsens the disease. They use immunosuppressive agents such as cyclosporine or cytotoxic agents as the drugs of first choice. This is frequently coupled with colchicine therapy, 1.0 mg PO bid, between attacks or during attacks in 16-week courses. Colchicine inhibits the enhanced polymononuclear cell migration noted in Behçet's disease. It appears to be useful in preventing recurrent attacks among Japanese but is probably of marginal use in whites. If cyclosporine A and colchicine fail, ozathioprine (2.5 mg/kg daily PO) for up to 2 years has proved effective in controlling progression of Behçet's, especially the eye disease. For acute exacerbations on azathioprine, 1000 mg IV of methylprednisolone every other day 3 times (or oral equivalent), may be added to the regimen and bring disease under control. Cytotoxic agents, particularly the alkylating agents cyclophosphamide or chlorambucil in dosages discussed in section **VI.C** may be tried and have been shown to be therapeutically effective in a number of patients. If disease is **unilateral** (rare), it is probably better just to observe or, if vision is being lost, to intervene only with colchicine and injected periocular steroids. Patients should be monitored closely for all the potential drug adverse side effects reviewed in section **VI.C.**

B. **Vogt-Koyanagi-Harada (VKH) disease** is a granulomatous panuveitis, with cerebral manifestations, depigmentation of the skin and hair, and ocular disease manifested clinically by bilateral diffuse vitritis and choroiditis beginning with bilateral visual failure, often accompanied by headache and nausea. In the fundus are multiple foci of unevenly elevated cloudy patches that form circumscribed oval detachments within a few days. Gradual sinking of the fluid results in bilateral inferior retinal detachment that tends to resorb spontaneously with resultant reattachment of the retina. Retinal and optic nerve neovascularization and papillitis are not uncommon. Anteriorly, mutton fat KP cells and flare, perilimbal vitiligo, pupillary nodules, and anterior chamber shallowing are often noted. The disease is identical to sympathetic ophthalmia, with the exception of a history of penetrating injury. The associated signs of exudative retinal detachment—**poliosis** (whitening of the eyebrows), **vitiligo** (depigmentation of the skin), **alopecia** (focal baldness), and **hearing difficul-**

ties, plus typical findings on fluorescein angiography—are useful diagnostically. Cranial neuropathy is demonstrated by optic neuritis, tinnitus, hearing loss, nystagmus, ataxia, vertigo, and extraocular muscle palsy. Other ocular complications of VKH are secondary glaucoma from peripheral anterior synechiae formation, cataracta complicata, and phthisis bulbi from severe involvement of the ciliary body. VKH is most common in Japanese and Latin American patients, and the clinical course is variable from mild and self-limited to severe and progressing to blindness. Systemic complications may be fatal, hence the need for an internist in evaluation and management with the ocular specialist.

1. **Differential diagnosis** is sympathetic ophthalmia and, in late cases, acute posterior multifocal placoid pigment epitheliopathy or sarcoid.

2. **Diagnosis** is based primarily on clinical findings. HLA-DR 4 testing is positive in 90% of Japanese but not white patients. There are high titers of antiretinal antibodies in the serum, total T-cell counts (helper and suppressor) are lower than normal, and there are high levels of circulating interferon gamma. Fluorescein angiography reveals various degrees of leakage, subretinal neovascularization, and, in some patients, AV anastomoses. ERGs and EOGs are abnormal.

3. **Treatment** of VKH is difficult but rewarding if carried out assiduously. It includes prednisone, 200 mg every morning with breakfast, plus periocular injections of soluble corticosteroid such as 4 mg of dexamethasone once or twice weekly during the acute phases. After 7–10 days, prednisone may be decreased to every other breakfast and 2 weeks later to 100 mg PO every morning for 1–2 weeks, with continuing decrease in every other day corticosteroid over the ensuing weeks. Length of therapy varies with severity, with some patients under gradually tapering treatment for a year. If there has been no improvement by 3 months, cyclosporine A in dosages discussed in section **VI.C** has been a successful alternative form of treatment and may be combined synergistically with systemic steroids, allowing lowering of the steroid dose. Some success has also been noted with cytotoxic agents. Laser therapy of neovascular nets is important adjunctive therapy.

XVII. Uveal trauma. Injury to the uvea may be either direct or contrecoup. Direct contusion of the cornea can produce a rather marked posterior displacement, first of the cornea and then of the iris-lens diaphragm. This displacement places great stress on the area of the iris root and the zonules. In addition, the sclera expands in circumference in the area of the ciliary body. The ciliary body follows suit, but with some lag, resulting in possible separation within the uveal tissues or between the uveal tract and the sclera. After trauma, the endothelium of the cornea may show a fine dusting of pigment, especially near the trabecular meshwork, on the lens capsule, on the iris surface, and occasionally in the vitreous. A **Vossius pigment ring** on the anterior surface of the lens gives evidence of previous ocular trauma. This ring is located at the site of pupillary margin at the time of injury. The following entities seen after uveal trauma are covered in Chap. 2 (see secs. **VIII** and **IX**): traumatic iritis, sphincter alterations (miosis and mydriasis), iridodialysis, angle recession, traumatic hyphema, choroidal trauma, traumatic chorioiditis, and uveal effusion (ciliochoroidal).

XVIII. Iris atrophy and degeneration. There is a generalized thinning of the iris stroma with a flattening of the architecture and disappearance of crypts, especially in the pupillary zone. The brown sphincter muscle becomes visible, and the entire pigment epithelial layer is easily seen. The pupillary ruff often develops a moth-eaten appearance; granules of pigment may seem to be scattered over the anterior iris surface and the anterior lens capsule as well as the back of the cornea and the trabecular meshwork.

A. Senile changes

1. So-called **senile miosis** is probably related to sclerosis and hyalinization of the vessels as well as of stroma, although preferential atrophy of the dilator muscle may play a role. Atrophy of both stroma and pigment epithelium occur as part of aging. The iris may become more blue or gray.

2. **Iridoschisis** is a bilateral atrophy affecting mostly patients over 65 years of age. The cleft forms between anterior and posterior stroma. Stromal fibers and blood vessels remain attached to a portion of the iris, with their loose ends floating freely in the anterior chamber. The avascular necrosis that may occur in angle-closure glaucoma predisposes to iridoschisis.

B. **Essential iris atrophy.** Multiple vascular occlusions may be responsible for essential iris atrophy, which is characterized by unilateral progressive atrophy of the iris. It is 5 times more common in women, commencing in the third decade and almost always complicated by glaucoma. The patient complains of a displaced pupil. The pupil is displaced away from the atrophic zone. This atrophy progresses over a period of 1–3 years. With dissolution of additional areas, a pseudopolycoria develops. Peripheral anterior synechiae develop on both sides of the holes, and the IOP starts to rise.

C. **Postinflammatory.** Although iritis can give rise to atrophy, it is seldom seen except in entities such as herpes zoster ophthalmicus.

D. **Glaucomatous.** Slight dilation and irregularity of the pupil as well as a more segmental atrophy may follow an acute angle-closure glaucoma, due to necrosis of the sphincter muscle.

E. **Neurogenic.** Depigmentation or focal hyperpigmentation may develop with an irregular pupil. This is seen in conditions such as neurosyphilis or lesions of the ciliary ganglion.

XIX. **Choroidal atrophies and degenerations.** Atrophy is a loss of tissue mass. Degeneration may be slight and possibly even reversible. The affected tissue may be viable, but the metabolism is disturbed and the end process is the death of the cells.

A. **Senile changes.** The most important senile changes occurring in the choroid, as in other parts of the uvea, occur in the blood vessels. These changes are especially evident at the posterior pole and about the optic disk. Associated hyperplasia and degeneration of the pigment epithelium may lead to an increase in deposition of hyaline material on Bruch's membrane. This deposition may result in small focal thickenings in the cuticular portion. These drusen or translucent colloid bodies are homogeneous, dome shaped, and sometimes calcified excrescences covered by damaged RPE. There is a diffuse thickening and basophilic staining of Bruch's membrane. Cracks of Bruch's membrane may develop.

B. **Choroidal sclerosis.** The clinical appearance of sclerosis of the larger choroidal vessels is mostly due to their prominence and easy visibility, with atrophy of the choriocapillaris and surrounding tissues. This process occurs in three regions: the extreme periphery of the fundus, the peripapillary zone, and the posterior polar region.

1. The **diffuse type of sclerosis** is rare. It usually commences in the fourth decade with an edematous appearance of the fundus, pigmentary migration, and small yellow or cream-colored spots. It slowly advances until the sixth decade, when the fundus develops a brownish tigroid appearance that is associated with extensive destruction of the RPE. The larger choroidal vessels are exposed and stand out as a prominent whitish network. The result is an exposure of the sclera, with complete atrophy. Transmission is usually autosomal dominant. Visual fields are contracted, but the visual acuity does not fail until the macula is involved. **Night blindness** is an early sign, and the ERG is subnormal. In the early stages the differential diagnosis is difficult, and in later stages it simulates choroideremia.

2. **Peripapillary choroidal sclerosis** begins around the optic disk and is similar to the senile peripapillary halo. In the early stages differential diagnosis includes senile peripapillary halo, central areolar sclerosis, senile macular degeneration, and posterior polar inflammation.

3. **Central choroidal sclerosis** begins in the macula and remains stationary or spreads. It may be seen as early as age 15 and may resemble uveitis because of the appearance of edema and exudation.

C. **Gyrate atrophy** of the choroid is characterized by a progressive atrophy of the choroid and retina, including the pigment epithelium. It usually begins in the third decade. Irregular atrophic areas develop, over which the retinal vessels appear normal, near the periphery. The atrophic areas enlarge, coalesce, and spread centrally. The macula is frequently preserved until late. **Night blindness** is a constant feature. The visual fields are usually concentrically contracted. Most of the hereditary patterns are recessive. Patients have an increased plasma, CSF, and aqueous humor ornithine concentration of from 10–20 times higher than normal. These findings suggest an inborn error of amino acid metabolism, possibly a defective activity in the enzyme ornithine ketoacid aminotransferase.

D. **Choroideremia** is a bilateral, hereditary choroidal degeneration characterized by **night blindness** from childhood. The typical and fully developed form with a progressive course toward blindness occurs in males, while females have a mild and nonprogressive course. It is transmitted in a recessive sex-linked manner. The earliest change is often seen in late childhood. In the male this change consists of degeneration of the peripheral RPE, giving a salt-and-pepper appearance. This is followed by progressive atrophy with exposure of the choroidal vessels, until the sclera is bared. The process continues both peripherally and centrally, leaving a small patch of retina and choroid in the macula. The retinal vessels and optic disk retain their normal appearance until late.

In female carriers the appearance resembles that seen in very young males, with a combination of pigmentation and depigmentation or salt-and-pepper atrophy most marked in the midperiphery. In females the condition is benign and does not progress. Night blindness begins in early youth in males and progresses to total night blindness after a period of about 10 years. The ERG shows an absence of rod (noncolor vision) scotopic activity and a progressive loss of photopic (color vision) activity.

E. **Angioid streaks** are reddish to dark-brown streaks of irregular contour, usually somewhat wider than retinal blood vessels. They extend outward from the disk toward the equator in a more or less circular pattern, and they lie underneath the retinal vessels. Later they may be bounded by a gray-white border representing proliferated fibrous tissue. Angioid streaks are almost always bilateral and are usually seen in middle-aged persons, more commonly in males. A stippled appearance of the fundus, resembling the cutaneous changes in pseudoxanthoma elasticum, has been called "peau d'orange." Several small, round, yellowish-white spots called "salmon spots" may also be seen in association with angioid streaks. Although the angioid streaks are asymptomatic, these breaks in Bruch's membrane allow the ingrowth of capillaries from the choroid that leak and produce a diskiform degeneration similar to that seen in senile patients. Angioid streaks signify the frequent association of widespread degenerative changes of a similar nature involving elastic tissue elsewhere, in **systemic conditions** such as pseudoxanthoma elasticum (Groenblad-Strandberg syndrome), osteitis deformans, Paget's disease, senile elastosis of the skin, sickle cell anemia, some hypertensive cardiovascular disorders, lead poisoning, thrombocytopenic purpura, and familial hyperphosphatemia. By far the most common association is that of pseudoxanthoma elasticum. Occasionally, photocoagulation of the neovascular net may be of value.

F. **Myopic choroidal atrophy.** In pathologic progressive myopia, a primary choroidal atrophy develops in which the sclera is thin and the choroid becomes atrophic. This degenerative myopia is usually associated with axial lengthening of the globe in the anteroposterior axis. The degree of myopia is usually genetically determined. It is more common in women and in some national groups, such as Chinese, Japanese, Arabs, and Jews.

Myopic degeneration often starts with the appearance of a temporal crescent at the optic disk that may spread to become a circumpapillary zone of atrophy. As the posterior eye enlarges, the sclera becomes thin and ectatic. The sclera may be exposed because the choroid does not reach the disk. Nasally, the choroid, Bruch's membrane, and RPE may overlap the optic nerve head. Clefts resembling lacquer cracks may develop in Bruch's membrane. These clefts are branching, irregular, yellow-white lines that take a horizontal course. Melanocytes disappear in the choroid, and there may be a widespread loss of the choriocapillaris. Breaks in Bruch's membrane may give rise to a Fuchs's spot at the macula that is similar to the maculopathy seen in angioid streaks and senile macular degeneration. The length of the eyeball should be determined with A-scan ultrasonography. If lengthening is documented, support for the stretching sclera can be gained by **surgical insertion of autographs** of fascia lata or homographs of sclera. This reinforcement surgery should be completed before severe degenerative changes take place.

G. **Pseudoinflammatory macular dystrophy of Sorsby** is a rare disease. To make the diagnosis, the physician should demonstrate dominant inheritance and lack of any signs of the presumed ocular histoplasmosis syndrome, angioid streaks, and high myopia. The onset is between the third and the fifth decade.

H. **Secondary atrophy and dystrophy**
1. **Ischemic.** Atrophy of choroidal tissues occurs when the blood supply to a given area is cut off or significantly diminished. Wedge-shaped areas of depigmentation are seen with their apices pointing toward the disk.
2. **Glaucomatous.** In chronic glaucoma, atrophy of the uveal tract may result. Atrophy may be so extensive that only a thin line of flattened pigmented tissue may be seen histologically.

XX. **Uveal tumors**
A. **Epithelial hyperplasia of the pigmented iris epithelium** is common in response to long-standing inflammation, degeneration, or glaucoma and consists of pigmented cells extending through the pupil over the anterior surface of the iris.
B. **Embryonal medulloepitheliomas (dictyomas)** arise from the nonpigmented epithelium of the ciliary body. Although distant metastasis has not been recorded, they are locally invasive. They occur in young children and appear as a grayish-white mass in the ciliary body, eventually presenting in the pupil. **Enucleation** is advised.
C. **Medulloepithelioma** in an adult form usually arises from the pigmented epithelium of the ciliary body but may also originate from the iris pigment epithelium. It occurs in previously traumatized or inflamed eyes, grows slowly, and appears as a dark mass. It is locally invasive and **enucleation** is suggested. **A- and B-scan ultrasonography and phosphorus-32 studies should be done prior to any surgical solution.**
D. **Nevi (freckles)** are a cluster of normal uveal melanocytes. A nevus is a highly cellular mass composed of "nevus cells" that are plump and that have few cytoplasmic processes. These cells are arranged in a nestlike manner. Although congenital, a nevus may not become recognizable until puberty, when it acquires pigment. It may be associated with ectropion uvea. Nevi may occasionally undergo malignant change. In the choroid they are bluish gray and flat with blurred margins, usually near the courses of the long posterior ciliary nerves. They are not usually associated with visual field defects.
E. **Malignant melanomas** are the most frequently occurring intraocular tumors in adults. The incidence in all eye patients is 0.4%. They are infrequent in blacks, occur usually after the fifth decade, and are rarely bilateral. The seriousness of the prognosis is directly related to their size and cell type. Spindle A cells are long cells with long, slender nuclei in which nuclear chromatin is arranged in a linear fashion along the long axis of the nucleus. There is some question as to whether these cells are malignant. Spindle B cells are oblong in shape; their nuclei are larger and plumper and have prominent nucleoli. Epithelioid cells are large and irregular in shape, and their nuclei are dense with prominent nucleoli. Usually there is a combination of cell types. Pigmentation can vary greatly from amelanotic to heavily pigmented lesions. The epithelioid cell type and pigmentation and larger size suggest greater malignancy. Malignant melanomas spread by direct extension, local metastasis, or generalized metastasis.

1. **Differential diagnosis** includes hemorrhagic detachment of the pigment epithelium or retina (or both), choroidal detachment (serous); ciliary body or retinal inflammatory disease (or both); pigment epithelial proliferation; hemangioma; and metastatic lesions.

2. **Clinical diagnosis** is based on several features. A small pigmented tumor **without retinal detachment** is most likely benign but should be photographed and reobserved for changes indicating growth in 3 months and every 6 months after that if no growth is detected. Localized **retinal detachment** in the macula causing loss of central vision may be caused by either benign or malignant melanotic tumor. Photopsia is a warning, however, that there may be acute retinal damage due to rapid tumor expansion. Visual field testing cannot differentiate between visual loss due to a chronic nongrowing tumor and acute damage from a rapidly growing one. **Tumor elevation** of 2 mm or more is indicative of an actively growing tumor. **Drusen** over the tumor surface are indicative of a minimally to totally inactive lesion. Scattered plaques and orange pigment **without drusen** suggest active growth. Serous **retinal detachment,** clear or cloudy, indicates toxic changes due to nutritional deficiency but not necessarily growth. Choroidal neovascularization, in the form of fine fan-shaped flat tufts over the tumor surface, suggests long-standing chronicity and lack of growth, whereas large-caliber vessels are seen in active tumors.

3. **Diagnostic tests.** If a lesion is classified as a dormant small melanoma (< 3 mm thick), baseline fundus photos, fluorescein angiography, and A- and B-scan ultrasonography should be done and repeated in 3–4 months. If there is no change, clinical observation and fundus photos should be repeated every 6 months and therapy started if changes appear. Medium size (< 10 mm thick), dormant-appearing melanomas have the same baseline examination, but because of greater tendency to growth, photos and ultrasound should be repeated every 3–6 months and evaluated for growth. **Fluorescein angiography** is useful in differentiating acute from chronic inactive lesions. Chronic signs are drusen, cystic retinal degeneration, and flat, fine neovascularization. More acute changes indicating growth are multiple pinpoint areas of dye leakage, widespread destruction of pigment epithelium, and an irregular pattern of moderate size vessels.

4. **Therapy** may be by laser photocoagulation for small melanomas not on the ciliary body and more than 2 mm from the macula or disk. More widely employed therapy currently is the use of surgically placed, low-energy, episcleral radioactive plaques. Isotopes used are cobalt 60, iridium 192, iodine 125, and ruthenium 106, depending on the size and virulence of the tumor. The plaques are left in place until 8000–10,000 cGy is delivered to the tumor apex and are then removed. Special plaques are used for peripapillary or subfoveal melanomas. Alternative radiotherapy is use of heavy ion bombardment using proton beam or helium ions. Treatment of choice is yet to be determined.
   Local resection may be used in some cases of ciliary body or small-medium ciliary-choroidal melanomas and, of course, iris melanomas. Plaques may also be used, however, for the ciliary body tumors. Enucleation is generally reserved for eyes with tumors too large to manage with radiotherapy in a patient with another seeing eye, eyes with hopeless visual loss (e.g., total retinal detachment), or eyes with invasion of the optic disk. If there is only one eye or the patient is old or already showing evidence of metastatic disease, surgery may be deferred in favor of radiotherapy, which may be palliative rather than curative. Exenteration is indicated only for extensive extraocular involvement, but no evidence of metastases at the time of initial evaluation, or if there is orbital recurrence after enucleation.

F. **Neurilemmoma** is a rare benign lesion that cannot be differentiated clinically from malignant melanoma but is extremely slow growing and, therefore, may be followed periodically for evidence of the notable growth indicative of melanoma.

G. **Neurofibroma** may appear only in the eye or may be a part of von Recklinghausen's disease. It is frequently associated with glaucoma, possibly because of chamber angle anomalies. It clinically resembles malignant melanoma and may be clinically confused with it.

H. **Leiomyoma** is a rare neoplasm and is difficult to differentiate from nevi and malignant melanoma of the iris. It appears as a grayish-white vascularized nodule, most frequently located in the inferior iris near the pupillary border. It is slow growing, and treatment is local excision.

I. **Hemangiomas** should be considered hamartomas and not true neoplasms. They can occur anywhere in the uvea, most frequently in the choroid. They may be associated with other angiomas and be a part of the **Sturge-Weber syndrome.** The choroidal lesions are usually in the posterior pole. The overlying retina shows microcystic changes. The lesions are not pigmented and are slow growing. They are usually associated with arcuate field defects. The tumors are endothelial-lined spaces engorged with blood and, because they lack a capsule, blend into the surrounding choroid. They are relatively flat and have a yellowish color. The diagnosis is improved with the use of fluorescein angiography, thermography, and ultrasonography. Photocoagulation can be used **therapeutically.**

J. **Secondary tumors.** Although any portion of the uveal tract can be the site of metastasis, the posterior choroid is the site of predilection because of its rich blood supply in the short posterior ciliary arteries. The breast is the most frequent primary site, with the lung second. The lesions clinically appear flat, diffuse, with an overlying shallow retinal detachment. The rapidity of growth is greater than that of malignant malanomas. **Radiation** may be used.

Glaucoma

Deborah Pavan-Langston and
David L. Epstein

I. **Definition and incidence.** *Glaucoma* is a condition in which the pressure inside the eye is sufficiently elevated ultimately to result in optic nerve damage and potential visual field loss via capillary microinfarction causing optic nerve ischemia. This combines with mechanical damage to the nerve by slippage of the lamina cribrosa. It is the second leading cause of blindness in the United States, with approximately 1 out of 50 Americans above the age of 35 having the condition. Approximately 1 million Americans have glaucoma and are unaware of it. Detection of glaucoma patients is, therefore, an important public health problem. There are over 40 different types of glaucoma. Glaucoma can also affect younger people, and measurement of eye pressure is an important part of a routine eye examination.

II. **Physiologic mechanisms of various glaucomas.** Aqueous humor is produced by the ciliary body and flows into the posterior chamber, then between the posterior iris surface and lens, around the pupil edge, into the anterior chamber. It exists from the anterior chamber at the angle of the anterior chamber, formed by the iris base and peripheral cornea, flowing through the trabecular meshwork of the sclera, into Schlemm's canal (Fig. 9-1F). Via the collector channels in the sclera, the aqueous is carried to the episcleral vessels, where aqueous mixes with blood. On slit-lamp examination, clear limbal aqueous veins can often be observed carrying aqueous into blood-filled episcleral veins. The latter can be identified by a laminated appearance of the blood-aqueous mixture. The level of intraocular pressure (IOP) at any time represents a balance between the rate of formation of aqueous humor and the amount of resistance to its flow out of the anterior chamber. In almost every case of glaucoma, increased IOP is due to an abnormality in outflow from the anterior chamber, rather than to above-normal rates of aqueous humor formation.

A. **In open-angle glaucoma** the aqueous humor has unimpeded access to the trabecular meshwork in the angle of the anterior chamber, but there is abnormally high resistance to the fluid flow through the trabecular meshwork and Schlemm's canal angle tissue. The peripheral iris does not interfere with the access of aqueous humor to the draining angle structures.

1. **Primary open-angle glaucoma** is the most common form of glaucoma. The underlying abnormality in the trabecular angle tissue causing abnormal resistance to fluid flow is not known. The disease is not secondary to another eye disease or condition. Primary open-angle glaucoma is a silent, surreptitious process. Usually there are no symptoms. Gradual loss of peripheral vision occurs. Loss of central vision is usually the last to occur. Only actual measurement of the IOP and inspection of the optic nerve head with an ophthalmoscope can detect primary open-angle glaucoma in its early stages.

2. **Secondary open-angle glaucoma** occurs as a result of or in association with another eye disease or condition such as uveitis or trauma, resulting in secondary blockage or damage to the canals and collector channels.

B. **In angle-closure glaucoma** the peripheral iris tissue covers the trabecular meshwork, preventing access of the aqueous humor to the trabecular meshwork. This type of glaucoma is often intermittent, with acute symptoms that are reversible when the peripheral iris is moved away from draining angle

Fig. 9-1. Anterior chamber angle depth and anatomic structures of the angle. **A.** Grade 0: Slit or closed angle. **B.** Grade 1: extremely narrow angle; closure probable. I-C (iris-corneal angle) = 10 degrees. **C.** Grade 2: moderately narrow angle; closure possible. I-C = 20 degrees. **D.** Grade 3: moderately open angle; no closure possible. I-C = 20–35 degrees. **E.** Angle wide open; no closure possible. I-C = 35–45 degrees. **F.** Anatomic landmarks of wide open angle as seen by gonioscopy. (Adapted from Anterior Chamber Angle Estimation Card, Allergan Pharmaceutical Co., Irvine, California. With permission.)

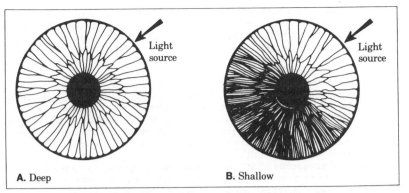

A. Deep   **B.** Shallow

Fig. 9-2. Estimation of anterior chamber depth by oblique illunination. **A.** Safe for dilation. **B.** Risk of acute angle closure, spontaneous or on dilation. (Adapted from D. Paton and J. Craig, *Glaucomas: Diagnosis and Management.* Clinical Symposia. Summit, N.J.: Ciba Pharmaceutical Co., 1976. With permission.)

structures. In pure angle-closure glaucoma, the trabecular meshwork and Schlemm's canal angle tissue have inherently normal resistance to fluid flow. The IOP is elevated only when the peripheral iris covers over the trabecular meshwork, preventing egress of the aqueous.

1. In **primary angle-closure glaucoma,** relative **pupillary block** is the mechanism of angle closure. This means that there is relative resistance to fluid flow of aqueous humor between the posterior iris surface and lens due to their close approximation at the pupil. This relative pupillary block increases the pressure of aqueous in the posterior chamber, forcing the peripheral iris forward over the trabecular meshwork (Fig. 9-1). The state of relative pupillary block depends greatly on pupillary size and rigidity of the peripheral iris. For example, relative pupillary block may be increased and angle-closure glaucoma produced by putting a patient in a dark room or by using dilating medications that move the pupil into a middilated state. Drug-induced miosis may produce a very small pupil, blocking posterior chamber aqueous passage and thus pushing the iris forward to close the angle. Most eyes subject to possible angle-closure glaucoma can be recognized by the shallowness of their axial anterior chamber depth.

2. **Secondary angle-closure glaucoma** occurs as a result of or in association with another eye disease or condition, such as a swollen cataract or diabetic neovascularization pushing or pulling the iris over the trabecular meshwork.

III. **Methods of examination**

A. **Flashlight.** After examining pupillary light reactions, the physician should direct the flashlight to the temporal side of each eye, perpendicular to the corneal limbus, and note the shadow produced by the nasal peripheral iris against the cornea. This technique allows a gross estimate of anterior chamber depth. In eyes with shallow anterior chambers that might be subject to angle-closure glaucoma, the relatively forward position of the iris will cause the nasal side to be in shadow. This flashlight examination should be performed in all patients prior to routine pupillary dilation. In eyes with shallow anterior chambers, the pupil should not be dilated until after gonioscopy is performed (Fig. 9-2).

B. **Slit-lamp examination**

1. The **axial and peripheral anterior chamber depth** should be measured and expressed in terms of corneal thickness. Anterior chamber depths less than three corneal thicknesses axially and one-fourth peripherally are suspect for the presence of narrow angles, and gonioscopy should be performed.

2. **Other diagnostic signs** during slit-lamp examination may be noted: the presence of inflammatory cell deposits (keratic precipitates [KPs]) on the corneal epithelium, anterior chamber cells and flare, iris heterochromia and transillumination (by placing the vertically narrowed beam coaxially in the pupil to create a red reflex back through the pupil), iris vessels, and lens surface exfoliation.

C. **Measurement of IOP** may be taken by finger tension (estimate), Schiötz, applanation, MacKay-Marg, or air-puff noncontact tonometry (see Chap. 1, II.F). **An IOP greater than 22 mm Hg should be considered suspicious,** if not frankly abnormal, and the patient should be followed. Considerable diurnal variation of IOP may occur in glaucoma patients (even down to normal levels); therefore, inspection of the optic disk cupping is just as important as the actual measurement of the IOP.

D. **Ophthalmoscopy of the optic nerve cup.** Atrophy of connective tissue associated with the hyaloid artery during embryogenesis results in a depression of the internal (vitrad) surface of the optic disk termed the *cup.*

1. **The normal physiologic disk cup** varies considerably. Large physiologic cups are always round in shape, unlike the vertical elongation that occurs in glaucoma. What are important are the amount and the contour of disk tissue present in the rim of the optic disk between the end of the cup and the edge of the disk proper (Fig. 9-3). Not until the cup extends toward the edge of the disk does frank glaucomatous field loss occur. It is important to recognize that many glaucomatous and normal patients have a circular halo around the optic disk in which the retinal pigment epithelium (RPE) and choroidal pigment is deficient, so that the physician is actually viewing the sclera underneath. The end of this peripapillary halo should not be misinterpreted as the edge of the disk in assessing the disk rim tissue. Statistically, **patients with very large, round physiologic cups are more at risk of developing glaucoma,** and they should be followed. Round cups with intact disk rim tissue, however, are not necessarily abnormal in the absence of other changes.

2. **The glaucomatous disk (nerve head)** may be recognized by certain changes in contour of the optic nerve cup.

   a. **Parallax** should be used in monocular (direct ophthalmoscope) examination of the optic disk in order to assess the contour of the disk tissue. **Stereo viewing** through a dilated pupil with a fundus contact lens or a + 90 d handheld lens at the slit lamp is very useful. With glaucomatous damage to the nerve there occurs actual loss of nerve tissue and its vascular and glial supporting tissue. Such atrophy results in both contour (cupping) and color (pallor) changes in disk appearance. In elderly people, however, nuclear sclerotic changes (early cataracts) often impart a rosy color to the disk and may be confusing. In primary optic atrophy, not due to glaucoma, pallor of the disk occurs with no change in contour.

   b. **In glaucoma, the cup usually enlarges vertically.** The increased cupping commonly progresses first toward the inferior pole of the disk and then enlarges superiorly, but there is considerable variation. Very rarely, the optic cup may extend straight temporally first rather than vertically. In such cases, **macular fibers may be affected early** in the course of the disease, with resulting **loss of central vision.** Cupping close to or at the inferior pole of the disk will, of course, result in superior field loss; cupping close to the superior pole of the disk, in inferior field loss. Occasionally, glaucomatous damage to the optic disk produces a shallower background bowing of disk tissue rather than excavation. The latter is called **saucerization.**

   c. **Asymmetry** in the appearance of the right and left optic disk cups may be an early sign of glaucoma, even though each is within normal limits.

   d. **Enlargement** in the size of the cup occurs before visual field loss results. Inspection of the appearance of the optic disk cup is an important part of glaucoma screening procedures. During long-term follow-up, the size

Fig. 9-3. Progressive glaucomatous atrophic cupping of the optic nerve head with commonly associated visual field defects. **A.** Early enlargement of physiologic cup. Field normal. **B.** Inferotemporal notching of cup. Field shows enlarged blind spot and superonasal Bjerrum scotoma. **C.** Increased notching, thinning of rim of cup, and visible lamina cribrosa. Field shows constriction of superonasal field and advancing superior Bjerrum scotoma. **D.** Advanced generalized thinning of rim of cup with nasalization of vessels. Field shows further superior constriction and new inferior field defect due to damage of superior retinal nerve fibers. **E.** Total atrophy of the rim; pale, deep cup. Vessels disappear under rim. Field shows small central and temporal island of vision remaining. (Adapted from D. Paton and J. Craig, *Glaucomas: Diagnosis and Management.* Clinical Symposia. Summit, N.J.: Ciba Pharmaceutical Co., 1976. With permission.)

and shape of the cup is noted in addition to the IOP and visual field. If enlargement of the cup occurs during follow-up, then, regardless of the absolute level of IOP, that pressure level is too high and additional glaucoma therapy is initiated. It is useful to record the appearance of the cup size and shape on a diagram (Fig. 9-3).

E. Visual fields

1. **Techniques** include confrontation (usually bedside examination), tangent screen, and various forms of automated static and kinetic perimetry (see Chap. 1, sec. II.I and Chap. 12, sec. I.A–F). Glaucoma patients are followed with visual fields every 6 months as a routine. This time period may be extended by a few months if the optic nerve is very healthy, if no field defect is present, and if the pressure is well controlled.

2. If **visual field loss progression** occurs while the patient is being followed, then, regardless of the level of IOP, that pressure is too high and glaucoma therapy should be adjusted and fields repeated every 3–4 months until stable. Similar considerations apply to progression of optic disk cupping. Except in myopes or in glaucoma patients with episodes of extremely high pressure elevation, visual field changes should correspond with optic disk cupping. For example, superior field loss does not occur unless the disk shows increased cupping to the inferior pole.

3. **Follow-up field examination** should be done with the pupil at the same size as in baseline examinations, so that a similar condition of retinal test object illumination exists for the follow-up fields added. Miotic glaucoma therapy may need to be reversed by dilation for field examinations with 2.5% phenylephrine or 1.0% tropicamide. Should the patient develop lens opacities, continued examination with the smaller test objects may produce artifactual field defects. The **size of the test object** should be graded to the visual acuity.

4. **Glaucoma field defects** characteristically respect the horizontal meridian (unlike chiasmal lesions, which respect the vertical). This is because glaucoma characteristically produces a nerve fiber bundle defect—an arcuate defect or Bjerrum scotoma, or a variant of these, such as a nasal step. The temporal nerve fibers in the retina sweep either superiorly or inferiorly around the macula and do not cross the horizontal raphe. Since it would be purely chance that exactly symmetric nerve fibers in the superior and inferior fields would be similarly affected, glaucoma defects characteristically show some discontinuity at the horizontal meridian, as a nasal step. The papillomacular fibers are usually relatively resistant to chronic pressure effects until late in the disease, and visual acuity changes do not occur early. After central vision is lost from glaucoma, typically all that is left is a temporal island of vision. Automated perimetry or Goldmann fields may be the first to detect early defects.

F. Gonioscopy. The angle is viewed at a slit lamp with a Goldmann lens or with the patient recumbent with use of a Koeppe-type lens and handheld microscope (see Chap. 1, II.P). It is assessed for shallowness and possible susceptibility to angle-closure glaucoma, as well as for other abnormalities such as pigment, synechiae, exfoliation, new blood vessels, inflammatory deposits, and evidence of old injury such as angle recession. Generally, if the scleral spur can be seen through the entire circumference and the iris is not excessively convex, the eye is not likely to be susceptible to angle closure and the pupil can be safely dilated. One commonly used **angle rating system** is depicted in Fig. 9-1. It should be noted, however, that narrow-angle eyes can look distinctly different at different examinations, perhaps reflecting different rates of aqueous production and differing relative pupillary block. Repeat examination in such narrow-angle eyes is usually indicated. The Zeiss gonioscopic lens is useful for rapidly viewing the angle, although it readily causes indentation of the eye and artificial deepening of the anterior chamber. The latter is deliberately utilized to look for peripheral anterior synechiae formation.

G. Tonography is the continuous recording of ocular pressures during several, usually 4, minutes while the eye is subjected to the indentation of the Schiötz tonometer, in order to determine how rapidly the pressure drops under this load. From this determination the facility of aqueous outflow from the anterior chamber is calculated (see Chap. 1, **II.F**). The indentation tonometers, such as the Schiötz, actually raise the level of true IOP at the time of indentation. This has all been back calculated in the tables that accompany the tonometer to give the true IOP before the indentation. This fact helps explain the falsely low Schiötz readings in myopes with glaucoma who have low scleral rigidity.

IV. **Principles of therapy. In all cases of glaucoma it is essential to establish whether the glaucoma is open or closed angle.** This is accomplished by placing a gonioscopic contact lens on the eye and actually viewing the angle structures.

   A. In the therapy of **open-angle glaucoma** the physician usually first treats the condition medically to lower the IOP. This pressure may be lowered by increasing the facility of aqueous outflow from the anterior chamber through the angle tissues or by decreasing the rate of aqueous humor formation by the ciliary body or both. Laser trabeculoplasty or surgery is required only when medical therapy fails to control IOP and when nerve cupping or visual loss is progressive.

   B. Angle-closure glaucoma may initially be treated medically, but it is primarily a surgical (laser) disease, requiring peripheral iridectomy (placing a hole through the peripheral iris) to relieve pupillary block permanently. Posterior chamber aqueous pressure is thus relieved by aqueous flowing through this extra opening, and the peripheral iris falls away from the meshwork.

V. **Medical treatments and side effects**

   A. Pilocarpine

     1. Mechanism of action. Pilocarpine is a direct-acting parasympathomimetic (muscarinic), **cholinergic** drug.

     2. Physiologic effects. The drug is used in chronic open-angle glaucoma to increase the facility of aqueous outflow. The mechanism of action is probably exclusively mechanical, via ciliary muscle contraction and pull on the scleral spur and trabecular meshwork. It is used in acute angle-closure glaucoma to move the iris away from the angle. Miosis is a side effect and is of no therapeutic benefit.

     3. Indications are chronic open-angle glaucoma, acute angle-closure glaucoma, chronic synechial angle-closure glaucoma (following peripheral iridectomy), and following cyclodialysis surgery.

     4. Contraindications are inflammatory glaucoma, malignant glaucoma, or known allergy.

     5. Available preparations are 0.5–10.0% eye drops, Ocusert P-20 and P-40 diffusion membranes, and 4% gel.

     6. Recommended dosage

       a. Eye drops. Except in very darkly pigmented irides, maximum effect is probably obtained with a 4% solution. In milder open-angle glaucoma, therapy is usually initiated with a 1% concentration. Duration of effect is 4–6 hours. It is usually prescribed for every 6 hours.

       b. Ocuserts are changed once weekly. P-20s are generally used in patients controlled with 2% drops or less, and P-40s in those requiring higher doses.

       c. The gel is a bedtime adjunct to daytime medication.

     7. Side effects

       a. Ocular

         (1) Contact allergy is fairly rare.

         (2) Contraction of the ciliary muscle results in accommodation and ensuing **fluctuating myopia.** In younger patients this is usually a disabling visual side effect that prevents use of pilocarpine. Continuous low-level, **constant delivery ocular insert devices,** such as the Ocusert, are very effective in young patients with glaucoma who require pilocarpine therapy. These low levels of continuous delivery result in small amounts of myopia that tend to be steady and correctable, if necessary, with spectacles. Most patients above the age of 50 do not develop such pilocarpine-induced myopia, presumably because of an inelasticity of their lens that is also responsible for their presbyopia.

(3) Pupillary **miosis** is a definite side effect of pilocarpine, which again exerts its antiglaucoma effect via ciliary muscle traction on the angle structures. This miosis results in **diminished night vision** and often some **contraction in peripheral visual field.** If the patient has early axial lens opacities, this miosis may result in **diminished visual acuity.** On the other hand, the miosis may result in a pinhole effect and an actual improvement in visual acuity.

(4) **Shallowing of the anterior chamber** may occur with higher doses of pilocarpine by forward movement of the lens-iris diaphragm subsequent to ciliary muscle contraction and relaxation of zonular tension. This shallowing may result in an increase in relative pupillary block, and it may convert an open-angle glaucoma with narrow angles into **partial angle-closure glaucoma.** This is true for all the standard miotic glaucoma therapies (carbachol, echothiophate iodide, demecarium bromide). In susceptible individuals, it seems to be dose related. There may be varying amounts of anterior chamber shallowing on miotic therapy. Similarly, in angle-closure glaucoma, lower concentrations of pilocarpine are used initially in order to minimize this axial shallowing and possible increase in relative pupillary block.

b. **Systemic side effects.** Occasional patients are peculiarly sensitive and may develop sweating and gastrointestinal overactivity with usual dosages. **Sweating, salivation, nausea, tremor, bradycardia,** and **hypotension** have sometimes been observed as results of too vigorous a treatment of angle-closure glaucoma with pilocarpine.

B. **Carbachol**

1. **Mechanism of action.** A **cholinergic** similar to pilocarpine.
2. **Physiologic effects.** Similar to pilocarpine.
3. **Indications.** Carbachol eye drops are longer acting than pilocarpine, thus having a greater stabilizing effect on diurnal pressure and myopia fluctuation. It may also be used in patients allergic to pilocarpine; otherwise, the indications are similar to pilocarpine. An intracameral preparation for intraoperative use induces miosis and inhibits postoperative pressure rise.
4. **Contraindications.** Similar to pilocarpine.
5. **Available preparations.** 0.75%, 1.5%, and 3.0% eye drops and 0.01% for intraocular use.
6. **Recommended dosage.** Carbachol 3% is approximately equivalent to pilocarpine 4% and 1.5% roughly equivalent to 2% pilocarpine. The effect is reported to last up to 8 hours. Dosage tid (compared to qid with pilocarpine) may be a distinct advantage in certain patients.
7. **Side effects.** Similar to pilocarpine.

C. **Anticholinesterase agents** (echothiophate iodide, demecarium bromide, physostigmine)

1. **Mechanism of action.** Indirect-acting parasympathomimetic activity by virtue of binding to the enzyme, acetylcholinesterase, allows endogenous acetylcholine to accumulate.
2. **Physiologic effects.** Ciliary muscle and iris sphincter muscle contraction occur similar to and possibly more marked than that occurring with other miotics, e.g., pilocarpine and carbachol. Miosis is a side effect of no therapeutic benefit.
3. **Indications** are chronic open-angle glaucoma (especially with aphakia), chronic synechial angle-closure glaucoma (following peripheral iridectomy), and following cyclodialysis surgery. These agents are more potent than pilocarpine or carbachol and should be used only when pilocarpine 4% is no longer effective.

4. **Contraindications.** Anticholinesterase agents should never be used in narrow-angle glaucoma because of the extreme miosis they produce, as well as possible forward lens movement, which may actually increase pupillary block. Similarly, open-angle glaucoma with open but narrow angles may worsen because of partial angle closure as a result of this therapy. Repeat gonioscopy on therapy is indicated. Other contraindications are inflammatory glaucoma or known allergy. These agents should be used cautiously in patients who are predisposed to **retinal detachment,** e.g., patients with lattice degeneration or family history of nontraumatic detachments.

5. **Available drop preparations** include echothiophate iodide 0.06–0.25%, demecarium bromide 0.12% and 0.25%, and physostigmine 0.25–0.5%. Physostigmine ointment is available for bedtime use.

6. **Usual dosage.** Anticholinesterase agents are administered twice a day. Since side effects are dose related, the lower concentration should be tried initially for pressure control. It may be of no added benefit to continue pilocarpine after anticholinesterase therapy is begun.

7. **Side effects**

   a. **Ocular**

      (1) Possible side effects include **accommodative spasm** and **shallowing of the anterior chamber** as well as **diminished night vision** and **peripheral field,** similar to and possibly more marked than that occurring with other miotics, e.g., pilocarpine and carbachol. It has been estimated that at least 50% of glaucomatous eyes treated with echothiophate over a period of 3 years will suffer some visual impairment owing to **cataractous lens changes** induced by the drug. These changes are related to drug concentration, frequency of dosage, age of the patient, and patient susceptibility. These agents should be used only when pilocarpine 4% is no longer effective, and the lower concentrations should be tried initially for pressure control. In phakic eyes, because of this potential for cataractous lens changes, these agents should be utilized only as a last resort prior to filtration surgery. The lens changes have been classically described as mossy anterior subcapsular opacities, but posterior subcapsular opacities and progression of nuclear sclerosis have also been described.

      (2) **Pupillary cysts** may occur with anticholinesterase therapy and may lessen with concomitant daily phenylephrine 2.5% eye drop therapy. These agents may induce a breakdown of the blood-aqueous barrier and **increase anterior chamber flare.** They should not be used in the presence of active uveitis. There seems to be some small risk of **retinal detachment** on this therapy, possibly due to traction and forward movement of the ora serrata as a result of intense ciliary muscle contraction. If feasible, glaucoma patients should have dilated indirect ophthalmoscopy with scleral depression prior to initiation of strong miotic therapy. **Lacrimal punctal stenosis, conjunctival goblet cell,** and **tear abnormalities** have been reported on occasion.

   b. **Systemic**

      (1) Anticholinesterase agents may cause **diarrhea, nausea,** and **abdominal cramps** if excessively absorbed. These toxic symptoms are cumulative and therefore appear only after many months of therapy. Patients should be instructed in lacrimal occlusion with digital pressure when taking drops to minimize systemic absorption and pharyngeal-alimentary passage of these agents. **Internists should be especially suspicious of gastrointestinal or systemic malaise complaints in glaucoma patients under chronic therapy with anticholinesterase or carbonic anhydrase inhibitor agents (see G.7). Since both of these agents frequently produce un-**

desired systemic effects only after months of therapy, the correct diagnosis is too frequently missed.

(2) **Serum pseudocholinesterase,** which hydrolyzes succinylcholine and procaine, is often **decreased** in patients on chronic topical anticholinesterase therapy, and therefore prolonged apnea may occur following use of succinylcholine in surgical procedures. It takes 4–6 weeks after cessation of topical anticholinesterase therapy for serum enzyme levels to return to normal, so **succinylcholine anesthesia should be avoided, if possible, in patients recently on these agents.**

8. **Contraindications** are uveitis and narrow-angle glaucoma.

D. **Epinephrine**
1. The **mechanism of action** is unclear but appears to be a function of both alpha- and beta-receptor stimulation.
2. **Physiologic effects.** Epinephrine both increases aqueous outflow (alpha and beta stimulation) and decreases aqueous humor formation (alpha stimulation in the ciliary body). It is additive to the cholinergics, anticholinesterases, and carbonic anhydrase inhibitors in pressure-lowering effects.
3. **Indications.** It is primarily used in open-angle glaucoma or in conjunction with miotics with mildly shallowed chambers. Certain patients show a greater pressure lowering following several weeks of epinephrine therapy than following a single, acute dosage.
4. **Contraindications** include narrow-angle glaucoma or known allergy.
5. **Available preparations.** Epinephrine is available in strengths 0.5–2.0% to treat open-angle glaucoma as a borate, bitartrate, or hydrochloride eye drop. There is no significant difference in the clinical efficacy of the preparations. The bitartrate has only 50% drug available as free base, however.
6. **Usual dosage** is epinephrine 1% bid–tid. There is some evidence that, at least in patients with dark irides, epinephrine 2% may be more potent than 1%. Epinephrine is also available in **combination with pilocarpine:** 1–6% pilocarpine with 1% epinephrine to be used bid–qid. Combined drug is of greater convenience to many patients.
7. **Side effects**
   a. Occasionally, paradoxic **pressure rise** may occur with epinephrine (with open angles); certain patients, for unknown reasons, have minimum pressure lowering on epinephrine therapy.
   b. Approximately 10–15% of patients are unable to tolerate long-term epinephrine therapy due to the development of **topical allergy.** This most often represents a true allergy to the epinephrine rather than to the preservatives in the solution. Therefore, switching brands of epinephrine is rarely effective, and usually epinephrine must be discontinued.
   c. Epinephrine has been documented to cause **cystoid macular edema** in certain aphakic patients. This is almost always reversible on cessation of epinephrine therapy.
   d. Oxidation products of epinephrine can result in **pigmented conjunctival deposits** as well as a **canalicular (tear duct) obstruction.**
   e. Occasional complaints of **palpitation, tachycardia,** and **faintness** have been recorded in patients after topical usage. Although theoretically a concern (one drop of epinephrine 2% = 0.1 mg), epinephrine can almost always be given safely to patients with cardiovascular disease, especially if patients are taught how to **perform punctal occlusion** following topical administration, in order to decrease systemic absorption, by pressing over the medial lid area.

E. **Dipivalyl epinephrine (dipivefrin hydrochloride [DPE])** is an epinephrine prodrug in which the two pivalic acids are cleared from an epinephrine molecule in the eye. It was synthesized for use on epinephrine-allergic as well as nonsensitized glaucoma patients.
1. The **mechanism of action** and **pharmacologic effects** are similar to epinephrine.

2. **Indications** are epinephrine-allergic patients plus all other indications for epinephrine use in the eye. Unfortunately, there is still some cross-allergenicity between epinephrine and DPE.
3. **Contraindications.** Similar to epinephrine.
4. **Available preparation** is 0.1% DPE solution.
5. **Recommended dosage.** 0.1% DPE is used once every 12–24 hours and is roughly equivalent to that of 2% epinephrine. DPE should probably not be used with anticholinesterases such as echothiophate iodide as they may inhibit the esterases necessary for cleavage of the pivalic acid groups. DPE should probably not be used until at least 4 hours after instillation of beta blockers, as noted under epinephrine.
6. **Side effects** are similar to epinephrine except that there have not yet been reports of adrenochrome deposit or aphakic cystoid macular edema.

F. **Apraclonidine** is a synthetic alpha-adrenergic agonist.
   1. The **mechanism of action** and **physiologic effects** are unclear but appear to be beta-2 receptor stimulation that results in decreased aqueous humor formation.
   2. **Indication** is for control of increase in IOP after anterior segment laser surgery (FDA-approved) or rarely for acute short-term pressure rises.
   3. **Contraindications** include known allergy to the drug and cardiac disease with untreated AV block or bradycardia.
   4. **Available preparations** 1% solution in a single-dose 0.25-ml container.
   5. **Usual dosage.** One drop 1 hour prior to laser surgery and 1 drop immediately after the procedure. This dose decreases the incidence of postlaser pressure spikes of 10 mm Hg or more to less than 2%.
   6. **Side effects** include possible transient upper lid retraction, conjunctival blanching, mydriasis, burning or itching sensation, and subconjunctival hemorrhage. Systemically there may be gastrointestinal reaction and cardiovascular effect such as bradycardia, vasovagal attack, palpitations, or orthostatic hypotension. CNS disturbance includes insomnia, irritability, and decreased libido, all of which are transient.

G. **Carbonic anhydrase inhibitors (CAIs)** (acetazolamide, methazolamide, dichlorphenamide)
   1. **Mechanism of action.** CAIs inhibit the enzyme, carbonic anhydrase.
   2. **Physiologic effects.** The ciliary body enzyme, carbonic anhydrase, is somehow related to the process of aqueous humor formation, most likely via the active secretion of bicarbonate. CAIs decrease the rate of aqueous humor formation.
   3. **Indications.** CAIs are additive therapy in the management of various acute glaucomas, but also in the chronic management of primary and secondary open-angle and angle-closure glaucomas not adequately controlled on topical medication.
   4. **Contraindications.** Because of the metabolic and possible respiratory acidosis effects, patients with significant respiratory disease should be given CAIs cautiously and in lower dosages. Patients with a history of calcium phosphate kidney stone formation should be given the medication cautiously and only after consultation with a urologist. Known allergy is a contraindication. Patients with allergies to other sulfonamides should be given these agents with caution.
   5. **Available preparations** include acetazolamide, methazolamide, dichlorphenamide, and ethoxzolamide (see Appendix A).
   6. **Recommended dosage.** Established dosages for near-maximum effect are: acetazolamide tablets, 250 mg q6h; methazolamide tablets, 50–100 mg bid-tid; acetazolamide sustained-release capsules, 500 mg q12h; dichlorphenamide tablets, 50 mg bid-qid; ethoxzolamide tablets, 125 mg bid-qid. For unclear reasons, these inhibitors must be given systemically but are under study topically. Since acetazolamide is excreted unchanged by the kidneys, patients with renal disease such as diabetic nephropathy should be started on lower than standard dosages.

7. **Side effects.** Unfortunately, 40–50% of glaucoma patients are unable to tolerate CAIs long term because of various disabling side effects. A symptom complex of **malaise, fatigue, depression, anorexia,** and **weight loss** is the most frequent side effect. **Loss of libido,** especially in young males, may also occur. These symptoms show some correlation with the degree of systemic metabolic acidosis on therapy. They may have a gradual, insidious onset over several months. Often neither the patient nor the physician relates these symptoms to the CAI therapy. **Frequently, patients erroneously undergo extensive medical evaluations searching for occult malignancies.**

   a. **Simultaneous CAI and chlorothiazide** systemic hypertensive therapy may develop frank **hypokalemia,** and the patient should have potassium (K^+) supplementation. In the absence of this concomitant chlorothiazide therapy, changes in serum potassium tend to be small and there is no symptomatic benefit from potassium supplementation.

   b. **Gastrointestinal** side effects occurring with CAI therapy tend to behave as local irritative phenomena, sometimes responding to administering the CAI with food, switching to a sustained-release preparation, or simultaneous mild alkali therapy.

   c. **Malaise** symptoms occur in some patients. Decreasing the dosage will sometimes improve tolerance. In particular, using one 500-mg acetazolamide capsule a day (which has an effect for over 18 hours) is very useful. In many of these patients this dosage will result in an undertreatment of their glaucoma, but in others, near-maximum effects will be maintained.

   d. **Kidney stones** developing during CAI therapy are believed to be a result of calcium precipitation secondary to a decrease of citrate or magnesium excretion or both in the urine. The former is felt to be a direct consequence of the drugs making normally acid urine alkaline, which, with reduced citrate, induces calcium carbonate stone formation. There is a far **lower incidence of kidney stone formation with methazolamide and dichlorphenamide** than with acetazolamide. Methazolamide has minimal action on citrate concentration or on the kidney, and dichlorphenamide does not induce a urine pH change to alkaline. Management of kidney stone patients involves use of methazolamide or dichlorphenamide in as low a dosage as the severity of the glaucoma permits, restriction of dietary calcium, and possibly concomitant use of chlorothiazide diuretics to alter the calcium-magnesium ratio in the urine. Electrolye imbalance should be watched for in patients on diuretics. Nephrologic consultation and measurement of urinary pH, calcium, and citrate should be obtained if stone formation is suspected.

   e. **Blood dyscrasias** are rare. Thrombocytopenia, agranulocytosis, and aplastic anemia may occur as idiosyncratic reactions. Periodic blood tests would not be expected to anticipate these reactions and are not routinely performed. A history of a mouth or body sore that does not heal may be a clue to the occurrence of a blood dyscrasia.

   f. **Myopia** occurs rarely as an idiosyncratic acute reversible phenomenon. It is felt to be due to a change in hydration of the lens, and it may be associated with a shallowing of the anterior chamber.

H. **Beta-adrenergic blockers** (timolol [Timoptic], betaxolol [Betoptic], levobunalol [Betagan])

   a. **Mechanism of action.** Timolol and levobunalol are nonselective beta-1 (cardiac) and beta-2 (smooth muscle, pulmonary) receptor blocking agents. Betaxolol has 100 times more affinity for beta-1 than beta-2 receptors.

   b. **Physiologic effects.** The drugs timolol and levobunalol lower IOP by blockade of beta-2 receptors in the ciliary processes, resulting in decreased aqueous production. The mechanism for betaxolol is unknown as there are so few beta-2 receptors in the eye, but there may be "spill over" to bind beta-2 as well. There is no effect on facility of outflow. The drug molecule timolol (and probably betaxolol and levobunalol) releases from the beta-receptor site as early as 3 hours after topical administration, yet clinical effect may last up to 2 weeks. This prolonged effect may result from re-release of beta blocker from depots in the iris pigment epithelial melanin.

   c. Indications are primary and secondary open-angle glaucomas including inflammatory glaucomas, acute and chronic primary and secondary angle-closure glaucomas, and childhood glaucomas (see sec. **g**). Timolol has been shown to have a significant protective effect against optic nerve and visual field damage in ocular hypertensives (22–28 mm Hg) over a several-year period.

   d. Precautions and contraindications include known drug allergy. These drugs should be used with caution or not at all, depending on severity of disease, in patients with asthma, emphysema, chronic obstructive pulmonary disease, bronchitis, heart block, congestive heart failure, or cardiomyopathy. While betaxolol is the blocker of choice in patients at risk for pulmonary reaction because of its greater beta-1 (cardiac) selectivity, the drug may induce bronchospasm in some patients.

   e. Available preparations. Timolol: 0.25–0.50% eye drops; betaxolol and levobunalol: 0.5% eye drops.

   f. Recommended dosage is 0.25% or 0.50% qd or q12h topically. All beta blockers may be used with significant additive effect in **combination** with miotic agents or carbonic anhydrase inhibitors. The combination with epinephrine or DPE is variable with only 2–5 mm Hg further lowering of pressure, but in some patients this may be sufficient. **Optimal effect** may be obtained by instilling epinephrine about 4 hours after timolol as the latter is releasing the same receptors to which the epinephrine must bind. Receptor release times for betaxolol and levobunalol are unknown but probably similar to timolol.

   g. Side effects

     (1) Bradycardia, cardiac arrest, acute asthma, and pulmonary edema have all been reported in susceptible individuals and result from systemic absorption of topical drug. **Lacrimal canalicular compression** should be practiced by patients at any risk, and the drug used with caution or not at all in those patients with moderate to severe cardiac or pulmonary disease.

     (2) Full adult dosage should be avoided in **children** as apnea may result; 0.25% qd-bid with canalicular compression is the lower advisable dosage.

     (3) Nursing mothers will excrete timolol in breast milk; timolol or other beta-blocker treatment of the mother should probably be discontinued if a woman is breast-feeding.

     (4) Other side effects are lethargy, depression, impotence, hallucinations, and gastrointestinal symptoms.

     (5) Ocular effects include allergy, punctate keratitis, and diplopia. Corneal anesthesia may result from the membrane-stabilizing effects of timolol but does not appear to occur with betaxolol or levobunalol.

I. Hyperosmotic agents (mannitol, glycerine, isosorbide)

  1. Mechanism of action. Lowering of IOP by increasing plasma tonicity sufficiently to draw water out of the eye.

  2. Indications. Additive therapy for rapid lowering of high IOP. Onset of action is 30 minutes and lasts 4–6 hours.

  3. Preparations and dosage

   a. Glycerin (Glyrol, Osmoglyn) dosage is 1.0–1.5 gm of glycerin/kg body weight PO. Osmoglyn is a 50%, lime-flavored solution with dosage 2–3 ml/kg (4–6 ounces/patient) and Glyrol 1–2 ml/kg (3–5 ounces/patient). Both are better tolerated served on cracked ice and may be given qd-tid.

Topical glycerin (Ophthalgan) is a viscous solution used to clear corneal edema for a better view of the intraocular structures.
   b. **Isosorbide** is a 45%, mint-flavored solution with dosage of 1-2 gm/kg (1.5-3.0 ml/pound body weight) given PO over ice qd-qid.
   c. **Mannitol** is a 5-25% hyperosmotic given warm (38-39°C to dissolve crystals) IV in dosage of 2 gm/kg body weight. Most common is 25-50 ml of 25% solution given by slow IV push.
   4. **Side effects** may include severe systemic hypertension aggravation, nausea, vomiting, confusion, congestive heart failure, pulmonary edema or diabetic hyperglycemia. The drugs are contraindicated in oliguria or anuria.
VI. **Argon, krypton, and Nd-YAG laser therapy** (see also Chap. 7, sec. **X**)
   A. **General considerations.** In the last several years there has been an important advance in the application of laser methods to glaucoma therapy as an alternative to surgical intervention. The **argon** and **krypton lasers** use the heating and disrupting effect of the laser energy to create tissue burns or openings. As the **krypton** laser has a **lower energy** output than the argon, the laser time for krypton should be increased to 0.2 second and initial power set at 400 mW with gradual increase. The remainder of the technique, complications, and management are similar for laser and krypton lasers. The neodinium **YAG laser** produces a sudden focal expansion with tearing and disruption of tissue by delivering high-powered near-infrared irradiances in small, focused spots in 30-nsec to 20-psec pulses. In open-angle glaucomas, application of nonpenetrating argon or krypton laser burns to the trabecular meshwork (TM) often results in improvement in the outflow of aqueous humor by an undetermined mechanism. Both mechanical and biologic effects have been postulated for this laser trabeculoplasty technique (LTP). In angle-closure glaucoma, the argon or YAG laser has been used to create a small opening in the peripheral iris, thus alleviating pupillary block, the mechanism for angle-closure glaucoma.
   B. **Argon laser trabeculoplasty**
      1. **Indications.** LTP should be attempted in almost all forms of open-angle glaucoma not adequately controlled on maximum tolerated medical therapy and prior to considering filtration surgery: phakic, aphakic, pseudophakic, pseudoexfoliative, pigmentary, and angle recession (50-90% success). Eyes with poor prognosis for beneficial laser effects (0-15% success) are steroid, juvenile, or inflammatory glaucomas. In the chronic treatment of open-angle glaucoma, evaluating the benefit-risk ratio, LTP should probably be employed prior to the use of cholinesterase inhibitors in phakic eyes. It is debatable at the present time whether LTP should be performed before or after the use of CAIs. Since LTP seems to be more effective in phakic eyes, it should be performed prior to cataract surgery in patients with borderline control. Some physicians have advocated early treatment of open-angle glaucoma with laser rather than medical therapy, but controlled studies are required before this can be advocated.
      2. **Technique.** An antireflective-coated Goldmann gonioscopic lens is utilized with 25 × ocular viewing power on the slit lamp. It is now standard practice to treat only half the angle (30-50 spots) at a treatment session. A 50-μ spot size and 0.1-second exposure are used. In general, 1000 mW power (or less) is initially chosen, but adjusted downward for pigmented meshworks and upward (to 1400 mW maximum) for "blank" meshworks without pigment. The end point for this power selection is "threshold" of bubble formation (tiny bubbles) in the treated TM. The aiming beam should be crisply focused midmeshwork on the anterior part of the posterior half of the TM, which is the filtering portion of the TM (see Fig. 9-1). By having the patient look toward the mirror of the gonioscopic lens, access into the angle is often improved.
      3. **Follow-up.** Acute pressure elevations (>10mm Hg) can occur in 10-15% of patients within 1-2 hours of LTP. Especially in patients with compromised optic nerves and visual fields, IOP rise should be prevented or lessened by prophylactic treatment with apraclonidine (see sec. **V.F**) and CAIs.

Current antiglaucomatous therapy is maintained and topical steroids tid–qid added and tapered over 2 weeks. The first post-LTP visit should be at 24 hours in patients who have shown a significant post-LTP pressure rise. For others the visit may be 5–7 days after treatment, and IOP and anterior segment inflammatory signs should be assessed. If notably inflamed, the patient should be gonioscoped (for which the Zeiss lens is convenient) to look for inflammatory deposits in the angle or beginning peripheral anterior synechiae, and the steroid dosage thereby adjusted. It is useful to examine the patient again 1 or 2 weeks later and, if the examination is uneventful, 1 month later, at which time the IOP lowering efficacy is assessed. Prior to this 1-month visit, IOP is often unchanged or slightly elevated, but this has little influence on the 1-month post-LTP IOP, following which completion of the LTP to the remaining half of the angle is performed.

4. **Complications** (see also sec. **3**)
   a. **Peripheral anterior synechiae**
      (1) Usually low and not functional, but if "high" can cause worsening of glaucoma (convert open-angle to combined chronic angle-closure glaucoma).
      (2) If observed, decrease number and power of applications for second half of treatment, and increase steroid dosage.
   b. **Corneal burns** (usually transient epithelial).
   c. **Hyphema**
      (1) Due to blood in Schlemm's canal or wandering vessel (rule out un-diagnosed neovascular glaucoma or increased episcleral venous pressure).
      (2) If encountered at time of LTP, increase pressure in eye by indent-ing with goniolens or decrease limbal compression in involved seg-ment by tilting goniolens.
   d. **Iritis,** especially in patients under 40 years of age. Use topical steroids.
   e. **Worsening of open-angle glaucoma,** about 3% incidence.
5. **Repeat LTP** is generally successful in eyes that have shown an excellent, prolonged initial response to LTP but have, with time, had return of in-creased IOP. Retreatment using argon blue-green laser, 50-μm spot, 700–900 mW power, 0.1-second duration, 40–50 burns/180-degree treated area has resulted in a second hypotensive response for at least a year in about 70% of patients.

C. **Laser iridectomy (LI)**
1. **Indications**
   a. Argon or YAG LI should always be attempted first, prior to considering surgical peripheral iridectomy. Osmotics, CAIs and beta blockers, for example, should be used to lower IOP and topical glycerin to clear the cornea. With the "chipping away" method, one is usually able to pen-etrate the iris, although these "acute" LIs may close more commonly than those done in quiet eyes, in which case a subsequent laser reopen-ing is similarly successful. If penetration of the iris is not achieved with attempted LI in an acute angle-closure eye, pupillary distortion induced by the laser often relieves pupillary block acutely.
   b. For combined-mechanism glaucoma, chronic open-angle glaucoma, and closeable asymptomatic narrow angles, LI is the preferred method of iridectomy.
2. **Technique of argon LI.** It is important to treat the patient with several applications of pilocarpine 1–2% 30 minutes prior to LI to stretch and thin the iris and to maintain miosis. Topical anesthetic is instilled 2 times, and a contact lens with a plus button such as the Abraham lens dramatically improves the ease of the procedure. On the slit lamp, 25 × ocular power should be used. Many methods involve pretreatment of the iris with low-power laser applications to stretch, thin, or "hump" it, but often the easiest method is the "chipping away technique," in which applications are super-imposed with 50-μ, 0.1-second, 1200-mW settings until the iris is pene-

trated (a puff of pigment debris heralds this). The power may be decreased and the exposure increased to 0.2 seconds for the deeper layers of the iris. The aiming beam must be crisply focused on the iris. If corneal endothelial clouding occurs, succeeding applications will have less effect, and laser applications must be immediately *stopped* in this area. When "pigment clouds" are dispersed into the anterior chamber, the treating surgeon should pause to allow its clearance before continuing with more laser applications. The lens capsule must be visualized to ensure that a full-thickness opening in the iris has been performed. Transillumination can be misleading. In enlarging the opening, the circumference of the opening should be treated rather than strands bridging across the opening. Less laser energy will thus be absorbed by the crystalline lens. The procedure should be performed ideally without causing any lens "whitening."

3. Technique of krypton LI. See sec. **A** for adaptations.

4. Technique of YAG LI. Topical pilocarpine and anesthetic are instilled as in argon LI and the specialized YAG contact lens with antireflective coating and plus add (Abraham lens) is placed on the eye to magnify the target site, converge the laser beam, and minimize blinking. Power settings are 2–8 mJ and bursts of 1–2 pulses/shot should create the iridotomy. Multiple pulses/shot may increase chance of lens damage. The beam is aimed on the iris in an area that will be covered by the upper lid and fired at a site between one-half and two-thirds of the distance between pupil margin and the visible periphery. Additional pulses should be delivered to the edge of the opening if enlargement is needed not directly over the lens capsule. Failure to penetrate the iris is usually due to poor focus (e.g., corneal edema), iris edema, or use of insufficient laser energy. Another area may be tried or the procedure terminated and retreatment performed later after additional therapy, as indicated, has been given.

5. Follow-up. An acute rise in IOP within 1–2 hours of LI may occur and should be managed as discussed under LTP (see sec. **B.**) LI can close anytime during a 6-week period. Therefore, it is best not to treat patients with dilating drops at home, but rather to dilate the pupil in the physician's office at follow-up visits. Topical steroids should be used approximately tid–qid for 1–2 weeks and then tapered. At follow-up visits the patency of the iridectomy should be documented by visualizing the lens capsule, and gonioscopy should be performed to document relief of pupillary block by observing deepening of the angle access. If iridectomy is observed to close, retreatment is necessary. At the 6-week office visit the pupil should always be dilated to conclude that the iridectomy is patent, to rule out plateau iris, and so forth.

6. Complications

    a. Lens injury. No long-term adverse effect on the lens has been documented, even in eyes with areas of lens whitening post-LI, but further long-term observations are required.

    b. Elevated IOP. IOP is often moderately elevated for weeks to several months following the procedure. This elevation is usually controlled with mild antiglaucomatous therapy. Occasionally, IOP can be elevated to very high levels, sometimes shortly after the procedure. This should be monitored and appropriately treated. Often increased steroid dosage is beneficial.

    c. Iritis, spontaneous angle closure from iridectomy closing, corneal burns (especially endothelial), and corectopia may all occur and require therapy as indicated.

VII. Surgical definitions

    A. General considerations. In **open-angle glaucoma,** when medical or laser therapy fails, surgery is performed that results in a bypass of the conventional outflow pathways and allows drainage of aqueous humor from inside the eye. These operations are generally called **filtration** or sometimes **fistulizing** operations. The name of a particular operation refers to the technique of the opening into the eye.

1. In a **trephine** operation, a piece of corneoscleral limbus is removed via a trephine.

2. In a **posterior lip sclerectomy,** an incision is made into the eye at the limbus, and portions of the posterior lip are removed with a punch.

3. In a **thermal sclerostomy,** cautery is applied to the lips of the limbal incision.

4. In a **trabeculectomy,** a partial-thickness portion of the corneoscleral limbus is removed under a partial-thickness scleral flap.

5. The **Molteno tube,** which drains aqueous from the anterior chamber to the subconjunctival space, is still under study.

B. **5-Fluorouracil (5-FU)** is an antimetabolite currently in use for the **prevention of postoperative scarring of filtering blebs** especially in the inflammatory glaucomas. At the conclusion of surgery, 5 mg of 5-FU in 0.5 ml of saline is injected subconjunctivally 180 degrees away from the filter site concurrent with subconjunctival steroids and antibiotics. Postoperatively patients receive 5 mg of 5-FU bid subconjunctivally on days 1–7 and qd on days 8–14 for a maximum total dose of 125 mg in 14 days. Intensive topical steroids are given during week 1 and then tapered. Lower postoperative doses of 5-FU with intensive topical steroids have also been successful (about 80% of patients), i.e., 5 mg of 5-FU subconjunctivally qd for 10 days or less if a corneal ulcer or wound leak developed. Adverse side effects are minimal and transient.

C. **Other operations sometimes performed**

1. In **cyclodialysis,** a spatula is passed via the suprachoroidal space into the anterior chamber, disinserting the ciliary body from the scleral spur. This may result in a lowering of IOP either by a decrease in aqueous humor formation from the now detached ciliary body or by increasing uveovascular scleral outflow of aqueous humor (which ordinarily contributes insignificantly to this egress).

2. **Cyclocryotherapy** refers to cryotherapy applied externally to the sclera over the ciliary body with the purpose of destroying the ciliary processes (in one-half the circumference) and thereby lowering aqueous production. It is especially useful in aphakic (postlens removal) patients.

3. **Goniotomy in congenital glaucoma** refers to an incision with a knife into the TM.

D. **Angle-closure glaucoma.** A surgical **peripheral iridectomy** is the removal of a peripheral portion of iris, alleviating pupillary block in angle-closure glaucoma by giving an extra opening for aqueous flow between chambers.

VIII. **Primary open-angle glaucoma**

A. **General considerations.** Primary open-angle glaucoma is the most common form of glaucoma, affecting 0.25–0.75% of the population. In most cases the disease develops in middle life or later and tends to be familial. The onset is usually gradual and asymptomatic and tends to become progressively worse. The angle remains open at all times. On gonioscopy the appearance of the angle structures is identical to, and cannot be distinguished from, that of normal patients. Despite this normal appearance on gonioscopy, the trabecular outflow channels are functionally abnormal, and the tonographic facility of aqueous outflow from the anterior chamber is constantly subnormal in most cases. The IOP may vary from normal to significantly elevated levels. This most likely represents variation in the rate of aqueous secretion, while the outflow facility remains subnormal. The facility of aqueous outflow usually becomes worse with the passage of time. Sometimes with age there is also a decline in the rate of aqueous production, and therefore this progressive impairment of outflow facility does not invariably result in further elevation of IOP. Nevertheless, in most cases, stronger medical therapy is required to control the IOP.

B. **Glaucoma detection**

1. A **spectrum** exists from normality to borderline abnormality to early glau-

coma to frank glaucoma. In the earliest stages of the disease it is sometimes difficult to know whether the patient is truly abnormal. The test of time is most useful in identifying patients with early glaucoma. Patients with an IOP of 22 mm Hg or greater, or those with optic disks with suspicious or asymmetric cupping regardless of the IOP (see sec. **XIV**), should be followed as **glaucoma suspects** or **ocular hypertensives.** Primary open-angle glaucoma differs from ocular hypertension in that the latter is a primary condition manifested by elevated IOP in the presence of open angles but with no evidence of optic nerve damage or field loss. Approximately 2% of the population has ocular hypertension. About 5% of ocular hypertensives with IOP of 25–30 mm Hg will go on to develop nerve damage and field defects within 10 years. The diagnosis is then changed to primary open-angle glaucoma and appropriate therapy started. Therapy may also be started in the absence of damage if the IOP is sufficiently high, i.e., high 20s to low 30s, as it is likely that damage is inevitable should treatment be withheld.

2. **Glaucoma suspects** should be followed 3–4 times a year with IOP measurements and with careful inspection and drawing of the optic nerve cupping. Stereo photographs are useful. Visual fields should be performed at least once a year.

3. **Monocular glaucoma.** Primary open-angle glaucoma always affects both eyes, although the disease may be more advanced in one eye. If glaucoma is truly monocular, other causes of secondary glaucoma must be investigated. Gonioscopy and tonography are useful aids in diagnosis.

C. **Symptoms.** Primary open-angle glaucoma is almost always a silent disease process. Occasionally, in younger patients, rapid rises in IOP may occur that result in corneal epithelial edema and symptoms of haloes, blurred vision, and pain, much as in pigmentary glaucoma (see sec. **XV**). The rapid rate of elevation of IOP determines the development of corneal edema. In usual primary open-angle glaucoma there is a slowly progressive elevation of IOP, and therefore such symptoms occur only rarely.

D. **Indications for treatment**

1. **Early stage** primary open-angle glaucoma may not require therapy. The optic nerves of different patients differ in their susceptibility to the same level of IOP. For example, certain patients with low-tension glaucoma will show progression of disk cupping at ostensibly normal IOP (< 22 mg Hg). Other patients with primary open-angle glaucoma and small physiologic cups will show no progression in disk cupping, tensions in the upper 20s to low 30s, and may not require treatment. It is generally felt that optic disks with small central physiologic cups tolerate a given level of IOP better than those with wider cups and glaucomatous damage. Patients followed off therapy generally require close follow-up. It is useful to check the IOP at different times in different visits, in order to detect significant diurnal peaks. A severe obstruction of outflow detected by tonography often may add to other indications for treatment.

Often in early glaucoma it is a borderline decision whether the patient should be treated or not. It is often useful to explain the situation and to let the patient have input into the decision. Often a trial of weak medical therapy to one eye is of value; if side effects occur, the patient may be followed off therapy a while longer. If therapy is efficacious and well tolerated, the patient often will prefer to have continued treatment, at least in one eye, often in both. In addition, by treating one eye initially, the efficacy of the therapy can be better evaluated.

2. **Change in disk cup appearance** indicates that medical therapy should be initiated. Different ophthalmologists have different cutoffs of IOP above which medical antiglaucoma therapy will be initiated regardless of disk appearance. With tensions above the low 30s, glaucoma therapy should be routinely begun provided there are not significant side effects. Certainly all patients with tensions in the upper 30s to 40s should be treated. Patients with wide cupping (even though it may be physiologic) with pressures in

the upper 20s should also be treated. Patients with some glaucomatous damage to the nerve are treated in order to lower their IOP into the normal range (at least initially below 22 mm Hg).

3. **Progressive disk cupping or field changes in follow-up,** regardless of measured IOP, indicate that pressure is too high for the optic nerve and that further medical therapy should be added. Similarly, patients who present with extreme glaucomatous damage and IOP in the low 20s require vigorous medical therapy to achieve as low a pressure as possible (10–12 mm Hg). Even if the IOP is subnormal with medical and laser therapy, should future progression occur (as often may happen in patients with totally cupped disks and extensive field loss) then glaucoma filtering surgery is indicated in order to achieve as low an IOP as possible.

4. **Medical therapy** is usually begun with pilocarpine, a beta blocker, epinephrine, or DPE. Beta blockers, DPE, or epinephrine is preferable in younger patients because of the accommodation and miosis produced by pilocarpine. Allergies may occur with epinephrine. Most but not all older patients tolerate pilocarpine well. With advancement of medical therapy, the strength of pilocarpine is increased, DPE, epinephrine, and/or a beta blocker may be added, and then carbonic anhydrase and anticholinesterase agents are added when needed and the weaker miotics discontinued. Laser trabeculoplasty may precede these latter two agents.

5. Should **maximum medical therapy** (i.e., that treatment the patient is able to tolerate locally and systemically) **fail** to control the IOP, laser trabeculoplasty should be performed; if this procedure fails, glaucoma filtering surgery is indicated.

IX. **Primary acute angle-closure glaucoma**
   A. **Clinical findings**
      1. **Symptoms.** In acute angle-closure glaucoma, the relative pressure in the posterior chamber is increased as a result of pupillary block, and the peripheral iris is forced forward over the TM. The IOP rises rapidly, due to the sudden blockage of aqueous outflow, resulting in the acute onset of severe pain, blurred vision, and perception of colored haloes about lights. The latter two symptoms are due to the corneal epithelial edema that results from the rapidity of the IOP rise. The pain is usually quite severe. Often it is not localized to the eye but involves the whole head and may be accompanied by nausea and vomiting. **The correct diagnosis may be missed by physicians who are not ophthalmologists, because they may misinterpret the headache and abdominal symptoms.**
      2. **Signs.** Corneal epithelial edema can be detected on flashlight examination as a fine, rough haziness in the light reflex. The pupil is usually middilated (4–5 mm) and nonreactive to light, and the eye is red. Slit-lamp examination reveals a shallowness of the axial and peripheral anterior chamber. There may be significant flare and a few cells as well in the anterior chamber. If the IOP has been elevated for a prolonged period during a previous attack, gray atrophy of the iris stroma and glaukomflecken (small white opacities in or under the anterior lens capsule) may be observed. Gonioscopy should be performed after clearing the corneal epithelial edema with topical glycerin (after a drop of topical anesthetic) and should confirm the angle closure (the peripheral iris covering over the TM).
   B. **Differential diagnosis**
      1. The physician should look carefully for the presence of new blood vessels on the iris and in the angle that would indicate a diagnosis of **neovascular angle-closure glaucoma** rather than primary angle-closure glaucoma. The differential diagnosis also includes **acute open-angle glaucomas** such as glaucomatocyclitis crisis or other uveitides, and pigmentary glaucoma. The physician should always gonioscope the fellow eye to confirm that it also is narrow and potentially closeable, with prominent iris convexity and the scleral spur not visible. If the fellow eye is not narrow, the physician should be careful that the correct diagnosis has in fact been made in the first eye

and should then consider the differential diagnosis of **true monocular angle-closure glaucoma.** This includes acute central retinal vein occlusion, dislocated lens, choroidal detachment or effusion, peripheral anterior synechiae secondary to uveitis, essential iris atrophy, and significant anisometropia (extreme difference in refractive error). In the emergency room, the diagnosis most commonly involves distinguishing primary angle-closure glaucoma from neovascular glaucoma.

2. **Inflamed red eyes** are always suspect of possible angle-closure glaucoma. In acute **conjunctivitis** there is usually a discharge with cells in the tear film, the cornea is clear, the vision is near normal, pupillary size and reaction are normal, and there is no true pain, unlike acute glaucoma. If the physician is suspicious of glaucoma in a red eye, it is important to measure the IOP. The Schiötz tonometer with a tonofilm cover is very valuable in these cases. In acute **anterior uveitis** the pupil is usually small (unlike the middilation in acute glaucoma), the redness is more prominent in the area about the limbus, and the anterior chamber usually contains significantly more cells and flare than in acute angle-closure glaucoma. The cornea in uveitis is usually clear except for the presence of KPs. The vision is usually blurred and there may be considerable pain. All patients with uveitis should have their IOP measured, both to rule out angle-closure glaucoma and to detect the secondary open-angle glaucoma that may accompany uveitis, especially in the later stages.

C. **Therapeutic implications of pupillary block.** A coincidence of various physiologic and anatomic factors is responsible for an increase in pupillary block of posterior chamber aqueous flow to the anterior chamber so that iris is pushed forward to cause angle closure. Pupillary size, rate of aqueous formation, rigidity of the iris, and axial position of the lens all influence the magnitude of pupillary block.

1. **Pupillary middilation** produces an increase in relative pupillary block. This middilated position may occur spontaneously due to changing illumination, e.g., an attack may occur when a patient visits a movie theatre, or it may result from either topical or systemic administration of a pupillary dilating agent such as cyclopentolate, phenylephrine, or atropine. Patients with narrow angles are asymptomatic before and after acute angle-closure attacks. The dilating agents must be used with care in patients found to have shallow anterior chambers on routine flashlight or slit-lamp examination (see sec. **III.A, B**). The importance of assessing anterior chamber depth in ostensibly normal patients before use of these agents needs to be emphasized. In suspicious cases gonioscopy should be performed. Although topical agents are more frequently involved, cases of angle-closure glaucoma have been precipitated by **systemic** use of **atropinelike drugs** and inhalation of **bronchodilators.**

2. **Maximum pupillary dilation** pulls the iris sphincter away from the lens, and this relieves pupillary block. Attacks of angle closure may actually be broken by maximum pupillary dilation, although for surgical and laser considerations this is less desirable than miosis. After use of a topical mydriatic, the pupil may rapidly pass through the stage of middilation without angle closure, only to have a full-blown attack occur as the pupil returns from the widely dilated state toward a more normal size.

3. **Treatment of acute angle-closure glaucoma with miotics** moves the pupil from the middilated state to a smaller size, where there is less relative pupillary block. With excessive miosis, however, as may occur with use of **anticholinesterase agents,** an increase in relative pupillary block may actually occur, and thus these agents are **contraindicated in angle-closure glaucoma.** Additionally, use of higher strengths of pilocarpine (4–6%) and other stronger miotics may move the lens forward due to zonular relaxation subsequent to ciliary muscle contraction, and this may actually increase relative pupillary block. For this reason, lower concentrations of pilocarpine (1–2%) are used initially to treat angle-closure glaucoma. Thus, in treat-

ment of angle-closure glaucoma, ciliary muscle contraction may be an undesired side effect of pilocarpine therapy, whereas in open-angle glaucoma the pupillary miosis may be.

4. By **decreasing aqueous production, beta blockers and CAIs** may decrease the relative pressure force in the posterior chamber and lessen relative pupillary block. It is important to perform gonioscopy in the fellow eye before administration of CAIs or osmotic agents, which dehydrate the vitreous, since these agents may effect a temporary deepening of the anterior chamber.

5. **Small attacks of angle-closure glaucoma** may be spontaneously arrested by spontaneous movement of the pupil and by decrease in the rate of aqueous formation. The latter may occur temporarily as a result of the sudden elevation of IOP. Following an attack the eye may become hypotonous, and with the presence of some cells and flare, a mistaken diagnosis of uveitis may be made. Clues to the presence of previous attacks are areas of gray iris stromal atrophy, glaukomflecken, and shallow anterior chamber depth (also in the fellow eye). A history of episodes of colored haloes, pain, and blurred vision should be sought. Provocative tests, such as the dark room prone test, should be performed (see sec. **X.C**).

D. **Treatment of acute angle-closure glaucoma**

1. **Systemic hyperosmotics** (glycerol or isosorbide PO, or mannitol IV [see sec. **V.I** for dosage]) and IV acetazolamide (250-500 mg) should be given initially to lower the IOP below 50-60 mm Hg. A beta blocker should be administered to lower the pressure further. At higher pressures the iris sphincter is ischemic and unresponsive to pilocarpine. Since miotics may allow forward lens movement by relaxation of zonular tension, a reduction in vitreous volume via the use of osmotics is probably useful in all cases. Pilocarpine 1% should be administered initially q15min. If the attack fails to respond to this therapy, higher strengths of pilocarpine, up to 4%, may be substituted.

   Once the IOP is lowered, it is important to gonioscope the patient to be sure the angle has opened. Use of osmotics, beta blockers, and CAIs may result in a temporarily lowered IOP despite persistent angle closure.

2. **Once the attack is broken,** LI should be performed. If this procedure is delayed, the patient is usually maintained on pilocarpine 1% q4-6h until LI. The fellow asymptomatic eye may also be treated prophylactically.

3. If medical therapy fails to break the attack, then LI should be performed as an emergency procedure. The use of osmotics almost always results in a temporarily sufficient IOP lowering and in less need for emergency surgery. The IOP, however, should not be allowed to remain above 60 mm Hg for more than a few hours, because permanent loss of vision from optic atrophy may result. If LI cannot be performed and if high pressure persists, surgical peripheral iridectomy should be performed.

4. **Prolonged attack** may result in permanent adhesions of the peripheral iris to the meshwork; i.e., **peripheral anterior synechiae** may form. In such cases, peripheral iridectomy will relieve pupillary block but will not restore normal IOP because of the residual chronic angle closure. LI with follow-up gonioscopy will help assess angle closure. If laser is unsuccessful, however, at the time of surgery a **chamber deepening technique** should be performed. The apparent angle closure viewed preoperatively may be due to a potentially reversible apposition of iris to TM or to true synechiae. In the chamber deepening technique, fluid is injected into the anterior chamber via a limbal paracentesis slit opening and gonioscopy performed to assess the extent of the peripheral anterior synechiae formation. If extensive peripheral anterior synechiae have formed (more than 90% of the angle), a filtering procedure rather than a peripheral iridectomy should be performed. (New techniques are being developed in which laser applications to the peripheral iris termed *iridogonioplasty* may break recently formed peripheral anterior synechiae with functional improvement in outflow.)

5. **Prophylactic laser peripheral iridectomy** should be performed on the fellow asymptomatic eye several days after surgery on the first eye, unless there are circumstances of true monocular angle closure.

X. **Subacute and chronic primary angle-closure glaucoma**
  A. **Subacute and chronic angle glaucoma** result if the iris does not cover the TM in the full circumference of the angle. This may cause intermittent moderate elevation of IOP that is roughly proportional to the extent of closure. These subacute episodes may occur with mild symptoms of colored haloes, blurred vision, and red eye. A condition of continuous chronic partial angle closure may occur and mimic open-angle glaucoma in its lack of symptoms and maintained elevation of IOP.
  B. **Differentiation** of chronic angle-closure glaucoma from open-angle glaucoma with narrow but open angles in which full width of TM can be seen is important. In cases of suspected partial chronic angle-closure glaucoma, the relative effects of bright light, thymoxamine (alpha blocker) drops, or weak (0.5–1.0%) strengths of pilocarpine on gonioscopic angle appearance and IOP may establish the correct diagnosis. **Thymoxamine** causes miosis but has no effect on facility of outflow.
  C. **The dark room prone test** should be done on patients with suspiciously narrow angles who are not seen during an acute attack and who do not have glaukomflecken or gray iris stromal atrophy. This test may be utilized to identify dangerously narrow (but open at the time of examination) angles. In this test, IOP is measured and the patient seated for 30–60 minutes in a darkened room with his or her head down on a cushioned table. The IOP is again measured in the darkened room. A rise of 8 mm Hg or greater or a significant asymmetric rise in pressure between the two eyes that is accompanied by gonioscopic confirmation of further angle closure is a positive test, and a prophylactic LI is indicated. It is important to perform all phases of this test in a darkened room. Miosis from external light or from the focal illuminator during gonioscopy may quickly reverse the angle closure. Placing the patient in a brightly lit room for 5 minutes after this test and observing a significant lowering of IOP will further confirm a positive test.
  D. **A pharmacologic mydriatic test** (2.5% phenylephrine) is sometimes used as a provocative test. Such a test is distinctly nonphysiologic and has significant false-negatives. Most important, the angle may not close during the pupillary dilation, but rather may close many hours later as the pupil contracts. If such a test is performed, the patient should be kept under observation for several hours until the pupil returns to normal size.
XI. **Plateau iris.** Very rarely, a mechanism of primary angle closure may be the direct expansion of the peripheral iris against the TM as the peripheral iris thickens during pupillary dilation. This mechanism is independent of, but may coexist with, pupillary block and is called a *plateau iris.*
  A. **Slit-lamp examination** reveals a discrepancy between the axial depth, which is good, and the peripheral depth, which is narrow. On gonioscopy the iris plane is somewhat flat, and the peripheral iris is very close to the TM with a characteristic small roll and trough just before the iris insertion on the ciliary body band.
  B. **Therapy** of patients with angle-closure glaucoma who have a plateau iris configuration includes an LI and, during convalescence, a provocative test with a weak mydriatic. A patient with true plateau iris will demonstrate a pressure elevation and gonioscopic angle closure. Such patients are managed successfully with long-term weak miotic therapy that prevents pupillary dilation and iris crowding of the angle. In those patients with a negative provocative test with pupillary dilation postiridectomy, it is believed that pupillary block was the mechanism of the preoperative angle closure despite the suspicious plateau configuration. The majority of plateau configuration patients fall into this latter category, which is why peripheral iridectomy should always be performed first in these patients.

XII. **Differential diagnosis of pressure elevation following surgical peripheral iridectomy for angle closure**
   A. **Plateau iris.** Treat with weak miotics.
   B. **Imperforate peripheral iridectomy.** Treat with a laser or repeat iridectomy.
   C. **Malignant glaucoma** is a condition in which there is maintained increase in total vitreous volume (or perhaps classically a pocket of aqueous trapped in or behind the vitreous) that results in flattening of the anterior chamber and closure of the angle. It occurs postoperatively after glaucoma or cataract surgery. Key to the diagnosis is a marked shallowing of the axial anterior chamber depth due to the vitreous expansion. **Treatment** consists of use of long-term daily mydriatic-cycloplegic drops used indefinitely, systemic osmotics, short term, beta blockers, and CAIs. If this is not successful, vitreous aspiration with puncture of the hyaloid is required. Aphakic eyes almost never respond to medical treatment.
   D. **Topical cycloplegic and steroid postoperative medications** may be responsible for elevated IOP through an ill-defined open-angle glaucoma mechanism. Such therapy may result in elevation of IOP in patients with primary open-angle glaucoma more characteristically. Axially, the anterior chamber is not flattened, and the glaucoma responds to cessation of the drops.
   E. **Extensive peripheral anterior synechiae** may occur if the wrong operation was performed. Filtering surgery should have been performed following the chamber deepening procedure.

XIII. **Combined open-angle and angle-closure glaucoma**
   A. **Angle-closure glaucoma** can occur occasionally in patients who have or subsequently develop **open-angle glaucoma.** Whether the latter is primary open-angle glaucoma or a result somehow of the episodes of high pressure elevation while the angle was closed is disputed. It has definitely been noted that some patients develop open-angle glaucoma several years after successfully treated angle-closure glaucoma.
   B. **Gradual, progressive partial angle-closure glaucoma** may occur in some patients with well-documented, long-standing primary open-angle glaucoma. With aging, most individuals, both those with and without glaucoma, will show some tendency toward shallowing of the angle, most likely due to an increase in size of the lens. The effect of miotic therapy on lens position may also be a factor. This partial angle closure will result in further chronic pressure elevation. Patients whose primary open-angle glaucoma worsens with therapy or age should always be **regonioscoped** to rule out coexisting additive partial angle closure (or other unusual glaucoma, such as occult KPs in the meshwork). When 4 hours or more of the angle is judged to be closed and the recent IOP course is consistent, LI is usually indicated.
   C. **Subacute or chronic angle-closure glaucoma suspects** may, with the application of bright light, thymoxamine, or weak pilocarpine, have a dramatic lowering of IOP and total opening of the angle, although the IOP is still definitely above normal. Such patients should be suspected of having combined open-angle and angle-closure glaucoma and residual glaucoma after an LI. **Tonography** when the angle is open will confirm the open-angle component.

XIV. **Low-tension glaucoma.** The optic nerves of different patients have differing susceptibilities to similar levels of IOP. In the extreme, there are certain patients who demonstrate progressive disk cupping and field loss with normal or mildly elevated IOP. Such patients are generally referred to as having low-tension glaucoma. About 20% of all primary open-angle glaucomas fall into the low-tension glaucoma category. Factors predisposing to progressive nerve damage include preexisting wide physiologic cupping and factors affecting nerve perfusion such as arteriosclerotic vascular disease, systemic hypotension, carotid artery disease, arrhythmias, and diabetes mellitus. A cardinal sign of **optic nerve ischemia** is **flame-shaped hemorrhaging on the disk** making treatment all the more urgent. **Medical therapy** is aimed at rapidly reducing the IOP to the lowest level possible, not just at treating on the basis of current extent of cupping and field loss. This is because the primary disease is in the vascular perfusion of the nerve, and every step should be taken to enhance its flow. As low-tension glaucoma is usually a disease of the elderly, miotics are usually the most effective and well-tolerated first therapeutic agents. To this may sequentially be added sympathomimetics and ultimately CAI. Beta blockers should be used with caution in the elderly because of potential vasogenic properties. A full medical evaluation should be carried out and systemic therapy, medical or surgical (e.g., carotid), to control problems relating to vascular perfusion initiated. **Laser trabeculoplasty** has not been fully evaluated in this condition but may have some beneficial effects as an adjunct to medical treatment of borderline success. Because of the low level of IOP that causes nerve damage, filtration **surgery** is frequently the only means of obtaining a low enough IOP.

XV. **Pigmentary dispersion syndrome and glaucoma** are the result of primary loss of pigment from the posterior surface (neuroepithelium) from the midperipheral iris. This pigment is disseminated intraocularly and deposited on various intraocular structures such as the corneal endothelium, where it may form a **Krukenberg's spindle,** and in the TM, where it forms a dense continuous band of pigment throughout the circumference. The latter may occur with inconspicuous corneal endothelial pigmentation—a reason the condition may often be missed.

   A. **Time of onset** is at a younger age than most other open-angle glaucomas; it appears in the 20- to 40-year group. The occurrence of this glaucoma in young myopic males is another good reason to perform routine applanation tonometry in all cooperative patients regardless of age.

   B. **Wide fluctuations in IOP** may result in crises of high pressure elevation with corneal epithelial edema. Gonioscopy always shows the angle to be open and to contain the characteristic pigment band. Liberation of large amounts of circulating pigment into the anterior chamber is sometimes associated with these pressure elevations and may be misinterpreted as cells of uveitis. In a few patients, exercise may induce such anterior chamber pigment liberation. During routine visits small numbers of circulating pigment particles can occasionally be seen in the anterior chamber in pigmentary dispersion syndrome patients. Because of the wide pressure fluctuations in this condition, a single normal IOP does not rule out the presence of pigmentary glaucoma. **Tonography** has been useful in identifying early pigmentary glaucoma patients. Although some authorities believe that all patients with pigmentary dispersion syndrome (even with normal tonographic facilities) will eventually develop pigmentary glaucoma, probably the majority of patients will not. Patients with borderline IOP or tonographic facilities need to be followed closely, but those with constantly normal IOP and outflow facilities need to be seen only once a year.

   C. **Examination** by viewing the iris stroma directly will not reveal the loss of posterior iris pigment (although occasionally pigment can be deposited on the anterior iris surface). **Transillumination** using a fiberoptic light source applied to the lower lid or sclera, or pupillary transillumination on the slit lamp will demonstrate typical linear slitlike defects in the midperiphery of the iris, which is the key to the diagnosis.

   D. **Treatment** is similar to that for primary open-angle glaucoma. Because of the patient's younger age and accommodation, however, there is poor tolerance to miotics, except perhaps the **pilocarpine Ocusert.**

XVI. **Exfoliation syndrome**

   A. **Clinical findings** in exfoliation syndrome include an amorphous gray **dandrufflike** material present on the pupillary border, anterior lens surface, posterior surface of the iris, zonules, and ciliary processes. This may represent basement membrane material from multiple ocular sites. The central area of the anterior lens capsule often has a dull lusterless appearance through the undilated pupil; when the pupil is dilated the gray membrane is seen to end in the midperiphery in a scalloped border, often with curled edges. **Transillumination** of the iris frequently reveals loss of pigment from the posterior iris surface adjacent to the pupil, in contradistinction to pigmentary dispersion syndrome, where defects occur in the midperiphery. This loss of pigment from the iris may result in an abnormal accumulation of pigment in the TM.

B. **Glaucoma may or may not occur in exfoliation syndrome.** Dandruff may be observed as an incidental finding during a routine examination in a patient with normal IOP. Such patients should be followed for possible future development of glaucoma, as exfoliation syndrome is often associated with a chronic open-angle glaucoma that may be initially monocular. Exfoliation glaucoma behaves similarly to and is **treated** like primary open-angle glaucoma. It may become more resistant to medical treatment with time than primary open-angle glaucoma, but fortunately is the type of glaucoma that usually responds best to laser trabeculoplasty.

XVII. **Glaucoma from contusion of the eye**

A. **Early onset**

1. **Acute glaucoma** may follow blunt trauma to the eye. This condition may be secondary to direct contusion injury to the trabecular angle tissue, or it may be because of the deposition of inflammatory or blood elements from traumatic hyphema in the outflow pathways. The obstruction of aqueous outflow may be masked by coexisting hyposecretion of aqueous humor that may occur for a variable period following the injury.

2. **Treatment** of acute contusion glaucoma consists of use of beta blockers and CAIs. Topical **miotics** should be **avoided** because of possibly promoting posterior synechiae and increasing the inflammation in the eye. **Epinephrine is avoided** because of the possibility of rebound bleeding. Should the IOP fail to be controlled with persistent pressures above the upper 40s, paracentesis and irrigation of the blood elements should be performed.

3. **Chronic erythroclastic (ghost cell) glaucoma** may be seen with prolonged hyphemas, but more commonly with vitreous hemorrhages in which the blood elements may remain in the vitreous for several days before passing into the anterior chamber. Red blood cells may degenerate into red cell ghosts with rigid cell membranes and **Heinz bodies** that are much more obstructive to aqueous outflow than the more pliable, fresh red cells, and a severe glaucoma may result. These red cell ghosts are khaki or off-white in color and must be distinguished from the white blood cells in inflammation. **Treatment** of chronic ghost cell glaucoma consists of use of beta blockers and CAIs and, these failing, paracentesis and anterior chamber irrigation. If the circulating cell and flare content of the anterior chamber is not marked (later in the course of ghost cell glaucoma), topical epinephrine and weak pilocarpine can be tried, although the effect is usually minimal. Again, in the immediate acute phase of the disease, these topical agents should not be used because of the possibility of rebound bleeding and synechiae formation. If significant increased IOP persists, vitrectomy to remove hemorrhagic debris may be necessary.

4. **Uveitis** usually accompanies the acute contusion injury and should be treated with topical cycloplegics and steroids. If there is a severe acute uveitis, the IOP is usually low due to hyposecretion. Occasionally, the glaucoma following within days of contusion injury may respond somewhat to topical steroids, and they should be attempted in this time period. In persistent glaucoma the physician should be careful to identify correctly the presence of ghost cell glaucoma, which does not respond to topical steroids.

B. **Late onset**

1. **Angle-recession glaucoma** may occur months to many years after blunt injury to the eye. It results from contusion to the trabecular angle tissue with associated tears in the uveal meshwork and ciliary muscle causing a more posterior, i.e., recessed, insertion of the iris onto the ciliary body band. This recession is not the cause of the glaucoma per se but is associated with the glaucoma-producing trabecular injury. It is subtle, and **simultaneous gonioscopy in both eyes** must be performed to identify it correctly. Although acute tears may be observed in the TM, these heal with time. In chronic angle-recession glaucoma, the TM itself may not appear abnormal.

2. **Evaluation of patients with significant blunt trauma** to the eye that results in hyphema should include gonioscopy several weeks after the injury to

identify possible angle recessions. Patients so identified, usually with greater than 180 degrees of recession, are at some risk of developing glaucoma in the future and should be so informed and followed. Fortunately, the majority of such patients will not develop glaucoma. Tonography may be of value in determining the frequency of follow-up.

3. **Differential diagnosis** of subtle angle recession must include other causes of true monocular glaucoma. Simultaneous gonioscopy must be performed to rule it out.

4. **Treatment** of angle-recession glaucoma is the same as that for primary open-angle glaucoma. It may become refractory in the later stages. It may also be associated with the development of a cuticular membrane in the angle histologically.

XVIII. **Glaucoma due to intraocular inflammation**
  A. **Anterior uveitis**
    1. In **acute anterior uveitis** there is probably some obstruction to outflow that is, however, masked at least initially by the more predominant hyposecretion of aqueous that results in hypotony. Later in the course when, with topical steroid treatment, aqueous production increases, this obstruction may become manifest with an elevation of IOP.

    2. **Steroid-induced open-angle glaucoma** may also be involved in certain patients. When faced with open-angle glaucoma in uveitis, it is usually unclear whether more or less topical steroid should be given. A brief trial of the former is usually useful to treat possible inflammation in the meshwork.

    3. **Angle-closure glaucoma** may also result from uveitis due to posterior iris-lens synechiae formation causing **pupillary block with iris bombé.** Peripheral anterior synechiae may also form from primary inflammatory adhesions in the angle without pupillary block.

    4. **Treatment** consists of using a beta blocker and CAIs and increasing or decreasing the steroid dosage. Epinephrine or DPE is also of value. Miotics are contraindicated. In treating inflammatory pupillary block, medications, usually intensive mydriatic-cycloplegic therapy, should be utilized to move the iris away from the lens into a dilated stage. If this fails, laser or surgical peripheral iridectomy will relieve the pupillary block.

  B. **Glaucomatocyclitic crisis**
    1. **Crises of intermittent unilateral acute open-angle glaucoma** that are associated with very minimum but definite signs of anterior chamber inflammation characterize this disease of unknown etiology. Usually only a few cells and one or two areas of smudginess on the corneal endothelium are observed. Corneal epithelial edema is present due to the sudden IOP rise. The eye is only mildly hyperemic and the patient has only slight discomfort. Repeated attacks may occur over the years and be benign. On the other hand, a patient may go on to develop chronic uveitis and open-angle glaucoma in later years. There is usually a great discrepancy between the acute glaucoma and the amount of anterior segment inflammation.

    2. **Gonioscopy** always reveals the angle to be open, although occasionally KPs are seen. The disease must be distinguished by gonioscopy from acute angle-closure glaucoma.

    3. **Treatment** consists of beta blockers, epinephrine, DPE, and/or CAIs and topical steroids. An attack may spontaneously abate without treatment within a few days to weeks.

  C. **Herpes simplex and zoster.** Open- or closed-angle glaucoma may occur in these diseases associated with uveitis. CAIs, epinephrine, or timolol (not miotics) should be utilized to treat the IOP in addition to adjustments in steroid dosage discussed above (see sec. **A.4,** Chap. 5, **IV.D, E,** and Chap. 8, **X.B, C).**

  D. **Fuchs's heterochromic iridocyclitis** is characterized by chronic anterior uveitis in a white and quiet eye with no synechiae formation, but with iris heterochromia (usually the lighter iris) and cataract formation. Filamentary precipitates on the corneal endothelium are also typical. This form of iridocyclitis is probably degenerative rather than inflammatory.

1. **Glaucoma** develops probably in a minority of such patients. It usually occurs late and develops gradually, although it often proves **refractory to topical medical therapy.** This may be due to a hyaline membrane histologically.
2. **Treatment** is standard anti–open-angle glaucoma therapy and then LTP. If this fails, patients do well with filtration surgery. Cataract surgery is also uncomplicated but does not influence the course of the glaucoma. Topical steroids do not influence the glaucoma.

E. **KPs** in the angle may occur occultly in a white and quiet eye with no apparent intraocular inflammation but with elevated IOP that may mimic primary open-angle glaucoma. This condition is another reason to gonioscope all glaucoma patients. The precipitates may be very subtle and are best seen by retroillumination. With time they may organize and result in irregular peripheral anterior synechiae and an uneven insertion of the iris in the angle. This occult disease responds well to **topical steroid therapy,** but not to conventional topical antiglaucoma therapy except perhaps timolol. Patients with presumed primary open-angle glaucoma who are placed on treatment and return with no apparent effect or even higher IOP should always be regonioscoped to rule out this (and other) causes.

XIX. **Neovascular glaucoma**
   A. **Clinical characteristics.** In certain patients with long-standing hypoxic retinopathy such as **diabetes, central retinal artery or vein occlusion, or carotid artery insufficiency,** a fibrovascular membrane will grow over the TM and ultimately result in total angle closure. Glaucoma may be present at a time when the membrane has not yet contracted and caused synechiae formation and the angle is still "open." Patients present with acute glaucoma that must be distinguished from primary angle-closure glaucoma by the presence of new blood vessels in the angle and almost always on the surface of the iris as well. Topical glycerin should be used to clear the corneal edema. A history of severe visual loss several months prior to the glaucoma may be helpful in identifying patients with central retinal vein occlusion. Other retinopathies and malignant melanoma may be associated with the development of neovascular glaucoma in rare cases.
   B. **Treatment.** In eyes with total angle closure, treatment consists of use of a beta blocker (if cardiac status allows) and CAIs (methazolamide if renal function impaired) to lower the IOP and topical steroids and cycloplegics for comfort. If the visual potential is good, filtration surgery, perhaps following laser treatment of iris neovascularization, sometimes succeeds. In eyes with early neovascular glaucoma, panretinal photocoagulation, perhaps supplemented with direct goniophotocoagulation of new blood vessels, will often lead to a regression or delay in the disease process.

XX. **Abnormal episcleral venous pressure**
   A. **Intracranial vascular malformations,** such as those seen in patients with carotid-cavernous sinus fistulas and dural shunts and in patients with Sturge-Weber disease, may produce an elevation of venous pressure that is transmitted back to the eye and results in a secondary open-angle glaucoma. This **elevated episcleral venous pressure** may also occur idiopathically in certain glaucoma patients. Usually a key to the diagnosis is the presence of prominent or abnormal episcleral vessels on slit-lamp examination. These prominent episcleral vessels may be misinterpreted as indicating episcleritis or other inflammatory disease.
   B. **Treatment** is standard open-angle glaucoma therapy, although the IOP cannot be lowered below true episcleral venous pressure, since the vessels constitute the draining bed for aqueous humor after it has passed through the angle tissue. Glaucoma filtering surgery may be successful, although these patients are at risk of developing **intraoperative choroidal effusions** due to the elevation of venous pressure. This should be anticipated and treated intraoperatively by a preliminary posterior sclerotomy.

XXI. Corticosteroid glaucoma

A. Clinical characteristics. Steroid glaucoma is anatomically indistinguishable from primary open-angle glaucoma: the pressure is elevated, angles open and appearing normal, outflow facility decreased, and, with time, the nerves progressively cupped and visual fields compromised. Increased IOP may develop within 2 weeks of initiating steroid use or after many months or even years of use. The more potent agents such as dexamethasone and prednisolone are more likely to induce pressure rises sooner and higher than weaker agents like hydrocortisone or fluorometholone. Patients who were formerly but no longer on steroids and who had steroid glaucoma may be misdiagnosed as having low-tension glaucoma because of the presence of glaucomatous cupping, visual field defects, and normal pressures. Successfully controlled glaucoma patients may go out of control if steroid therapy is added to their drug regimen, and infants treated with steroid may develop a picture similar to that of primary congenital open-angle glaucoma. Close relatives of patients with primary open-angle glaucoma stand a significantly greater chance of developing steroid glaucoma (20%) than the rest of the population (4%). **The history of patient steroid drug therapy is essential to making the correct diagnosis.**

B. Medical therapy is first and foremost to stop or at least reduce the steroids if possible. Discontinuing the drug will almost invariably result in spontaneous resolution of increased IOP within 2–6 weeks. If IOP does not return to normal but is reduced simply by discontinuing the steroid, it is likely that an underlying undiagnosed primary open-angle glaucoma was simply unmasked or aggravated by steroid usage. There is no definitive proof that these drugs cause permanent alterations in the ocular outflow channels. If steroids cannot be stopped or if the IOP is unacceptably high while waiting for spontaneous resolution, therapy as for primary open-angle glaucoma may be initiated to prevent progression of ocular damage. Miotics, beta blockers (except in asthmatics on steroids), sympathomimetics, and CAIs all may have a beneficial effect in this form of glaucoma.

C. Surgical therapy is rarely used for this condition and only in those cases where IOP does not return to acceptable levels despite stopping steroids and initiating antiglaucoma medical treatment. Subconjunctival depot injections may have to be resected, although they have usually washed out by 2 weeks. The effect of laser trabeculoplasty is not established.

XXII. Crystalline lens-induced glaucoma (see also Chap. 6, **V.G,** and Chap. 8, sec. **XIII**)

A. Clinical characteristics. An acute secondary open-angle glaucoma **(phacolytic glaucoma)** may result from a leaking hypermature or mature (rarely immature) cataract. There is usually rapid onset of ocular pain and redness with often very high pressures and corneal epithelial edema. Light projection may be faulty. Gonioscopy reveals the angle to be open, which distinguishes this disease from acute angle-closure glaucoma. Cellular reaction in the anterior chamber is usually minimum to moderate, although there is usually a heavy flare. Circulating white particles, which are larger than white cells and probably represent small portions of lens material, aggregated lens protein, or swollen macrophages can be seen frequently in the aqueous. The cataract often has patchy white deposits, which are probably macrophages, on the anterior lens capsule.

B. Mechanism. Phacolytic glaucoma is most likely due to direct mechanical obstruction of the outflow pathways by the liberated lens proteins that leak from the cataract. Macrophages that act to clear lens material from the eye may also be involved in the obstruction to outflow. The **diagnosis** of phacolytic glaucoma is made by paracentesis and aspiration of aqueous humor, microscopic examination of which usually reveals the presence of engorged macrophages. Biochemical analysis for lens proteins may be also useful (see Chap. 1, **III.G**).

C. Dislocated lenses. In cases of cataractous lenses that are dislocated into the vitreous, the findings in phacolytic glaucoma may be quite subtle. The **differential diagnosis** includes angle-recession glaucoma, primary open-angle glaucoma, and an idiopathic type of chronic open-angle glaucoma apparently not related to lens reaction or obvious signs of angle recession.

D. Retained lens cortex. Glaucoma may result from the obstructive properties of liberated lens particles on the outflow pathways following extracapsular cataract surgery or lens injury. An inflammatory component may be additive.

E. Differential diagnosis. Phacolytic glaucoma must be distinguished from inflammatory glaucoma. Some KPs may be present on the cornea in phacolytic glaucoma. Consideration of the above factors will usually lead to the correct diagnosis but, especially in the rare cases of phacolytic glaucoma with immature cataracts, a trial of topical steroids may be useful. In phacolytic glaucoma such steroid therapy will not result in a lasting improvement of IOP, and cataract surgery should then be contemplated. Again, diagnostic paracentesis will usually establish the correct diagnosis.

F. Treatment is cataract extraction. In general, the eyes show short-lived response to topical antiglaucoma or anti-inflammatory therapy. There is usually significant lowering of IOP with use of a beta blocker, CAIs, and osmotic agents, but the pressure frequently continues to rise again to high levels (40–80 mm Hg). All patients with presumed phacolytic glaucoma should be hospitalized and have urgent cataract extraction the same day if the pressure continues to rise to these high levels. In the case of retained lens cortex, medical therapy with a beta blocker, epinephrine, DPE, CAIs, cycloplegics, and possibly topical steroids should be tried, but if the glaucoma remains severe, the remaining lens material must be surgically removed.

XXIII. Intraocular lens (IOL)–associated glaucoma may stem from any of the previously mentioned causes such as exacerbation of preexistent primary open-angle glaucoma, pupillary block, malignant glaucoma following pupillary block, viscoelastic substance (see sec. **XXIV**) or vitreous herniation into the anterior chamber blocking trabecular meshwork, or chronic peripheral anterior synechiae (PAS). Additionally, IOLs uniquely predispose to three other causes of glaucoma: smouldering chronic iridocyclitis, anterior chamber (and TM) mechanical distortion, and pseudophakic pigmentary dispersion.

A. Therapy of all but the last three has already been discussed. For these three a decision must be made as to whether the IOL should be removed or medical therapy will suffice. IOL iritis is often associated with mechanical distortion of the anterior chamber due to improper lens sizing or placement. Steroid and, if needed, antiglaucoma therapy may control the process. If progressive adhesions or cystoid macular edema develop, however, the lens should probably be removed in the absence of other contraindications. In pigment dispersion (seen with iris plane and posterior chamber IOLs), the pupil and iris may be immobilized with longer-acting miotics to minimize mechanical rubbing against the lens. The IOL usually does not have to be removed.

XXIV. Viscoelastic substance–induced glaucoma is a secondary open-angle glaucoma seen postoperatively after use of these vitreous-stimulating materials.

A. Clinical characteristics. Viscoelastic gels, although a great boon to anterior and posterior segment surgery, have the undesirable side effect of transiently blocking the aqueous outflow system occasionally with resulting severe rise in IOP. Pressure rise may begin within an hour or two of closing the eye in the case of residual anterior chamber material and at 72 hours in situations where viscoelastic substance has been left in the posterior segment and has then moved forward. Symptoms may be absent or similar to acute IOP rise with ocular pain, steamy cornea, nausea, and vomiting. Posterior segment viscoelastic substance usually must be removed to control the glaucoma.

XXV. Perforating injuries may produce glaucoma as a result of peripheral anterior synechiae from the loss of the anterior chamber or may be due to inflammation, lens material, or pupillary block. It is important to restore the anterior chamber in the treatment of such injuries.

XXVI. Unusual secondary angle-closure glaucomas

A. Malignant glaucoma. See sec. **XII.C.**

B. A dislocated lens that is incarcerated in the pupil may cause angle-closure glaucoma by pupillary block. Treatment consists of dilating the pupil, lying the patient on his or her back, and attempting to force the lens back into the posterior chamber, following which the pupil is made miotic. If medical therapy fails, an LI (rather than lens extraction) should almost always be done. An exception would be a lens dislocated into the anterior chamber, close to or touching the cornea, which cannot be moved into the posterior chamber. Cataract extraction of dislocated lenses is usually accompanied by vitreous loss and significant complications.

C. Essential iris atrophy is almost always a monocular condition of progressive iris atrophy with **distortion of the pupil** and **iris hole formation** with glaucoma, due to progressive peripheral anterior synechiae often extending anterior to Schwalbe's line. Corneal endothelial dystrophy and iris nodule formation may be observed. The disease may be due to progression and contraction of an endothelial cell membrane. In **Chandler's syndrome,** corneal endothelial dystrophy is a predominant feature with corneal edema and haloes at mild elevations of IOP. Only mild iris atrophy without hole formation is characteristic of Chandler's syndrome, although there is a disease spectrum. In addition to the iris and corneal changes, **diagnosis** is made on gonioscopy by the observation of peripheral anterior synechiae extending anterior to Schwalbe's line (unlike almost all other peripheral anterior synechiae). **Standard medical therapy** is employed, but this is a progressive disease and, especially in Chandler's syndrome where a very low IOP is required, filtering surgery is frequently required.

D. Multiple iris and ciliary body cysts is a rare condition, though often familial, in which the cysts may directly push the iris over the TM and close the angle. They may be discovered after LI for angle closure. An uncommon bumpy contour of the peripheral iris on gonioscopy is characteristic. If accessible, the cysts may be ruptured by application of laser therapy through an iridectomy.

E. Retinal detachment surgery. Indentation of the eye by the buckle or suprachoroidal fluid or both may act as a force pushing the vitreous forward and increasing pupillary block. Rotation of ciliary processes forward against the iris with direct secondary angle closure may also be a factor. **Medical therapy** of cycloplegics to tighten the zonules and osmotics to dehydrate the vitreous may be tried, but most frequently **surgical therapy** of suprachoroidal fluid drainage and peripheral iridectomy is required.

F. Central retinal vein occlusion may rarely result in a reversible secondary angle-closure glaucoma, presumably due to increased fluid volume in the vitreous or retina. The key to the diagnosis is the presence of true monocular angle closure and the severe impairment of vision due to the vein occlusion. Since it is reversible after a few weeks, **standard medical therapy** for angle-closure glaucoma should be employed, except that maintained cycloplegics should be tried rather than miotics initially in order to tighten the zonules and reverse forward lens movement, as well as to dilate the pupil away from the lens.

XXVII. Glaucoma in children (see Chap. 10, sec. **XV**). Congenital glaucoma must be suspected in all babies with photophobia and excessive tearing. The cornea becomes hazy, and the eye often enlarges in size. In addition to this acute glaucoma, glaucoma in children may develop silently, as in adults. Whenever possible, measurement of IOP and inspection of the optic nerve head should be performed as a routine part of all ophthalmologic examinations.

XXVIII. Nonophthalmologic systemic medication in glaucoma patients. The physician must first differentiate between open-angle glaucoma and angle-closure glaucoma patients.

A. Angle-closure glaucoma. If a systemic medication causes the pupil to dilate, angle-closure glaucoma can be precipitated. Therefore, both systemic adrenergic and systemic anticholinergic medications can precipitate angle-closure glaucoma. Most patients who have diagnosed angle-closure glaucoma, however, will have been treated with a peripheral iridectomy in both eyes, and therefore the pupillary dilation that ensues from systemic medication will not cause the angle to close (unless the patient has the rare condition of plateau iris).

The **risk group** includes those patients with shallow anterior chambers and undiagnosed, asymptomatic, narrow, closeable angles. In these patients, pupillary dilation from systemic medication could cause the angle to close; therefore, the physician should routinely examine the depth of the anterior chamber in all patients with a flashlight projected tangential to the cornea. Cerebral vasodilators can be used with impunity in patients with narrow-angle glaucoma on the basis of all present data.

B. Open-angle glaucoma

1. **Systemic anticholinergics.** If a systemic medication paralyzes the ciliary muscle (cycloplegic effect), then, theoretically at least, this medication may worsen open-angle glaucoma because of the effect of ciliary muscle contraction on aqueous outflow. Those open-angle glaucoma patients who respond to topical anticholinergic drugs with a significant increase in IOP (highest risk group) demonstrate only a slight increase in IOP when given systemic anticholinergic drugs. This increase is easily controlled by standard glaucoma therapy. Therefore, if open-angle glaucoma patients need systemic anticholinergic therapy, it is possible for them to have it, provided there is ophthalmologic consultation so that the ophthalmologist can adjust the glaucoma therapy, if necessary.

2. **Systemic adrenergic drugs.** Administration of systemic dextroamphetamine sulfate (Dexedrine) to patients with open-angle glaucoma does not affect the IOP one way or the other. From this it can be assumed that systemic adrenergic agents are safe to give to open-angle glaucoma patients; vasodilator drugs are also safe. Systemic corticosteroids can increase IOP, and therefore ophthalmologic consultation should be requested. There is no absolute contraindication to their use in open-angle glaucoma patients, however, and most likely the effect of systemic corticosteroids on IOP can be managed by adjustment of the glaucoma therapy.

Pediatric Ophthalmology

William P. Boger III and
Robert A. Petersen

Many of the methods of examination and ocular disorders relevant to adults pertain also to children. This chapter emphasizes the examinations, ocular disorders, and therapies that are especially relevant to pediatric patients. Strabismus is very prevalent in childhood, and the development of amblyopia is a problem up to age 9 or 10. (See Chap. 11 for many issues that often must be considered simultaneously in the care of pediatric patients.)

I. **Vision testing and clinical examination of the young patient**
   A. **Well-baby examinations.** Evaluation of visual function and the structural integrity of the ocular structures should be an integral portion of the pediatrician's routine examinations. The well-baby examination should include the following:
      1. **Newborn period**
         a. Pupillary responses to light.
         b. Size and clarity of cornea.
         c. Eye movements full in response to passive head turning.
         d. Red reflex with ophthalmoscope. (This maneuver screens for opacities in the media such as cataract as well as for gross fundus lesions.)
      2. **Infancy**
         a. Visual function (see sec. **B**).
         b. Pupils round and reactive.
         c. Size and clarity of cornea.
         d. Eye movements full in following objects.
         e. When the child looks attentively at a flashlight, does the light reflex on the cornea fall in the middle of both corneas?
         f. Red reflex with ophthalmoscope.
      3. **Childhood**
         a. Formal visual acuity testing with verbal or matching responses from child after age 2 or 3.
         b. Glimpse of fundus details, especially the optic nerve, with direct ophthalmoscope.
         c. Remainder of examination as in sec. **2**.
   B. **Evaluation of visual acuity.** The physician should concentrate on each eye separately when assessing visual acuity. A child may have a blinding disorder that needs attention or a life-threatening tumor in one eye and yet function normally with the other eye. Therefore, the examiner must **put an adhesive patch over one eye to ensure that the child is not peeking when assessing the visual acuity in the fellow eye.**
      1. **Newborn period.** Pupillary responses to light.
      2. **Infancy.** By 4–6 weeks of age most infants will follow a light or large objects over a short range. By 3 months they should fix on an object and follow it over a wide range and evidence social response to mother's face. If one eye is constantly deviated (inward with esotropia, outward with exotropia), the examiner must assume that its acuity is abnormal. A child with an eye deviation but with equal vision in the two eyes will alternately fixate with one eye and then the other. If available, preferential looking tests for infant vision such as the Teller acuity cards are quantitative and helpful.

251

3. Childhood. At 2 or 3 years of age most children are sufficiently verbal that a subjective visual acuity can be obtained using picture cards, such as Allen cards or matching games, such as HOTV. **Each eye must be tested separately, and the child must not be able to peek.** A year or two later most children will be able to identify Es in various positions after another year or two letters or numbers can be used. It is easiest to identify isolated figures, but by 5 or 6 years of age children should be able to read rows or clusters of letters. Visual acuity assessment should be checked annually.

C. Indications for referral to an ophthalmologist

1. Newborn period. Some referrals at this age are dictated by abnormalities noted by the pediatrician during the examination prior to discharge from the maternity unit. The panoramic view of the fundus provided by the indirect ophthalmoscope through the dilated pupil can provide important information not otherwise obtainable. Critically ill newborns who may have a congenital infection (see sec. **II**), those with multiple congenital anomalies, and those suspected of having a chromosomal abnormality (see sec. **VI**) should have indirect ophthalmoscopy. Very premature infants (see sec. **XII**) should have an ophthalmic examination prior to or shortly after discharge from the hospital.

2. Infancy. During the first few months of life, many youngsters have brief periods when the eyes do not appear to be aligned. It is abnormal at any age, however, to have a constant ocular deviation. An infant with a constant ocular deviation should be promptly and thoroughly evaluated by an ophthalmologist. The referral should not be delayed in the hope that the deviation will improve spontaneously. Most constant deviations do not improve with time; more important, a constant deviation may be the first sign of a serious ocular disorder, such as a **retinoblastoma** (see sec. **XI**).

If an intermittent deviation of the eyes persists past 6 months, the child should be referred to an ophthalmologist for evaluation. Infants with physical abnormalities such as asymmetric or large corneas, cloudy corneas, or a dark fundus reflex with the ophthalmoscope should be promptly referred for evaluation. Delay in referring a youngster with a large cornea due to glaucoma (see sec. **XV**) may contribute to irreparable loss of vision.

3. Childhood

a. Visual acuity should be comparable in the two eyes and should be testable to at least 20/40 in both eyes by the age of 3. If the vision is less than 20/40 in either eye or if there is more than one line difference on the Snellen chart between the two eyes, the child should be evaluated by an ophthalmologist.

b. Identification of the cause of visual asymmetry is important. Serious ocular disease may be the cause, or there may be a marked difference in the refraction of the two eyes. In the latter case, glasses (perhaps with patching) may fully correct the situation if instituted in the early years. Amblyopia from asymmetric refractive errors discovered several years later may be irreversible or much more difficult to treat (see Chap. 11, sec. **VI.D**). **An adequate refraction cannot be done in infancy and early childhood without cycloplegic medication.**

c. Age at examination. The question is often raised, "What is the best time to have my child's eyes checked?" If the child has an evident ocular abnormality, it should be evaluated by the ophthalmologist regardless of the age of the child. Although the child has no evident ocular problem and the pediatrician has found no abnormality on routine well-baby examination, some parents still request a routine eye examination. Three years of age is an ideal time for this kind of screening examination. At this age the child is old enough to give a subjective response to visual acuity testing and yet still young enough for effective amblyopia therapy if such an abnormality is discovered.

D. Medications in the young patient. Medications administered as eye drops may be absorbed through the mucous membranes in significant amounts and exert systemic effects. This fact is particularly important in infants and small children when multiple eye drops are administered. Adequate cycloplegia and mydriasis are usually achieved within 30 minutes after one drop of cyclopentolate 1% is instilled into each eye along with one additional drop 5 minutes later. If dilation is insufficient after 30 minutes, an additional waiting period is advisable. The use of additional cycloplegic drops runs the risk of toxic side effects with disorientation and ataxia. Alternatively, atropine 1% *ointment* can be used for 3 nights preceding the next office visit to obtain adequate mydriasis and cycloplegia.

Some ophthalmologists routinely use atropine and accordingly defer the fundus examination and refraction until the patient's second visit. The use of the shorter-acting cycloplegic-mydriatic agents such as cyclopentolate allows the examiner to rule out the presence of a serious ocular disorder such as retinoblastoma and makes possible a more thorough evaluation at the first visit. Cyclopentolate administered as described in the preceding paragraph provides satisfactory and reproducible cycloplegia for refraction. Appropriate glasses can therefore be prescribed for a refractive error or for strabismus therapy after the first visit.

E. **Differential diagnosis of clinical presentations in childhood**
   1. **Cloudy cornea**
      a. **Unilateral**
         (1) Infantile glaucoma.
         (2) Trauma with rupture of Descemet's membrane (forceps injury).
      b. **Bilateral**
         (1) Infantile glaucoma.
         (2) Corneal endothelial dystrophy.
         (3) Mucopolysaccharidoses (Hurler's, Scheie's, Morquio's, and Maroteau-Lamy's syndromes).
         (4) Mucolipidoses.
         (5) Interstitial keratitis.
   2. **Tearing**
      a. Infantile glaucoma.
      b. Dacryostenosis.
   3. **Large cornea**
      a. Infantile glaucoma.
      b. Megalocornea (less likely).
   4. **Photophobia**
      a. Keratitis (herpes simplex).
      b. Infantile glaucoma.
      c. Uveitis.
      d. Achromatopsia.
   5. **Red eye in newborn period (rule out trauma, uveitis, keratitis)**
      a. Chemical conjunctivitis (usually mild with onset 1–2 days after birth).
      b. Gonorrhea (purulent conjunctivitis, usual onset 1–3 days after birth).
      c. Chlamydial infection (usual onset 5–14 days after birth).
      d. Bacterial infection (staphylococcal, pneumococcal, usual onset 3–30 days after birth).
   6. **Strabismus.** All eye deviations should be assumed to be due to an organic lesion in the deviating eye (e.g., retinoblastoma) involving the macula until proved otherwise (see Chap. 11).
   7. **Nystagmus**
      a. Sensory nystagmus (associated with poor visual acuity):
         (1) Macular scars, e.g., toxoplasmosis.
         (2) Macular hypoplasia, e.g., albinism, aniridia.
         (3) Achromatopsia.
         (4) Retinal degeneration, e.g., Leber's congenital amaurosis.
         (5) Optic nerve hypoplasia.
      b. Motor nystagmus (visual acuity is maximum in position of least nystagmus—the null point).

   c. Latent or occlusional nystagmus (nystagmus is induced or aggravated by covering one eye).
   d. Spasmus nutans (uniocular or markedly asymmetric nystagmus, often associated with head nodding, head cocking, and strabismus).
8. **Unusual, gross, or chaotic eye movements**
   a. Opsoclonus:
      (1) Neuroblastoma.
      (2) Encephalitis.
   b. Diencephalic ("happy waif") syndrome.
   c. Subacute necrotizing encephalomyelopathy (Leigh's disease).
9. **Optic atrophy**
   a. Associated with CNS degenerative disorders, such as multiple sclerosis, adrenoleukodystrophy, metachromatic leukodystrophy, subacute necrotizing encephalomyelopathy.
   b. Associated with CNS tumor, such as pituitary adenoma, craniopharyngioma.
   c. Hereditary optic atrophies may be inherited in an X-linked fashion (Leber's optic atrophy) or in a recessive fashion (Behr's optic atrophy); dominantly inherited forms have also been reported.
   d. Secondary to retinal degeneration, as seen in Tay-Sachs disease, Niemann-Pick disease, G_{M1} gangliosidosis, mucopolysaccharidoses, retinitis pigmentosa, and allied disorders.
10. **Cherry-red maculae**
   a. Commotio retinae (following blunt trauma to the eye).
   b. Central retinal artery occlusion.
   c. Metabolic storage diseases
      (1) Tay-Sachs and Sandhoff disease (G_{M2} gangliosidosis) (100% of individuals evidence this macular change).
      (2) Niemann-Pick disease (50% of affected individuals evidence this macular change).
      (3) G_{M1} gangliosidosis, infantile form.
      (4) Farber's lipogranulomatosis (subtle grayness around fovea, difficult to distinguish from normal).
      (5) Metachromatic leukodystrophy (subtle grayness around fovea, difficult to distinguish from normal).
      (6) Sialidosis.
11. **Subluxed or dislocated lenses**
   a. Marfan's syndrome.
   b. Homocystinuria.
   c. Weil-Marchesani syndrome (short stature, brachycephaly, stubby fingers and toes with joint stiffness, spherophakia, myopia).
   d. Sulfite oxidase deficiency.
   e. Traumatic.
   f. Familial idiopathic.
12. **White pupil (leukocoria)**
   a. Retinoblastoma.
   b. Cataract.
   c. Retinal detachment.
   d. Severe posterior uveitis from any cause.
   e. Severe retrolental fibroplasia (RLF).
   f. Persistent hyperplastic primary vitreous.
   g. Retinal dysplasia (Norrie's disease).
   h. Coats' disease.
13. **Proptosis**
   a. Rhabdomyosarcoma.
   b. Orbital cellulitis.
   c. Pseudotumor of the orbit.
   d. Optic nerve glioma.
   e. Retrobulbar hemorrhage.

    f. Thyroid ophthalmopathy.
    g. Chloroma (granulocytic sarcoma).
    h. Neuroblastoma.
    i. Histiocytosis.

14. Lid ecchymosis
    a. Trauma.
    b. Neuroblastoma.

15. Hyphema
    a. Trauma.
    b. Juvenile xanthogranuloma.
    c. Tumor (retinoblastoma, rare presentation).
    d. Herpes simplex uveitis (uncommon presentation).

16. Microphthalmus
    a. Developmental anomaly.
    b. Persistent hyperplastic primary vitreous.
    c. Chromosomal anomaly.
    d. Congenital rubella syndrome.

II. Congenital and neonatal infection. (TORCH titers: *t*oxoplasmosis, *o*ther (syphilis and others), *r*ubella, *c*ytomegalovirus, *h*erpes simplex)

    A. Infections that are usually congenital

        1. Congenital toxoplasmosis. Although ocular lesions may rarely be acquired during a primary infection in adulthood, the vast majority of ocular toxoplasmosis lesions are due to congenital infections. The characteristic lesion is a focal necrotizing retinitis. It may be solitary or in small clusters and is commonly in the posterior pole. Juxtapapillary lesions are not uncommon.

            a. Physical findings. Classic findings of congenital toxoplasmosis are focal necrotizing retinitis, intracranial calcification, and hepatosplenomegaly, but there is a wide spectrum of presentations. **Severely affected children** have massive inflammation of the retina, choroid, and vitreous, cataract, strabismus, microphthalmus, and petechial hemorrhages in the newborn period. **Mildly affected children** may be left with only small inconspicuous retinal scars and positive serologic titers.

            b. Treatment (see Chap. 8, sec. XI.G).

        2. Congenital syphilis. The introduction of penicillin dramatically reduced the incidence of syphilis in general with a concomitant reduction in the incidence of congenital syphilis. There has in recent years, however, been a resurgence of syphilis in the population as a whole, and in 1988 crude rates of primary and secondary syphilis reached their highest levels in 40 years. Reported rates of congenital syphilis in 1988 were also the highest for the past several decades. In contrast to the stages of acquired syphilis, congenital syphilis has no primary stage.

            a. Early congenital syphilis. The sequelae of focal inflammation in the intrauterine and early formative years become apparent in bony and structural malformation. Manifestations of the first 2 years of life are as follows:

                (1) Inflammatory manifestations
                    (a) Dermal eruption, vesicular or pustular.
                    (b) Mucous membrane involvement:
                        (i) Purulent snuffles.
                        (ii) Conjunctivitis (treponemes can be isolated).
                    (c) Periostitis ("pseudoparalysis" of limb).
                    (d) Generalized lymphadenopathy.
                    (e) Severely affected infant may have
                        (i) Hepatosplenomegaly.
                        (ii) Hyperbilirubinemia.
                        (iii) Anemia.
                    (f) Chorioretinitis
                      (i) More common: widespread, small, focal yellowish-white

exudates leading to "salt and pepper" fundus—tends to be bilateral, heals spontaneously, and is said not to recur.

    (ii) Less common: isolated peripheral circumscribed lesions.

  (g) Rhagades (cracks or fissures about the mouth or nose resulting from infantile syphilitic rhinitis).

(2) Sequelae of focal inflammation

  (a) Bone deformities:

    (i) Frontal bossing of skull.
    (ii) Saber shins.
    (iii) Scaphoid scapulas.
    (iv) Saddle nose.
    (v) Scoliosis.
    (vi) Perforation of hard palate.
    (vii) Clutton's joints (painless hydroarthrosis, usually of the knees).

  (b) Teeth deformities:

    (i) Hutchinson's teeth (notched and barrel-shaped central incisors).
    (ii) Mulberry or Moon's molars (maldeveloped cusps of first molars).

  (c) Psychomotor retardation.

  b. Late congenital syphilis is more analogous to latent forms of acquired syphilis. Manifestations include

(1) Neurosyphilis

  (a) Optic atrophy.
  (b) Pupillary abnormalities.
  (c) Eighth nerve deafness.

(2) Interstitial keratitis (IK). This condition is usually due to congenital syphilis but may occur after acquired syphilis. When due to congenital syphilis, the onset is usually between 5 and 20 years, although it has been observed at birth. Although IK often appears in later life, treponemas have been isolated from clear corneas in newborns. The pathogenesis of IK may be immunologic. IK has occasionally been reported after adequate treatments with penicillin in early years of life.

3. Congenital rubella syndrome (CRS). Approximately 50% of mothers with clinical evidence of rubella infection during the first month of gestation will bear offspring with malformations at birth. Slightly lower rates of malformation follow rubella infections during the second and third months of gestation. The **classic physical findings** are as follows:

  a. Ocular findings

    (1) Nuclear cataract in newborn period with surrounding zone of clear cortex; gradual progression so lens becomes pearly white.
    (2) Microphthalmus closely associated with presence of cataract.
    (3) Congenital or infantile glaucoma. The infant may or may not have cataract as well; the cataracts and the infantile glaucoma are independent variables.
    (4) Corneas transiently hazy without increased intraocular pressure (IOP), possibly due to a keratitis or to an endothelial dysfunction.
    (5) Speckled retinitis of posterior pole "like a piece of coarse Scotch tweed over which pepper has been strewn."

  b. Nonocular findings

    (1) Congenital heart disease.
    (2) Neurosensory deafness, which may be acquired in early childhood years and is not necessarily congenital.

  c. Current knowledge about CRS was greatly increased by intensive study of the United States epidemic in 1964 and 1965. It is now clear that affected youngsters actively shed virus up until 2 years of age. Virus has been recovered from lens material as late as 3 years of age. It is still unclear how long virus persists within the congenitally infected individual. The persistence of virus in these individuals is not a matter of immunologic tolerance, since the rubella child's serologic and cell-mediated responses have been appropriate. During the 1960s a multisystem disease, the **expanded rubella syndrome,** was identified during the first months of life. Signs of this expanded rubella syndrome include

(1) Thrombocytopenia and consequent purpura (blueberry muffin baby).

(2) Bone lesions.

(3) Hepatitis.

(4) Hemolytic anemia.

(5) CNS involvement.

d. Late-onset disease. From 3 months of age until the end of the first year several other clinical problems may arise. These problems include a generalized rash with seborrheic features, an interstitial pneumonitis that is responsive to corticosteroids, and lymphocytic infiltration of the pancreas. These manifestations of late-onset disease have been difficult to explain, and the question of an immunologic mechanism stimulated by the rubella virus has been raised.

e. Intrauterine infection with rubella does not act simply as a teratogenic agent. It clearly stimulates an ongoing process that has neonatal features but may also cause continuing disease. Some youngsters with the congenital rubella syndrome have measurable hearing in early childhood, but when they are tested 2 years later they have become entirely deaf. The mechanism of this progressive loss is uncertain. A handful of youngsters born with maternal rubella syndrome have developed a panencephalitis at 10 or 12 years of age, with rubella virus recoverable from the brain at that time.

f. Ophthalmologic care of these children starts with attention to cataracts and glaucoma in infancy. The glaucoma is treated as described under infantile glaucoma (see sec. **XV.A**). When cataracts are bilateral they should be aspirated in the first few months of life. As much lens material as possible should be removed during the operation.

Infants with congenital rubella syndrome who have had surgery for glaucoma or cataract *must* be followed regularly throughout life. The onset of intraocular inflammation or glaucoma (or both) has occurred even 10 or 15 years after initial successful and uneventful surgery. Late retinal detachment is also a complication of cataract surgery.

4. Cytomegalovirus (CMV) belongs to the herpes group and is a common virus. Many women have complement-fixation titers to CMV by their childbearing years. Approximately 4–5% of pregnant women actively excrete CMV in their urine. Postnatal infections are also possible, since 25% of women with positive antibody to CMV have the virus in breast milk. Most neonates with congenital CMV are asymptomatic. Now that these youngsters can be identified serologically and followed longitudinally, it appears that there is an increased incidence of psychomotor retardation and microcephaly. A small subgroup of neonates with congenital CMV are very sick with hepatosplenomegaly, hyperbilirubinemia, thrombocytopenia, and petechiae. Intrauterine growth retardation and microcephaly may be evident at birth, and there may be encephalitis with or without hydrocephalus. Chorioretinitis similar to that seen with congenital toxoplasmosis has been reported. Intracranial calcification, hydrocephalus, hepatosplenomegaly, and focal chorioretinitis due to CMV may mimic congenital toxoplasmosis. The chorioretinitis reported in **congenital** CMV has been focal, in contrast to the widespread retinal necrosis and "smeary" hemorrhage described in adults in the context of an **acquired** CMV infection in an immunologically compromised host, e.g., following renal transplant. **No specific treatment** for congenital CMV currently exists, although ganciclovir is FDA approved for use in progressive retinitis in immunocompromised patients (see Chap. 8, sec. **X.D**).

B. Ophthalmia neonatorum. These hyperacute infections are generally acquired after rupture of the membranes during the time the child is in contact with the mother's cervix and vaginal tract. They may occur anytime in the first month of life and be considered neonatal. Potential **etiologic agents** include chemical conjunctivitis from 1% silver nitrate antimicrobial instilled prophylactically at birth, *Chlamydia trachomatis* (inclusion blenorrhea), *Staphylococcus aureus, Streptococcus pneumoniae, Haemophilus* sp., *Pseudomonas* sp., *Neisseria gonorrhoeae,* and herpes simplex virus. (See Chap. 5, sec. **III.B.2** and **IV.C,** Table 5–2, and Chap. 8, sec. **X.B** for additional discussion).

1. **Herpes simplex.** Rarely, a youngster may be born with evidence of infection acquired during pregnancy. Such evidence includes microcephaly, cerebral calcification, chorioretinitis, and mental retardation. The more usual form is acquired at the time of birth.

   a. **Neonatal herpes simplex**

      (1) **Cutaneous** manifestations may be present without systemic involvement. Cutaneous vesicles may be present with or without **conjunctivitis,** and with or without **keratitis.** The keratitis may present as a **classic dendrite.**

      (2) **The disseminated form** has an average onset of 1 week of age. The neonate may be severely ill with jaundice, fever, hepatosplenomegaly, encephalitis, and disseminated intraocular coagulopathy. There may be few or no skin lesions to help with the diagnosis.

      (3) The more localized form of **CNS involvement** without systemic visceral involvement has an average onset of 11 days. It is more likely to have herpetic skin vesicles. Apparently the virus is rarely isolated from the CNS in this form.

   b. Neonatal systemic infection with herpes simplex virus is almost invariably symptomatic and often lethal; only rare cases of inapparent infection have been documented despite large-scale attempts to identify these patients. The role of brain biopsy for early diagnosis is controversial. The availability of antiviral agents such as vidarabine and acyclovir has provided new possibilities for systemic therapy. The risk of transmission to offspring when maternal genital lesions are present at birth has been estimated at 40%. Transmission to the offspring is common when delivery follows rupture of the membranes by more than 6 hours, whereas abdominal delivery within 4 hours of membrane breaking appears to reduce the risk of intrauterine spread.

2. **Gonorrhea.** It is wise to consider **all purulent conjunctivitis in the first few days of life as gonococcal until proved otherwise.** The rapidity with which gonococcus can penetrate the cornea has been well documented, and gonococcal conjunctivitis presents a true ophthalmic emergency.

   a. Once the diagnosis is made by Gram's stain of conjunctival scraping, the child should be hospitalized and **treated** with high-dose parenteral penicillin and topical antibiotics (penicillin or erythromycin). Confirmatory cultures should be planted on Thayer-Martin medium. Although prophylaxis with silver nitrate drops or antibiotic ointment is helpful against the organism, the current epidemic of gonococcal disease makes it prudent to maintain a high suspicion for gonococcal conjunctivitis not only in the newborn period but at all ages. The parents should be treated as well as the neonate.

   b. **The 1990 Centers for Disease Control (CDC) treatment guidelines for gonococcal disease** are as follows:

      (1) **Infants born to mothers with untreated gonococcal infections** are at high risk of infection, e.g., ophthalmia and disseminated gonococcal infection and should be treated with a single injection of **ceftriaxone** (50 mg/kg IV or IM, not to exceed 125 mg). Ceftriaxone should be given cautiously to hyperbilirubinemic infants, especially premature infants. Topical prophylaxis for neonatal

ophthalmia is not adequate treatment for documented infections of the eye or other sites.

(2) Neonates with clinical gonococcal ophthalmia should be evaluated by a careful physical examination, especially of the joints, blood, and CSF cultures. Infants with gonococcal ophthalmia should be treated for 7 days (10–14 days if meningitis is present) with one of the following regimens:

- **(a) Ceftriaxone,** 25–50 mg/kg/day IV or IM qd **or**
- **(b) Cefotaxime,** 25 mg/kg IV or IM q12h.

 Children > 8 years of age should also be given **doxycycline,** 100 mg bid for 7 days. All patients should be evaluated for coinfection with syphilis and *C. trachomatis.* Follow-up cultures are necessary to ensure that treatment has been effective.

(3) Alternative regimens

- **(a)** Limited data suggest that uncomplicated (no corneal involvement) gonococcal ophthalmia among infants may be cured with a single injection of **ceftriaxone** (50 mg/kg up to 125 mg). A few experts use this regimen for children who have no clinical or laboratory evidence of disseminated disease.
- **(b)** The quinolones, **ciprofloxacin** and **norfloxacin** are highly active against gococococcus and may be given PO to children or adults, including the penicillin allergic. Dosage is 1.5 gm PO for ciprofloxacin or 1.2 gm PO for norfloxacin once if no corneal involvement or q12h for 7–14 days with corneal involvement.
- **(c)** If the gonococcal isolate is proved to be susceptible to penicillin, **crystalline penicillin G** may be given. The dosage is 100,000 units/kg/day given in 2 equal doses (4 equal doses/day for infants more than 1 week old). The dosage should be increased to 150,000 units/kg/day for meningitis.
- **(d)** Infants with gonococcal ophthalmia should receive **eye irrigations** with buffered saline solutions until discharge has cleared. Topical antibiotic therapy alone is inadequate.
- **(e) Simultaneous infection** with *C. trachomatis* and syphilis has been reported and should be considered for patients who do not respond satisfactorily. Therefore, the mother and infant should be tested for chlamydial and syphilitic infection.

3. Inclusion conjunctivitis (blenorrhea, chlamydial infection) is caused by *Chlamydia trachomatis.* Credé's 1% silver nitrate prophylaxis is not effective against inclusion blenorrhea. The conjunctivitis usually commences 5–12 days after birth.

- **a.** The **diagnosis** is made by seeing cytoplasmic inclusions on a Giemsa stain of conjunctival scrapings. There is a mixed cellular response in these scrapings with both mononuclear cells and polymorphonuclear cells present. Culture and nonculture methods for diagnosis of *C. trachomatis* (Microtrak) are also now available. Results of chlamydial tests should be interpreted with care. The sensitivity of all currently available laboratory tests for *C. trachomatis* tests is substantially less than 100%; thus, false-negative and false-positive tests are possible.
- **b. Therapy.** Since the presence of chlamydial agents in the conjunctiva implies colonization of the upper respiratory tract as well, systemic erythromycin (125 mg PO qid for 3 weeks) should be given. Sulfisoxazole is the alternative drug (see Appendix B). The infant should also receive topical sulfonamide, erythromycin, or tetracycline qid for 3 weeks. Both parents should be treated (see Chap. 5, sec. **IV.C**).
- **c. Long-term follow-up** has indicated that poorly treated individuals may develop a trachomalike corneal pannus or vascularization. Appropriate **topical** antibiotic therapy appears to prevent this. Some children born to mothers with chlamydial infections do not have conjunctivitis but

still develop antibodies to the organism, and the agent of inclusion ble-norrhea has recently been implicated as the cause of a severe pneu-monitis in infancy.

4. **Prevention of ophthalmia neonatorum.** Instillation of a prophylactic agent into the eyes of all newborn infants is recommended to prevent gonococcal ophthalmia neonatorum and is required by law in most states. Although all regimens listed below effectively prevent gonococcal eye disease, their ef-ficacy in preventing chlamydial eye disease is not clear. Furthermore, they do not eliminate nasopharyngeal colonization with *C. trachomatis.* Prophy-laxis of gonococcal and chlamydial disease is
   a. **Erythromycin** (0.5%) ophthalmic ointment, once, **or**
   b. **Tetracycline** (1%) ophthalmic ointment once, **or**
   c. **Silver nitrate** (1%) aqueous solution, once.
   One of these should be instilled into the eyes of every neonate as soon as possible after delivery and definitely within 1 hour after birth. Single-use tubes or ampules are preferable to multiple-use tubes.

III. **Infections of childhood**
   A. **Orbital cellulitis versus periorbital cellulitis**
      1. **Periorbital cellulitis.** Facial cellulitis that happens to involve the lids may produce alarming swelling and closure of the lids. The eye itself, however, retains full range of movement, is not proptotic, and has good visual acuity and normal pupillary reactions. Like cellulitis elsewhere, staphylococcal or streptococcal etiology is most likely, and parenteral antibiotics are indi-cated. *Haemophilus influenzae* must also be considered, especially in young children.
      2. **Orbital cellulitis** denotes the infection of tissues behind the orbital septum, involving orbital structures, to produce proptosis, chemosis, limitation of eye movement, and possible loss of vision. The orbit is usually infected from a contiguous structure; often sinusitis is the cause, and in a young child *Haemophilus* infection must be considered. Blood cultures and consultation with an otolaryngologist are indicated. This is a life-threatening condition and requires emergency treatment. Exploration of the orbit itself is not usually indicated immediately but may be necessary later if an abscess forms. In addition to parenteral antibiotics, surgical drainage of the contiguous abscess or sinus infection by an otolaryngologist may be indicated.
   B. **Toxocara canis** is a nematode infestation that may present as a large vitreo-retinal mass. Pica has been implicated in the etiology, particularly when dirt has been contaminated by animal feces. Covers for sandboxes are highly rec-ommended as a prophylactic measure. The diagnosis is difficult to establish conclusively on clinical grounds. Eosinophilia of the peripheral blood may be helpful. A serologic test, Enzyme-Linked Immuno Serum Assay (ELISA), is available at the CDC in Atlanta, Georgia and in many state laboratories. Active systemic infestation with *Toxocara canis* is almost never present when ocular involvement is noted. Presumably the ocular lesion is a late sequela of systemic infestation (see Chap. 8, sec. XI.G.2).
   C. **Subacute sclerosing panencephalitis (SSPE)** presents as an intellectual and behavioral deterioration in school-age children. There may be rhythmic my-oclonic jerking. A focal chorioretinitis may be present. The chorioretinitis fre-quently but not always affects the macular region. Since SSPE is a panen-cephalitis, cortical blindness, optic atrophy, nystagmus on a neurologic basis, and papilledema may occur. SSPE is a slow virus disease that occurs after naturally acquired measles infection in 5-10 cases/million. It may more rarely follow live measles vaccination (0.5-1.1 cases/million). No specific therapy for the chorioretinal lesions is indicated.

IV. **Inflammations of childhood**
   A. **Juvenile rheumatoid arthritis (JRA)**
      1. The basic **ocular** lesion is iridocyclitis. In contrast to most other forms of iridocyclitis, ocular inflammation associated with JRA is chronic and in-sidious with minimum symptoms until complications have already set in.

Cataract, glaucoma, band keratopathy, and synechiae are all consequences of the basic inflammation.

2. **Nonocular** aspects of JRA can be subdivided into (1) systemic disease with arthritic disease and (2) two forms of joint disease with less prominent systemic manifestations: polyarticular arthritis and pauciarticular arthritis. Ocular disease is extremely rare in systemic disease with arthritic disease. It is uncommon in the polyarticular variety and is most often seen in youngsters, especially girls, with only a few joints involved. It is associated with ANA positivity and HLA class II antigens, e.g., HLA-DR5. The ocular inflammation may come long after the arthritis has completely resolved or may precede the onset of arthritis. Since the early stages of ocular inflammation are asymptomatic in JRA, it seems wisest to examine these youngsters routinely every 4–6 months. Therapy of the iritis involves the use of topical steroids and topical mydriatics (see Chap. 8, sec. **VIII.D**).

B. **Ankylosing spondylitis**

1. **Iridocyclitis** of ankylosing spondylitis is usually highly symptomatic. When the inflammation begins, the patient has photophobia and discomfort in the eye, and the eye has a "ciliary" or limbal injection. The iridocyclitis is acute and remits with topical steroids and mydriatic-cycloplegics, but it may be recurrent (see Chap. 8, sec. **VIII.B**).

2. **The tissue-type antigen HLA-B27** is relatively uncommon in the normal population (6%) but is very prevalent in the population with ankylosing spondylitis (90%). Fifty percent of all patients with acute anterior uveitis, regardless of cause, have positive HLA-B27. Patients with JRA do not differ significantly from the population with anterior uveitis in general, 42% of them being HLA-B27 positive.

C. **Peripheral uveitis** is a chronic inflammation that may present as iridocyclitis. The diagnosis does not become apparent until a careful examination of the peripheral retina is performed and until cellular debris is found in "snowbanks" along the vitreous base. The etiology is not clear. Systemic corticosteroids or periocular steroid injections can reduce the inflammation, but in view of the chronic nature of the disorder, these therapies are usually reserved for microcystic edema of the macula or intense vitreous involvement that reduces vision (see Chap. 8, sec. **IX**).

D. **Erythema multiforme.** The conjunctiva along with other mucous membranes may become inflamed in severe erythema multiforme. Cleansing of the lids and lubrication with bland antibiotic ointments are recommended. Topical steroids and sweeping of the fornices have been advocated as therapies and have some theoretic justification, but conclusive evidence for their efficacy has not been presented. **Herpes simplex** must be thoroughly excluded in the differential diagnosis before topical steroid administration is considered.

E. **Pseudotumor of the orbit** is a poorly understood cause of recurrent orbital inflammation and proptosis. The diagnosis is generally made only by exclusion of other causes. Regression of the orbital mass after systemic corticosteroids has been helpful diagnostically and therapeutically.

V. **Principles of genetics and genetic counseling**

A. **Basic genetic principles.** Hereditary characteristics are carried on loci on the chromosomes called *genes.* The normal number of human chromosomes is 46, one-half being inherited from the father and one-half from the mother. There are 22 pairs of autosomes plus, in the female, two X chromosomes and, in the male, an X and a Y chromosome. Deviations from the normal number of chromosomes, either extra chromosomal material or deficient chromosomal material, cause severe abnormalities.

1. **Alleles.** The alternative forms that genes in a particular locus on a chromosome may take are called *alleles.* An individual who inherits the same gene from both parents is called *homozygous.* If the two allelic genes are different, the individual is said to be *heterozygous.* The sex chromosomes are paired in the female (two X chromosomes), and the male has an X and a Y chromosome. The X chromosome contains much more genetic material

than the Y. In the male, the genetic material on his single X chromosome is not paired. The male is said to be *hemizygous* for the characteristics represented by the genes on his single X chromosome.

2. **Inheritance and expression of genetic traits.** The individual's genetic makeup as inherited from his or her parents is known as the *genotype.* These inherited characteristics may or may not be expressed in a way that affects the individual's appearance or functioning. The outward expression of the genotype is called the *phenotype.* The phenotype depends on the mode of inheritance of various characteristics. It may also be affected by the environment.

3. **Modes of inheritance.** The three modes of inheritance are dominant, recessive, and X-linked.

   a. In **dominant inheritance,** the expression of a specific trait is determined by only one of the pair of genes and is not affected by its allele. Therefore, an individual with a dominantly inherited disease will be affected when one of the allelic genes is abnormal even if the other one is normal. Examples of dominantly inherited disorders are Marfan's syndrome and neurofibromatosis. Both alleles may be expressed simultaneously, in which case they are called *codominant.* An example would be in the hemoglobinopathies, in which both members of the pair of genes will be expressed phenotypically. Thus, an individual may be AA (normal), SA (sickle trait), SS (sickle cell disease), or SC (sickle-C disease). Dominantly inherited diseases are not expressed in all individuals who carry the gene but may still be passed on to the offspring of unaffected carriers.

   b. In **recessive inheritance,** the expression of the trait determined by a recessive gene is masked by the presence of its allele. An innocuous example would be a gene for blue eyes being masked by the gene for brown eyes, so that an individual who is heterozygous for eye color would have brown eyes. Many metabolic disorders are inherited recessively (see sec. **VII**). Individuals who are heterozygous for recessively inherited disorders (carriers) generally have a normal phenotype but may be identifiable biochemically. For example, individuals heterozygous for Tay-Sachs disease may be identified because they have less than the normal concentration of the enzyme hexosaminidase-A, but this partial deficiency is not enough to cause abnormal function. The homozygote is severely and fatally affected by an almost total absence of the enzyme.

   Patients who are homozygous for a recessively inherited disease may be protected by their environment from phenotypic expression of the disorder. This protection may, in fact, form the basis for treatment. Patients with galactosemia (deficiency of the enzyme galactose-1-phosphate uridyl transferase) who are not exposed to galactose in the diet will remain normal.

   c. In **X-linked inheritance,** affected males manifest traits carried on the X chromosome, i.e., they are hemizygous. Carrier females have the normal allele on one of the paired X chromosomes. A classic example of X-linked inheritance is red-green **color blindness.** Carrier females, with only one abnormal gene for color blindness and a normal allele on the other X chromosome, have normal color vision. Affected males, having only the gene for protanopia (red blindness) or deuteranopia (green blindness), are color blind. Heterozygote female carriers of X-linked disorders may sometimes be phenotypically identified or may express the disease in milder form than their hemizygous sons. An explanation of this phenomenon is the **Lyon hypothesis.** Each cell of a female acts as if one or the other of her X chromosomes is inactivated, so that only one of each of the allelic genes on the chromosomes can be expressed. This would make each female a mosaic in which about one-half of the cells have one X chromosome active and the other one-half have the other X chromosome active. Heterozygous females in Fabry disease exhibit the ocular findings, but not such severe and ultimately fatal systemic manifestations as their hemizygous male relatives suffer (see sec. **VII.B.7**).

B. **Genetic counseling.** The psychosocial aspects of genetic counseling are important. When an abnormal child is born to a set of parents, there is psychic trauma, including feelings of guilt, which may be aggravated if the disorder is inherited. If the parents want more children, they will need to be advised about the chances of producing another affected offspring. The physician's role is to advise the parents what the chances are of having further affected offspring and to explain ways of preventing the birth of an unwanted affected offspring, if the parents so desire. The physician must refrain from advising the parents whether or not to have more children. The parents should make the decision, based on the best information the physician can give. In some straightforward cases, the ophthalmologist can provide the genetic counseling; in more complicated situations, the parents should be referred to a clinical geneticist.

1. **Autosomal recessive disorders.** If a child has a disorder recognized to be recessively inherited, each of the parents must be phenotypically unaffected carriers of the abnormal recessive gene; i.e., each parent must be heterozygous for the abnormality. Chances of future offspring being affected can be calculated by recognizing that one-half of the mother's eggs and one-half of the father's sperm will contain the normal gene and the other one-half the abnormal allele. There is a 25% chance that both normal genes will be present in the offspring, a 25% chance that both abnormal genes will be present in the offspring, producing an individual homozygous for the disease, and a 50% chance that the offspring will be heterozygous for the abnormal gene (25% of the offspring will get a normal gene from the father and an abnormal gene from the mother, and 25% will get an abnormal gene from the father and a normal gene from the mother). These heterozygotes will be phenotypically normal; therefore, it can be predicted that **each** future offspring will have a 25% chance of being abnormal and a 75% chance of being normal. It will depend on the family situation and the nature of the disorder whether the parents will find these odds acceptable or unacceptable for having further children.

Fortunately, in a few instances of recessively inherited diseases, diagnosis of the disease can be made antenatally in the fetus through **amniocentesis.** The classic example is **Tay-Sachs disease.** Genetic counseling may begin even before marriage. This gangliosidosis has a much higher incidence in individuals with Ashkenazic Jewish ancestry (4%) than in the general population. The deficiency of hexosaminidase-A can be identified in the heterozygous carriers, so Ashkenazic Jewish populations can be screened and individuals advised of their genotype for this illness. Heterozygous individuals may decide not to marry each other or to refrain from having children. In families where such premarital screening has not occurred, with the birth of a child affected with Tay-Sachs disease, **amniocentesis** can provide a way of avoiding the birth of future affected offspring. If further children are desired, cells from the fetus can be obtained by amniocentesis and grown in tissue culture so the level of hexosaminidase-A can be measured. If the fetus is identified as lacking the enzyme, the parents may elect therapeutic abortion. If the fetus is a heterozygote, or homozygous normal, the pregnancy can be carried to term. Unfortunately, biochemical assays that may be performed after amniocentesis are currently limited to only a few inherited diseases.

2. **Dominantly inherited disorders.** An individual who is affected with a dominantly inherited disorder is known to be carrying an abnormal gene that is presumably paired with a normal allele. Fifty percent of the gametes, i.e., eggs or sperm, of the affected individual will have the abnormal gene and 50% will be normal. Since all gametes from the other parent will presumably be normal, each offspring has a 50% chance of being born with the domi-

nantly inherited gene. Because of partial penetrance of most dominant genes, somewhat less than 50% of the offspring will be phenotypically affected.

3. **X-linked recessive disorders.** Female carriers of X-linked recessively inherited disorders can often be identified because they have some phenotypic characteristic. They may also be identified by tracing the family tree. The daughter of a man affected with an X-linked recessive characteristic must be a carrier, since one of her X chromosomes to make her a female must have come from her father. Since a male must get his single X chromosome from his mother, he cannot inherit an X-linked recessive characteristic from his father. An affected maternal uncle may help to identify a mother as a carrier. Each of a female carrier's sons will have a 50% chance of inheriting the X-linked recessive characteristic. When a woman is known to be a carrier of a severe X-linked recessive disorder, amniocentesis and therapeutic abortion may be used to prevent the birth of male offspring, each of whom has a 50% chance of being affected. Chromosomal analysis can be performed on the fetal cells to determine the sex of the fetus.

If the parents are opposed to therapeutic abortion on religious grounds, amniocentesis should not be offered since the information gained would be of no therapeutic significance. Since the procedure carries a small risk to the mother and to the possibly normal fetus, it should be performed only if the information gathered will be used.

VI. **Chromosomal abnormalities**

A. **Basic principles.** Chromosomes are classified according to their microscopic morphology into eight groups, A through G, and numbered from 1 through 22, plus the X and Y chromosomes. Different chromosomes and different regions of each chromosome may be distinguished by staining techniques called *banding.* The centromere of each chromosome divides it into long and short arms. The short arm is represented by "p" and the long arm by "q." Chromosomes are prepared for analysis by culturing tissues, most commonly skin fibroblasts or leukocytes, arresting the cell division in metaphase by use of colchicine, and staining the chromosomes appropriately for microscopic examination.

Two kinds of abnormal occurrences during meiosis (cell division leading to gamete formation) may lead to chromosomal abnormalities: **nondysjunction** and **translocation.** In normal meiosis, each pair of chromosomes contributes one chromosome to each daughter cell so that each egg or sperm has 23 single chromosomes (the haploid number).

1. In **nondysjunction,** the two chromosomes of a specific pair remain together; as a result, one of the daughter cells gets both chromosomes and the other gets neither. If the gamete (daughter cell) receiving both chromosomes of a pair combines with a normal gamete during fertilization, the resulting zygotes will contain an extra chromosome. This is called **trisomy.** If the gamete that is missing the chromosome in question entirely combines with a normal gamete during fertilization, the resulting zygote will have only a single chromosome of the pair in question. This deletion produces **monosomy.**

2. **Translocation** can produce partial trisomies or deletions. During formation of the gamete, chromosomal breakage may occur and genetic material may be exchanged between chromosomes. If this exchange is uneven, part of the original chromosome will be duplicated in one of the new chromosomes, and part will be missing in the other. This leads to a **partial trisomy** or partial deletion. Trisomy 13 and trisomy 21 are usually due to nondysjunction but sometimes may be due to translocation. Except for Turner's syndrome, which is caused by deletion of an entire X chromosome, the major chromosomal deletion syndromes are due to partial deletion secondary to translocation.

3. **Chromosomal mosaicism** is the condition in which some of an individual's cells contain the trisomy or the deletion and others contain the normal number of chromosomes. These individuals may be less severely affected phenotypically.

B. The most common **trisomies that produce ocular abnormalities** are trisomy 13 (D trisomy or Patau syndrome), trisomy 18 (E trisomy or Edwards syndrome), and trisomy 21 (G trisomy or Down syndrome).

1. Trisomy 13 (D trisomy, Patau syndrome). The life expectancy is only a few months, so even though the eyes are severely affected, the ophthalmologist's role is limited mainly to help in diagnosis.

  a. The **ocular findings** of trisomy 13 are

    (1) Microphthalmus.

    (2) Colobomas (almost 100%).

    (3) Communication of extraocular connective tissue with intraocular hyaloid system via ciliary body coloboma.

    (4) Intraocular cartilage.

    (5) Retinal dysplasia.

    (6) Cataracts.

    (7) Corneal opacities.

    (8) Optic nerve hypoplasia.

    (9) Cyclopia.

  b. The **systemic findings** are

    (1) Failure to thrive, death within first few months of life.

    (2) Congenital heart disease.

    (3) Hernias.

    (4) Cryptorchidism in males.

    (5) Bicornuate uterus in females.

    (6) Scalp defect.

    (7) Arrhinencephaly.

    (8) Mental retardation.

    (9) Wide fontanelles.

    (10) Apneic spells.

    (11) Seizures.

    (12) Deafness.

    (13) Microcephaly.

    (14) Cleft lip and palate.

    (15) Polydactyly.

    (16) Simian crease.

    (17) Hyperconvex, narrow fingernails.

    (18) Posterior prominence of heel.

2. Trisomy 18 (E trisomy, Edwards syndrome). These patients survive less than 1 year, so the ophthalmologist's role is limited mainly to help in diagnosis.

  a. The major **ocular findings** are

    (1) Epicanthal folds.

    (2) Blepharophimosis.

    (3) Ptosis.

    (4) Hypertelorism.

    (5) Corneal opacities.

    (6) Microphthalmus.

    (7) Congenital glaucoma.

    (8) Uveal colobomas.

  b. The major **systemic findings** are:

    (1) Death within first year.

    (2) Mental deficiency.

    (3) Decreased growth.

    (4) Congenital heart disease.

    (5) Cryptorchidism.

    (6) Hernias.

    (7) Hypoplasia of muscle and subcutaneous fat.

    (8) Prominent occiput, narrow bifrontal diameter.

    (9) Low-set, malformed ears.

    (10) Micrognathia.

      (11) Microstomia, narrow palatal arch.
      (12) Hypertonicity.
      (13) Camptodactyly.
      (14) Overlapping of index finger over third and fifth finger over fourth.
      (15) Rocker-bottom feet, prominent heels.
      (16) Hypoplasia of nails.
3. Trisomy 21 (Down syndrome). Patients with trisomy 21 have nearly normal life spans, and the ophthalmologist will be called on to follow the patients and to intervene when necessary. Correction of high refractive errors, treatment of blepharitis and amblyopia associated with esotropia, and surgical treatment of cataracts may all be necessary to help these patients function optimally.

  a. The major **ocular findings** are
      (1) Upward slanting palpebral fissures.
      (2) Almond-shaped palpebral fissures.
      (3) Epicanthus.
      (4) Telecanthus.
      (5) Narrowed interpupillary distance.
      (6) Esotropia (35%).
      (7) Blepharitis.
      (8) High refractive errors.
      (9) Cataracts.
      (10) Brushfield's spots.
      (11) Iris hypoplasia.
      (12) Keratoconus.

  b. The major **systemic findings** are
      (1) Mental deficiency.
      (2) Small stature.
      (3) Defective, awkward gait.
      (4) Congenital heart disease.
      (5) Dry, rough skin.
      (6) Brachycephaly.
      (7) Small nose.
      (8) Small, round external ears.
      (9) Thick, protruding tongue.
      (10) Dental hypoplasia.
      (11) Short, thick neck.
      (12) Hypotonia.
      (13) Small, broad, stubby hands and incurved little finger.
      (14) Simian crease.
      (15) Short, broad feet with gap between first and second toes.
      (16) Renal hemangiomas.
      (17) Infertility.
      (18) Undescended testes.
      (19) Duodenal atresia.
      (20) Cleft lip and palate.

C. The major **chromosomal deletions** that have been associated with ocular abnormalities include 5p− syndrome (**cri-du-chat** syndrome), in which part of the short arm of the 5 chromosome is missing; 11p− syndrome, in which part of the short arm of the 11 chromosome is missing; 13q− syndrome, in which part of the long arm of the 13 chromosome is deleted; 18q− syndrome (**De-Grouchy** syndrome), in which the long arm of the 18 chromosome is deleted; and XO syndrome (**Turner** syndrome), in which an entire X chromosome is missing. The ocular and systemic abnormalities of these syndromes are listed in Table 10-1.

Patients with 5p−, 13q−, and 18q− syndromes are almost always severely retarded and require institutionalization. The ophthalmologist may help in the identification and diagnosis of these patients. (Rarely, patients with 13q− have **retinoblastoma** as the only finding and are of normal intelligence.) Patients

Table 10-1. Chromosomal deletion syndromes

Syndrome	Chromosome	Ocular signs	Systemic signs
Cri-du-chat	5p-	Hypertelorism, epicanthus, antimongoloid slant, strabismus	Retardation, mewing cry, microcephaly, hypotonia, failure to thrive, low ears, round face, micrognathia, high palate, simian crease
	11p-	Aniridia, glaucoma, foveal hypoplasia nystagmus, ptosis	Wilms' tumor, genitourinary anomalies, retardation, prominent bridge of nose
	13q-	Retinoblastoma, hypertelorism, microphthalmus, epicanthus, ptosis, coloboma, cataract	Retardation, microcephaly, trigonocephaly, low-set malformed ears, micrognathia, congenital heart disease, hypoplastic or absent thumb, foot anomalies
DeGrouchy	18q-	Hypertelorism, epicanthus, ptosis, strabismus, myopia, glaucoma, microphthalmus (with or without cyst), coloboma, optic atrophy, corneal opacity	Retardation, microcephaly, low birth weight, midface hypoplasia, prominent forehead and jaw, fish mouth
Turner	XO	Antimongoloid slant, epicanthus, ptosis, strabismus, blue sclera, eccentric pupils, cataract, male incidence of red-green color defects, coloboma, retinitis pigmentosa–like fundus	Short, webbed neck, low posterior hairline, broad chest, widely spaced nipples, nevi, congenital heart disease, genitourinary anomalies

with Turner syndrome, however, are generally of normal intelligence and will benefit from treatment of their ophthalmologic defects.

D. Genetic counseling in chromosomal anomalies. Most trisomies are sporadic in their occurrence, although the chance of a future sibling of a child with Down syndrome being affected is slightly increased. The chance of giving birth to a child with Down syndrome increases with maternal age, approaching 1% by age 40. In translocation Down syndrome, chromosomal analysis on the parents may identify one of them as having a balanced translocation, with material missing from a 21 chromosome and attached to another chromosome. This greatly increases the chances of an offspring being affected. Similarly, parents of patients with partial deletions may be identified as having balanced translocations, making the risk for their future offspring great. Parents with such translocations may decide to have no more children. Alternatively, parents may elect **amniocentesis** with chromosomal analysis on fetal cells to identify an affected fetus.

VII. Inherited metabolic disorders

A. The mucopolysaccharidoses (MPS) are caused by deficiencies of enzymes responsible for the turnover of mucopolysaccharides. These enzymopathies cause abnormal tissue accumulation and urinary excretion of certain mucopolysaccharides and a variety of systemic and ocular abnormalities. The mucopolysaccharidoses are classified by number and eponym. All but one are inherited as autosomal recessive disorders.

1. **MPS I-H (Hurler syndrome)** is an autosomal recessively inherited disorder with skeletal and facial dysmorphism, mental retardation, and corneal clouding. Retinal pigmentary degeneration and optic atrophy have been reported. Activity of the enzyme alpha-L-iduronidase is deficient, and the patients excrete increased amounts of heparan sulfate and dermatan sulfate in the urine.

2. **MPS I-S (Scheie syndrome,** formerly MPS V) is inherited as an autosomal recessive with the gene at the same locus as the gene for Hurler syndrome. The major difficulty in these patients is corneal clouding, which is accompanied by very mild facial and skeletal dysmorphism and usually normal intelligence. Retinal pigmentary degeneration and optic atrophy have been reported. Deficiency of alpha-L-iduronidase (the same enzyme as in Hurler syndrome) is less severe, and the same mucopolysaccharides are excreted in the urine. MPS I-H/S is a genetic compound of MPS I-H and MPS I-S genes. The phenotype is intermediate.

3. **MPS II (Hunter syndrome)** is an X-linked recessive disorder that occurs in two phenotypes: A and B. In severely affected boys (MPS II A), the skeletal and facial dysmorphism is milder but reminiscent of that in Hurler syndrome, but there is no corneal clouding. Mental retardation is present. In the milder phenotype (MPS II B), there is less severe dysmorphism, and the intelligence is less handicapped. These patients have rarely been reported to develop mild corneal clouding later in life. Retinal pigmentary degeneration and optic atrophy have been reported in both phenotypes. The enzyme L-iduronosulfate sulfatase is deficient, and heparan sulfate and dermatan sulfate are excreted in excessive amounts in the urine in both types.

4. **MPS III (Sanfilippo syndrome)** occurs in four forms: A, in which heparan N-sulfatase is the deficient enzyme; B, in which alpha-N-acetylglucosaminidase is the deficient enzyme; C, in which acetyl coenzyme A–alpha-glucosaminide-N-acetyltransferase is deficient; and D, in which N-acetyl-alpha-D-glucosaminide-6-sulfatase is deficient. They are recessively inherited, but they are not allelic and are classified together because of their phenotypic similarity. These children have normal appearance with mild dysmorphism, but they are severely retarded and may have seizures. Corneal clouding has not been described in either, but retinal pigmentary degeneration and optic atrophy have been reported. There is excessive excretion of heparan sulfate in the urine in all four types.

5. **MPS IV (Morquio syndrome)** occurs in two autosomal recessively inherited forms, A and B. Skeletal dysplasia is a major feature in type A. Facial dysmorphism is unusual, and the patients are generally of normal intelligence. These children have corneal clouding that is generally less severe than that in the MPS I disorder. Retinal pigmentary degeneration has not been reported, but optic atrophy has been seen rarely. The deficient enzyme in type A is galactosamine-6-sulfate sulfatase. Patients with MPS IVB are deficient in the enzyme beta-galactosidase. They have mild skeletal dysplasia and corneal clouding. Patients of both types excrete an excessive amount of keratan sulfate.

6. **MPS V** classification is vacant now that Scheie syndrome has been reclassified (see sec. **2**).

7. **MPS VI (Maroteaux-Lamy syndrome)** occurs in three allelic phenotypes: severe, intermediate, and mild. All are inherited as autosomal recessive characteristics. Facial and skeletal dysmorphism is prominent in the first two types and mild in the last. Patients with all types are generally of normal intelligence, and corneal clouding is a prominent feature. Optic atrophy is rare in the severe phenotype and has not been reported in the others, and retinal degeneration has not been reported. There is a deficiency of

arylsulfatase B activity, and an excessive amount of dermatan sulfate is excreted in the urine.

8. **MPS VII (Sly syndrome)** is a rare autosomal recessively inherited disorder with facial and skeletal dysmorphism, mental retardation, and corneal clouding. The enzyme beta-glucuronidase is deficient, and dermatan sulfate, heparan sulfate, and chondroitin sulfate are excreted in the urine.

9. In summary, **corneal clouding** is a prominent feature of MPS I-H and I-S and is less severe in MPS IV, VI, and VII. (It may occur to a mild degree in older individuals with MPS II B.) Keratoplasty has been performed successfully in patients with Scheie syndrome. Pigmentary degeneration of the retina occurs in MPS I-H, I-S, II, and III, but not in IV or VI. Optic atrophy occurs in all types except VI B. Facial dysmorphism is prominent in MPS I-H, II, and VI; skeletal dysplasia is present in all these as well as in MPS IV. Patients with MPS I-H, II A, and III are severely mentally retarded, whereas patients with MPS I-S, II B, IV, and VI are generally of normal or near-normal intelligence.

B. The **sphingolipidoses** are characterized by enzyme deficiencies that interfere with the normal hydrolysis of certain sphingolipids. Because of this lack of ability to metabolize the lipid, it accumulates in abnormal amounts in the CNS or the viscera or both. Metachromatic leukodystrophy, often considered with the sphingolipidoses, and G_{M1} gangliosidosis are discussed under the mucolipidoses (see sec. **C**).

1. G_{M2} **gangliosidosis type I (Tay-Sachs disease)** is the best known of the sphingolipidoses. Approximately 65–80% of the patients are of Ashkenazic Jewish ancestry. With the exception of unusual sensitivity to sound, infants with Tay-Sachs disease develop normally until the age of 6 or 7 months. A **cherry-red spot** in the macula can be seen as early as 2 months of age. It is caused by a deficiency of hexosaminidase A, which leads to accumulation of G_{M2} ganglioside in the ganglion cells of the retina. These cells occur in greater numbers around the macula. Severe CNS manifestations, including dementia, spasticity, blindness, and deafness, are caused by similar accumulation in the large neurons of the gray matter. As the ganglion cells die from the effects of excessive lipid accumulation, the cherry-red spot gradually fades and the optic disk develops atrophy. The patients are generally blind by 18 months of age and die by age 3.

2. A similar clinical course may be expected in G_{M2} **gangliosidosis type II (Sandhoff disease).** In this disorder both globoside and G_{M2} ganglioside accumulate, due to a lack of both hexosaminidase A and B enzymes. There is no specific ethnic predisposition in Sandhoff disease.

3. In G_{M2} **gangliosidosis type III** there is no cherry-red spot in the macula, but there may be pigmentary retinopathy, and optic atrophy is usually present. These children become blind later in the course of the disease than in Tay-Sachs disease and Sandhoff disease.

4. **Type A (infantile) Niemann-Pick disease.** This recessively inherited disease is characterized by accumulation of sphingomyelin and cholesterol in the viscera, causing hepatosplenomegaly, and in the brain, causing severely retarded psychomotor development. The enzyme sphingomyelinase is deficient. The cornea is slightly cloudy and there is a brown discoloration of the anterior lens capsule as well as a macular cherry-red spot in most cases. Patients with this infantile form of Niemann-Pick disease have a life span about the same as Tay-Sachs, i.e., 2–3 years. The other three or more phenotypes of Niemann-Pick disease are either much less common or do not become manifest in childhood.

5. **Globoid cell leukodystrophy (Krabbe's disease)** is a recessively inherited deficiency of beta-galactosidase that causes accumulation of galactocerebroside. It produces an early and rapidly progressive CNS degeneration and optic atrophy with blindness. A cherry-red spot is not a feature of Krabbe's disease. The life span is about 2 years.

6. **Gaucher disease,** also recessively inherited, occurs in at least three types.

A defect in beta-glucosidase causes accumulation of glucocerebroside in the viscera and probably the nervous system. The infantile variety usually leads to death within a year or two of age. The eyes are normal in the infantile type and in the extremely rare juvenile type.

7. **Angiokeratoma corporis diffusum universale (Fabry disease)** is distinguished from the other sphingolipidoses by being inherited as an X-linked recessive, by having normal intelligence without the severe CNS effects of other sphingolipid accumulations, and by having systemic manifestations. Characteristic skin lesions (angiokeratomas) are present on the trunk, and hemizygous males are subject to recurrent fevers and episodes of severe abdominal and limb pain. The lipid accumulation in blood vessels causes severe renal disease and may cause cerebrovascular disease. The most characteristic eye manifestation, seen best with the slit lamp, is a striking whorl-like corneal epithelial opacity radiating out in curved lines from a spot just inferior to the center of the cornea. Characteristic star-shaped radiating lines of opacity are found in the posterior lens as well as strikingly kinky conjunctival and retinal blood vessels. Heterozygous female carriers usually manifest these ocular findings. They may also suffer from the systemic manifestations, though much less severely than the hemizygous males.

C. **The mucolipidoses** present some phenotypic and chemical features that overlap the mucopolysaccharidoses on one hand and the sphingolipidoses on the other. The various disorders in this group may have the facial and skeletal dysmorphism of the mucopolysaccharidoses and accumulate mucopolysaccharides in the viscera, as well as exhibiting corneal clouding in some of the disorders. With the exception of juvenile sulfatidosis and G_{M1} gangliosidosis, however, these patients do not excrete excessive amounts of mucopolysaccharide in the urine. Features overlapping with the sphingolipidoses include early progressive neurologic deterioration and, in some of the disorders, a cherry-red spot in the macula. The mucolipidoses are all recessively inherited.

1. **G_{M1} gangliosidosis,** infantile form, is somewhat reminiscent of Hurler syndrome, with corneal clouding, facial and skeletal dysmorphism, but also usually a cherry-red spot and optic atrophy. Both keratan sulfate and G_{M1} ganglioside accumulate in the tissues because of a deficiency of lysosomal beta-galactosidase.

2. **Metachromatic leukodystrophy** may rarely have corneal clouding but commonly has a pigmentary change in the macula and optic atrophy. Because of the lack of the arylsulfatase enzymes, both sulfated acid mucopolysaccharides and sphingolipid sulfatide accumulate.

3. **Sialidosis** (formerly mucolipidosis I) exhibits a deficiency in alpha-neuraminidase.

   a. **Type I.** The patients have a cherry-red spot and myoclonus but somatically appear normal.

   b. **Type II.** There are coarse features, cherry-red spot, myoclonus, and ataxia.

4. Two disorders of lysosomal synthesis have failure of acid hydrolase incorporation into lysosomes. **I-cell disease** exhibits Hurler-like features and mild corneal clouding and **pseudo-Hurler polydystrophy** has stiff joints and mild peripheral corneal clouding later. These disorders were formerly classified as mucolipidosis II and III.

5. **Farber lipogranulomatosis** may produce ocular inflammation as well as macular pigmentary change. It is characterized most dramatically by arthropathy and subcutaneous swellings caused by formation of histocytic granulomas. An intracellular accumulation of a ceramide occurs in and around joints, viscera, retinal ganglion cells, and brain caused by a deficiency of acid ceramidase.

D. **Neuronal ceroid lipofuscinosis (Batten-Mayou disease)** is characterized by mental deterioration and by a pigmentary retinopathy involving most severely the macula, with loss of central vision. Optic atrophy also occurs. Cherry-red spots are not seen. The onset is usually in the first decade, less commonly in the second decade. The peripheral leukocytes in both affected homozygous patients and unaffected heterozygotes may have characteristic abundant azurophilic granules. The pathologic changes include loss of the outer segments and pigment epithelium of the retina and accumulation of ceroid-lipofuscin in various tissues (histologic examination of ganglion cells on rectal biopsy may help make the diagnosis), including the retinal pigment epithelium and CNS. No specific enzyme defect has been identified, but there are lysosomal inclusions on electron microscopy. This disease occurs in four types:

1. **Infantile,** with blindness by age 2 and death by age 5.
2. **Late infantile.**
3. **Juvenile,** with optic atrophy and macular degeneration by age 4–8 and death in adolescence.
4. **Adult,** with severe CNS deterioration, often with blindness, without clinical ocular signs.

E. **Aminoacidurias.** Most aminoacidurias are recessively inherited.

1. **Homocystinuria** is inherited as an autosomal recessive and is due to the absence of the enzyme cystathionine synthetase. Some affected individuals are helped by **pyridoxine therapy.** Subluxed lenses (ectopia lentis) are characteristic. Patients may also have myopia, retinal detachment, glaucoma, and optic atrophy. Patients are frequently hypopigmented and are usually mentally retarded or have a peculiar affect. They may suffer from osteoporosis. Special care must be taken if a patient requires ocular surgery with general anesthesia because of the tendency to arterial and venous thromboses.

2. **Cystinosis** is inherited as an autosomal recessive disorder. A lysosomal transport defect causes intracellular accumulation of cystine. The deposition of cystine crystals in the cornea causes photophobia. Such crystals are also deposited in the conjunctiva and choroid. They may be readily seen on slit-lamp examination. Pigmentary and degenerative changes may occur in the retinal periphery. The disease has severe systemic manifestations of renal tubular acidosis, with renal rickets and eventual renal failure leading to death. Benign cystinosis is an unrelated adult disorder.

3. **Oculocerebrorenal syndrome (Lowe syndrome)** is an X-linked recessive characteristic with an unknown enzyme defect. It may be due to deficient amino acid transport. The eye involvement is very severe and includes cataract, microphakia, and severe congenital glaucoma. The glaucoma is due to malformation of the filtration angle or to subluxed lenses. The systemic abnormalities include metabolic acidosis (which makes anesthesia more difficult, complicating surgery of the cataracts and glaucoma), rickets, mental and growth retardation with hypotonia, and, usually, early death.

4. **Cerebrohepatorenal syndrome (Zellweger syndrome)** is autosomally recessively inherited. The specific enzyme defect is unknown, but aminoaciduria is a prominent feature. The eye involvement includes a characteristic hypoplasia of the superior orbital margins, with resultant flat brow and prominent eyes. The patient may also have a characteristic "leopard spot" peripheral retinal pigmentation, as well as cataracts, congenital glaucoma, and optic nerve hypoplasia. Patients are severely retarded secondary to cerebral dysgenesis, and they have microcystic kidneys and hepatic dysgenesis. Life expectancy is less than 1 year; therefore, ophthalmologic treatment is moot.

5. **Galactosemia** is an autosomal recessive deficiency of galactose-1-phosphate uridyltransferase. It is included here because aminoaciduria is a prominent part of the picture. Accumulation of galactose causes sugar cataracts in infancy that, in their early stages, can be reversed by a galactose-free diet. The severe systemic manifestations include failure to thrive, vomiting, hepatomegaly, jaundice, and aminoaciduria, all of which can also be reversed by a galactose-free diet.

6. **Galactokinase deficiency** is an autosomal recessively inherited deficiency of the enzyme galactokinase. There are no systemic manifestations; the

cataracts that form when the child is exposed to galactose are the presenting finding. If the problem is recognized early enough, the **cataracts are reversible** by a galactose-free diet.

F. Miscellaneous disorders of connective tissue

1. **Arachnodactyly (Marfan syndrome)** is inherited as an autosomal dominant. Patients exhibit skeletal abnormalities including arachnodactyly, laxity of the joints, tall stature, scoliosis, and sternal deformities. They may suffer from dissecting aneurysms of the thoracic aorta and aortic and mitral valvular disease. They are of normal intelligence. No chemical abnormality has been identified; therefore, no confirmatory laboratory tests are available. The most important ocular manifestation is ectopia lentis, which occurs in about 80% of the patients. The usual direction of dislocation is upward, but the lens may be dislocated in any direction. In contrast, dislocation of the lens in homocystinuria is usually downward. Other ocular abnormalities include strabismus, myopia (sometimes with retinal changes), glaucoma, filtration angle anomalies, retinal detachment, and blue sclerae. The subluxation of the lens may cause high degrees of astigmatism, and patients require frequent refractions. There is some **risk in dilating the pupils,** especially chronically, because of the danger of dislocation of the lens into the anterior chamber. Generally, the lens should not be extracted unless it becomes cataractous or unless it is dislocated into the anterior chamber and cannot be made to return posteriorly by dilating the pupil and positioning the patient supinely.

2. **Osteogenesis imperfecta** may be inherited as either an autosomal dominant or autosomal recessive disorder. Recessive inheritance generally is associated with more severe skeletal anomalies. The bones are fragile and fracture easily, sometimes spontaneously, causing deformities, especially of the long bones. Blue sclerae are characteristic because of the thinness of the sclerae. The corneas are also thin and vulnerable to laceration and rupture from relatively minor trauma. Keratoconus, megalocornea, embryotoxon, and glaucoma may occur. Protective spectacles with safety glass and sturdy frames should be prescribed for patients who are not bedridden.

3. **Disorders associated with angioid streaks of the retina. Angioid streaks** are cracks in Bruch's membrane of the retinal pigment epithelium (RPE). They may interfere with visual acuity if they involve the macular area. Generally, **no treatment** is indicated, but **photocoagulation** has been advocated for neovascularization in an angioid streak not yet involving the macula. The most common disorders associated with angioid streaks are listed below:

   a. **Pseudoxanthoma elasticum** is a recessively inherited disorder. Affected areas of the skin have small yellow papules and plaques. Eventually, affected skin may hang in loose folds. The most commonly affected skin is in the axillae, the antecubital and popliteal fossae, and the sides of the neck. Similar papules and plaques in the stomach may cause gastrointestinal bleeding.

   b. **Ehlers-Danlos syndrome** is an autosomal dominant condition with hyperelasticity of the skin, hyperextensibility of the joints, and fragility of the tissue, sometimes resulting in bleeding. Keratoconus, microcornea, blue sclera retinal hemorrhages, angioid streaks, and retinal detachments may occur.

   c. **Paget's disease of the bone** is dominantly inherited. Its major manifestation is thickening of the bones, most prominently of the skull. Angioid streaks usually occur relatively late in adult life.

   d. **Sickle cell anemia** is a codominantly inherited disease that causes severe anemia and multiple thromboembolic crises. Other eye manifestations are more prominent than the angioid streaks (see sec. **XVII.E**).

G. Hepatolenticular degeneration (Wilson's disease) is inherited as an autosomal recessive. In children it usually presents as hepatic disease. In older adolescents and young adults a more common presentation is progressive neurologic disease and ataxia from deposition of copper in the CNS, especially in the basal ganglia. Its major manifestation in the eye is the Kayser-Fleischer ring in the cornea. This is a brownish or golden deposition of copper in the peripheral portion of Descemet's membrane. In early cases it may be visible only on slit-lamp examination. A brownish discoloration of the anterior lens capsule in a petallike distribution (the sunflower cataract) may also be seen. Copper is deposited in many other tissues as well. Liver biopsies from affected homozygous individuals have 20–30 times the normal concentration of copper. Usually the level of ceruloplasmin, which binds copper in the serum, and the level of copper in serum are low. **Treatment** is necessary to avoid irreversible liver damage and basal ganglion damage. It consists of a low-copper diet and treatment with a chelating agent, penicillamine. As treatment progresses, the Kayser-Fleischer rings may diminish.

H. **Albinism.** The three most common and important types of albinism from an ophthalmologist's point of view are (1) tyrosinase-negative oculocutaneous albinism, (2) tyrosinase-positive oculocutaneous albinism, both of which are inherited as autosomal recessives, and (3) X-linked ocular albinism. Other, much rarer forms of albinism may be associated with a variety of other anomalies. All types are associated with abnormal crossing of nerve fibers in the chiasm.

1. **Tyrosinase-negative oculocutaneous albinism.** These patients are generally almost completely devoid of pigment. They have pink skin and white hair, including the eyelashes and eyelids. Irides are light blue and transilluminate markedly. Transillumination is best accomplished by making the room completely dark and placing the tip of a shielded transilluminator against the lower eyelid with the patient's eye open. In normal individuals the light will come through the pupil only, but in albinos a red reflex will be seen through the iris as well. Patients with oculocutaneous albinism have macular hypoplasia or aplasia and generally have very poor vision and sensory nystagmus. They also have a tendency toward high refractive errors, especially myopia. They require correction of their refractive errors and help with low-vision aids. Their lack of pigmentation makes them sensitive to bright light, and they may require sunglasses for comfort. The skin is also sensitive to sun damage. Parents of affected children should be warned to avoid exposure of their children to sunlight.

2. **Tyrosinase-positive oculocutaneous albinism** is nonallelic with the tyrosinase-negative variety. A mating between these two types of albinos would produce a normally pigmented child, since the child would be heterozygous for each form of albinism. The two forms can be distinguished by a simple test in which hairs epilated from the scalp are incubated in tyrosine solution. Tyrosinase-negative albinos will show no darkening of the hair bulb. In contrast, the hair bulbs of tyrosinase-positive albinos will become much darker when incubated in tyrosine. Patients with tyrosinase-positive oculocutaneous albinism tend to show some increasing pigmentation as they grow older, and there may be some improvement in visual acuity with time. There is no good evidence, however, that the decreased pigmentation per se is directly related to the decreased visual acuity. Rather, the poor vision and nystagmus seem to be associated with macular hypoplasia.

3. **Ocular albinism** is inherited as an X-linked recessive. The affected males have normal skin and hair pigmentation, but deficient pigmentation in the eyes and macular hypoplasia with poor visual acuity. The carrier females are not entirely unaffected; they have abnormal iris transillumination and a blotchy pigmentary abnormality in the peripheral retina. They have normal visual acuity, however.

I. **Miscellaneous disorders**

1. **Achromatopsia** is an autosomal recessive difficulty. Patients have absent or markedly abnormal cone function with poor visual acuity, sensory nystagmus, and virtually complete color blindness. These patients characteristically avoid bright lights. This is not true photophobia, but an attempt to keep their rods dark-adapted so they can see. The appearance of the

fundus is normal. Achromatopsia can be diagnosed by the clinical picture and electroretinogram (ERG). **Treatment** consists of (1) correcting any refractive error, (2) fitting the patient with extra-dark sunglasses with side shields, (3) and the use of low-vision aids as required.

2. **Protan and deutan color blindness.** These two forms of color blindness are both X-linked recessive. The loci for the two forms are closely linked on the X-chromosome but are not allelic. Approximately 8–10% of the male population is hemizygous for one of these two forms of color blindness. Homozygous females are rare. Each form of color blindness can exist in a relatively mild deficiency in red sensitivity (protanomaly) or green sensitivity (deuteranomaly) or in a more complete lack of sensitivity to red (protanopia) or green (deuteranopia). The eyes of these individuals are otherwise normal, with normal visual acuity. They should be counseled to avoid occupations that require good color vision, but otherwise they will suffer no disability.

3. **Norrie's disease** is inherited as an X-linked recessive. Boys with this disorder are usually born with bilateral complete detachments of severely dysplastic or undifferentiated retinas. Occasionally, the retinal detachment may occur in early infancy rather than being congenital. The affected males are normal mentally at birth, but about 25% of them become demented or psychotic sometime during life. **Amniocentesis** and therapeutic abortion of male fetuses may be offered to carrier females.

4. **Incontinentia pigmenti** is an X-linked trait that is lethal in affected male fetuses, resulting in spontaneous abortion; consequently, the disease is seen only in females. Its name comes from the whorls of pigmented lines in the skin of the trunk and limbs. Patients may also have skeletal, dental, cardiac, and CNS anomalies. About 25% of affected individuals have eye problems, including cataracts, strabismus, optic atrophy, intraocular inflammation, microphthalmus, and retinal detachment in infancy.

5. **Aicardi's syndrome** is another disorder that is found only in females and is probably lethal in males. Its mode of inheritance is uncertain, since no familial cases have been described in the 120 cases so far reported. The fundus picture is quite striking, with lacunas of depigmented and pigmented areas of varying sizes in the fundus, mostly in the posterior pole. These lacunas may be confused with chorioretinal scars of toxoplasmosis, which they somewhat resemble, or with colobomas in atypical locations. The optic disk often exhibits a dark gray discoloration. These patients have infantile spasms with hypsarrhythmic electroencephalogram (EEG) and are severely mentally retarded. The corpus callosum is absent, and there are ectopic projections of abnormal brain tissue into the ventricles.

6. **Familial dysautonomia (Riley-Day syndrome),** an autosomal recessive, is almost exclusively seen in individuals of Ashkenazic Jewish ancestry. A deficiency in the enzyme dopamine-beta-hydroxylase interferes with the synthesis of norepinephrine and epinephrine from dopamine. Affected individuals have marked vasomotor instability with paroxysmal hypertension, abnormal sweating, relative lack of sensation, and absent fungiform papillae on the tongue. Intradermal histamine injection produces less than the normal pain and erythema. Patients suffer also from recurrent fevers and have an increased susceptibility to infection. The eyes are involved with decreased tear production and corneal hypesthesia, which may lead to drying, exposure, and corneal scarring. Because of this susceptibility to exposure keratopathy, care must be taken to protect the corneas during the periodic crises of these patients. The pupil exhibits denervation **supersensitivity to parasympathomimetic drugs.** Methacholine 2.5% or pilocarpine 0.25% will cause pupillary constriction in a Riley-Day patient but not in the normal patient. The ophthalmologist can help in the **diagnosis** of Riley-Day syndrome with this pharmacologic test.

VIII. **Phacomatoses.** The term *phacomatosis* was first introduced to unify the diverse manifestations of **tuberous sclerosis** and **neurofibromatosis.** The tumors of these two disorders arise in different organs and were recognized to be congenital aberrations.. They were called *phakomata* from the Greek *phakos,* meaning *mother spot.* The tumors may be present in the newborn child or may appear later. **Angiomatosis retinae** and **encephalotrigeminal angiomatosis** have subsequently been included in the classic phacomatoses. The concept is sufficiently vague that a large number of other diseases have been proposed to be included among the phacomatoses. **Ataxia-telangiectasia** and the **Wyburn-Mason syndrome** are often included in current discussions of phacomatoses. Some authors also include the Klippel-Trenaunay-Weber syndrome (a rare condition in which soft tissue and bony hypertrophy of an extremity is associated with a cutaneous vascular abnormality). There has also been a tendency to designate a large number of diseases as neurocutaneous disorders.

All of the classic phacomatoses are multisystem diseases. They all have at least ocular and CNS lesions, and in most of them the cutaneous manifestations are prominent. The basic lesions are **hamartomas;** that is, they are tumors consisting of those tissue components that are normally found at the involved site. This is to be contrasted with a **choristoma,** which is a tumor, such as a dermoid, composed of elements not normally found at the involved site. In some families there is evidence for autosomal dominant inheritance of tuberous sclerosis, angiomatosis retinae, and neurofibromatosis, although tuberous sclerosis and neurofibromatosis have high spontaneous occurrence rates as well. The hereditary influence is uncertain for the Sturge-Weber syndrome, although there have been reports suggesting dominant inheritance. Ataxia-telangiectasia has an autosomal recessive inheritance.

A. **Tuberous sclerosis (Bourneville disease)**
   1. **Ocular lesions.** Retinal lesions may be either large with white concretions within their substance ("mulberry" lesions) or flat and gelatinous in appearance. Pathologically, they are astrocytic hamartomas of the nerve fiber layer. They may enlarge over the years.
   2. **Cutaneous manifestations** include
      a. "Adenoma sebaceum," usually developing between 2 and 5 years of age; this is actually a misnomer since the lesion does not involve the sebaceous glands and is an angiofibroma.
      b. Ash-leaf spots of depigmentation, particularly evident under ultraviolet illumination, which may be present at birth.
      c. Periungual and subungual fibromas, often appearing after puberty.
   3. **Systemic manifestations** include
      a. CNS involvement with variable mental deficiency, seizures, and intracranial calcifications.
      b. Hamartomatous lesions of heart and kidney.
B. **Neurofibromatosis (von Recklinghausen disease)**
   1. **Ocular lesions** include
      a. Plexiform neuromas of the eyelids that may produce a characteristic S-shaped configuration of the lid margin.
      b. Optic nerve gliomas of optic nerve and chiasm.
      c. Nevoid hamartomas of the iris (Lisch nodules).
      d. Glaucoma (in some cases abnormal tissue in the filtration angle is the cause).
      e. Deficiency in sphenoid development, leading to pulsating exophthalmus.
      f. Retinal lesions (rarely).
   2. **Cutaneous manifestations** include
      a. Café au lait patches.
      b. Pedunculated skin lesions (fibrous molloscum)
      c. Plexiform neuromas.
   3. **Systemic manifestations** include
      a. CNS neurofibromas, gliomas, meningiomas, and ependymomas.
      b. Neurofibromas of the viscera.
      c. Skeletal deformities.

d. Phenochromocytomas.

e. The gene has been localized to chromosome 17 by linkage analysis.

C. Angiomatosis retinae (ocular lesion described by **von Hippel**, systemic aspects of the disease described by **Lindau**).

  1. Ocular manifestation is retinal hemangioma.

  2. Systemic manifestations include

  a. Cystic cerebellar hemangiomas.

  b. A wide variety of visceral manifestations, such as renal cysts, association with renal cell carcinomas, tumors and cysts of the epididymis, pancreatic cysts, and pheochromocytomas.

D. Encephalotrigeminal angiomatosis (Sturge-Weber syndrome). Although port-wine stains may occur anywhere on the body, Sturge observed that patients with unilateral **facial** port-wine stains (nevus flammeus) regularly had seizures and hemiparesis of the contralateral side and speculated correctly that this was due to an intracranial hemangioma. Weber described the characteristic linear calcifications seen on skull x rays.

  1. Ocular manifestations include

  a. Lid nevus flammeus.

  b. Conjunctival and episcleral vascular lesions.

  c. Glaucoma (both abnormal angle structures and increased episcleral venous pressure are possible etiologies).

  d. Choroidal hemangiomas, which give the fundus a "tomato-ketchup" appearance (suprachoroidal serous detachments may develop in these eyes during the hypotony of intraocular surgery).

  e. Heterochromia iridis.

  2. Cutaneous manifestation is nevus flammeus or the port-wine stain.

  3. Systemic manifestations include Jacksonian seizures, hemiparesis, hemianopia, and, at times, mental deficiency.

E. Ataxia-telangiectasia (Louis-Bar syndrome)

  1. Ocular lesions. Bulbar conjunctival telangiectasis is an essential component of the disorder. It is not present at birth, but is usually noted between 4 and 7 years of age. Abnormalities of eye movements are consequent to the CNS abnormalities.

  2. Cutaneous manifestations have been reported but are not pathognomonic of the disorder.

  3. Systemic manifestations

  a. CNS. Progressive ataxia in childhood was the striking feature initially reported in 1941. At autopsy, degeneration of the cerebellar Purkinje cells is a prominent finding.

  b. Immune deficiency. Thymic hypoplasia is associated with a profound defect in cell-mediated immunity (T cells) and a selective humoral deficiency of IgG_{21}, IgG_4, IgA, and IgE. This immune deficiency appears to be the reason for frequent pulmonary infections.

  c. More random chromosomal rearrangements and the inability to repair radiation-induced damage to DNA. Chromosomal breaks occur at sites responsible for the assembly of genes required for the synthesis of antibodies and T-cell antigen receptors, sites at which "cutting and splicing" of DNA naturally occur.

  d. Chromosome localization of the genes. The gene responsible for ataxia-telangiectasia has been localized to 11q22–23.

F. Wyburn-Mason syndrome

  1. Ocular lesions. Racemose hemangioma of the retina is present on the ipsilateral side of midbrain involvement with racemose hemangioma.

  2. Cutaneous lesions. On occasion, these may be pulsatile vascular nevi in the distribution of the trigeminal nerve.

  3. Systemic manifestations. The racemose hemangioma of the midbrain is congenital and nonprogressive. Neurologic consequences develop as a result of direct-compression hemorrhage infarction.

IX. Developmental disorders by anatomic region

A. Abnormalities of the lacrimal drainage apparatus: lacrimal duct obstruction, dacryocystitis, congenital dacryocele

1. **Background.** The watery component of tears is produced largely by the lacrimal glands in the conjunctival fornices. Tears are distributed across the cornea by the lids during blinking and then pass through the lacrimal drainage apparatus. Tears enter the puncta of the upper and lower lids, pass through the canaliculi, through the common canaliculus, and into the lacrimal sac. The lacrimal sac drains through the nasolacrimal duct into the nose. Lacrimal duct obstruction may occur at the lower end of this nasolacrimal duct where it enters the nasal cavity. In the presence of lacrimal duct obstruction, tears and mucus pool in the lacrimal sac above the obstruction. The mucoid material may reflux through the puncta when pressure is placed over the nasolacrimal sac. The stagnation of tears in this situation leads to chronic discharge on the eyelashes, and **dacryocystitis** (infection of the lacrimal sac itself) may occur.

   In rare instances the obstruction at the lower end of the nasolacrimal duct is associated with distention of the nasolacrimal sac (congenital dacryocele). The infant is born with a distended nasolacrimal sac full of a mucoid material but does not have an active infection in the lacrimal sac.

2. **Physical findings**

   a. **Congenital lacrimal duct obstruction** will cause tearing. Characteristically, there will be some mucous discharge on the lashes, but the conjunctiva will be white and uninflamed. Injection of the conjunctiva indicates a concurrent conjunctivitis. Digital pressure over the nasolacrimal sac often produces a reflux of mucoid material.

   b. **Tearing without discharge** on the lashes or reflux from the nasolacrimal sac should make the clinician suspicious that **congenital glaucoma** rather than lacrimal duct obstruction may be causing the tearing.

   c. **Dacryocystitis** will produce redness, tenderness, and swelling medial to the inner canthus. It may be present at birth but characteristically develops after a period of stagnation and obstructed tear flow.

   d. A **congenital dacryocele** will produce swelling and bluish or purplish discoloration of the soft tissues medial to the inner canthus but is not inflamed. It is usually present at birth and occasionally may wax and wane in size if untreated.

3. **Treatment**

   a. **Congenital lacrimal duct obstructions.** Eighty percent of congenital lacrimal duct obstructions will remit during the first 6–9 months of life. It becomes increasingly rare after 6–9 months of life for the situation to clear spontaneously.

      (1) During those first 6–9 months, **antibiotic ointment** (e.g., erythromycin or tobramycin ointment qid) and **digital compression of the nasolacrimal sac** (qid initially and then as frequently as necessary to keep the sac empty of mucoid material) should be prescribed. The effort is to avoid infection and to minimize stagnation.

      (2) If tearing persists after 6 months of age, **probing of the nasolacrimal sac** may be indicated. Although probing can sometimes be done in the office, a brief general anesthesia gives the surgeon better control and may be preferable. Endotracheal intubation is not required, so the procedure can be done under mask insufflation anesthesia in an ambulatory surgery unit. Although there is no controversy with regard to the efficacy of probing, there is some variation in the recommended timing of the probing. Some ophthalmologists if presented with a family unhappy with a child's purulent, recurrently infected eye, probe at presentation regardless of age. An advantage of probing early is that youngsters are smaller and therefore weaker and require less restraint for probings done in the office. Most ophthalmologists who do office probings will tend to probe

children early (e.g., 6 months of age), whereas most ophthalmologists who wait 9–12 months or longer to see if the child's problems will remit spontaneously will tend to use brief general anesthetics on an outpatient basis for the probing of the older child. If tearing persists or occurs after probing, another probing is indicated. If several probings have failed, the physician is dealing with an unusual situation, and intubation with Silastic tubing or a dacryocystorhinostomy may be indicated.

b. Dacryocystitis should be treated with systemic antibiotics. The systemic antibiotic choice keeps changing and for these small infants needs to be calculated on a per weight basis (see Appendix B). Once the infection has cleared, the obstruction and cause of the problem can be relieved by probing the nasolacrimal duct.

c. Congenital dacryocele can be relieved by probing in the newborn period. At this age probing can be done without general anesthesia.

B. Ptosis. A ptosis may be present as an isolated anomaly, but there may be associated abnormalities. As soon as the diagnosis of ptosis is made, a complete ophthalmologic examination is indicated, even though surgical intervention to lift the lid may not be undertaken for several years.

1. Isolated congenital ptosis. Even if it is severe, congenital ptosis rarely threatens visual development by covering the pupil. Children usually hold their heads back and peer out below the ptotic lid. Visual development may be threatened, however, by the astigmatism that may be present in the eye with a ptotic lid. These children are at risk for anisometropic **amblyopia** (see Chap. 11, sec. **VI.D**). They should be seen early and given glasses and patching as indicated.

Generally, it is best to wait for ptosis surgery until the child is 4 or 5 years old and until reliable measurements of levator function are obtainable.

2. Differential diagnosis. In the evaluation of ptosis, special attention should be paid to pupillary size. A small pupil associated with ptosis may indicate **Horner's syndrome.** A larger pupil associated with ptosis and appropriate extraocular muscle weakness would indicate a **third nerve palsy.** Occasionally, the amount of ptosis may be influenced by chewing through a synkinesis known as the **Marcus-Gunn "jaw-winking"** syndrome. As the patient chews or moves the jaw from side to side, the ptotic eyelid elevates, sometimes to a level higher than the normal position.

C. Colobomas along the optic fissure. A number of congenital anomalies appear to derive from localized failure of the optic fissure to close during intrauterine development. These anomalies may be of no visual consequence, as is the case with isolated inferior iris colobomas or small choroidal defects seen inferior to the disk. Although iris colobomas per se are of no visual consequence, they may be associated with more extensive colobomas in the back of the eye that are visually significant, or they may be associated with other systemic anomalies. Large chorioretinal colobomas may cause profound visual dysfunction if they involve the macula or the optic nerve. One of the more extreme examples of failure in fissure closure is microphthalmus with cyst. In this condition substantial portions of intraocular tissue are found in a colobomatous cyst, and useful vision is not possible.

D. Optic nerve anomalies (see Chap. 12, sec. **II**). All visual information generated by the retina must pass through the optic nerve, so anomalies of the optic nerve may have profound effects on visual function. **Severe colobomas** and anomalous configurations such as **"morning glory"** anomaly and **profound hypoplasia** of the optic nerve may cause profound and irreparable defects in visual function and in pupillary reactions. Regional defects in the optic nerve such as **segmental optic nerve hypoplasia** or **optic nerve drusen** may give rise to visual field defects but leave good central vision and good visual acuity. **Optic nerve pits** are congenital defects that may be associated later in life with serous detachments of the macula and an acquired diminution of vision. One of the most common anomalies of the optic nerve is the presence of **medullated**

nerve fibers in the nerve fiber layer of the retina. These featherlike white patches do not interfere with visual function except for localized visual field scotomas that correspond to their location. (The medullated nerve fibers are opaque and prevent light from stimulating the outer segments behind them.)

E. **Macular hypoplasia.** The embryologic defect that gives rise to macular hypoplasia is not known. In some cases it is inherited in association with albinism or aniridia. Macular hypoplasia may, however, also occur in isolation without other ocular or systemic findings. The diagnosis is made on the basis of clinical examination in the context of poor vision. No foveal reflex is seen, and blood vessels may course through the normally avascular macular region.

F. **Hyaloid system.** During embryologic life the hyaloid vasculature extends from the optic nerve through the vitreous and nourishes the developing lens. It normally regresses completely in later development, but in some individuals remnants remain at the surface of the optic disk as **Bergmeister's papilla.** More rarely, a loop of vascular tissue extends some distance into the vitreous from the optic disk. Sometimes the hyaloid vascular system regresses completely at the optic disk, but a small opacity at the posterior surface of the lens (a Mittendorf dot) reminds one of its anterior location. These anomalies do not interfere with function and require no therapy.

If the hyaloid system does not regress at all and if glial tissue **(persistent hyperplastic primary vitreous [PHPV])** persists between the optic nerve and the posterior surface of the lens, the eye does not develop normally. These eyes are small, and the glial tissue behind the lens gives the eye a white pupil. Vision is poor because of occlusion by the glial tissue and anomalous development. Surgery is indicated to prevent angle-closure glaucoma caused by progressive shallowing of the anterior chamber and to avoid recurrent vitreous hemorrhages. An occasional patient has achieved useful vision after clearing of the visual axis followed by aggressive amblyopia therapy. The term *posterior PHPV* has been used for a glial contracture of the retina **(falciform fold)** without a retrolental mass. These eyes also have evidence of anomalous development and are microphthalmic.

G. **Anterior chamber dysgenesis.** A spectrum of congenital malformations involve the iris, the iridocorneal or filtration angle, and the cornea. The etiology of these disorders is unclear. The most peripheral edge of Descemet's membrane of the cornea terminates at the upper edge of the trabecular meshwork (TM). This most peripheral edge is called Schwalbe's line. If Schwalbe's line is unusually thickened or prominent, it is called **posterior embryotoxon** (on the posterior surface of the cornea, it is a curved line; from the Greek work *toxon,* meaning *bow*). The term *Axenfeld's anomaly* has been given to a prominent Schwalbe's line when it is associated with large peripheral anterior synechiae from the iris. **Reiger's syndrome** includes the prominent Schwalbe's line, peripheral iris anomalies, iris atrophy, glaucoma, as well as nonocular skeletal and structural abnormalities. Although **Peter's anomaly** is sometimes classified with these chamber angle anomalies, the characteristic features include (1) a central corneal opacity (leukoma) apparently due to an absent corneal endothelium, and (2) iridocorneal adhesions at the edge of the central leukoma. Glaucoma is frequently associated with these anomalies. **Therapeutic** efforts involve treatment of glaucoma when present and penetrating keratoplasty when Peter's anomaly is bilateral (see Chap. 5, Fig. 5-2).

H. **Dermoids.** A rubbery, firm, subcutaneous mass along the orbital rim present since birth is most likely a dermoid tumor. Although dermoids are most common along the superotemporal orbital rim, they occur not infrequently in other quadrants. They may enlarge slowly. A dermoid is a choristoma and is composed of tissues not normally present in that region of the body. Dermoids can be removed satisfactorily by local dissection. In children this is best done with endotracheal intubation and general anesthesia. On occasion, a dermoid that appears to be localized to the orbital rim may have a significant posterior extension into the orbit or may extensively involve the bone of the orbital rim. It may be advisable to consider radiologic studies of the involved area prior to surgery if the extent of the mass cannot be determined with certainty by palpation alone.

I. **Hemangiomas.** "Strawberry" hemangiomas that involve the eyelids pose special problems. Infants with such hemangiomas should be followed by an ophthalmologist from the earliest possible age. The mass of the hemangioma may cause total occlusion of the eye and produce irreparable **deprivation amblyopia.** Like hemangiomas elsewhere on the body, those that involve the lids have a tendency to grow during the first year of life and then tend to regress spontaneously. In terms of minimizing scarring and side effects of **therapy,** the physician should delay intervention as long as possible, but if the eye is completely occluded by a hemangioma, the physician must intervene however young the infant. Favorable results have been obtained by injecting triamcinolone directly into the tumor with a "tuberculin" needle and syringe. It is noteworthy that the doses of injected steroids commonly used are quite substantial when calculated on a per weight basis. Infants may have a period of slower growth right after their lid injection. In addition to occlusion amblyopia, these eyes are at risk for anisometropic amblyopia, since the mass effect of the hemangioma produces an astigmatism in the involved eye. The involved eye may also develop high myopia. Whether or not the eye is completely occluded, it is essential that the child be refracted at an early age and appropriate attention be given to glasses and patching.

X. **Developmental disorders by syndromes**

A. **Branchial arch syndromes versus Tessier's clefting classification.** Specific ocular anomalies are regular features of certain syndromes with facial anomalies. Overlapping classification schemes have been proposed for these disorders, but knowledge of underlying mechanisms is still lacking. Tessier's comprehensive classification of facial clefting syndromes based on morphology can be used for the **Treacher Collins and Goldenhar syndromes,** but the cause of the clefts is unknown. Another classification is based on the embryologic origin of many of the affected tissues (the branchial arch syndromes). Heredity plays a strong role in many families with Treacher Collins deformity but appears to play less of a role in Goldenhar syndrome.

1. **Mandibulofacial dysostosis: Treacher Collins (Franceschetti-Klein) syndrome.** Maxillary hypoplasia and downward displacement of the lateral canthi give these individuals a highly characteristic appearance. Prominent ocular findings include notching of the inferior lids, deficient lashes on the lids medial to the notching, and astigmatism that seems to correlate with the clefting axis. Corneal irritation may result from misdirected lashes caused by lid notching. Deafness and ear anomalies often accompany the ocular and facial deformities.

2. **Oculoauriculovertebral dysplasia: Goldenhar syndrome.** Usually the ocular features (limbal corneal dermoids, orbital lipodermoids, and notching of the superior lid) and the preauricular skin tags are the prominent features in childhood. The most frequent vertebral anomalies include fused cervical vertebrae, hemivertebrae, spina bifida, and occipitalization of the atlas. Occasionally, however, the associated systemic abnormalities (cardiovascular, renal, genitourinary, and gastrointestinal defects) may be so severe that they dominate the clinical picture. The limbal dermoid is amenable to local excision with a partial keratectomy, but the orbital lipodermoid should not be treated surgically. The orbital lipodermoid is much less disfiguring, and attempted excision may lead to scarring involving the extraocular muscles.

3. **Hallerman-Streiff-François syndrome.** Mandibular hypoplasia and feeding problems are prominent in the neonatal period. The characteristic ocular lesions are cataracts that mature rapidly in infancy, are quite fluid, and may absorb spontaneously if left untreated. In general, however, it is advisable to proceed with cataract aspiration as soon as the child can tolerate general anesthesia, since the rate and completeness of spontaneous absorp-

tion cannot be predicted and the process of spontaneous absorption may be a causative factor in the late development of secondary glaucoma.

4. **Pierre Robin anomalad.** Mandibular hypoplasia with upper airway obstruction and feeding problems may be prominent in the neonatal period. Most are sporadic, but some have Stickler disease (see sec. **XVII.C.4**) and may have high myopia, glaucoma, and retinal detachment, so a complete ophthalmic examination at an early age and follow-up are advisable.

B. **Craniofacial dysostosis.** The most commonly seen disorders of this type are **Crouzon** syndrome and **Apert** syndrome. The syndactyly of Apert syndrome is the most clear-cut distinction between these two disorders, both of which have craniofacial deformities due to craniosynostosis. Both disorders have markedly shallow orbits with prominent globes, and the globes may prolapse in front of the lids with minimum trauma. This prolapse usually appears to do no harm to the globes, and the eyeball can be gently repositioned with the lids held open. Most if not all cases of optic atrophy in these disorders are due to hydrocephalus. Youngsters with both Apert and Crouzon syndromes have highly characteristic eye movements. They regularly have V patterns with eyes most divergent in up gaze, closer together in gaze straight ahead, and closest together in down gaze. They regularly have markedly underactive superior rectus muscles. They may also have underactive superior oblique muscles and overactive inferior oblique muscles. These individuals may have a V pattern **esotropia,** a V pattern **exotropia,** or mixed strabismus with a V pattern (exotropia in up gaze, esotropia in down gaze). Some individuals with Apert syndrome also have irides that transilluminate.

Although children with craniostenosis were thought in the past to develop optic atrophy from bone encroachment on the optic nerve, this mechanism must be exceedingly rare. When these children with craniostenosis do have optic atrophy, it generally appears to be secondary to their hydrocephalus. In contrast, optic atrophy from abnormal bony overgrowth is a prominent feature of the rare disorder **craniometaphyseal dysplasia.** This dominantly inherited disorder appears to be due to a deficiency in bone resorption and causes gradual narrowing of all cranial foramens. There is a characteristic facial disfigurement.

C. **Hypertelorism.** The term *hypertelorism* has somewhat different meanings, depending on whether the clinician is considering **ocular hypertelorism** or **orbital hypertelorism;** for this latter determination craniofacial surgeons refer to the distance between the medial walls of the orbits as determined by CT scan. The distance between lateral orbital walls (outer orbital distance) is a traditional ophthalmic measurement. Interpupillary distance gives a clinical measure of **ocular hypertelorism.** The distance between medial canthi, if it is excessive, gives a measure of **telecanthus.**

Orbital hypertelorism may be part of a large number of craniofacial syndromes, but it also occurs in an isolated form. There is a high association of exotropia with isolated orbital hypertelorism. After craniofacial surgery, the degree of exotropia is often markedly reduced, and the patient may even be esotropic. If a patient with orbital hypertelorism is a candidate for craniofacial surgery, it would be prudent to postpone strabismus surgery until after the craniofacial surgery.

XI. **Tumors of childhood**

A. **Retinoblastoma** is the most frequent ocular tumor of childhood. The incidence is about 1 in every 20,000 live births. It has one of the highest cure rates of any malignant tumor. Untreated, it is almost invariably fatal.

1. **Heredity.** Retinoblastoma acts like an autosomal dominant trait with greater than 90% penetrance. In fact, it is really recessively inherited since both retinoblastoma genes at the 13q14 locus must be abnormal before the cell becomes malignant. Individuals with the hereditary form have one abnormal gene in all their cells. A mutation in the other gene allows expression of the tumor. In the nonhereditary form, both mutations occur only in the retinal cell that has become malignant. Of all cases of retinoblastoma, 60%

are nonhereditary and 40% are hereditary. Since there is a high spontaneous mutation rate in retinoblastoma, even most of the hereditary, bilateral cases will have no previous family history of the tumor. Such sporadic,
bilaterally affected individuals will nevertheless still have a 50% chance of
passing the disease on to each offspring. All bilateral cases and about 10-20%
of unilateral cases of retinoblastoma are hereditary. Again, because of the
high spontaneous mutation rate, 94% of all cases of retinoblastoma are
sporadic, i.e., there is no **previous** family history of the tumor.

The risk estimates are important for **genetic counseling.** If one parent is
affected with familial retinoblastoma or bilateral sporadic retinoblastoma,
each of the offspring will have a 50% chance of inheriting the tumor. The
risk of the offspring of healthy siblings or healthy children of a patient with
familial retinoblastoma is 1 : 15. Once an affected child is born to such an
individual, the chance becomes one in two since she or he is then known
to be an unaffected carrier. Since unilateral sporadic cases of retinoblastoma are usually not hereditary, the risk to the offspring of such individuals
is much less, variously estimated at between 1 and 8%. The risk to siblings
of sporadic cases of being affected has been revised downward over the years
from 15 to 1%. That there is any risk at all stems from the fact that the
first mutation may have occurred in one of the parents without being expressed rather than in the affected child. Fortunately, risk estimation and
genetic counseling have become much more accurate in most families through
the use of DNA sequence analysis and polymorphisms.

2. **Presentation.** In families known to harbor retinoblastoma, the diagnosis
should be made within a few days of birth by routine examination. In sporadic cases, those who are bilaterally affected usually present by the age of
15 months and those who have unilateral retinoblastoma by 20-30 months
of age. The most common presenting sign is a **white reflex** in the pupil,
detected by the parents or the pediatrician. **Strabismus** is the second most
common mode of presentation. Apparent intraocular inflammation and
glaucoma secondary either to the tumor pushing the lens iris diaphragm
forward or to tumor cells clogging the TM are also seen. Much less common
modes of presentation include proptosis (secondary to retrobulbar extraocular extension), the appearance of a pseudohypopyon of tumor cells in
the anterior chamber, and evidence of distant metastases. These all indicate
a poor prognosis for life.

3. **Appearance.** The tumor may be a single or multifocal, smooth, pinkish,
rounded mass in the retina. It may grow in, on top of (endophytic), or under
(exophytic) the retina. The tumor may seed into the vitreous and grow back
into the optic nerve. As mentioned, it may extend to the anterior segment.

4. **Mode of spread.** The tumor most commonly metastasizes to the bone
marrow or extends back through the optic nerve into the subarachnoid
space and spreads, via the CSF, throughout the CNS. Less commonly, distant metastases may occur to bone, and direct extension through the sclera
into the orbit may occur.

5. **Pineal malignancies,** histologically similar to the ocular tumors, ("trila-
teral retinoblastoma") have been uniformly fatal.

6. **Survivors** of familial retinoblastoma are very prone to develop other malignancies, most notably osteogenic sarcoma.

7. **Treatment**
   a. If it is thought that the eye be saved with useful vision, then **radiation
      therapy** is the treatment of choice. With external beam irradiation us-
      ing supervoltage x ray, the local control rate is about 85-95%. With this
      sharp-edged beam, the entire retina can be treated without irradiating
      the lens. Contraindications to the use of radiation therapy as a primary
      mode of treatment include invasion of the optic nerve, invasion of the
      anterior segment of the eye, extensive vitreous seeding, and irreversible
      loss of vision in the eye. The total tumor dose is about 4000-5000 cGy.
      All bilateral tumors that are favorable to radiation therapy should be

subjected to this mode of treatment. Because of the risks of radiation therapy, including a 4% incidence of malignant tumors in the field of radiation, the use of radiation for unilateral retinoblastoma, even in favorable cases, is somewhat controversial. The traditional treatment is enucleation of the unilaterally affected eye. With small, solitary tumors, except those in the fovea, photocoagulation or cryotherapy may be justified (see sec. **d**).

b. If the tumor is unfavorable for radiation therapy, then **enucleation** is the treatment of choice. Especially if the optic nerve is involved ophthalmoscopically, a long piece of optic nerve should be included with the enucleation of the globe. The prognosis is poor when the tumor has extended beyond the lamina cribrosa, and even poorer if it extends to the cut end of the optic nerve, on the histologic examination. Local orbital spread and the detection of tumor at the end of the optic nerve in an enucleated specimen are indications for radiation therapy to the orbit and remaining optic nerve back to the chiasm. Evisceration is probably not of value.

c. The role of **chemotherapy** in retinoblastoma is uncertain. As an adjunct to radiation therapy, it seems to have no benefit. If the choroid is massively involved with tumor on histologic examination of the enucleated specimen, prophylactic chemotherapy with antitumor agents may be beneficial. If the tumor has spread to bone marrow or viscera, systemic chemotherapy is, in most cases, of only palliative value. Until recently, no patient with retinoblastoma had survived the spread of tumor outside the orbit. Multiagent chemotherapy such as that used for neuroblastoma offers hope for long-term survival.

d. **If individual tumors recur** or if new tumors appear in an eye after radiation therapy, they may often be successfully treated with **cryotherapy** by repeated freeze and thaw cycles or by **photocoagulation.** Since retinoblastoma is usually multicentric, cryotherapy and photocoagulation should not be depended on as the primary mode of therapy, except in the case of a small, solitary, unilateral, extrafoveal tumor.

B. Rhabdomyosarcoma is a rare tumor, but it is the most common primary orbital tumor in childhood. It usually presents with rapidly progressive proptosis and displacement of the globe either upward or downward depending on the location of the tumor. It may mimic inflammation because of its rapid course and attendant signs of inflammation. The **diagnosis** is made by biopsy. In the past, **therapy** involved radical evisceration, sometimes with removal of bones around the orbit, with a 35–40% long-term survival. Radiation therapy with chemotherapy offers a 65% long-term survival with 90% local tumor control, and the treatment is much less disfiguring. No attempt is made to shield the lens or cornea from the effects of radiation therapy in this situation, and about 5000–6000 cGy are given to the orbit with supervoltage x ray through an anterior port. With this dose of radiation, a cataract always develops, and radiation retinitis is frequently seen. Radiation keratitis sometimes is a problem that must be dealt with. Before radiation therapy, the child, if old enough to understand, and the parents should be informed of the inevitable loss of vision.

C. Neuroblastoma is a common childhood tumor, usually originating in the paraspinal sympathetic chain or in the adrenal glands. It often metastasizes to the orbit. It frequently first presents as proptosis of the globe or ecchymosis of the eyelids or both. These presentations must be distinguished from trauma. The **treatment** consists of local radiation therapy and systemic chemotherapy, both of which are primarily of palliative value, though some young infants survive.

D. Optic glioma is thought by some to be a relatively stable hamartoma of the optic nerve. It may occur anywhere along the length of the nerve, including the optic chiasm. Optic glioma is commonly associated with neurofibromatosis (see sec. **VIII.B**). If it is in the intraorbital portion of the nerve, it may produce loss of vision and unilateral optic disk swelling. In the optic chiasm it may produce visual field defects (which may remain stable over long periods of time) and optic atrophy. Some tumors in this area behave aggressively, invading the third ventricle, causing hydrocephalus, or they may involve the hypothalamus. It is unclear in some of these instances whether the tumor originates in the optic chiasm or in the hypothalamus itself. Because of the benign course of many of these tumors, some clinicians have advocated simple observation. If an intraorbital optic glioma is causing marked proptosis and is endangering the cornea, the optic nerve containing the tumor can be excised either from an orbital or intracranial approach. Chiasmal gliomas generally do not respond well to surgical treatment and may be subjected to radiation therapy. There are conflicting opinions about the effectiveness of this mode of treatment of optic glioma.

E. **Leukemia.** The most common form of leukemia in childhood is acute lymphoblastic leukemia that, with modern techniques of chemotherapy, has a greater than 70% 5-year survival and apparent cure rate. Acute myelogenous and monocytic leukemias are less common and have a worse prognosis, with survival of about 50%. The ocular manifestations are similar. The most common manifestation in the eye is retinal hemorrhage, which generally occurs when the patient is quite anemic and thrombocytopenic. These hemorrhages often have white centers **(Roth spots).** The central white area is not evidence that the retina is involved with leukemic cells. The retina can be massively infiltrated with leukemic cells, but this is rare and usually occurs in a patient who has a relapse of his leukemia. Leukemic infiltration of the optic nerve is an emergency situation, because vision may be lost within a period of a few hours. The optic nerve is swollen and infiltrated with leukemic cells and may resemble papillitis. Radiation therapy to the posterior globes and orbit on an emergency basis is indicated to preserve vision. Leukemic cells may infiltrate the iris and circulate in the anterior chamber, resembling iritis. Secondary glaucoma may ensue. Sometimes the anterior segment involvement will respond to topical steroid treatment, but usually a small dose of radiation therapy to the anterior segment is required. In acute myelogenous leukemia, local large infiltrates of leukemic cells may rarely occur in the orbit, causing proptosis. This uncommon manifestation has been called **chloroma.** It responds dramatically to radiation therapy.

F. **Craniopharyngioma** is a tumor arising from the anterior pituitary in children. Posterior pituitary tumors occur only rarely in children. A craniopharyngioma frequently presents with visual field loss or loss of vision in one eye secondary to pressure on the optic chiasm or an optic nerve or tract. It may also involve the third ventricle, causing increased intracranial pressure or hydrocephalus. Calcification in the suprasellar region is seen on x ray. Sometimes the tumor can be completely excised surgically. More commonly, the cysts that form in the tumor are decompressed neurosurgically and then the tumor is treated with radiation therapy. Patients who have rapidly evolving visual field loss sometimes have complete restoration of visual function if treatment is undertaken quickly. Another complication of craniopharyngioma is hypopituitarism, from damage to the posterior pituitary by tumor, surgery, or radiation therapy.

G. **Medulloepithelioma (diktyoma)** is a rare embryonic epithelial tumor usually involving the ciliary body and sometimes the optic nerve. It may be benign or malignant and may contain heterotopic mesodermal elements (teratoma). The presentation in the ciliary body may grow into the pupillary area, becoming visible to the parents or interfering with the child's vision. Sometimes it presents as cysts in the pupil. Those in the optic nerve may cause proptosis. **Treatment** is enucleation.

H. **Juvenile xanthogranuloma** is a benign dermatologic disorder in which yellowish skin lesions ranging in size from a few millimeters to several centimeters in diameter appear in the first few months of life, increase in size gradually, and then gradually fade spontaneously, by age 5. The iris may be involved with xanthomas, which may cause a spontaneous hyphema. Generally, the blood absorbs without causing permanent damage, although secondary glaucoma and other complications of hyphema may occur. Sometimes the hyphemas are recurrent. The iris xanthomas usually resolve spontaneously as the child grows older, and the problem resolves. On rare occasions topical steroids or a small dose of radiation therapy to the iris may be required.

XII. **Retinopathy of prematurity (ROP,** formerly **retrolental fibroplasia)**

   A. **Background.** ROP was the leading cause of blindness in children in the 1940s and 50s. After oxygen was identified as an etiologic factor, ROP became relatively rare. The severe oxygen restriction that prevailed from the mid-1950s to the mid-1960s, however, resulted in a striking increase in neonatal death and brain damage in premature infants. Therefore, the use of oxygen was liberalized in the late 1960s. Very small premature infants, who previously had died, now survive in large numbers. These tiny infants are at great risk, and ROP has become more common again.

   B. **Etiology.** Excessive oxygen in the newborn period in premature infants certainly seemed to be the important factor in ROP in the 1940s and 50s. The etiology now is not so certain. The occurrence of ROP correlates with the length of time in an increased oxygen environment but not with levels of partial pressure of oxygen in the arterial blood or by continuous transcutaneous oxygen monitoring. The danger of ROP increases with short gestational age and low birth weight. ROP has been reported rarely, however, in full-term infants and in premature infants who never received added oxygen.

   C. **Pathophysiology.** Normal retina is gradually vascularized from the optic disk to the periphery during the final half of gestation, the temporal periphery finally becoming vascularized shortly after term. The earlier in the gestational period an infant is born, the less the vessels have grown out. The developing vessels may be arrested in their growth by poorly understood factors, which obliterate the newly forming vessels. When normal blood vessel growth is interrupted in this way, the vanguard of mesenchymal tissue builds up and forms a ridge that may be interrupted or continuous. The capillaries posterior to this ridge are obliterated, and the ridge forms an arteriovenous (AV) shunt. Microaneurysms may form posterior to the ridge. In more severe cases, neovascular proliferation on the surface of the retina and in the vitreous may occur. In milder cases, capillaries may bud from the anterior edge of the ridge, resuming the normal vascularization of the retina with complete regression of the ROP. In more severe cases, scarring takes place, which may produce traction on the retina. This scarring may be localized to the previous area of the ridge or may produce distortion of the posterior retina, including the macula, with fixed folds, and, in the most severe cases, may produce total retinal detachment. Even in cases where the posterior retina is relatively intact, there may be persistent AV shunts and avascular peripheral retina. Up to the point at which scarring occurs, it is possible for acute, active ROP to regress, leving no abmormalities or only minimum peripheral changes and normal function.

   D. **Stages of ROP.** A generally accepted international classification of ROP has been developed to standardize communication and criteria for evaluating treatment.

   1. **Stage 1** is the appearance of a distinct demarcation line separating the peripheral avascular retina from vascularized posterior retina.

   2. **Stage 2** involves the formation of a ridge that is elevated and has width.

   3. **Stage 3** includes extraretinal fibrovascular proliferative tissue growing off the posterior edge of the ridge into the vitreous or onto the surface of the retina.

   4. **Stage 4** exhibits a subtotal retinal detachment without involving the fovea (4A) and a retinal attachment involving the fovea (4B).

   5. **Stage five** is a total retinal detachment.

   6. Any of the stages of ROP may exhibit **dilation** and **tortuosity** of the posterior retinal blood vessels, in which case a + is added to the number of the stage.

   E. **The location and extent of ROP** is described by dividing each retina into three zones with the disk, where the retinal blood vessels begin, at the center of concentric circles.

1. **Zone 1** has a radius that extends from the disk about twice as far as from the disk to the macula.
2. **Zone 2** extends all the way to the ora serrata on the nasal side and a little bit anterior to the equator on the temporal side.
3. **Zone 3** is a crescent that involves the remaining superior, inferior, and temporal retina. The retina is divided also into clock hours.

F. **Examination and Treatment.** Premature infants who are born with a birth weight of less than 1250 to 1500 gm should be examined beginning around 4 weeks of age and every 2–3 weeks thereafter until the vessels have reached the ora serrata. If ROP is discovered, the patient should be followed more closely, depending on the activity and severity of the abnormalities. If stage 3+ ROP is reached, involving 5 hours or more of the circumference of the retina, one should consider treating with confluent cryotherapy to the entire avascular retina. When ROP has reached this stage, about 25% will still regress spontaneously without loss of central vision, but with cryotherapy about 50% will regress. If the severe ROP occurs in zone 1 or posterior zone 2, the prognosis is much poorer with or without treatment. In stage 4A and 4B ROP, scleral buckling with drainage of subretinal fluid may be indicated, and with stage 5 ROP, vitrectomy with lensectomy and peeling of preretinal membranes will be necessary in an attempt to reattach the retina. The retina can be reattached in 50–60% of eyes that have reached stage 5 ROP, but useful vision may be obtained in only about 20–30%.

G. **Late complications of cicatricial ROP** include angle-closure glaucoma from anterior displacement of the lens iris diaphragm and late rhegmatogenous retinal detachments from traction of the peripheral scarring causing retinal holes. Patients with cicatricial ROP also have an increased incidence of high myopia, and those with visual disabilities may require low vision aids and referral to special education programs for the visually handicapped.

XIII. **Toxicity of systemic medications to ocular structures**

A. **Chloramphenicol** may cause **optic neuritis** as well as **peripheral neuritis.** Because the toxicity appears after chronic use, most of the children in whom it occurs have **cystic fibrosis** of the pancreas, since this is the major use of chronic chloramphenicol in childhood. The toxic effect of the drug acts like retrobulbar neuritis, with loss of visual acuity of varying severity and development of a **central scotoma.** In the vast majority of patients, the visual acuity returns to normal when the chloramphenicol treatment is discontinued. If treatment is resumed in order to control pulmonary infection, many patients will not suffer a recurrent attack of toxic optic neuritis. Papillitis with swelling of the optic nerve has not been noted in chloramphenicol toxicity. Optic nerve swelling in a patient with cystic fibrosis secondary to hypercapnia causing papilledema does not interfere with vision. It should not be confused with the chloramphenicol optic neuritis.

B. **Systemic steroids**

1. **Cataracts.** Prolonged treatment with high-dose systemic steroids will eventually lead to posterior subcapsular cataract. The opacity may progress to involve the rest of the lens if the dose cannot be decreased. Steroid cataract may regress if the patient can be kept on a very low dose of systemic steroids or if the steroids can be stopped entirely. Cataracts will develop in most patients after the equivalent of 15–20 mg of prednisone a day for a period of 2 years. In children, two diseases that commonly require systemic steroids for periods long enough to produce cataracts are asthma and systemic lupus erythematosus. Other entities in which the use of long-term steroid therapy has caused cataracts include Crohn's disease, nephrotic syndrome, renal transplantation, scleroderma, and leukemia.

2. **Glaucoma** can be caused by long-term systemic corticosteroid therapy as well as by topical steroids in susceptible individuals (see Chap. 9, sec. **XXI**).

XIV. **The management of cataract in infancy and childhood.** The etiology of cataract and associations with other disorders and syndromes are discussed in preceding sections of this chapter. The development of amblyopia when the vision is blurred or completely obscured by a cataract in infancy or childhood introduces additional factors into the management of these youngsters.

Even when it is opaque with cataract, the crystalline lens in infancy and childhood is soft compared with an adult lens. The lens in childhood can be readily broken up and aspirated through a needle. A variety of techniques are available to aspirate the lens while fluid is irrigated into the eye to maintain its normal configuration (see Chap. 6, sec. **VII.B**). In childhood the lens should not be removed intact (intracapsularly) since the vitreous is adherent to the back of the lens, and the loss of vitreous may lead to serious ocular complications. Phacoemulsification and other techniques that have been introduced to break up the hard nucleus of the adult lens are not necessary and are contraindicated for the removal of childhood cataracts (see also Chap. 6, sec. **VII.B**).

A. **Dense bilateral cataracts in infancy.** Dense cataracts early in life obscure vision and produce sensory nystagmus. Review of systems and systemic pediatric examinations may reveal additional abnormalities. These cataracts should be removed as early in infancy as possible, preferably within the first few days or weeks of life, the second eye being done within days after the first. If the 3-mm central axis is opaque, amblyopia will occur without surgical correction.

B. **Dense unilateral cataracts.** Marked asymmetry in the visual input to the CNS from the two eyes will lead to a dense amblyopia in the more handicapped eye. Unilateral cataracts may also be associated with other ocular abnormalities. The therapy of a unilateral cataract includes prolonged and vigorous amblyopia therapy after the surgical removal of the cataract within the first few days or weeks of life.

C. **Traumatic cataracts.** A cataract after trauma in childhood may produce dense amblyopia. Deprivation of vision in this way may lead to loss of steady fixation in only a few months. Once the cataract is removed, continued attention is required to provide appropriate optical correction and vigorous amblyopia therapy with patching of the better eye. With an injury in early childhood, management of the amblyopia requires very close supervision at least until age 10 or 12. Late complications from severe trauma and cataract surgery, such as glaucoma or retinal detachment, may not manifest themselves until adult life, so the patient needs to be followed indefinitely.

D. **Zonular (or lamellar) developmental cataracts.** Developmental cataracts are present at birth and have a highly characteristic appearance (see Chap. 6, sec. **V.B**). Usually they are present in both eyes and remain unchanged year to year. If they are quite symmetric in the two eyes and if the child's visual development seems to be satisfactory, it is often possible to delay surgery indefinitely or until the child has difficulty with school work or some other specific visual task. Marked asymmetry in the opacities in the two eyes, however, may create amblyopia in the eye with the denser cataract, and might require intervention at an earlier age.

E. **Visual rehabilitation** after cataract surgery is achieved by fitting the infant or child to a **daily-wear contact lens(es).** There is **no indication** for **intraocular lenses** (IOLs) in congenital cataracts and only limited and questionable experience with their use in traumatic cataracts. An IOL may be justified in an older child who had normal vision prior to acquiring the cataract and an otherwise normal eye.

F. **Amblyopia** is treated or prevented by patching the unaffected eye for 80% of the waking hours in an infant or for 4–5 hours daily up to full time in an older child. Once strong fixation is achieved with the contact lens–bearing aphakic eye, occlusion of the normal eye should be continued in young children, varying the length of time as necessary until vision can be measured (age 3–4 years) and occlusion times adjusted appropriately. Although not entirely comparable to Snellen (recognition) acuity, grating acuity tests, e.g., Teller acuity cards, are helpful in following the treatment of amblyopia in preverbal and preliterate infants.

XV. Glaucomas of infancy and childhood.* Public awareness of glaucoma has increased to the point that most people know that it affects a significant proportion of the adult population over 40 years of age (variably estimated as between 2 and 5%). Regrettably, there is not the same awareness that glaucoma exists in childhood. It is crucial to make this diagnosis early in life before vision has already been irreparably damaged or lost. To make the diagnosis it is important to maintain a high index of suspicion and to consider it routinely in the differential diagnosis of ocular problems of childhood.

A. Infantile glaucoma

1. **Signs.** Tearing, photophobia, cloudy cornea, and corneal enlargement in one or both eyes are the classic signs of infantile glaucoma. The signs may be present at birth (truly congenital), they may develop early in the newborn period, or they may develop in the first few years of life. Only one sign may be present initially, and it is important not to wait for the full constellation before making a complete evaluation for glaucoma. It is worthy of note that after 2 years of age the corneas generally do **not** enlarge even if the intraocular pressure (IOP) is elevated.

2. **Differential diagnosis of cloudy cornea**

   a. **Congenital glaucoma.** Cloudy corneas from **congenital glaucoma** may be diffusely hazy with epithelial edema or may have more intense opacification of the cornea over a break in the corneal endothelium (Haab striae). Characteristically, this break due to increased IOP and stretching will be circumferential or sometimes horizontal.

   b. **Forceps injury.** In contrast to Haab striae, an endothelial break due to **forceps injury** will usually be vertical in its orientation, there may be other signs of facial injury in the newborn period, and IOP will not be elevated.

   c. **Corneal endothelial dystrophy.** Infants with **corneal endothelial dystrophy** also have diffusely hazy corneas with epithelial edema. The endothelial surface of the cornea may have marked irregularities to help localize the difficulty at this level, but these changes are not always present. The IOP and the optic nerves are normal in corneal endothelial dystrophy.

   d. **Mucopolysaccharidoses (Hurler, Scheie, Morquio, and Maroteaux-Lamy syndromes) and mucolipidoses.** The corneas are hazy but there is no epithelial edema. The IOP is normal and the optic nerves do not have glaucomatous cupping.

   e. **Interstitial keratitis (IK).** Although it has been reported at birth, IK rarely presents at such an early age.

   f. **Congenital rubella syndrome.** The corneas may be transiently or permanently hazy with normal IOP, or a true infantile glaucoma may be present.

3. **Examination.** Complete ophthalmologic examination includes assessment of IOP, inspection of the optic nerves, gonioscopic examination of the filtration angle, and examination of the cornea under magnification. In many infants all of these examinations can be done in the office. Although some information may have to be obtained during anesthesia, especially in older children, the physician can usually narrow the differential diagnosis substantially at the time of the initial thorough examination in the office.

   a. **Assessment of IOP.** Measurement of IOP in the office is greatly facilitated if the infant is hungry at the time of examination and is given a bottle.

   After the infant is involved in feeding, a combination topical anesthetic and fluorescein (Fluress) can be applied and IOP measured. A handheld applantation device (e.g., Perkin's tonometer) is very helpful in this

---

* Examination and therapy of this disorder has been greatly benefited by the work and teachings of W. Morton Grant, M.D., and Davis S. Walton, M.D. The authors gratefully acknowledge that their work draws heavily on the work of these two men.

situation. Several readings are taken, and it is the lowest consistent unsedated IOP that is usually the most relevant. Struggling or lid squeezing will tend to erroneously elevate the IOP.

IOP measurements in the office are much more satisfactory than those under general anesthesia. General anesthetics, including barbiturates and halothane, all lower the IOP, so that measurements in the operating room are helpful in diagnosis only if they are elevated.

   b. Inspection of the optic nerves. Optic disk cupping in childhood is a very sensitive indicator of IOP, especially in the stages prior to permanent visual field loss. Asymmetry in optic nerve cupping may be helpful in making the initial diagnosis, and evaluation of cupping may also be helpful in the postoperative management and long-term follow-up of the glaucoma patient. The optic cup may become smaller within hours of successful goniotomy.

   c. Gonioscopic examination of the angle. Koeppe lens examination is often possible in the unsedated infant without discomfort or struggling. In an older child this may have to await general anesthesia. Gonioscopy is an important initial step in making the differentiation between infantile glaucoma and other forms of angle anomalies such as Reiger's syndrome. In follow-up, gonioscopy is helpful in understanding the success or failure of previous trabecular operations.

   d. Examination of the cornea under magnification. In cases of corneal cloudiness, close inspection is essential for proper diagnosis. With the Koeppe lens in place, close inspection of the cornea may be done with the Barkan light and handheld microscope. Even small children can be held up to the slit lamp if sufficient personnel are mobilized. Standard slit-lamp examination in the operating room with the anesthetized child lying on his or her side can also be helpful.

4. **Special studies.** If the office ophthalmologic examination indicates infantile glaucoma, a prenatal and birth history, review of systems, and careful pediatric evaluation are worthwhile. It may be very helpful to identify a syndrome such as congenital rubella syndrome that up to age 2 years requires isolation during hospitalization. A systemic metabolic disorder such as Lowe syndrome will require considerable medical attention in addition to the ophthalmologic evaluation. Special studies are selected on the basis of the history and systemic examination.

5. **Treatment.** Once the diagnosis of infantile glaucoma has been made by office examination, acetazolamide, 15 mg/kg/day in 3 or 4 divided doses, is started. A cloudy cornea may clear significantly after a few days of acetazolamide therapy. Examination under anesthesia completes the diagnostic procedures. Surgery is directed to the trabecular tissues in the form of either goniotomy or trabeculotomy, both of which result in an incision into the TM. Goniotomy (or internal trabeculotomy) was the first major advance in therapy of this condition and remains a straightforward, low-risk procedure. Trabeculotomy (or external goniotomy) has advantages when the cornea is hazy, and apparently also develops filtration in some patients. Trabeculotomy scars the conjunctiva, making future filtration surgery in that area more difficult. Barkan's observations regarding the effectiveness of trabecular surgery remain the major clues to the etiology of infantile glaucoma.

Goniotomies and trabeculotomies are not always successful, even when repeated several times. Long-term management of youngsters in whom surgery has not been successful is difficult and involves the use of chronic medications, including miotics, carbonic anhydrase inhibitors (CAIs), and beta-adrenergic blocking agents (see Chap. 9, sec. **V**). Although miotics do not appear to be very effective in untreated infantile glaucoma, a youngster who has had a partially effective goniotomy or trabeculotomy procedure may subsequently be benefited by miotic agents. Filtration surgery can be tried, but it is more difficult to maintain filtration in children than in adults.

Cyclocryotherapy may also be effective, but if undertaken it is essential to leave several hours of the circumference unfrozen to avoid hypotony.

6. Follow-up. Even if initial trabecular surgery appears to be effective, these youngsters must be followed indefinitely (several times a year initially and then at least annually for their lifetime) since the elevated pressure may return even years after successful surgery. If the glaucoma recurs, another goniotomy or trabeculotomy may be effective.

B. Aniridia

1. Physical findings. The term *aniridia* is used for a multifaceted ocular disorder that involves much more than the underdevelopment of the iris. In spite of the term, the iris is not totally absent, a small stump being visible 360 degrees by gonioscopy and sometimes by slit lamp. Also present at birth is the macular aplasia that correlates with the markedly diminished vision and sensory nystagmus. Congenital lens opacities are frequent. During the first and second decades these patients often develop a characteristic peripheral corneal pannus, readily seen at slit-lamp examinations. Indirect ophthalmoscopy of the far peripheral retina may reveal small yellow dots circumferentially.

These children may or may not develop glaucoma. Since glaucoma does develop in a significant number of aniridia patients, close examination from infancy onward is warranted. The occurrence of glaucoma correlates with adhesion of the peripheral iris to the TM. The mechanism of this adhesion is not well understood. Once the peripheral iris covers the outflow channels and glaucoma is present, the condition is difficult to treat. Walton has advocated the use of prophylactic goniotomy when the peripheral iris starts to cover the TM and before the IOP is elevated.

2. Heredity. Aniridia may be inherited in a dominant fashion, or it may appear as the result of a spontaneous mutation. The eponym **Miller syndrome** has been given to the close association of spontaneously appearing aniridia and **Wilms' tumor.** Accordingly, thorough evaluation of the abdomen should be done when the diagnosis of aniridia is first made in a child without family history of the condition. Studies of the abdomen should probably be repeated once or twice a year during the first few years of life. Some patients with aniridia and Wilms' tumor apparently have a deletion of the short arm of the eleventh chromosome, 11p⁻ syndrome. It appears that a more extensive deletion involving the aniridia locus gives rise to the association of aniridia and Wilms' tumor with mental retardation and hypogonadism.

C. Juvenile open-angle glaucoma. On occasion, open-angle glaucoma may have its onset in the first decades of life. The diagnosis may be overlooked because the disorder is asymptomatic until irreversible visual damage has occurred. Certainly a family history of glaucoma, particularly early-onset glaucoma, is a strong indication to take routine IOP measurements in childhood. The only way to make this diagnosis in the very early stages is to check IOP routinely even in children. **Large cups** or **asymmetric cupping in childhood** is as valuable an early sign of glaucoma as it is in adults. Juvenile-onset open-angle glaucoma is treated with the same medications and the same principles as adult open-angle glaucoma (see Chap. 9, sec. **V**).

D. Childhood glaucomas secondary to inflammation. Untreated ocular inflammation (uveitis may cause glaucoma by producing an adhesion between the iris and the anterior surface of the lens (seclusion of the pupil). When the aqueous is no longer able to pass through the pupil into the anterior chamber, iris bombé and glaucoma result. Mydriatic therapy during episodes of uveitis is designed to avoid this.

Chronic iritis such as that associated with pauciarticular JRA or sympathetic ophthalmia, or following extracapsular cataract extraction, on occasion can produce a secondary open-angle glaucoma with markedly diminished outflow facility. The exact nature of the damage to the TM is not known. Although rare in occurrence, **open-angle glaucoma secondary to inflammation is difficult to treat.** Miotic agents are often contraindicated because of the ongoing inflammation. Other glaucoma medications include carbonic anhydrase inhibitors and beta-adrenergic blocking agents; the latter should be used with caution in children (see Chap. 9, sec. **XVIII**). If these medications cannot control the IOP, filtering surgery must be considered, but both the young age of the patient and the presence of active inflammation are adverse factors for achieving effective filtration. Trabecular surgery by goniotomy or a modified goniotomy "trabeculodialysis or trabeculotomy" has helped some individuals over short periods, but long-term successes from these procedures have not been reported.

The influence of steroid therapy on the IOP has to be evaluated in each patient. Steroids employed in the management of the uveitis may cause glaucoma in some individuals (steroid-induced glaucoma). In contrast, steroid therapy lowers the IOP in the condition of keratic precipitates in the angle (see Chap. 9, sec. **XXI**). Iridocyclitis usually causes a reduction in aqueous production by the ciliary body, and therefore in some critical situations the decision may be made to reduce the steroid therapy and allow the inflammation to worsen. If it has been decided to do filtration surgery, however, it is important to suppress inflammation with steroids as much as possible in the pre- and postoperative periods.

   E. **Glaucoma following trauma.** Glaucoma following ocular trauma in childhood may occur promptly or years later by the same mechanisms as in the adult (see Chap. 9, sec. **XVII**). In childhood it is important to include assessment of IOP in the initial and follow-up examinations of the traumatized eye because of the possibility of permanent trabecular damage following blunt trauma or hyphema.

XVI. **Special issues concerning trauma in childhood**
   A. **History taking** from traumatized children is notoriously unreliable. Not infrequently, the child feels guilty about the circumstances of the injury and gives an inaccurate or incomplete account of the accident. The physician must not be misled by an innocuous sounding history, but should be guided by the **physical findings** and entertain a high degree of suspicion that the injury involves more than the presenting signs. For example, lid laceration must be assumed to involve an intraocular injury until specifically proved otherwise.
   B. **Penetrating ocular trauma.** A full-thickness lid laceration should be fully evaluated and repaired by an ophthalmologist. The likelihood of an accompanying penetrating injury to the globe is great; if any doubt remains after examination in the emergency room, it is best to treat the eye as if it were penetrated and resolve the issue in the operating room (see Chap. 2, sec. **VI**). Although several routines for inducing sedation in the emergency room are available (pedimixes for IM injection or "soothing syrups" for drinking), the child is usually not sufficiently sedated for repair in this sensitive area. Heavy sedation runs the risk of serious respiratory depression, so it is generally safest and best to make the repair in the operating room with the aid of general anesthesia.
   If careful examination establishes the fact the injury causing a lid laceration has not caused a penetration of the globe, it may still have involved sufficient force to have caused intraocular damage.
   C. **Blunt ocular trauma.** Despite the slight, even jocular, attention often given to a "shiner," a black eye may be the prominent initial feature of serious ocular injury. Blowout fracture of the orbital floor, retinal detachment, hyphema, dislocated lens, traumatic iritis, and other ocular injuries may be overlooked because the lids are so swollen that insufficient attention is paid to the globe itself. All black eyes should be evaluated by an ophthalmologist. If there is any other sign of ocular abnormality such as conjunctival infection or diminished visual acuity, ophthalmic examination with dilated fundus examination is definitely indicated (see Chap. 2, sec. **VIII**).
   D. **Patching in young children.** Young children often need an eye patch applied for a day or two after **treatment** of an ocular condition such as corneal abrasion, removal of a corneal foreign body, or an ultraviolet sunlamp burn. A pressure patch of this sort is sometimes prescribed for several days consecu-

tively. In a very young child (especially in the first year or two), this may be a significant period of visual deprivation. In some cases, a patch has induced **strabismus** or **amblyopia.** Therefore, indications should be carefully weighed against risk when patching of very young children for more than a few days is being considered.

XVII. Retinal diseases in children

A. Retinal degenerations. Retinitis pigmentosa and its allied disorders constitute a diffuse group of disorders in which the mechanism of retinal degeneration is not known. Early loss of night vision, followed by loss of peripheral vision and eventual difficulty with central vision is characteristic. In classic retinitis pigmentosa, family history is prominent; the pattern of inheritance may be recessive, dominant, or X-linked. Some allied disorders, such as **albipuncuate dystrophy,** have a distinctive fundus appearance; others, such as choroideremia, have characteristic fundus features and characteristic hereditary patterns (X-linked in the case of choroideremia). **Leber's congenital amaurosis,** recessively inherited, may have little morphologic abnormality of the retina on fundus examination but presents with severe visual loss in the newborn period or early childhood. Confirmation of this diagnosis is provided by a markedly abnormal ERG.

Although it is not currently possible to treat most retinal degenerations, it is nevertheless important that efforts be directed toward identifying affected individuals early in their diseases. One should rule out potentially correctable disorders as well as give genetic counselling. Therapeutic interventions cannot hope to recover vision from the damaged retinas of adults already blind from the disorders. **Therapy** should be directed toward individuals who are still functioning, in the hope of avoiding further retinal degeneration. Systemic biochemical abnormalities have recently been identified with **gyrate atrophy,** and treatment with vitamin B_6 seems to have been beneficial in some patients. Previously, systemic biochemical abnormalities had been identified only in multisystem disorders that happened also to include retinal degeneration, e.g., **abetalipoproteinemia (Bassen-Kornzweig syndrome),** neuronal ceroid **lipofuscinosis (Batten-Mayou disease)** (see sec. VII.D), and **Refsum's disease.** The finding of a specific biochemical disorder in an isolated retinal degeneration such as gyrate atrophy is particularly encouraging and gives hope of similar discoveries with regard to retinitis pigmentosa and its allied disorders.

B. Childhood macular degenerations. A number of dominantly inherited macular degenerations, such as **Best's vitelliform dystrophy** and **butterfly dystrophy,** present in childhood. Family history is helpful in identifying these conditions.

Stargardt's macular degeneration (fundus flavimaculatus) may cause considerable reduction in central visual acuity with minimum fundoscopic changes. These youngsters have on occasion been erroneously considered to be malingering, and only years later when the process had reached an advanced stage was it properly recognized. There is **no** specific **therapy** for these disorders, but fundoscopic, psychophysic, and electrophysiologic testing should at least help characterize the disorder and improve early **diagnosis.**

C. Vitreoretinal degenerations

1. Juvenile retinoschisis. Strabismus, poor visual acuity, nystagmus, or a "cart wheel" (spokelike) macular region may be the presenting features of juvenile retinoschisis. Although the macular areas resemble microcystic edema on ophthalmoscopy, there is no leakage on fluorescein angiography. Schisis in the peripheral retina and X-linked heredity complete the clinical picture. Careful documentation of the fundus findings may be helpful since some of these youngsters subsequently lose vision acutely because of hemorrhaging from a retinal vessel or a retinal detachment. The family may benefit from genetic counseling.

2. The Goldmann-Favre syndrome is a rare disorder that might be considered if peripheral retinoschisis were seen in a young girl or in a boy in whom autosomal recessive inheritance seemed more likely than X-linked inheritance. There are preretinal membranes and a retinitis pigmentosa fundus picture.

3. **Wagner's vitreoretinal degeneration** has a dominant inheritance. Cataracts occur at an early age, and the vitreous contains dense membranes. Characteristic retinal pigmentation parallels the retinal vessels. Retinal detachments are frequent so periodic indirect ophthalmoscopic examinations to identify retinal breaks or early detachment is recommended.

4. **Sticker's disease,** dominantly inherited, has high myopia, liquefied vitreous, retinal pigmentary changes, and retinal detachment, which may be very difficult to treat. Systemic manifestations include skeletal dysplasia, cleft palate, and characteristically flattened facies.

D. **Coats' disease (Leber's miliary aneurysms).** The basic anomaly appears to be a congenital malformation of the retinal blood vessels leading to aneurysmal dilations that look like "light bulbs" in the peripheral retina on indirect ophthalmoscopy. The aneurysmal dilations are "leaky," so exudate accumulates in the subretinal space. This exudate tends to accumulate initially in the macular area, so a peripheral lesion should be considered when an unexplained macular star figure is seen. Obliteration of the peripheral vascular anomalies by **cryotherapy** or **photocoagulation** may be beneficial at this stage. With more exudation the retina may be completely detached. Total retinal detachment with fat and cholesterol in the subretinal fluid may create a white pupil (leukokoria). By that point vision is irretrievable, but it is very important to differentiate Coats disease from retinoblastoma as the cause of the white pupil.

E. **Sickle cell anemia.** Although sickle cell SS disease is the more severe systemic disorder, sickle C and sickle thalassemia disease are the more frequent causes of retinal neovascularization. Perhaps the anemia of sickle cell disease partially protects the flow through the small vessels of the retina. Retinal detachment may follow neovascularization; patients with sickle cell, sickle C, and S thalassemia disease as a group do poorly with retinal detachment surgery. Prophylactic treatment of retinal breaks seems particularly prudent in these patients. Since retinal changes can be seen even in the first decade, it is advisable to begin periodic ocular examinations when the diagnosis of SC or S thalassemia is made.

Extraocular Muscles, Strabismus, and Nystagmus

Deborah Pavan-Langston

I. Normal anatomy and physiology of the extraocular muscles

A. Innervation and action. All four recti muscles and the superior oblique muscle originate at the orbital apex (Fig. 11-1).

1. The **medial rectus** (MR) muscle runs forward along the medial side of the globe to insert 5.5 mm medial to the limbus. Innervation is by the third cranial nerve. Contraction of the muscle causes the eye to **turn inward (adduct)** toward the nose.

2. The **lateral rectus** (LR) muscle courses along the lateral side of the eye to insert 7 mm temporal to the limbus. Innervation to this muscle is by the sixth cranial nerve. Contraction causes the eye to **turn outward (abduct)** horizontally.

3. The **superior rectus** (SR) muscle runs over the dorsal aspect of the eye to insert 7.5 mm superior to the limbus. Innervation is via the third cranial nerve. Contraction produces various combinations of **vertical, horizontal,** and **rotary** movement, depending on the angle of gaze of the eye. As the muscle runs forward at an angle of 23 degrees to the medial wall of the orbit and inserts anterior to the center of rotation of the eye, the movement produced by contraction of the muscle would be pure elevation if the eye were at a horizontal starting position of 23 degrees abduction. If the eye is adducted inward to a position of 67 degrees, the only movement on contraction of the SR would be intorsion of the globe. With the eye in the primary position of straight-ahead gaze, contraction of the muscle produces combined elevation and intorsion with slight adduction.

4. The **inferior rectus** (IR) muscle courses along the ventral side of the eye to insert 6.5 mm inferior to the limbus. Innervation to this muscle is also via the third cranial nerve. Contraction produces various combinations of **vertical, horizontal,** and **rotary** movement, depending on the horizontal position of the eye. With the eye at a position of 23 degrees abduction, the only movement is depression. If the eye is adducted inward to a position of 67 degrees, the only movement is extorsion as the muscle inserts anterior to the center of rotation of the globe. When the eye is in the primary position, contraction of the IR produces depression and extorsion with minimum adduction.

5. The **superior oblique** (SO) muscle runs forward along the superomedial wall of the orbit to pass through the cartilage ring, the trochlea, where it turns backward temporally, traveling at an angle of 51 degrees from the medial wall of the orbit over the dorsal aspect of the globe but ventral to the SR muscle. It inserts on the posterotemporal surface. Innervation to this muscle is by the fourth cranial nerve. Contraction results in various combinations of **vertical, horizontal,** and **rotary** movements, depending on the location of the eye horizontally. With a starting position of 39 degrees of abduction, the only movement is intorsion. With a starting position of 51 degrees of adduction, the only movement is depression. If the eye is in the primary position of straight-ahead gaze, the motion is combined intorsion and depression with minimum abduction. Abduction is secondary to

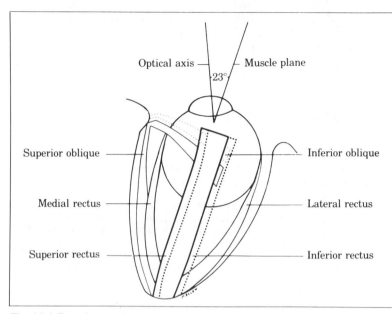

Optical axis — / — Muscle plane

23°

Superior oblique ——— / ——— Inferior oblique

Medial rectus ——— / ——— Lateral rectus

Superior rectus ——— / ——— Inferior rectus

Fig. 11-1. Dorsal view of extraocular muscle attachments to the eye. Dotted lines are muscles inferior to the globe. (Adapted from G. vonNoorden and A. E. Maumenee, *Atlas of Strabismus*. St. Louis: Mosby, 1967. With permission.)

the muscle insertion being posterior to the ocular rotation center when the eye is in the primary position.

6. The **inferior oblique** (IO) muscle originates at the anterior nasal orbital floor and runs backward and temporally at an angle of 51 degrees from the nasal orbital wall to insert under the LR muscle in the macular area. Innervation to this muscle is by the third cranial nerve. Contraction produces various combinations of **vertical, rotary,** and **horizontal** movements. Starting from a 39-degree position of abduction the only movement is extorsion. If the starting position is 51 degrees of adduction, the only movement is elevation. Contraction of the muscle with the eye in the primary position produces a combined extorsion and elevation with minimum abduction secondary to the insertion being posterior to the center of rotation when the eye is in the primary position.

7. The **spiral of Tillaux** is a theoretic line connecting the insertions of the four rectus tendons.

B. **Hering's law of equal innervation** states that equal and simultaneous innervation is given to synergistic muscles or muscle groups concerned with a desired direction of gaze. The law is applicable to voluntary and some involuntary muscle movement.

1. In **practical application,** during left gaze the right MR and left LR muscles receive equal innervation. During convergence the right and left MR muscles receive equal and simultaneous innervation. If the head is tilted to the right, the muscle groups concerned with cycloduction (intorsion) of the right eye and excycloduction (extorsion) of the left eye will receive equal and simultaneous innervation.

2. **Diagnosis of paralytic strabismus** is aided by knowledge of Hering's law in determining **primary and secondary deviation.** As the amount of innervation to both eyes is determined by the fixating eye, the angle of deviation will vary depending on the eye used for fixation. Primary deviation

occurs with fixation using a normal eye; secondary deviation occurs if fixation is with the paretic eye. The examiner may detect a paretic muscle or muscle group in **noncomitant** (unequal in different directions of gaze) **strabismus** by measuring the deviation of the eyes in diagnostic positions of gaze with each eye fixating in turn. As a case in point, in paralysis of the right LR, normal innervation moves the normal left eye in adduction during right gaze. The paretic right eye does not follow outward beyond the midline, however, as the normal amount of innervation required by the paretic eye is not sufficient to overcome the paresis of the right LR. The resulting horizontal deviation is primary. When the paretic eye fixates, however, and an excessive amount of innervation is released in attempt to perform abduction on right gaze, by Hering's law, the same increased amount of innervation will be transmitted to the normal MR of the contralateral eye, resulting in an excessive adduction of that eye. This is secondary deviation and is greater in magnitude than the primary deviation. It points to the right LR as the paretic muscle.

C. **Sherrington's law of reciprocal innervation** states that increased contraction of an extraocular muscle is associated normally by diminished contractile activity of its antagonist muscle. Therefore, on right gaze there is increased contraction of the left MR and the right LR accompanied by decreased tone of the antagonistic left LR and right MR. During convergence there is increased activity of both MR muscles with associated decreased activity of both LR muscles. When the head is tilted to the right shoulder there is contraction and relaxation of antagonistic muscle groups on levocycloversion. **Retractory nystagmus** and **Duane's retraction syndrome** are pathologic examples of cocontraction of medial and lateral recti in the same eye.

D. **Ductions** refer to the movement of just one eye. The horizontal ductions have been referred to under actions of the extraocular muscles (see **A**). **Abduction** is horizontal movement lateral to the midline vertical axis and is a function of LR contraction and MR relaxation. **Adduction** is horizontal movement medial to the midline vertical axis and is accomplished by the contraction of the MR muscle and relaxation of the lateral muscle. **Infraduction** is a vertical movement or depression inferior to the horizontal axis of the eye and results from combined contraction of the IR and SO muscles. **Supraduction** is a vertical movement or elevation superior to the horizontal axis of the eye and results from the combined contraction of the SO and IO muscles and the combined relaxation of the IR and SO muscles. **Incycloduction** or **intorsion** is a rotary movement of the eye about the anteroposterior (AP) axis such that the superior pole of the cornea is displaced medially and results from combined contraction of the SO and SR muscles with relaxation of the IO and IR muscles. **Excycloduction** or **extorsion** is a rotary movement of the eye around the AP axis displacing the superior pole of the cornea laterally and results from the combined contraction of the IO and IR muscles with concomitant relaxation of the SO and SR muscles.

E. **Binocular movements** are divided into two categories: **versions** and **vergences.**

1. A **version** refers to the simultaneous movement of both eyes in the same direction. Versions, like ductions, normally adhere to Hering's and Sherrington's laws, and include right and left lateral horizontal and vertical gaze.

   a. **Dextroversion** and **levoversion.** Dextroversion is the result of contraction of the right LR and left MR muscles. Levoversion is accomplished by contraction of the left LR and right MR with simultaneous relaxation of the left MR and the right LR.

   b. **Vertical versions** are supraversion or infraversion. **Supraversion** or **upgaze** is the result of bilateral contraction of the SR and IO muscles with simultaneous relaxation of the inferior recti and SO muscles in the primary position. **Infraversion** or **downgaze** in the primary position is the result of increased innervation to the IR and SO.

   c. **Cycloversion** is the simultaneous and equal tilt of the superior corneal

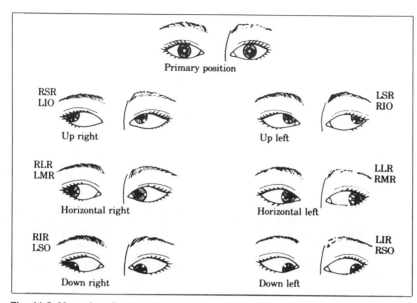

Fig. 11-2. Normal cardinal positions of gaze and extraocular muscles involved as primary movers in a given field of gaze. R = right; L = left; SR = superior rectus; IO = inferior oblique; LR = lateral rectus; MR = medial rectus; IR = inferior rectus; SO = superior oblique.

poles to the right or left. **Dextrocycloversion** is the result of contraction of the extorters of the right eye (IR and IO) and the intorters of the left eye (SR and SO) with concomitant relaxation of their antagonist muscles. **Levocycloversion** is the mirror image of this action, with increased innervation to the extorters of the left eye and the intorters of the right eye and decreased innervation to their antagonistic muscle groups.

2. A **vergence** is the equal simultaneous movement of the eyes in opposite directions. **Convergence** is inward movement; **divergence** is a simultaneous outward movement. Convergence is the result of contraction of both medial recti and relaxation of the lateral recti; divergence results from contraction of the lateral recti with concomitant relaxation of the medial recti. **Vertical vergences** result in contraction of the elevators of one eye and the depressors of the contralateral eye with subsequent opposing vertical movements. **Cyclovergence** is simultaneous equal tilting of the corneal superior poles inward or outward.

F. The **primary position of gaze** is the position assumed by the eyes when fixating a far distant object directly ahead. This position may be maintained with the head erect or with it tilted to either side. **Secondary positions** are any eye positions other than primary and include near-fixation, the cardinal positions, and midline vertical positions.

   a. The **near-fixation position** is usually taken at 0.33 m from the eyes. This reflex involves convergence and accommodative action.

   b. The **cardinal positions** are six positions of gaze that compare the horizontal and vertical eye alignment resulting from action by the six extraocular muscles (Fig. 11-2).

   c. The **midline positions** are vertical positions up and down from the primary positions.

II. **Single binocular vision** is a conditioned reflex, the prerequisites for which are straight eyes starting in the neonatal period and similar images presented to each retina. Patients with congenital strabismus lack single binocular central vision, but early elimination of the strabismus may result in peripheral single binocular vision. The age at which congenitally strabismic patients may develop single binocular vision after surgical straightening is unknown, but the current maximum estimate is 2 years. **Simultaneous perception, fusion,** and **stereopsis** are three different perceptual phenomena comprising single binocular vision. They may function simultaneously or in decreasing degrees, with stereopsis being the most highly developed and simultaneous perception the least developed in normal eyes. **For each retinal point in one eye there is a corresponding area in the opposite eye, within which the same image must project if the two are to be fused into a single image.** The further this retinal point is from the fovea, the larger the corresponding area in the opposing eye. If the retinal sites are anatomically identical, **normal retinal correspondence** (NRC) is present (see sec. **VI.C**).

A. In **simultaneous perception** all objects projecting their images outside of corresponding retinal areas are not fused, but they may be perceived simultaneously. This may result in double vision or diplopia unless the patient is inattentive to these images.

B. **Fusion** is the result of all objects projected onto corresponding retinal points, with their two images fused at the level of the CNS into one perception.

C. **Stereopsis** is the perception of the third dimension, i.e., the relative nearness and distance of object points as obtained from fused but slightly disparate retinal images. The **Titmus test** for stereopsis is described under tests for retinal correspondence (see sec. **VI.C.3.a**).

III. **Strabismus classification**

A. **The general order of examination** for strabismus is as follows:

1. **History**
   a. Deviation: age of onset, description of deviation, frequency and duration, symptoms, previous treatment.
   b. Personal: pre- and postnatal factors, course of pregnancy, delivery, growth and development, medications, surgery.
   c. Family: strabismus in blood relatives.

2. **General observation**
   a. Abnormal head posture or nodding.
   b. Spontaneous closure of one eye (squint).

3. **Visual acuity**
   a. Without glasses and with glasses, if worn.
   b. Near and distance vision (oculus dexter [OD], oculus sinister [OS], oculus uterque [OU]).
   c. Amblyopia testing.

3. **Motor**
   a. Extraocular muscle function, cardinal positions of gaze, ductions, versions.
   b. Phoria or tropia (cover test).
   c. Near point of convergence.
   d. Near point of accommodation, where indicated.

4. **Measurement of deviation**
   a. Distance and near, without and with glasses, if worn; with +3.00 add at near; with eyes in primary position, up, down, and, if indicated, in cardinal positions
   b. Accommodative convergence–accommodation (AC/A) ratio.

5. **Sensory tests** (depending on age and cooperation)
   a. Worth four-dot near and distance, without and with glasses, if worn.
   b. Stereopsis.
   c. Amblyoscope: after image, Bagolini lenses where indicated.
   d. Fusional vergence reserves.

6. **Fixation**
   a. Monocular, alternating, binocular.
   b. Nystagmus type.

      c. Visuscope: foveal, eccentric viewing, or fixation.
    7. Slit-lamp examination.
    8. Fundic examination.
    9. Cycloplegic refraction and dilated fundus examination on first or second office visit.
  B. Pseudostrabismus
    1. Pseudoesotropia or apparent **turning in** of the eyes may result from a prominent **epicanthal** skin fold that obscures part of the normally visible nasal aspects of the globe, thereby giving a false impression that esotropia is present. As the infantile flat nasal bridge develops, this excessive epicanthal skin is raised and the condition self-corrects.
    2. Pseudoexotropia is seen in hypertelorism, where there is an abnormally wide separation of the eyes as a result of disproportionate growth of the facial bones, or as a primary deformity. Despite the physical appearance, the eyes are aligned normally.
    3. Pseudohypertropia may result from facial asymmetry simulating a vertical ocular deviation.
    4. Angle kappa is the angle between the visual line that connects the point of fixation with the nodal points at the fovea and the pupillary axis with the line through the center of the pupil perpendicular to the cornea. The angle is **positive** when the corneal light reflex is displaced nasally and **negative** when it is displaced temporally. A positive angle kappa up to 5 degrees is considered physiologic in emmetropic (straight) eyes. The angle kappa is **measured on a perimeter** with the patient fixating on the central mark. A light is moved along the perimeter until its reflex is centered on the cornea. The difference in the position of the light and the center mark is indicated in degrees of arc on the perimeter and constitutes the angle kappa. This angle is significant in that a positive angle kappa may **simulate an exodeviation.** This is particularly common in arrested retrolental fibroplasia (RLF) of the retina where a positive angle kappa causes pseudoexodeviation and usually **masks a significant esotropia.** A negative angle kappa may **simulate esodeviation.** These deviations may be missed clinically if a positive angle kappa is associated with a small angle esotropia or a negative angle kappa with a small exotropia.
  C. Orthophoria indicates that the eyes are perfectly aligned with no deviation even when fusion is artificially disrupted by the examiner.
  D. Heterophoria is a misalignment in which fusion keeps the deviation latent. It may be detected by the tests described in sec. **IV.** Basically, however, in the cover-uncover test, **if only one eye moves when the cover is removed, a phoria is present.**
  E. Heterotropia is the manifest misalignment of the ocular axis. In the cover-uncover test, when the cover is removed, **if neither eye moves or if both eyes move and stay moved, a tropia is present** (Fig. 11–3).
    1. Horizontal deviations include **esophoria** and **esotropia,** which are convergent (inward) deviations of the visual axis, while **exophoria** and **exotropia** are divergent (outward) deviations of the visual axis.
    2. Visual deviations include right hyperphoria or hypertropia, in which the right visual axis is higher than the left, and left hyperphoria or hypertropia, in which the left visual axis is higher than the right.
    3. Torsional deviations include incyclophoria or incyclotropia, in which the superior poles of the corneas are tilted medially, and excyclophoria or excyclotropia, in which the superior poles of the corneas are tilted temporally.
IV. Diagnostic tests in strabismus are many. The most commonly used tests fall into four basic categories: (1) the cover tests, which depend on the fixation reflex, (2) the corneal reflex tests, which are based on the ability of the corneal surface to reflect the examining light, (3) the dissimilar image tests, which are based on patient response to double vision produced by converting an isolated object of regard into separate images on each retina, and (4) the dissimilar target tests, which are based on patient response to dissimilar images when different targets

Left esotropia

Left exotropia

Over action LIO
Left hypertropia

Over action LSO
Right hypertropia

Fig. 11-3. Common heterotropic muscle imbalances. LIO = left inferior oblique; LSO = left superior oblique.

are presented to each eye. Many of these tests involve eliciting **diplopia (double vision)** as a means of evaluation.

A. **Cover tests.** During these tests the patient must fixate on a small target designed to control accommodation. The first two tests are **qualitative** only; the simultaneous prism and cover test is **quantitative**.

1. **Cover-uncover tests for heterophoria detection.** Phoria deviations are kept latent by the fusion mechanism as long as both eyes are in simultaneous use. Tests for fusion will be positive when fusion is disrupted by covering one eye; i.e., deviation of the covered eye occurs if heterophoria is present. Each eye is covered separately in turn for 2–3 seconds and the occluder then quickly removed. The examiner must note whether or not the eye **under cover** makes a movement inward or outward to pick up fixation again. If there is no movement of either eye when it is covered and then uncovered, there is either no latent phoria present or a microtropia syndrome is present and must be tested for (see sec. **X.A.**). If, when uncovered, an eye moves outward to fixate, esophoria is present. If the eye moves inward to fixate, exophoria is present. A movement down to fixation reveals hyperphoria, and a movement upward to fixation reveals hypophoria. A disadvantage of this test is that small-angle phorias may be missed, but these may be picked up later with the Maddox or base-out prism tests (see secs. **B** and **C**). **Phorias** of any type may be **quantitated** by Maddox rod testing or by placing **prisms** of increasing strength before the deviating eye until no fixation movement occurs on uncover: **base-out for esodeviation, base-down for hyperdeviation, base-up for hypodeviation, and base-in for exodeviation** (Fig. 11-4).

2. **Cover tests for detection of heterotropias.** If heterotropia is present, tests for fusion are negative because one eye is not aligned with the fixation target. Covering the fixing eye will require the deviated eye to move to take up fixation, and this movement in the **uncovered eye** is looked for by the observer. If the nonfixating deviated eye is covered, however, there will be no movement of the fixating eye. Consequently, each eye must be covered in turn and the fellow eye watched for a fixation shift to determine whether tropia is present or not. If the eye moves outward to fixate, esotropia is present; if the eye moves inward to fixate, exotropia is present. If the uncovered eye moves downward, a hypertropia exists. If the uncovered eye moves upward, a hypotropia exists.

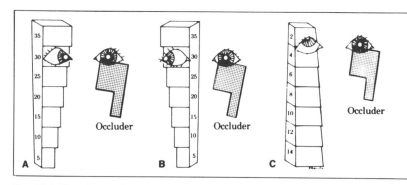

Fig. 11-4. Use of prism bar. **A.** Horizontal prism bar run base-out to measure esodeviations. **B.** Horizontal prism bar run base-in to measure exodeviations. **C.** Vertical prism bar base-down over hypertropic right eye (or base-up over hypotropic left eye alternative).

   3. **Simultaneous prism and cover test** is a quantitative measure of strabismic deviation. This is most useful in patients with **small-angle heterotropias** and is commonly used in esotropia. This test measures the actual heterotropia present while both eyes are uncovered. The examiner covers the fixating eye and simultaneously slips a prism of known power and appropriate base direction to compensate for the heterotropia in front of the uncovered eye. When the prism power selected equals the heterotropic angle, no movement occurs as the eye behind the prism takes up fixation.

  B. **Quantitative measurement of strabismic deviation by corneal reflex tests.**

   1. **Hirschberg's test.** A fixation light is held 33 cm from the patient, and the deviation of the corneal light reflex from the center of the pupil in the nonfixating (turned) eye is estimated. **Each millimeter of decentration corresponds to 7 degrees of ocular deviation.** Therefore, a 3-mm **inward** deviation of the light reflex corresponds roughly to a 21-degree **exotropia**, while a 4-mm **outward** deviation of the light reflex corresponds roughly to 28 degrees of **esotropia. One degree equals two prism diopters of deviation.**

   2. **Krimsky method.** Dissimilar positions of the corneal reflex in the pupils of each eye are indicative of strabismus, which may be measured by placing successively increasing prism power before the deviating eye until the reflection is similarly positioned in both eyes. Base-out prism is used for esotropia, base-in prism for exotropia (Fig. 11-4). This is a direct reading of the estimated squint angle.

   3. **In the corneal reflex test,** the prism is placed before the fixating eye with the examiner on the side of the deviated eye to avoid parallax error in observation. The prism power is increased to center the corneal reflection in the deviated eye.

   4. **Perimeter method** requires that the patient steadily fixate the 0 mark on the perimeter with the preferred eye as the examiner moves a light along the back side of the perimeter arc until the corneal reflex of the light appears located in the pupillary center of the deviated eye. The angle of deviation may be read in degrees from the perimeter arc at the point where the flashlight is stopped. **One degree equals approximately two prism diopters of deviation.**

   5. **The major amblyoscope** is a haploscopic device that consists of a medial septum between the two eyes with angled mirrors that reflect separate targets for each eye. These targets are set at the focal distance of the lenses in the eye piece; thus, viewing the targets simulates optical infinity or distance

fixation. The addition of −3 spheres into the eye piece stimulates accommodation and near convergence, so that a reading of the deviation at near can be made. Adjusting the tubes so that the corneal reflexes of illumination are centered in each pupil gives the examiner an approximation of the angle of deviation. By occluding the light sources alternately and having the patient fixate on the lighted target, the alternate cover test can be performed and the angle of deviation can be read directly.

C. **Dissimilar image tests**

1. **Maddox rod testing for heterophoria or tropia** is diplopia testing with dissimilar images of the same object. The Maddox rod is a red- or white-ribbed lens. A point source of light shined through this lens is seen as a red or white streak 90 degrees away from the axis of the multiple cylinders of the rod. Horizontal alignment may be checked by orienting the rod so that the streak is vertical, and vertical alignment checked by orienting the rod so that the streak is horizontal. The patient views the fixing light with both eyes open. If the streak appears to run through the center of the light both vertically and horizontally as the lens is turned, orthophoria is present in both directions. If the streak is displaced away from the light, misalignment is present. **A phoria cannot be distinguished from a tropia by this test.**

   a. **Horizontal deviations.** If the patient sees the vertical rod streak on the same side of the light as the eye that has the rod in front of it, **uncrossed** images are present and are indicative of esodeviation. If the patient sees the streak on the other side of the fixation light from the eye behind the Maddox rod, **crossed** images are present and are indicative of exophoria or exotropia. The degree of phoria or tropia may be **measured** directly by increasing the amount of prism power presented before one eye with **base-out for esodeviation** and **base-in for exodeviation** until the streak is aligned in the center of the light. The measurement may then be read directly from the prism power producing this effect.

   b. **Vertical deviation** may be measured by presenting **base-down prism to a hypertropic** eye or **base-up prism to a hypotropic** eye until the horizontal streak is aligned with the fixation light.

   c. **Cyclodeviations** may be checked by placing Maddox rods, one red and the other white, before each eye at the same axis setting for each eye. The axis settings of the rods are then adjusted until they appear parallel to the patient. The difference in degrees in cyclodeviation may then be measured directly from the trial frame in which the rods are set.

2. **The red glass test** is straightforward diplopia testing utilizing the image seen by the fovea of the fixating eye and the extrafoveal image of the deviated eye. It is performed by placing a plain red lens in front of one eye. This test is similar to the Maddox rod tests in horizontal and vertical deviations but is of no value in cyclodeviation measurement. Prisms with bases oriented toward the appropriate direction for the types of deviation (see sec. **1**) are used to eliminate the horizontal or vertical diplopia of white light and red light when the patient is viewing the fixation bulb, thereby yielding a direct measure of the deviation in the presence of normal retinal correspondence. The Maddox rod and red glass tests can be used to measure deviations in the diagnostic positions of gaze.

D. **Separate image tests.** In the presence of NRC, the point at which two separate images, one presented to each eye, appear superimposed provides a direct reading of the patient's alignment.

1. **Lancaster red-green projection.** The patient wears glasses with a red filter before one eye and a green filter before the other and views a white screen marked with a grid calibrated in squares of 7 degrees (14 **diopters [d]**) from a distance of 1 m. A linear red light and a linear green light are shined on the screen simultaneously, one light held by the patient and the other by the examiner (light held by the examiner determines the fixing eye), and adjusted until they are seen as superimposed by the patient. Any actual

disparity between the location and angle of the red and green lights gives the examiner a direct reading in centimeters of any deviation—horizontal, vertical, and torsional.

   2. The **major amblyoscope** is used to show the patient dissimilar objects that are simultaneously seen, one with each eye. The patient is asked to adjust the angle of the tubes so that one image is superimposed on the other. In the presence of NRC, horizontal, vertical, and torsional deviations may be read directly from the scales on the instrument, which indicate the deflection of the tubes away from 0 in these three planes.

V. **Measurement of fusional reserves (vergences).** Patients with heterophoria and microtropia may be asymptomatic by virtue of their relative fusional reserves. These reserves may be measured using accommodative targets at near and distance or a major amblyoscope. To **measure divergence reserves,** the examiner increases base-in prism over one eye until the patient reports blurring or diplopia of the target. To **measure convergence reserves,** base-out prism is increased to a similar end point. Vertical fusional reserves, positive, are determined by placing prism base-down before OD and, negative, by placing prism base-down before OS. **Normal divergence reserves** are in the range of 6 d with rapid recovery at distance, 10–14 d at near. **Normal convergence reserves** are 20–30 d at distance with rapid recovery and slightly more at near. Vertical reserves average 2–4 d at near or distance.

VI. **Sensory evaluation**

   A. **Visual acuity. Early determination of visual acuity is critical in evaluation of any patient with strabismus.** An estimation of visual acuity may be obtained in infants by observing behavior as each eye is alternately covered. If vision is equal or nearly equal in either eye, an infant or very young child will not object to having either eye covered. If visual acuity is reduced in one eye, however, the child will cry or push the occluder away when the normal eye is covered. If this occurs, ocular disease, **amblyopia** (nonorganic visual loss), or high refractive error should be suspected.

      1. **The preferential looking technique** permits reliable measurements of visual acuity to be made in infants from birth to age 1. At present this technique, as well as **evoked potential estimates of acuity,** is still available at specialized university medical centers. Before assuming that amblyopia is present (see **D**), it is essential that the examiner establish that visual loss is not due to organic disease. This is done by taking a **past medical history** on the child, including any circumstances during or after pregnancy that may have contributed to ophthalmic disease in the child. An examination of the **ocular anterior segments under magnification** is essential. A dilated **fundus examination,** preferably with the indirect ophthalmoscope, to rule out retinal pathology is an essential part of every examination.

      2. **Visual acuity** may be determined in the **illiterate and in preschool children** (age 36–60 months) using the E game. The parent instructs the child at home to indicate with the hand, or with a test letter that he or she holds, the direction in which the three bars of a test letter E held by the examiner are pointing. The illiterate Es can also be projected. An alternate means is the use of Allen preschool vision test on cards or projected Allen figures, which are small animals and common images that the child age 18–36 months is asked to identify. Once the child understands the test, vision may be determined by finding the smallest letter E or Allen figure read with each eye at 20 feet or, alternately, if vision is very poor, designating the optotype read at a distance closer than 20 feet.

   B. **Suppression testing.** Suppression **scotomas** are present both in eso- and exotropic patients. The esotropic patient has an area of suppressed vision extending nasally to the hemiretinal line, while the exotropic patient has an area of suppressed vision extending over a large area temporal to the hemiretinal line. These scotomas protect the patient from double vision (diplopia) when both eyes are open.

      1. **The Worth Four-Dot test** will detect fusion, suppression, and anomalous

retinal correspondence (see sec. **C**). The patient wears a red filter before one eye and a green filter before the other, mounted in the glasses frame, and views four lights at near and distance—two green, one red, and one white. Normally the white light is seen through both filters, the green lights are seen through only the green filter, and the red light through only the red filter. A patient who is fusing reports four lights, with the white light usually seen as a mixture of red and green. A patient suppressing the eye with the red filter will see only green, and the patient suppressing an eye with the green filter will see only red. The examiner may test the **macular area** by using very small Worth dots held at 0.33 m from the patient. This projects only a 6-degree angle, and the macular area is approximately 3 degrees. Fusion at this distance reveals normal bimacular or central fusion. Extramacular fusion (peripheral fusion) is detected by projecting larger Worth lights at a distance 6 meters from the patient. Patients with an esotropia of 10 d or greater will not fuse the distance Worth four dots. **NRC** will be identified in strabismic patients if they report that they see five lights (two red and three green), if the position of the lights corresponds to the angles of deviation. The dots seen by the fixating eye will be clear, whereas those seen by the deviating eye will be blurred. **Anomalous retinal correspondence** is present if the patients report that they see four dots while displaying a manifested deviation or if they have a microstrabismus (see sec. **C**).

2. **The red glass test for suppression and detection of retinal correspondence.** A heterotropic patient with normal vision in each eye but no diplopia (double vision) may be suppressing or ignoring the image received by the retina of the turned eye. With the patient fixating on a bright white light, a red glass placed before the deviated eye will make the second image visible to the patient if it has been ignored. If there is deep suppression present, only the white light will be seen despite the presence of the red lens over the deviated eye. Some examiners prefer holding the red glass over the fixating eye to make the patient aware of diplopia more easily, thereby evaluating the depth of suppression. If NRC is present, the patient sees the red light on the same side as the eye behind the red glass; **uncrossed diplopia** is present, indicating esodeviation. In **crossed diplopia** the red image is seen on the opposite side of the eye behind the red glass and indicates an exodeviation. If the red image falls on a suppression scotoma in the deviating eye of an exotropic patient, it is not seen. If the red filter is then placed before the fixating eye, diplopia may be elicited despite the presence of deep suppression. **Suppression may be differentiated from anomalous retinal correspondence** by holding a prism base-down before the red glass, thereby displacing the retinal image upward and beyond the suppression scotoma. With NRC the image will appear superiorly and to the right or left of the light. If anomalous retinal correspondence is present, the image will appear horizontally aligned but separated vertically from the fixation light.

3. **The 4-diopter base-out test** is used to determine whether central fusion (bifixation) or absence of central fusion (monofixation) is present in a patient whose **eyes appear straight.** With the patient reading letters on the distance vision chart, a 4-d, base-out prism is slipped alternately before one eye and then the other. The prism-covered eye is watched for movement. If the prism is placed before the fixating eye and both eyes move toward the apex of the prism and **stay moved,** a microtropia is present. If the prism is placed before the nonfixating eye, **neither** eye will move. The absence of movement by one eye is proof of a relative macular scotoma on that side. Bifixation may be recognized by each eye moving inward to refixate in response to displacement of the image produced by the prism. Occasionally, a bifixating patient will not make the necessary convergence movement to pick up the moved image, thereby making the test variable in its accuracy.

4. **Blind spot syndrome** may be found in patients with an esotropia persistently between 25 and 35 d at near and distance fixations. These patients are utilizing the blind spot of the deviated eye as a mechanism of avoiding diplopia in binocular vision. The image of the deviated eye falls on the optic nerve head scotoma. This phenomenon may be detected by placing a **base-out prism** before the deviating eye, thereby moving the visual image to an area between the optic disk and the fovea. The patient will suddenly experience uncrossed diplopia.

C. **Retinal correspondence**

1. **NRC** is the occipital cortical integration of similar images projected onto anatomically corresponding areas of each retina into a single perception, producing normal single binocular vision. Once binocular vision of this nature is established, it will be retained as long as there is functional vision in both eyes.

2. **Abnormal retinal correspondence (ARC).** If there is a disruption of the alignment of the eye, normal binocular vision may produce an annoying diplopia or **visual confusion.** Very young children are able to adapt to this disturbed state of alignment by compensatory CNS occipital cortex adjustment such as suppression, or by development of anomalous retinal correspondence. ARC is the occipital cortical adjustment in the directional values that permit fusion of similar objects projected onto noncorresponding retinal areas. It may develop whether the strabismus is vertical or horizontal. ARC may be present whether there is foveal fixation in both eyes or eccentric fixation present in one eye. It is **manifest only during binocular viewing.** There is no abnormality in the directional values of the retina in either eye during monocular viewing. A patient who has developed ARC may be made aware of diplopia or may experience visual confusion again after surgical correction of strabismus. A new angle of ARC may be developed to rid the patient of these annoying symptoms.

3. **Tests for retinal correspondence.** All tests commonly used for retinal correspondence involve some degree of alteration in the normal conditions of seeing. With the exception of the Bagolini lenses, the eyes are dissociated in the tests, thereby creating an apparatus-induced situation that will influence the result.

   a. **The Titmus stereotest** for three-dimensional vision and retinal correspondence allows the examiner to quantitate a patient's ability to fuse similar images projected onto slightly noncorresponding retinal areas. The patient wears polarized glasses and views pictures of a large fly, three lines of animals, and nine 4-circle sets, all with increasing refinement of projection on the noncorresponding retinal areas. Patients with NRC, good vision, and fusion will appreciate all nine sets of circles for three dimensions; patients with ARC may appreciate the three-dimensional aspect only of the large fly using their peripheral fusion mechanisms or up to six circles with microtropia.

   b. **The Bagolini striated lenses** are optically plano lenses with barely perceptible striations that do not blur the view but do produce a luminous streak when the wearer looks at a point source of light. These lenses are mounted in a spectacle or trial frame with the patient's visual corrective lenses in place behind. The Bagolini lenses should be placed so that the axis variation is oriented at 45 degrees in the right eye and 135 degrees in the left eye. The test is carried out at 33 cm and at 6 m (20 ft) from the eye. If patients see only one line running down hill from left to right, they are suppressing their left eye. If they see an X and the cover test reveals no shift, fixation is central and NRC is present. If the cover test reveals a shift and they see an X, ARC is present.

   c. **The Hering-Bielschowsky afterimage test.** With the fellow eye occluded, the better eye views a horizontal glowing linear filament for 20 seconds or an electronic flash in a darkened room. The better eye is then occluded and the contralateral eye views a vertically oriented glowing filament or an electronic flash for 20 seconds. Patients will continue to see these **afterimages** for some time after they have been turned off. They are asked to indicate the relative position of the two gaps in the center of each afterimage. These gaps correspond to the visual direction of each fovea in the presence of central fixation. The interpretation of the test, however, is dependent on the result of previously determined fixation behavior. If central fixation is present by Visuscope examination, the patient may have NRC and will see a perfect cross with the two gaps superimposed. In the presence of ARC, the vertical line will be displaced nasally in an esotropic patient and temporally to the horizontal in an exotropic patient.

D. **Amblyopia** is impaired foveal vision in the absence of organic disease and is most likely due to lack of continuous use of one or both foveas for visual fixation. It is basically a deprivation phenomenon caused by nonuse of fixation reflex. **The fixation must be developed early in life and used until a child is approximately 5 years old, or amblyopia may develop.**
1. **Types of amblyopia**
   a. **Strabismic amblyopia** is most frequently encountered in the esotropic patient but also may occur less frequently in exotropia. As a compensation to avoid diplopia from foveas oriented in two different directions, the patient will inhibit the foveal region of the deviating eye, which in turn will result in strabismic amblyopia of disuse.
   b. **Anisometropic amblyopia** is the result of a marked disparity in the refractive error. Small differences are tolerated, but a difference in refraction greater than 2.5 d between the eyes may disturb binocular function and cause a patient to develop either alternating vision, using the near-sighted eye for near vision and the contralateral eye for distance vision, or to suppress the blurred image of one eye, thereby causing amblyopia in that eye.
   c. **Organic amblyopia.** Damage to the foveal receptors may occur at birth or subsequently, causing interference with fusion due to blurring in one eye. This may be further enhanced by superimposition of disuse of the fovea in the damaged eye, thereby causing amblyopia over the level of blurring due to organic disease. This may be referred to as **relative amblyopia.**
2. **Diagnostic tests in amblyopia**
   a. **The visual acuity** of the amblyopic eye is greater for isolated letters than for whole lines of letters. The acuity drops according to the degree that the letters are crowded together and is called the **crowding phenomenon.** The etiology is unexplained but is thought to be retinal rather than cortical. As amblyopia responds to therapy this phenomenon will be reduced or disappear altogether. Since the visual acuity obtained on the reading of entire lines of letters is a more sensitive indicator of the depth of amblyopia than the acuity obtained with isolated letters, the crowding of letters is a more accurate indicator of the depth of amblyopia and is of therapeutic importance.
   b. **The neutral density filter test** is used to differentiate between functional and organic amblyopia. Combined neutral density filters, such as Kodak No. 96, N.D. 2.00 and 0.50, of sufficient density to reduce vision in a normal eye from 20/20 to 20/40 are slipped before the amblyopic eye. Vision will be decreased by one or two lines, be unaffected, or be slightly improved if the impairment is functional and, therefore, reversible. If organic amblyopia is present, the vision is often markedly reduced.
   c. **Fixation behavior** should be determined in patients with amblyopia. Central viewing is foveal; **eccentric viewing** is a stage intermediate between central and eccentric fixation. Either abnormal phenomenon may be present in one or both eyes. In eccentric viewing the patient uses extrafoveal retinal elements for fixation as foveal vision is impaired

by suppression or organic disease; however, the principal visual direction is normal and still associated with the fovea, thereby giving the patient the impression of looking beyond the image. In **eccentric fixation** the principal visual direction and motor orientation have shifted to become associated with the eccentric retinal area rather than the fovea and patients feel that they are looking directly at the image. Eccentric viewing has a better prognosis for visual recovery than eccentric fixation. The following tests are commonly used to differentiate these phenomena:

(1) **Visuscope motor test.** The Visuscope is a modified ophthalmoscopic device that projects an asterisk onto the patient's retina. The untested eye is occluded and the patient is requested to look directly at the asterisk while the examiner observes the fundus. In **eccentric viewing** the asterisk will initially stop on the fovea, and then the eye will make a second shift so that the asterisk falls onto the nasal peripheral retina. The initial movement to the fovea reflects the normal fixation reflex present in eccentric viewing, followed by the second motor shift to move the image to an area of clearer vision. In **eccentric fixation** the eye will shift so that the asterisk moves immediately to the extrafoveal area of retinal fixation.

(2) **Visuscope sensory test.** The examiner places the Visuscope asterisk nasal to the fovea in the amblyopic eye. In **eccentric viewing** the patients will respond that the asterisk is localized in the temporal periphery and they feel as though they are looking past it. In **eccentric fixation** patients will have the impression that they are looking directly at the asterisk.

(3) **Alternate cover test for bilateral eccentric fixation** reveals that either eye remains in its exotropic position when the contralateral eye is covered and makes no attempt to pick up what appears to be refixation of the image. The Visuscope test will be that of eccentric fixation in both eyes.

(4) **Hering-Bielschowsky afterimage test in eccentric viewing and fixation.** In eccentric viewing the foveas retain their common visual direction, and the afterimage result will be similar to that in an esotropic patient with ARC. In eccentric fixation the fovea of the better eye has a common visual direction with a noncorresponding retinal area in the contralateral eye, so the patient will see a perfect cross, as if NRC were present. The Visuscope must be relied on for diagnosis of eccentric fixation.

3. **Therapy of suppression** should be carried out only in selected cases, by an orthoptist under the direction of an ophthalmologist, as elicited awareness of diplopia may be the one result, producing new annoying symptoms in patients unable to fuse.

a. **Suppression** may be treated by placing a red filter over one eye to produce dissimilarly colored objects when the patient fixates on white light. The patient is then asked to fixate either the red or the white image but at the same time to try to view the other image. The deviated eye is then rapidly covered and uncovered with an occluder, so that the previously suppressed image may be seen alternately with the first. If the patient is unable to achieve diplopia using this method, a 4-d prism may be placed base-down before the deviating eye to lift the image out of the suppression scotoma. Diplopia will then be apparent. Once the patient learns to recognize the diplopia, he or she must concentrate on maintaining it. The red filter is removed and the patient will, with good fortune, continue to see two different white lights alternately flashing on and off. When the occluder cover-and-uncover motion is stopped, the patient should see two sustained white lights. If a vertical prism is used, it may be withdrawn either abruptly or gradually. Once the two lights are maintained without alternate cover, the patient is taught to transfer fixation of the light from eye to eye, maintaining double vision while either eye fixates. Once this is accomplished the patient may practice on other objects, such as a ball or matchbox. Between practice sessions, occlusion on the nonsuppressed eye is continued to prevent renewal of the suppression habit. **Other techniques** involve the use of the major amblyoscope rather than fixation light, red filter, occluder, and vertical prism to perform antisuppression treatment.

b. **After a patient has been taught to recognize diplopia** and ARC is present, attempts are made to restore NRC, either by correcting for the angle of deviation with prisms or by placing the amblyoscope tubes at the objective setting. The patient is asked to try to fuse the identical targets or to superimpose larger dissimilar targets. The patient may experience monocular diplopia or binocular triplopia, which represents a transient stage in passage from ARC to NRC as retinal areas view with one another to localize the image in the nonfixating eye. Once the patient has achieved fusion with NRC, occlusion of one eye is maintained to prevent recurrence of ARC between practice sessions. The eyes may then be aligned by surgical means or by use of prisms.

4. **Treatment of amblyopia** is based on forcing the patient to depend on the amblyopic eye for vision.

a. **Occlusion therapy with patching** of the preferred eye is the treatment of choice. Adhesive patches should be used to discourage removal by the patient and to prevent peeking. Elastoplast eye occluders and Opticlude orthoptic eye patches are most commonly used. **A general rule of thumb is 1 week of patching for each year of age between acuity checks of both eyes.** Very young children should be seen every few weeks and vision or at least preferred fixation tested in **both eyes** to ascertain that **occlusion amblyopia** is not developing under the patch and that progress is or is not being made visually in the amblyopic eye. Once good visual acuity or alternating fixation is achieved, the patient may be put on part-time patching, such as 6 hours daily, and then followed every 2–3 months until time for cosmetic surgery, if any is required. Postoperatively, the patient should be followed as frequently as during the part-time patching phase because **amblyopia may recur** despite cosmetically satisfactory surgical correction.

b. **Lens occlusion** of the preferred eye by taping the back of a spectacle correction to force use of the amblyopic eye through the other lens may be used in children who are reliable and will not pull the spectacles down to peek over the covered lens. In general, the acuity in the amblyopic eye must be better than 20/60 (6/18) for this form of therapy to be successfully used.

c. **Occluder contact lenses** have been used more frequently in patients with aphakia or high **anisometropia;** however, the hard lens is not of practical use in controlling strabismic amblyopia.

d. **Atropinization** of the preferred eye may be effective only if acuity in the amblyopic eye is 20/50 (6/16) or better. If vision is less than this the patient will prefer the blurred image in the atropinized eye and continue to use it in favor of the amblyopic eye. Atropine 1% is instilled each morning in the preferred eye or may be coupled with part-time occlusion of the preferred eye, in which case atropine is instilled at weekly intervals. Atropine in the good eye and miotic therapy of the amblyopic eye is an acceptable combination.

e. **Eccentric fixation** is usually treated with adhesive patching of the normal eye. Occlusion of the eccentrically fixated eye for a month or so to interfere with the established pattern of vision before initiation of occlusion of the better eye has **not** been found to be of significant clinical use.

VII. **Motor evaluation**

A. **Comitant esodeviations** may be defined as those in which the convergent angle of the eyes remains unchanged in any given direction of gaze within 5 d, using fixed accommodation. These deviations may be caused by seemingly unrelated factors, such as the near convergence reflex, congenital overaction of the medial recti, acquired hypotony of the lateral recti, and monocular loss of useful vision in infancy or childhood. **Noncomitant deviations** (horizontal or vertical) are unequal in different fields of gaze and are usually seen in situations where there is paresis of one or more muscles or in A-V deviation (see sec. **IX**).

1. **Accommodative esodeviations** are associated with overaction of the convergence reflex in its association with near accommodation. If this deviation is within the fusional range, it is **accommodative esophoria**; if the esodeviation is beyond fusional possibility, it is **accommodative esotropia.**

   a. The **etiology** of accommodative esodeviation may be one of two unrelated causes that may occur together or alone. The first is seen in the **hypermetropic** or farsighted patient in whom the retinal image remains blurred unless the patient clears it by increased accommodative effort. This is associated with an increased convergence of the eyes in the accommodation convergence reflex. The second cause is an abnormally high **AC/A ratio.** This may occur even in patients with no refractive error and represents an abnormal relationship between accommodation and the accommodative-convergence reflex elicited with focus at the near point. The amount of convergence associated with each diopter of accommodation may be minimum to marked.

   b. The **average age of onset** of accommodative esotropia regardless of etiology is 2.5 years but ranges between 6 months and 7 years. If a high AC/A ratio is associated with hypermetropia, esotropia will be present both at near and distance fixation. If the patient is emmetropic (no refractive error), esotropia will be present only on near fixation. Frequently, there is a familial history of esotropia in these patients.

   c. **Clinical evaluation**

      (1) A **cycloplegic refraction** is an integral part of the evaluation of any strabismic patient, but is of critical value in the patient with accommodative esodeviation. A patient may be prepared for cycloplegic refraction with one drop of 1% cyclopentolate q10min times 3 within an hour of retinoscopic examination. Similarly, 1% atropine drops tid OU or 0.5% atropine ointment in each eye qhs for 3 days immediately prior to retinoscopic examination is sufficient and preferable in preschool children. By paralyzing accommodation the examiner may usually detect nearly the full amount of hypermetropia, although subsequent cycloplegic refraction may disclose more hypermetropia than detected during the first refraction. It is not uncommon for patients with a normal AC/A ratio to have more hypermetropia than those with a high AC/A ratio. The greater the degree of hypermetropia, the greater the tendency to accommodate to clear vision and secondarily to overconverge to an esodeviation state.

      (2) **The AC/A ratio** may be most easily determined with the gradient method by measuring the eso- or exodeviation with full glasses correction at distance using an accommodative target, e.g., as esotropia 10 d. A −1 sphere is then placed over both eyes to stimulate 1 d of accommodation and the deviation remeasured. For example, the esotropia may now be 16 d. The AC/A in this example is 6 d of accommodative convergence to 1 d of accommodation. This is one of many ways of measuring AC/A.

      (3) **Sensory complications** seen in accommodative esotropia are those mentioned earlier (see sec. **VI**). In addition, a motor complication that may occur is secondary to apparent hypertrophy of the frequently contracted medial recti. A nonaccommodative esotropia may

be superimposed on the accommodative component as a result of this buildup of MR strength.

(4) Therapy of accommodative esotropia includes **glasses** or the instillation of **miotic** (parasympathomimetic) drugs in both eyes (or both).

    (a) Bifocals are the treatment of choice in the accommodative esotropic child with a high AC/A ratio causing esotropia at near despite a full correction for any existing hypermetropia at distance. A child given his or her full cycloplegic refraction should be examined at 1-2 monthly intervals to ascertain that the glasses control the accommodative esotropia. If the esotropia persists at near despite the eyes being straight at distance, an additional +2.50-d bifocal segment should be prescribed. This may be glued on or ground into the distance correction. This lower segment should be set higher for children than is routinely done for adults, as segments that are too low will be overviewed by the child, or the child will raise his or her chin in order to depress the eyes to see through the additional plus lens. The ideal level for the top of the bifocal segment is 3 mm above the 6:00 limbus position with the eyes in primary position.

    (b) Miotic therapy. Echothiophate (Phospholine Iodide) is the most commonly used miotic in accommodative esotropia. Concentrations of 0.06-0.12% may be used with one drop in each eye each morning. The drug will cause pupillary miosis and may be associated with pupillary cysts. These cysts may be prevented by instilling phenylephrine hydrochloride 2.5% daily to 3 times a week. This diminishes the miosis but does not interfere with the function of the miotic in "tricking" the eye into thinking that it is maximally accommodated, thereby preventing the convergency reflex. Occasionally, children, particularly older children, may be controlled with every other day miotic therapy. Side effects of echothiophate such as cataracts are rarely if ever seen in children. **If surgery is anticipated, echothiophate must be discontinued** 2-3 weeks prior to any general anesthesia to allow restoration of the normal plasma and erythrocyte cholinesterase levels, thereby avoiding the **risk of prolonged postoperative apnea.** Since this drug cannot be considered harmless because of its systemic and possible cataractogenic effect, dosage should be reduced as soon as the accommodative esotropia is brought under control. This should be a progressive decrease to every other day and possibly to 2 or 3 times weekly dosage, with the final levels being determined by the minimum dosage necessary to control the deviation and to allow fusion.

    (c) In children under 4 years of age the full cycloplegic plus refractive correction is prescribed as glasses. If the child initially refuses to wear the glasses, the instillation of atropine 1% drops in each eye each morning (see sec. **VI.D.4**) for a month may be useful in encouraging use of the glasses, but miotics should not be used as alternative permanent therapy in place of the glasses.

    (d) Children 4-8 years of age need to wear only that amount of plus lens power required to maintain fusion and provide maximum visual acuity rather than wearing the full cycloplegic refractive correction. **The examiner should be able to demonstrate some esophoria by alternate cover tests with glasses on.** This indicates a high degree of tone and that the fusional divergence is being maintained. If orthophoria is maintained for several years with glasses without any stress on the patient's fusional divergence, eventual withdrawal of the glasses will cause only symptoms of asthenopia or blurred vision.

(e) **Children over 8 years of age** may begin to show signs of spontaneous improvement. The hypermetropia usually decreases and the severity of the AC/A ratio diminishes spontaneously well into the teens. The power of the plus lenses may be decreased, and if bifocals were used to correct a condition that was due primarily to a high AC/A ratio rather than hypermetropia, these may be discontinued as well. The other factors of concern in total withdrawal of the glasses, e.g., astigmatism and severity of hypermetropia, must be taken into account. Many children with high hyperopia who manifest an accommodative esotropia ultimately exhibit an exodeviation in their early teens. This may be controlled, in part, by reduction of the plus lens condition, but many children come to surgery for the basic exodeviation previously masked by the accommodative convergence.

2. **Nonaccommodative esodeviations** are the varying convergent forms of strabismus not associated with accommodation. The **etiology** may be either neurogenic or anatomic. Patients may have **partially accommodative** and **partially nonaccommodative** deviations, and therapy (surgical and medical) should be adjusted accordingly. The nonaccommodative deviation is that amount that remains when full therapy of the accommodative component is in effect.

a. **Congenital esotropia** is usually noted shortly after birth but may not become clinically apparent for 1–2 months. The angle of deviation is usually greater than 30 d with little variation in measurement in the non-brain-damaged child.

(1) **Diagnosis** of congenital esotropia is assisted not only by the time of discovery but also by the finding of alternate fixation in the primary position and **crossed fixation** on lateral gaze such that the patient uses the right eye to view objects in the left field and the left eye to view objects in the right field. Those few who do not alternate are amblyopic in the nonpreferred eye and may have eccentric fixation. Nystagmus blockage syndrome is discussed in sec. **XIII.D.7.**

(2) The **differential diagnoses** of congenital esotropia are the abduction limitation syndromes and lateral rectus paralysis problems including Duane's and Möbius' syndromes (see sec. **X**).

(3) **Tests for abduction**

(a) **Spinning.** If the child is held and spun around the examiner's head, the labyrinth stimulation will create a nystagmus causing abducting movements of the eye on the side opposite to the direction of head acceleration. In this manner the examiner may determine if there is, in fact, abduction potential of each LR. **Doll's head** movement may serve a similar purpose.

(b) **Occlusion.** An alternate method of inducing abduction in the cross-fixating eye of a congenital esotrope is occlusion of one eye for several hours. Abduction will appear in the contralateral eye if true crossed fixation is present.

(c) **Forced ductions** are of use in determining whether or not an ocular deviation is secondary to mechanical obstruction. It is most commonly used in congenital esotropes with crossed fixation who cannot be made to abduct despite the foregoing tests. Under general anesthesia the conjunctiva and episclera are grasped with forceps near the muscle in question, and the globe is moved in the direction away from that muscle. If the eye moves freely away from the location of the muscle, no mechanical obstruction exists. If the eye is moved only with difficulty, it is likely that there is scarring or fibrosis of the muscle that is the source of the deviation. This test may also be performed with local anesthesia in adults, but voluntary eye movement may affect the results. It is used in children and adults in **differentiating such entities** as traumatic paralysis of the IR muscle from an orbital floor fracture with entrapment of the muscle, a tight LR muscle after excessive surgical resection, CNS from peripheral fibrosis as an etiology of Duane's retraction syndrome, and thyroid myopathy from IR muscle or elevator paralysis.

(4) The **esotropia angle is measured** by techniques discussed earlier (see sec. **IV**).

(5) **Therapy of congenital esotropia** in the absence of amblyopia involves surgical straightening of the eyes, botulinum injection of the medial recti, or both (see sec. **XII**). If amblyopia is present or suspected, occlusion therapy should be carried out **prior to any surgical correction.** In the nonamblyopic child, surgery is performed early in life in an attempt to achieve at least peripheral fusion. A new and experimental approach to oculomotor imbalance is to make use of the muscle-paralyzing effect of botulinum toxin. This toxin is injected into a functioning eye muscle to prevent contraction and consequent tightening of the muscle. The long-term effects of this remain to be determined, and it is not clear just how it might fit into the more conventional treatment of strabismus.

b. **Esotropia secondary to monocular impaired vision.** Any anomaly either preventing development of normal sight or interfering with normal sight once developed may produce an esotropia, usually about 6 months after the anomaly appeared.

(1) The **esotropic angle** is not usually as large as that encountered in congenital deviation, but fixation is irretrievable in the involved eye, thereby making measurements of the angle of deviation impossible using prism and cover alternates. The Krimsky or prism reflex test must be used for evaluation of the angle of deviation.

(2) **Management** includes careful ophthalmoscopy to elicit the etiology of decreased vision; i.e., retinoblastoma or chorioretinitis can be ruled out if no disease is apparent in the anterior segment. If the etiology is not life-threatening and the visual anomaly cannot be corrected, surgical correction of the esodeviation is indicated for cosmetic purposes. This may be done at any age but usually before the child is 4 years old. The object of cosmetic surgery is to correct the angle of deviation to approximately 15 d of esotropia to prevent the ultimate development of a secondary exotropia. The eyes tend to drift outward as a child matures, and the initial esotropic correction may have to be reversed in subsequent years.

c. **Divergence insufficiency** is an acquired comitant esodeviation that is maximum at distance, decreases to orthophoria on near fixation at 1 m or less, and remains unchanged in angle of deviation on lateral gaze. **Onset** may be at any age, and the initial symptom is homonymous diplopia at distance. Abduction is normal in each eye. The **etiology** is often obscure but may be rarely associated with intracranial disease. This must be ruled out. **Treatment** of divergence insufficiency is supportive, with the object being only to relieve diplopia using occlusion therapy or prisms after neuroophthalmologic evaluation has been completed. If the condition persists for more than 6 months without change, surgical intervention may be justified. The prognosis is good.

B. **Concomitant exodeviations.** An outward divergence of the visual axis is an exodeviation. If this divergence is kept latent by singular binocular vision, thereby maintaining stereopsis, the condition is termed **exophoria.** A gross manifestation of misaligned visual axis outward, often with associated suppression scotoma and loss of stereopsis, is termed **exotropia**. Patients may fluctuate between the two. The **etiology** is considered to be a disturbance in the tonic horizontal vergence that may be neurologic in origin or secondary to anatomic factors such as hypertrophic lateral recti.

1. **Exophoria** of less than 10 d is often asymptomatic in adults. Even larger degrees of deviation may be asymptomatic in children.

   a. **When symptoms become manifest** they are characterized by vague asthenopia that worsens with prolonged visual tasks, transient diplopia, or momentary blurred vision when the fusional convergence fatigue threshold has been exceeded or exhausted. In compensation a patient may overaccommodate to increase convergence, thereby blurring out visual detail. The symptoms of exophoria will predominate in the field of gaze where the deviation is greatest; i.e., they will be greatest at distance visual tasks if the deviation is greater for distance viewing, and greater for near visual tasks if **convergence insufficiency** is the predominant problem. A common solution to this latter problem is closing one eye during near visual tasks. Exophoric patients have good fusional vergence amplitude and no amblyopia.

   b. **Measurements** of the deviation are discussed in sec. **IV.**

   c. **Treatment** of exophoria is nothing if it is asymptomatic. Symptomatic exophoria is often helped by convergence exercise to increase fusional convergence amplitude. For deviation greater at distance, therapy consists of the reading of small detailed distance targets with increasing base-out prism; for near, small print to enhance the stimulus of fusional convergence. Overcorrection of any existing myopia will also stimulate accommodative convergence to assist the patient with convergence insufficiency problems. This is useful in younger patients, but adults may suffer asthenopia. Base-in prism spectacles are of greater use in reducing symptoms in older presbyopic patients and in prepresbyopic patients unable to increase their fusional convergence with orthoptic training. The degree of exophoria may be measured at near and distance with Maddox rod and prisms. One-half of this measurement may then be placed as base-in prism in a spectacle correction (one-half of the amount to be put in each lens) along with the normal hypermetropic or myopic correction. When all else fails, surgery may be the answer for exophoria but may lead to overcorrection.

2. **Intermittent exotropia,** like exophoria, is associated with normal fusional vergence and amplitudes, no amblyopia, and bifixation. Stereopsis is normal during the exophoric phases but absent when the patient becomes manifestly exotropic.

   a. **Sensory adaptation** in intermittent exotropia is extremely rare but includes suppression scotomas in the temporal fields and ARC to avoid the symptoms of diplopia and visual confusion during exotropic phases. As soon as the patient returns to an exophoric phase, however, NRC recurs and bifixation functions at peak level with normal stereopsis. These sensory adaptions must be developed before the age of 10 or frank diplopia will occur when the exotropia becomes manifest.

   b. **Measurement of exodeviation** must be at near and distance **using a reading chart rather than fixation light** to prevent the patient from using extra accommodative convergence to reduce the exodeviation. A blurred fixation light will not bother the patient, but blurring of print due to overaccommodation will cause the patient to back down on the accommodative effort until vision is clear, thereby revealing the accurate levels of exodeviation. A high AC/A ratio is more frequently found in intermittent exotropia than a low AC/A ratio. Deviations measuring up to 35 d at distance and 10 d at near are common in young children but will increase with age at near, causing the near and distance deviation measurements to approximate each other. It is useful to have the patient view the near accommodative target through +3-d lenses to reduce accommodative-convergence and more accurately measure the near exodeviation. The alternate cover test is used to measure the exodeviation at near and distance. If it is found that the **distance deviation is significantly greater than the near,** a patch should be placed over one eye for 2–3 hours or overnight to dissociate thoroughly the eyes because the convergence mechanism at near may be artificially reducing the true amount of exodeviation. Before the patch is removed the contralateral eye is covered with an occluder. After the patch is removed it is critical to prevent the patient from using both eyes together even momentarily, as this brief exposure may be sufficient to reestablish binocular vision and reobscure the near deviation by fusional convergence. The alternate cover test is performed again at near and prism measurements taken. If the angle of deviation at near has now increased to approximate that of the distance measurement, it has been established that convergence is being used to overcome the near deviation. If the measurements at near are still significantly less than distance exodeviation measurements, it has been established that there is a **divergence excess.** Establishing the difference between divergence excess and simulated divergence excess is critical in decisions concerning surgical management.

    c. **Treatment of intermittent exotropia** is botulinum injection of the lateral recti (see sec. **XII**) or surgery and is justified if, in the presence of corrected refractive error (anisometropia or myopia), there is still a manifest exodeviation. Surgery of divergence excess is recession of both lateral recti; surgery of a basic exotropia where near and distance measurements are approximately the same is resection of the MR and recession of the LR on the same eye. If the patient is older than 10 years of age and has not developed suppression or ARC elimination of the divergence angle, surgery will prevent any such sensorial adaption. **Patients under the age of 10 are at risk for suppression and possible ARC so long as exotropia exists.**

3. **Exotropia** is constant divergence of one eye and is commonly associated with a normal or low AC/A ratio. Fixation is commonly alternating between the two eyes, thereby preventing amblyopia, although constant exotropia in a patient less than 10 years of age causes a significant increase in the risk of development of amblyopia, suppression, or ARC, as there is no binocular vision present to prevent development of sensorial adaption.

    a. **The measurement of exotropia** is similar to that described in sec. **IV.**

    b. **Amblyopia.** If, after appropriate refraction and vision testing, amblyopia is found in an exotropic patient, therapy is similar to that described in sec. **VI.D** and should be undertaken prior to any surgical correction of the deviation. Patients 10 years of age or younger usually respond to such therapy. The congenitally exotropic child should undergo surgery early in life, if possible. Older patients undergo surgery as described in sec. **2.c.** If one eye has irreversibly reduced visual acuity, surgery should invariably be a recession of the lateral rectus and resection of the medial rectus on the amblyopic eye.

C. **Concomitant vertical deviations** of up to 4 d are not uncommon and are often associated with horizontal deviation. In the absence of horizontal deviation, good fusional vergence is present and associated with normal fusion and binocular vision.

    1. **Skew deviations.** Vertical deviations should be differentiated from skew deviations, which are associated with CNS disorders or labyrinthitis. In skew deviation the onset is often abrupt, and the vertical deviation is large and either constant or variable in various positions of gaze.

    2. **Therapy of concomitant vertical deviations** is usually vertical prisms with one-half the correction ground into each lens of a spectacle, base-down over the hypertropic eye, base-up over the hypotropic. Optical correction should also be incorporated; if prisms fail, surgical correction may be undertaken. Botulinum injection is rarely used in vertical deviations because of potential lid complications or lack of effect (see sec. **XII**).

VIII. Dissociated hyperdeviation is characterized by an upward turn of the nonfixating eye. If bilateral, it is "double hyperdeviation"; if unilateral, "right or left dissociated hyperdeviation." Alternating sursumduction elicited during the cover-uncover test is identical to dissociated double hyperdeviation. The condition is particularly common bilaterally and should not be confused with other imbalances in the vertical muscles. These deviations may be present either as phorias or tropias, depending on whether or not single binocular vision is found.

A. **Clinically** dissociated hyperdeviation is recognized by an upward turn of the covered eye on alternate cover testing. Either eye turns up when covered, and the covered eye moves down to fixate as the occluder is moved from side to side. This occurs in all fields of gaze. Radial limbal vessels may be observed to pick up the **cyclodeviation** that occurs simultaneously with the hyperdeviation in these patients.

B. **The Bielschowsky phenomenon** is found in dissociated hyperdeviation. This is manifested as a downward movement of the elevated eye, which may infraduct to a level lower than the fixating eye. This is observed by reducing or increasing the light entering the fixating eye only by passing a series of filters of decreasing or increasing density in a filter rack before the fixating eye. When the stimulus threshold is reached in the fixating eye, the downward movement will occur in the contralateral eye.

C. **Therapy of dissociated hypertropia** is rarely necessary. Patients are asymptomatic, as there is no binocular vision during the tropic phase. If the patient suffers asthenopic symptoms, however, surgical correction may be considered.

IX. A-V patterns in horizontal strabismus are manifested by a change of ocular alignment that occurs on up, midline, and down gaze as the eyes move from the primary position. In an **A** pattern the eyes will move from being relatively close together in up gaze to splay relatively outward in down gaze. In the **V** pattern the eyes will be relatively closer together on down gaze and move outward as they progress toward up gaze. These patterns may be seen in orthophoric patients or patients with eso- or exodeviation. Compensatory head postures to provide sufficiently good alignment for single binocular vision are often found in these patients.

A. **The V pattern**
  1. The **etiology** of **V** esotropia or exotropia is most frequently associated with overaction of the IO muscles or a primary underaction of the SO muscles (or both). As the IO muscles act as abductors in upward gaze, the esodeviation decreases and an exodeviation increases on upward movement of the eyes. Alternate mechanisms that have been suggested and that have affected surgical management include overaction of MR muscles. These muscles are most effective in midline down gaze particularly due to their role in convergence. Overaction of the LR muscles has also been proposed as an alternate etiology of **V** exotropia. These muscles are most effective in midline up gaze, since divergence is normally accomplished by looking upward from the downturned near seeing position to view a distant object.
  2. **Measurements.** The extent of a **V** pattern may be measured using the alternate cover test and prisms with the patient gazing at a distant fixation object in up gaze, primary midline gaze, and downward gaze. Testing of versions may reveal overaction of one or both IOs, underaction of one or both SOs, or overaction of a horizontal rectus muscle.
  3. **Head position** in patients who fuse is characteristically chin held down when doing close work in **V** esodeviation. Conversely, a chin-up position may be seen in patients with **V** exodeviation.
  4. **Treatment of V esotropia** is recession or disinsertion of the IOs if they are found to be overactive or recession and downward transposition of the MR muscle(s) if the obliques are normal. Similarly, in **V exotropia**, disinsertion or recession and upward transposition of the lateral recti is indicated if the IOs are overactive. **The principle of upward or downward transposition**

of horizontal muscles is that the insertions are always moved in the direction in which the surgeon wishes to reduce the action of the muscle.

B. **The A pattern**

1. **The etiology** is most frequently found to be associated with overaction of the SO muscles with or without underaction of the IOs. As the SOs act in abduction in downward gaze, esotropia decreases and exotropia increases in that field of view. In the absence of overaction of the oblique muscles, underaction of LR muscles is suspected.

2. **Measurements.** An A tropia is measured by alternate cover tests and prisms held base-in or base-out, according to the form of horizontal deviation, with the patient looking upward, midline, and downward at both distance and near. Versions will often reveal the overacting muscles.

3. **Treatment of A esotropia** is not indicated if the deviation is 10 d or less in primary position and below. In the presence of symptoms such as asthenopia, diplopia, or blurred vision, overacting SO muscles may be modified in their action by bilateral tenectomy in combination with any indicated horizontal surgery. If the oblique muscles appear normal, horizontal muscle surgery may be combined with upward displacement of the MR. In **A exotropia,** an overactive SO should undergo tenectomy in combination with horizontal surgery. If the obliques appear normal, horizontal surgery should be carried out alone or in combination with downward transposition of the LR muscles.

X. **Strabismic syndromes**

A. **Microstrabismus** should be suspected when heterophoria is present on the uncover test but there is an absence of shift on the cover test. The index of suspicion should be raised by the finding of moderate degrees of amblyopia, parafoveal fixation, **harmonious ARC** (ARC adapted to the angle of deviation), and reduced but present stereopsis. In microstrabismus there is a sensory and motor adaptation to a primary **small central suppression scotoma** that is rarely found in patients without either anisometropia or a history of esotropia. Clinically, the eyes appear straight and the cover test fails to reveal fixation movement. The Visuscope, however, reveals fixation as much as 2–3 degrees nasal to the fovea.

B. **Monofixation syndrome** is characterized by consistent findings of a deviation of 8 d or less, good fusional vergence amplitudes, and a scotoma within the deviating eye that prevents diplopia. Many patients have no history of manifest strabismus but frequently have significant anisometropia. The presence of the central scotoma precludes bifixation but allows active peripheral binocular vision. **Etiologic factors** include small-angle strabismus, anisometropia, unilateral macular lesions, and inherent inability to fuse similar images perceived by the maculas. Strabismic monofixation syndrome is more frequently seen in esotropia than in exotropia, as the constant tropia more frequently seen with the former prevents the establishment of visual bifixation. Anisometropia induces monofixation secondary to a clear image on one macula and a blurred image on the other. The refractive error is often discovered too late to correct the macular image discrepancy and allow for the establishment of bifixation. A unilateral macular lesion produces an organic scotoma precluding binocular vision. Inherent inability to fuse identical macular images is still poorly understood.

1. The **diagnosis** of monofixation syndrome can be made by determining the **area of scotoma** within the binocular field and detecting peripheral fusion and fusional vergence amplitudes. The **cover-uncover test** may reveal a small fixation movement in the nonfixating eye, but the diagnosis of the syndrome can be truly made only by **sensory testing.**

a. **Fusion** may be evaluated with the Worth Four-Dot test at near and distance (see sec. **VI.B**). A bifixating patient will fuse the dots, but the monofixating patient possesses a scotoma in the nonfixating eye that will obscure the dots projected onto that eye. Until the dots are projected onto a retinal area larger than the scotoma, the patient will report either three green dots or two red dots. As the Worth dots are moved farther into the distance, the retinal projection area will increase and the patient will suddenly report fusing the four dots.

  b. The 4-diopter base-out prism test may also be used to reveal the central scotoma (see sec. **VI.B**). A shift of both eyes toward the apex of the 4-d prism placed base-out before a fixating eye is a positive test, but a significant number of monofixation patients will not respond to this form of prism testing.

  c. The Bagolini striated glasses may also disclose the scotoma (see sec. **VI.C**). The glasses are positioned so that the light streak is seen by the right eye at 135 degrees and by the left eye at 45 degrees. Patients with monofixation syndrome will see a scotoma as a gap surrounding the light in the streak in the nonfixating eye.

2. Amblyopia is found in the majority of patients with monofixation syndrome, but this will vary with the etiology of the syndrome. A minority of the congenital exotropes, most of the primary monofixating patients, most patients with a microstrabismus, and almost all anisometropes with monofixation syndrome will have amblyopia.

3. Treatment of monofixation involves occlusion therapy for improvement of the vision in the amblyopic eye if the decreased vision is nonorganic in origin. Improvement of the motor problems, i.e., the deviation, is usually not necessary because the strabismus is 8 d or less in angle. Orthoptic therapeutic approaches for overcoming monofixation are less than encouraging, as these patients have great difficulty in recognizing other than physiologic diplopia, possibly because the scotoma is not due to active cortical suppression but is a manifestation of the patients' ability to acknowledge the image from just one macula at a time. Anisometropic patients may be treated by appropriate spectacle or contact lens correction.

C. Convergence spasm may simulate esotropia at near fixation in an otherwise orthophoric patient. A sustained convergence is usually associated with spasm of accommodation. The condition may be seen in hysteria. Clinically, the patient will be orthophoric or possibly exotropic at distance. The syndrome classically includes induced myopia, miosis of accommodation, esotropia, and diplopia that increases at near. This spasm may persist for up to 10 minutes after the visual target is removed. **Diagnosis** is made by cycloplegic refraction to rule out true myopia. **Treatment** includes plus lenses in the hyperopic patient or weak minus lenses in the emmetrope, to be used during times of spasm, and psychotherapy to reassure the patient that he or she is not going blind.

D. Retraction syndrome (Duane's syndrome) is characterized most commonly by the absence of abduction of one eye with some restricted adduction and retraction while attempting to adduct that eye. There may be an associated up or down shooting of the adducted eye, simulating overaction of an IO or SO muscle. The palpebral fissure is simultaneously narrowed during attempted adduction. Duane's syndrome may be unilateral or bilateral and is often hereditary. The **etiology** is felt to be fibrosis of the LR muscle(s) or paradoxic innervation due to anomalous connections at the nuclear level in the CNS. In the latter instance it is felt that there is cocontraction of the MR and LR muscles on attempted adduction that results in retraction of the globe. The LR muscle is not innervated on attempted abduction. Other forms include defective abduction only with or without esodeviation, adduction more defective than abduction with or without exodeviation, and vertical retraction syndrome with retraction seen mainly in elevation.

E. Strabismus fixus is an extremely large esotropic deviation in both eyes seen in patients with bilateral rectus paralysis and maximum contracture of the MR muscles, secondary to replacement by fibrous tissue. Neither eye may be abducted across the midline even on **forced duction** testing. A similar condition may occur in which the eye is anchored in an abducted position, a fibrous band replacing or present in addition to the LR. **Vertical strabismus**

fixus may be unilateral or bilateral. The affected eye is anchored in depression and appears to be associated with a fibrotic IR.

F. **Möbius' syndrome** is a multisystem problem. Ocular examination reveals that horizontal versions are congenitally absent and that esotropia is frequently present. The presence of an **A** or **V** pattern is not uncommon, and a compensatory head posture up or down may be used by the patient in an effort to avoid diplopia symptoms. This congenital **inability to adduct** either eye may result in a patient maintaining fixation on the lateral target by voluntarily converging. Associated with the **lack of lateral horizontal eye movement,** probably due to sixth nerve palsy, is a **seventh cranial nerve palsy,** manifested by relaxation of the orbicularis muscle, sagging of the lower lids, and pooling of the tears in the lower fornix. There are other associated facial abnormalities, vestibular nystagmus cannot be elicited, and the pupils are normal.

G. **Syndromes inducing limitation of ocular elevation**

1. **Brown's syndrome—superior oblique tendon sheath syndrome—**is manifested by an inability to elevate the adducted eye above the midhorizontal plane. The restriction of elevation decreases as the eye moves laterally, but some restriction may persist even in full abduction. There may be slight downshooting of the adducted involved eye mimicking SO overaction. Palpebral fissure widening is associated with elevation restriction on attempted adduction. The **etiology** of this syndrome is probably variable, but the true congenital syndrome is felt to be due to restricted action of a shortened and fibrous sheath of the homolateral SO tendon. The syndrome may also be acquired postoperatively following the tucking of the SO muscle. **Forced ductions** are positive in that there is an inability to elevate passively the adducted involved eye. There is often a compensatory head posture. **Surgical procedures** directed at the SO tendon have not produced good results in resolving either the ocular problem or the head position. A related group of patients have increased resistance to elevation in adduction. These patients may report abrupt elevation after attempted adduction associated with an **audible snap,** which may be palpated in the superonasal orbit. In general, no surgery is indicated in Brown's syndrome except in cases of extreme head turn. Patients should be advised of the poor prognosis associated with incision of the SO tendon sheath in such attempts to improve head posture.

2. **Congenital fibrosis syndrome** is usually familial. It is characterized by bilateral ptosis, chin elevation, absence of elevation of both eyes, limited if any depression of both eyes, overconvergence in attempted upward gaze, exotropia or divergence in attempted downward gaze, and limited horizontal eye movements. Most patients have hyperopic astigmatism and amblyopia. The best cosmetic correction comes with freeing up the IR muscles plus ptosis surgery.

3. **Orbital floor fracture** (see sec. **VII.A.2** and Chap. 4, sec. **VIII**).

4. **Double elevator palsy** is rare and is due to the combined weakness of contraction of both the IO and SR muscles in the same eye. There is complete inhibition of eye movement in upper field of gaze. **Treatment** involves transposition of the insertions of both medial and lateral recti to the insertion of the SR muscle.

5. **Thyroid ophthalmoplegia** associated with the exophthalmus of thyrotoxicosis is secondary to hypertrophy of the extraocular muscles, reducing the motility of the eyes. Elevation is particularly limited, probably secondary to fibrosis of the IR muscles. During the toxic state, excessive amounts of mucin are deposited in the extraocular muscles. As the hypertrophy resolves with therapy of the basic disease, the IR muscle may cicatrize, leaving the patient permanently unable to elevate the eye. **Forced ductions** are positive for restricted movement of this muscle. Patients frequently develop a **chin-up** compensatory head posture. **Treatment** is carried out after the basic disease is stabilized and is usually a generous recession of fibrotic IR

muscle or appropriate movement of any other extraocular muscle involved. Botulinum injection of the IR has been a useful adjunct or alternative to surgery in acute or fairly recent onset Graves' disease.

6. **Parinaud's syndrome.** Paralysis of upward and downward gaze may develop secondary to lesions of the subcortical brain centers for vertical gaze. There may be associated absence of convergence and pupillary reaction to light. Tumors of the pineal gland are the most common **etiology** of this syndrome.

H. **Marcus Gunn ("jaw-winking") syndrome** is a congenital abnormality characterized clinically by unilateral ptosis. On opening the mouth or moving the jaw to the noninvolved side of the head, there is a momentary lid retraction of the ptotic eye. The **etiology** is felt to be an anomalous connection between the nuclei of the external pterygoid muscles of the jaw and the levator muscle of the lid.

I. **Cyclic esotropia (clock mechanism alternate-day squint)** is an unusual form of esotropia that follows a regular circadian rhythm of 48 hours. During this period the patient is orthophoric for 24 hours and manifestly esotropic for the following 24 hours. Spasm of accommodation is not involved, as demonstrated by normal vision throughout the cycle, and no phoria is present during the orthophoric phase. The cycles continue a few months to years before the esotropia becomes constant. Bimedial surgical recession is successful and does not lead to overcorrection on orthophoric days.

J. **Ophthalmoplegias** are a group of ocular motility disorders associated with temporary or permanent changes at the myoneural junction or within the muscle fiber itself.

1. **Progressive external ophthalmoplegia** is a bilateral myopathy of the extraocular muscles. It may progress asymmetrically, but end-stage disease is identical in both eyes. The condition may be sporadic or inherited as an autosomal dominant. The initial **sign** is acquired ptosis, followed some years later by progressive paresis of the extraocular muscles, usually starting with the MR. Elevation weakness precedes depression paresis, causing the patient to take on a compensatory **chin-up** posture. As the condition progresses and the eyes become progressively more frozen in primary gaze, the head will return to normal position. There is no involvement of the intraocular muscles of the eye.

2. **Myasthenia gravis** is a chronic neuromuscular disease characterized primarily by fatigue of muscle groups, usually starting with the small extraocular muscles before involving other larger muscle groups. **Initial findings** usually include ptosis, which becomes progressively more severe as the day wears on. Weakness of convergence and upgaze are seen. Infrequently, isolated paresis of the inferior or lateral rectus may be noted. The latter may simulate a sixth nerve palsy. **Diagnosis** is by electromyogram; the myogram becomes silent as action potentials drop during fatigue. A second important diagnostic test is the injection of **edrophonium bromide (Tensilon)** or **neostigmine IV.** Their injection causes a transient reversal of clinical findings. **Therapy** of myasthenia is usually pyridostigmine bromide (Mestinon), 60 mg PO tid, but should be managed by a neurologist.

XI. **Cranial nerve palsy** may involve a single or all three nerves in varying degrees of paresis. It may be congenital, due to developmental defects in the nuclei of the CNS or peripheral motor nerve fibers, or it may be acquired. **Lyme disease** may cause a variety of extraocular muscle palsies and other inflammatory and neurophthalmic disorders (see Chap. 5, sec. IV.L.2).

A. **Third nerve palsies** are characterized as congenital and acquired, although some authorities feel that they are virtually all acquired.

1. **Congenital third nerve palsy** may variably affect the medial superior and inferior recti and IO **but never involves** the intraocular muscles (pupil, ciliary body). The levator muscle may also be involved, producing a variable form of ptosis.

a. **Clinically,** the patients usually have ptosis and exotropia with intact pupillary and accommodative reflexes. There are varied degrees of limitation, of elevation, adduction, and depression of the involved eye. By use of a compensatory head turn, many patients develop normal singular binocular vision. In the absence of binocular vision, amblyopia will develop in one eye if the patient does not maintain a compensatory torticollis to avoid the symptoms of diplopia.

    b. The **etiology** is unknown but is presumed to be developmental.

    c. **Forced ductions** are negative, ruling out adhesive problems as etiologic. Because of the hypotropia of the affected eye, an apparent ptosis may in fact be a **pseudoptosis** as the lid position follows eye position. If the hypotropic eye is allowed to fixate, the pseudoptosis will disappear.

    d. **Treatment** requires surgery for the exotropia, hypotropia, and ptosis. Hypotropia is treated by disinsertion of the SO tendon, while maximum recession of the LR and resection of the MR aid in moving the eye to a satisfactory location in the horizontal plane. A frontalis sling is usually indicated for the ptotic lid. The patient should be evaluated for the presence or absence of Bell's phenomenon (see Chap. 5, sec. **V.E.**) before any lid evaluation procedure is carried out or the **risk of exposure keratopathy** may be significant postoperatively.

  2. **Acquired third nerve palsy** may be partial or complete, involving intraocular and extraocular muscles together or alone.

    a. **Clinically,** the appearance is similar to congenital third nerve palsy, but if the intraocular muscles are involved, there is a **fixed dilated pupil with paralysis of accommodation.**

    b. **Onset** is usually rapid and maximum with recovery, if any, usually complete by 6 months.

    c. The **etiology** is variable and often ominous. **Diabetic third nerve palsy** never involves the pupil and usually recovers 100% of function.

    d. **Other causes of acquired third nerve palsy** may involve both intraocular and extraocular muscles. These include brainstem lesions; inflammatory disease such as meningitis, encephalitis or toxic polyneuritis; vascular lesions **(painful third nerve palsy with pupillary involvement** is a particularly ominous sign of an **intracranial aneurysm); intracranial tumors** (commonly associated with **aberrant regeneration of the third nerve**); and demyelinating diseases such as multiple sclerosis and trauma.

    e. **Treatment** involves therapy of the underlying disease as an initial step, if warranted. Diplopia is often not a problem if significant ptosis is present; however, elevation of the lid surgically will **produce diplopia** unless the corrective surgical procedures (see sec. **1**) are carried out.

B. **Fourth nerve palsy** is most commonly caused by the involvement of the fourth cranial nerve, but it must be differentiated from paresis of other cyclovertical muscles manifesting a cyclovertical tropia.

  1. **Clinically,** a patient with isolated fourth nerve palsy usually presents with a **head tilt to the opposite shoulder** in compensatory movement against the torsion of the affected eye. Paralysis of the fourth nerve allows the antagonistic IO muscle to extort the eye. The patient will therefore tilt the head to the opposite shoulder to bring the vertical alignment of the affected eye parallel with the vertical alignment of the normal contralateral eye in an effort to avoid tortional diplopia.

  2. **The diagnosis of any isolated cyclovertical muscle palsy** such as a fourth nerve paresis necessitates **three evaluative steps:**

    a. **Which eye is hypertropic?** Is it due to a weak depressor or a weak contralateral elevator, e.g., to a weak IR or SO or to a weak contralateral SR or IO?

    b. **Determine whether the vertical deviation increases to the right or left gaze.** A weak right SO or left SR results in a right hypertropia increasing in left gaze, the field of action of these two muscles.

    c. **Determine whether vertical deviation increases on tilting the head toward the right or left shoulder,** using the alternate cover test. **For example,** step 1, an alternate cover test, may reveal a right hypertropin implicating a paretic RSO, RIR, LSR, or LIO. Step 2, evaluating the effects of levoversion and dextroversion, may reveal that vertical deviation increases on dextroversion, thereby implicating now only the RIR and the LIO. Step 3 indicates that vertical deviation increases with tilting the head to the right, due to a downward movement of the left eye secondary to the unopposed action of the LIR. The paretic muscle, therefore, is the left IO. If a paretic right IR had been present, vertical deviation would have increased in tilting the head to the left due to the upward movement of the right eye secondary to the unopposed action of the RIO.

3. **Head tilt** in patients with fourth nerve palsy will be in the direction of least disparity. **The disparity will increase markedly if the head is forced to be tilted toward the shoulder on the side of the paretic SO (Bielschowsky's sign).**

4. **In the presence of a third nerve paralysis** evaluation of fourth nerve function may be carried out by asking the patient to look down; the iris crypt markings or the radial limbal vessels will reveal a conspicuous intorsion as the SO turns the globe. On attempted superduction there will be a conspicuous extorsion, noted by examining movements of the iris marking or radial limbal vessels.

5. The **etiology** of congenital fourth nerve palsy is developmental in the nucleus or motor portion, and the etiology of acquired fourth nerve palsy is most commonly closed head trauma. Intracranial tumors and aneurysms must be ruled out, however.

6. **Treatment of congenital palsy** is surgery on the cyclovertical muscle as soon as possible after diagnosis is firmly established. This is done to prevent a permanent torticollis, facial asymmetry, and scoliosis. **Treatment of acquired fourth nerve palsy,** after underlying disease is ruled out, is watchful waiting to assess the degree of spontaneous recovery until 6 months after onset. The object of surgery is to improve cyclo and vertical deviations. If there is obvious contraction of the direct antagonist of the paretic muscle, recession of this antagonist should be the first procedure. In the absence of contraction, weakening of the yoke muscle of the palsied muscle or tucking the palsied muscle may be a first procedure.

C. **Sixth nerve palsy** may be congenital or acquired. It produces an esotropia in the primary position that increases on attempted lateral gaze in the direction of the involved muscle. Patients may establish and maintain normal binocular vision by compensatory **head turn** toward the side of the paretic eye. Patients with congenital or recently acquired sixth nerve palsy have a greater primary gaze esotropia due to **secondary deviation** when they fixate with the palsied eye than when they fixate with the sound eye **(primary deviation).**

1. **Congenital sixth nerve palsy** is rare and must be distinguished from congenital esotropia and Duane's and Möbius' syndromes. Trauma to the LR and abducens nerve may be the cause. Primary hypoplasia of the sixth nerve motor nucleus may also be the cause.

2. **Acquired sixth nerve palsy** may be due to multiple etiologies because of the long intracranial course taken by the postnuclear portion of the nerve. Sixth nerve palsy is not uncommon in diabetes but may also be seen in heavy metal poisoning, a variety of viral diseases inducing intracranial inflammation, intracranial tumors and aneurysms, and middle ear infection with secondary meningeal irritation and edema affecting the nerve as it passes through the petrospinous area in Dorello's canal of the dura.

3. **Treatment** of unilateral sixth nerve palsy after etiologic evaluation is supportive for the first 6 months. Recovery is often noted by 3 months after onset. If there is no improvement after 6 months, surgery involving maximum recession of the ipsilateral MR muscle, which is usually quite con-

tracted by this time, is the primary procedure. If persistent primary position esotropia remains and if **forced ductions** of the palsied eye are normal following recession of its MR, recession of the contralateral MR muscle may be helpful. Resection of the paretic LR will provide some mechanical benefit and may be done as either a primary or a secondary procedure. The **Hummelsheim operation** is used as an alternative procedure to assist the LR by dividing the superior and inferior recti in half and transposing half of each muscle to the superior and inferior folds of the LR muscle insertion. The MR muscle in the involved eye is recessed at the same time. Botulinum injection of the MR is useful in acute sixth nerve palsy or as an adjunct to surgery in chronic paresis (see sec. **XII**).

XII. **Botulinum A toxin injection for strabismus**
   A. **Mechanism of action.** *Clostridium botulinum* exotoxin potently blocks release of acetylcholine and functionally denervates muscle for several weeks. Injection of the toxin into an extraocular muscle, usually under the guidance of an electromyogram, produces temporary paralysis with consequent slight atrophy and stretching of the muscle and simultaneous functional shortening of the antagonistic muscle, thus moving the globe toward realignment.
   B. **Indications.** Botulinum A injection has been most successful in reversing surgical overcorrections, small to medium comitant esodeviations (20–30 d), and acute sixth nerve palsies with diplopia. Chronic sixth nerve palsy may also benefit from surgical transposition of the vertical rectus muscles to the LR muscle with injection of toxin into the ipsilateral MR muscle. If esotropia recurs, MR recession or reinjection with toxin may be used effectively. Accommodative esotropia in children with high AC/A ratio is frequently responsive to injection of both medial recti. Similar treatment in infantile esotropia reduces a mean of 35 d preinjection to a mean of 5 d postinjection. Conversely, large-angle exotropia is usually only transiently responsive to injection of the lateral recti, and restrictive forms of strabismus such as Duane's syndrome are minimally to unresponsive. Vertical deviations are more difficult to treat by injection both because of technical considerations and because of a very high incidence of blepharoptosis in SR injection. Dissociated vertical deviations may be treated with IO or IR toxin, although IR injection may leak to affect the IO adjacent to it. Injection of the IR in **Graves' disease** may be effective in acute disease and a surgical adjunct in the chronic state.
   C. **Dosage.** Vertical and horizontal deviations less than 20 d are treated initially with 1.25–2.5 units and horizontal deviations greater than 20 d with 2.0–5.0 units initially in volumes of 0.05–0.15 ml. The saline reconstituted lyophylized powder must **not be shaken** or the protein will denature. Rejections may be titrated down depending on effect achieved from the original injection.
   D. **Complications.** No adverse systemic side effects have been reported. Diplopia is very common due to transient overcorrection but resolves in a few weeks; permanent overcorrection is extremely rare. Blepharoptosis occurs in 25% of children and 16% of adults after horizontal muscle injection (toxin spillage in the orbit) but resolves in 2 months or less. No amblyopia has been noted in children. Vertical deviations after horizontal muscle injection occur 17% of the time, but only 2% of these persist. Very rare complications are perforation of the globe and vitreous, retrobulbar, or subconjunctival hemorrhage.

XIII. **Nystagmus.** There are more than 38 classifications of nystagmus. The more common forms are discussed in this section.
   A. **Congenital nystagmus** is a lifelong condition beginning during the neonatal or early childhood years and includes the horizontal forms classified as latent, pendular, jerk, and spasmus nutans. The etiology is poorly understood but appears to be related to a malfunction of the visuomotor systems of fixation.
      1. **Latent nystagmus.** Steady binocular fixation is present with both eyes open. Occlusion of one eye results in a jerk nystagmus with the fast component away from the covered eye and consequent diminution in visual acuity. There are many **methods to test vision monocularly** without eliciting this nystagmus. One method is to mount a high plus lens before the

nonfixing eye without reducing the amount of light entering the eye but blurring vision in that eye. Binocular vision should always be checked to indicate the best possible vision, although this will not reveal whether one eye sees better than the other.

2. **Pendular nystagmus** is usually but not always associated with sensory deprivation due to reduced central visual acuity such as that associated with macular scarring (toxoplasmosis), macular hypoplasia (albinism, aniridia), achromotopsia, retinal degeneration (Leber's congenital amaurosis), or optic nerve hypoplasia. This horizontal nystagmus is a slow pendular movement in primary gaze but may change to jerk nystagmus in lateral gaze. It decreases on convergence, persists in the dark with eyes open but eases on closure of the eyes under any lighting. The primary visual complaint is blurring.

3. **Jerk nystagmus** is a bidirectional phenomenon with the fast component toward the side of lateral gaze. Somewhere between far levoversion and dextroversion is a **null point,** at which the nystagmus is decreased or absent. If this point is outside primary gaze, the patient will maintain a head turn to maintain gaze in the position of least eye motion.

4. **Spasmus nutans** is a combination of symmetric or asymmetric horizontal pendular nystagmus combined with **head nodding** and occasionally torticollis. Rarely, the nystagmus is rotary or vertical. Onset is in infancy, and the condition self-resolves by childhood.

B. **Acquired pendular nystagmus** may be seen in the only seeing eye of monocular adults who develop decreased visual acuity in that eye or in patients with brainstem dysfunction or the drug toxicity of sedatives or anticonvulsants.

C. **Acquired jerk nystagmus** may generally be classified as gaze-paretic or vestibular.

1. **Gaze-paretic nystagmus** is a slow horizontal beat due to upper brainstem dysfunction. Compression of the brainstem produces a nystagmus characterized by a slow gaze-paretic movement with eyes toward the side of the lesion and a fast jerk nystagmus with eyes away from the side of the lesion.

2. **Vestibular nystagmus (VN)** is due to malfunction or overstimulation of the eighth nerve vestibular apparatus or its connections, producing a horizontal or rotary jerk nystagmus in the primary position of gaze or any nystagmus associated with **vertigo. Peripheral VN** is never purely vertical or rotary but is reduced by visual fixation. **Central VN** is purely vertical or rotary and not affected by fixation.

   a. **Cold water irrigation test.** Such stimulus of the tympanic membrane mimics a **destructive** lesion of the vestibular system, e.g., Ménière's syndrome, viral labyrinthitis. A normal response to cold irrigation is a horizontal nystagmus with the fast component away from the side of the stimulus **(COWS—cold: opposite; warm: same),** vertigo, postpointing, and a positive Romberg test.

   b. **Warm water irrigation test.** This stimulus mimics an **irritative** lesion. A normal response to warm irrigation is horizontal nystagmus with the fast component toward the side of the stimulus (COWS), vertigo, postpointing, and a positive Romberg test.

D. **Other nystagmus forms**

1. **End-gaze (physiologic) nystagmus** is a small-amplitude, nonsustained horizontal nystagmus seen in normal patients on far right or left gaze.

2. **Upbeat nystagmus** may be congenital, drug induced, or indicative of posterior fossa disease. In primary position the fast component is upward.

3. **Downbeat nystagmus** is characterized by the fast component in the downward direction and associated with posterior fossa disease. Compression at the foramen magnum results in marked downbeating on lateral gaze.

4. **Rotary nystagmus** is a torsional jerk movement around the anteroposterior axis of the eye and is usually seen with horizontal or vertical nystagmus. It

may be congenital or acquired, as in brainstem lesions or in acute vestibular disease.

5. **Dissociated nystagmus** is a horizontal, markedly asymmetric nystagmus most commonly seen in the abducting eye in **internuclear ophthalmoplegia** (medial longitudinal fasciculus lesions). Sixth nerve paresis should be ruled out as an alternate cause of the eye movement pattern.

6. **See-saw nystagmus** is a conjugate pendular torsional motion such that the intorting eye rises and the extorting eye falls. It is associated with expanding lesions in the area of the third ventricle or with upper brainstem vascular disease.

7. **Nystagmus blockage syndrome** is seen in patients with discordant nystagmus. This nystagmus is characterized by horizontal increased oscillations on abduction and by decreased oscillations on adduction. To obtain clearest vision many patients damp or block the nystagmus by fixing with the adducted eye or by converging both eyes, but they will still fix with just one eye and turn the head in the direction of the fixing eye at both near and distance. Many patients with this syndrome have crossed fixation. Some appear orthophoric unless clear vision is required and the focusing mechanism is called into effect. Preferential surgery is on the fixating eye.

8. **Other nystagmoidlike oscillations**
   a. **Ocular myoclonus** is a rhythmic pendular motion, usually vertical, associated with synchronous rhythmic movements of other parts of the body, particularly around the oropharynx and diaphragm. Midbrain lesions are commonly associated with this acquired oscillation.
   b. **Ocular bobbing** is characterized by rapid downward jerks of both eyes followed by slow drift back to midposition. Patients are usually comatose and have massive lesions in and around the pontine area.

9. **Optokinetic nystagmus** is a physiologic jerk nystagmus elicited by presenting to gaze objects moving serially in one direction, horizontally or vertically, such as the stripes on a spinning optokinetic drum. The eyes will follow a fixed stripe momentarily and then jerk back to reposition centrally and pick up fixation on a new stripe. Clinically, this test may be used as a gross estimate of visual acuity in infants and poorly cooperative patients including malingerers by varying the size of the fixation stripes or pictures. It is also useful in localizing lesions causing homonymous hemianopic field defects. Disease of the parietooccipital region diminishes the optokinetic response when the drum is rotated to the side of the cerebral lesion.

Neuroophthalmology: Visual Fields, Optic Nerve, and Pupil

Shirley H. Wray

I. The visual fields

A. Nerve fiber anatomy. To examine the visual field efficiently yet quickly, the diagnostic features of a suspected disease must be known. A knowledge of these features is sound only when based on the anatomy of the visual system (Fig. 12-1).

1. The retina. In the retina the axons of the ganglion cells are arranged in three basic patterns: the papillomacular bundle from the macula, the superior and inferior arcuate nerve fiber bundles from the temporal retina, and radial fibers from the nasal retina (Fig. 12-2).

    a. The macula, which lies approximately 3–4 mm lateral to the optic disk, contains a disproportionately large number of nerve fiber axons. The axons, the papillomacular bundle, stream medially across the retina and layer out thinly along the lateral margin of the optic disk. They comprise more than 90% of all axons in the optic nerve. The papillomacular bundle subserves the area of central fixation. Its situation corresponds to a spindle-shaped area of the visual field known as the centrocecal area, which lies between the fixation point and the blind spot. Damage to the papillomacular bundle produces two types of visual field defects: central or centrocecal scotoma (Fig. 12-3D, E).

    b. The nasal and temporal half of the retina is divided by an imaginary vertical line drawn through the fovea. It is projected on the visual field on the vertical meridian. The horizontal raphe acts as the boundary between the functional superior and inferior halves of the retina, and it is projected on the visual field on the horizontal meridian.

        (1) Fibers from the temporal, superior, and inferior zones of the retina crowd together, sweep over and under the papillomacular bundle, and wedge themselves into the remaining superior and inferior poles of the optic disk. Because of their arcuate course above and below the papillomacular axons, they are referred to as the superior and inferior arcuate bundles, respectively. The arcuate nerve fiber bundles from the temporal retina respect the horizontal raphe (see Fig. 12-2A). Consequently, arcuate field defects have a sharp border on the horizontal meridian (Fig. 12-3B).

        (2) Fibers from the nasal retina course in a radial pattern directly to the nasal margin of the optic disk (see Fig. 12-2A).

2. The papilla and **optic nerve.** The arrangement of the nerve fibers at the disk is maintained in the immediate retrobulbar segment of the optic nerve. The papillomacular bundle occupies the temporal wedge, the arcuate bundles occupy the superior and inferior poles, and the nasal retinal fibers occupy the remaining nasal margin of the papilla (see Fig. 12-2A). It is useful to remember this architecture when evaluating optic atrophy. Further posteriorly in the intracanalicular and intracranial segments of the optic nerve, the cross-sectional anatomy of the nerve changes. The papil-

This chapter is taken in part from Shirley H. Wray, Harvard Medical School, Department of Continuing Education, Neuroophthalmology, 1979.

Fig. 12-1. The nerve fiber anatomy of the visual pathways from retina to occipital cortex. Cross sections on right show location of fibers at various levels in the pathway. OS = oculus sinister; OD = oculus dexter. (Modified and reproduced with permission from D. D. Donaldson.)

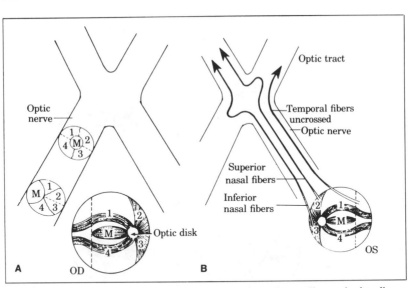

Fig. 12-2. The three basic patterns of retinal nerve fibers: the papillomacular bundle (M), the superior (1) and inferior (4) arcuate nerve fiber bundles from the temporal retina, and radial fibers from the nasal retina (2 and 3). **A.** Right fundus and cross-sectional anatomy of the fibers in the right optic nerve. **B.** Left optic nerve and decussation of the crossing nasal retinal fibers in the chiasm.

lomacular bundle migrates inward toward the core of the nerve. The axons from the nasal and temporal halves of the retina diverge and segregate. The nasal fibers come to lie in the lateral perimeter of the nerve (see Fig. 12-2A).

3. **The chiasm.** The precise nerve fiber arrangement of the chiasm is not known. It is known, however, that the nasal retinal fibers cross the chiasm and the temporal fibers remain uncrossed. This anatomy is important in relation to chiasmatic field defects (Fig. 12-4). The ratio of crossed to uncrossed fibers is 3:2. Four points to remember about the **decussation of the nasal retinal fibers** are

   a. **Inferior peripheral nasal fibers** cross in the inferoanterior part of the chiasm and arch first into the medial aspect of the opposite optic nerve for a short distance. This loop is called the anterior knee of von Willebrand. The fibers then course backward into the opposite optic tract (see Fig. 12-2B).

   b. **Superior peripheral nasal fibers** cross to the opposite optic tract in the superoposterior part of the chiasm but arch first for a short distance into the optic tract of the same side. This loop is called the posterior knee of von Willebrand (see Fig. 12-2B).

   c. **Fibers arising from the nasal half of the macular area** of the retina fan out into a broad band to cross in the central superior and posterior portions of the chiasm and move upward to lie in a superior wedge of the optic tract.

   d. **Uncrossed temporal retinal fibers** from corresponding upper and lower retina eventually find their mates from the crossing nasal group in the respective medial or lateral portion of the optic tract.

4. **The optic tract.** In the optic tract, nerve fibers from corresponding areas in the two retinas become more closely associated. At the termination of the tract and in the lateral geniculate body, the nerve fibers that started in a superior position in the optic nerve are medial in situation, and the lower

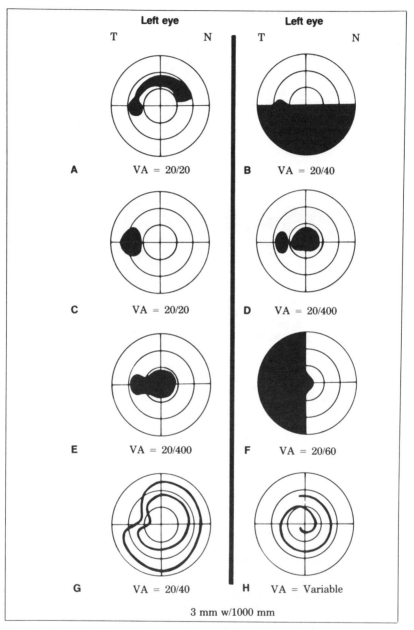

Fig. 12-3. Types of monocular visual field loss in left eye (3-mm white object at 1000 mm). **A.** Superior arcuate scotoma (inferior nerve fiber bundle defect). **B.** Inferior altitudinal field defect respecting the horizontal meridian (superior nerve fiber bundle defect). **C.** Enlargement of the blind spot in the left eye. **D.** Central scotoma, normal blind spot. **E.** Centrocecal scotoma. **F.** Temporal hemianopia respecting the vertical meridian but with involvement of central vision. **G.** Generalized constriction of the visual field to 2 isopters. **H.** Nonorganic "corkscrew" field defect (hysteria, malingering) to 1 isopter. VA = visual acuity.

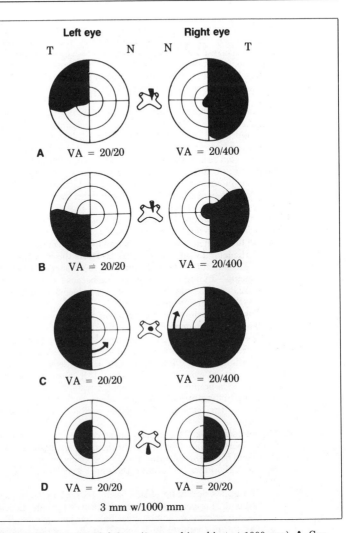

Fig. 12-4. Types of bitemporal field defects (3-mm white object at 1000 mm). **A.** Central visual fields of a lesion anterior and inferior to chiasm with compression of the optic nerve. **B.** Lesion located anterior and superior to the chiasm affecting predominantly the right side. **C.** Progressive lesion inferior to the chiasm. **D.** Lesion posterior to the chiasm causing bitemporal hemianopic scotomas. VA = visual acuity. (Adapted from D. Vaughan, R. Cook, and T. Asbury, *General Ophthalmology.* Los Altos, Calif.: Lange Medical Publications, 1974. With permission.)

fibers in the optic nerve become lateral in the tract and lateral geniculate body (see Fig. 12-1). This rotation results in a medial location for fibers from the corresponding upper quadrant of each retina and a lateral location for fibers from the corresponding lower quadrant of each retina. A **central wedge of macular fibers** is insinuated between the lateral lower and the medial upper extramacular fibers in both the tract and the lateral geniculate body.

5. **The lateral geniculate body** consists of six layers, numbered from ventral to dorsal. The lateral geniculate body receives crossed retinal fibers in layers 1, 4, and 6 and uncrossed retinal fibers in layers 2, 3, and 5. There is a vertical alignment of corresponding points of the visual field. The **right side of the brain receives its sensory input from the left side of the visual environment;** thus, the right optic tract and right lateral geniculate body get their input from the left visual field, which must perforce be from the right half of each retina, i.e., the temporal retina of the right eye, and the nasal retina of the left eye.

6. **The optic radiation.** The nerve fibers of the optic radiation arise from all six layers of the lateral geniculate body.
   a. **All fibers** then sweep laterally and inferiorly around the temporal horn of the lateral ventricle (see Fig. 12-1). As the radiation sweeps laterally it ascends for a short distance in the posterior limb of the internal capsule—an important relationship because a vascular lesion of the internal capsule may be expected to produce a **hemiplegia** and a **homonymous hemianopia.**
   b. **The most anteroinferior fibers** of the optic radiation form Meyer's loop. Meyer's loop, which contains projections of the inferior retinal fibers, sweeps forward toward the pole of the temporal lobe. Amputation of the temporal pole in excess of 4 cm produces a homonymous superior quadrantanopia (**"pie in the sky"**). The defect is always adjacent to the vertical meridian (Fig. 12-5A). If 8 cm of the temporal lobe tip is excised, a homonymous hemianopia results.
   c. **Deep in the parietal lobe,** the radiations lie external to the trigone and pass to the medial surface of the occipital lobe (the striate calcarine cortex).

7. **The visual cortex.** The primary visual cortical area lies on the medial surface of each occipital lobe in the interhemispheric fissure. It is situated both above and below the calcarine and postcalcarine fissures. These two fissures represent the junction between the upper and lower halves of the visual fields (see Fig. 12-1).
   a. **The upper dorsal lip** of this fissure receives projections from the corresponding upper quadrant of both retinas that are associated with the lower quadrant of the binocular field on the opposite side.
   b. **The inferior ventral lip** is related to the superior quadrant of the binocular field of the opposite side.
   c. **The periphery of the retina** is represented most anteriorly in the deep rostral aspects of the visual cortex near the splenium of the corpus callosum.
   d. **The macula** is represented posteriorly by an extensive area of visual cortex that extends onto the posterolateral aspect of the occipital lobe. This anatomy is important when considering bullet wounds and similar **traumatic lesions** of the occipital lobe.
   e. **In the evaluation of occipitocortical lesions,** it should always be remembered that there is accurate localization in the occipital cortex, that areas 17, 18, and 19 are interconnected in each hemisphere, and that area 18 may be responsible for pursuit eye movements.

B. **The monocular visual field**
   1. **The visual field** is that area of one's surroundings that is visible at one time. The normal monocular visual field extends approximately 100 degrees laterally, 60 degrees medially, 60 degrees upward, and 75 degrees downward.

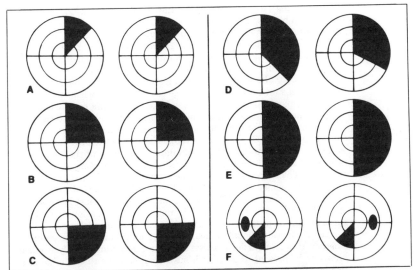

Fig. 12-5. Types of homonymous field defects. **A.** Superior right homonymous quadrantic defect ("pie in the sky") due to a lesion of the most antroinferior fibers of the optic radiations in the left temporal lobe (Meyer's loop). **B.** Complete right superior homonymous quadrantanopia due to a lesion of the optic radiations in the left temporoparietal lobe. **C.** Complete right inferior homonymous quadrantanopia due to a lesion of the superior fibers of the optic radiations in the parietal lobe ("pie on the floor"). **D.** Incongruous right homonymous hemianopia due to a lesion in the anterior optic radiations. **E.** Complete right homonymous hemianopia due to a lesion in the left temporoparietal optic radiations or left visual cortex. **F.** Homonymous hemianopic congruous scotoma abutting fixation in the left inferior quandrant due to a lesion in the right visual cortex.

It is divided into nasal and temporal halves by an imaginary vertical line drawn through the fovea, into superior and inferior altitudinal halves by the horizontal raphe that runs from the fovea to the temporal periphery. Situated in the temporal half field is the normal blind spot, 15 degrees temporal to fixation and 1.5 degrees below the horizontal meridian.

2. **The blind spot** is represented by an absolute scotoma corresponding to the scleral canal through which the retinal nerve fibers leave the eye at the optic disk.

C. **Visual field tests**

1. **When is a visual field test indicated?** The ideal is to include a visual field test in every ophthalmic examination, but time is a precious commodity. Thus, the consensus seems to be that perimetry is mandatory only when indicated by the clinical history, the eye examination, or radiologic or CT scan findings.

2. **Indications for field testing**

   a. **History**

   (1) **A medical history** of headache or amenorrhea-galactorrhea (or both).

   (2) **A neurologic history** of seizures, migraine with visual defects, amaurosis fugax with residual deficit, hemiplegia, head injury, or multiple sclerosis.

   (3) **An ophthalmic history** of blurred vision or loss of vision, bumping into objects, difficulty in reading, exertional amblyopia (Uhthoff's syndrome), unexplained failure to pass a routine eye test (school,

driving), loss of depth perception, loss of color vision, recognition of a blind spot, or double vision.

b. Several ocular signs may require perimetry or elucidation. These signs include optic disk pallor, cupping of the optic disk, papilledema, ischemic optic disk swelling, and retinal diseases such as infarction, degeneration, or detachment.

c. Radiologic changes. Visual field testing is essential when an x ray of the skull shows enlargement of the sella, J-shaped sella, tumor calcification, particularly suprasellar, enlargement of the optic canals, displacement and calcification of the pineal gland, hyperostosis of the sphenoid bone, or multiple skull fractures, or when a CT scan or MRI documents an orbital or intracranial lesion. See Chap. 1.

3. Selection of the method of examination. The choice of the best method of visual field examination and the most suitable equipment for plotting the visual field depends on the clinical condition of the patient, the corrected visual acuity, the type of visual field defect suspected, and the purpose of the examination. The method and equipment must be selected so as to allow the most accurate and reproducible examination in as short a space of time as possible to avoid patient and examiner fatigue.

A clear distinction should be made between an examination to determine whether or not a field defect exists and an examination to analyze a defect known to be present. If a defect is suspected, no more than 5 minutes are required to detect and plot its form with one or two targets. From the simple chart thus produced a diagnosis may often be confirmed. Every defect, however, must be analyzed and as many techniques as necessary used for this analysis, inclusive of dynamic or static perimetric tests. Since this may take 30 or more minutes, it is often advisable to do the locating and the analysis at separate sittings, or to refer the patient to a skilled perimetrist for further testing. In this way, the more complicated field chart, resulting from the analysis of a defect, may be compared on serial examinations of the field and thus provide vital information about the advance or recovery of disease.

D. Methods. The opinion persists among some ophthalmologists that the examination of the visual field is not only a complicated, time-consuming procedure, but that it is also frequently unrewarding. It is the aim of this brief review to present a simple account of the techniques used for the examination of the visual field and to show that visual field testing may be both rapid and of great diagnostic value. All visual field tests are performed with each eye covered in turn.

1. The monocular confrontation field test. Almost all types of visual field defects can be detected with a few colored pins by the monocular confrontation test. Yet, the value of this simple method is not universally appreciated. It is highly recommended for use in the emergency room. Moreover, it is the technique of choice in the bedridden, in those who lack the ability to concentrate, and in children. Sometimes it is the only attainable form of field examination.

a. Visual observations by the patient. In the monocular confrontation field test the examiner compares the patient's visual field with her own. The examiner, sitting face to face with the patient, asks the patient if he can see the examiner's face clearly or if some area is missing (face-to-face confrontation). Frequently, an intelligent patient will describe blurring or loss of certain facial landmarks, indicating that he has a specific type of field loss. For example, with an inferior altitudinal defect there is loss of clarity of the lower half of the examiner's face. The observation is an invaluable guide to the examiner.

b. The peripheral field. The field is then charted to moving targets. The patient is asked to fixate on the examiner's eye. A white pinhead is moved inward from the periphery. The pin, a 3-, 5-, or 10-mm white hatpin (not a pearl pin), is held about 30 cm from the patient's and examiner's eyes. The patient calls "yes" when he catches a glimpse of it without wavering fixation. This is repeated around the circumference of the field, and any defect of the periphery can be detected. Each eye is tested in turn. A homonymous hemianopia is quickly discovered by this method.

c. **Central fields.** A red pin (5 or 10 mm) is best for exploring the central 20 degrees, particularly on either side of the vertical meridian. If in one spot the red appears pale or hazy, a relative scotoma is present. The central scotoma in optic neuritis is rapidly detected this way. The results are conventionally recorded in the chart as the patient views the world.

d. **When visual acuity is seriously impaired,** confrontation is limited to a 40-mm white target, to finger counting, to finger or hand movement, or to a flashlight if necessary. When a defect is found, if possible it should be further analyzed and recorded by using the tangent screen or a perimeter. Both techniques provide a better method of documenting progressive change. Further examination is also necessary when no defect is discovered by confrontation, especially in patients with visual complaints.

2. **The tangent screen (Bjerrum screen)** is a black felt screen on which radial lines and 5-degree concentric circles are inconspicuously marked. It is used to examine the central field within 30 degrees from the fixation point and to determine the size of the blind spot. By increasing the distance of the patient from the screen, the size of the field defect increases and allows evaluation in greater detail. The hysterical constricted field characteristically remains the same size when charted at different distances. Screens are therefore made for use at 1 or 2 m. A 1-m screen can be accommodated on the wall of most consulting rooms and evenly illuminated.

a. The **method** is simple. The field is charted for each eye alone to one or two sizes of round white targets and occasionally to red or other colors. The traditional method is to fit the colored disk onto a black wand and move the target in from the periphery. The examiner stands in front of the patient to observe fixation and works from each side of the screen in turn. Targets on wands have now largely been replaced by the use of a flashlight especially designed to project a light spot of precise size and luminosity on the screen. Greater versatility is obtained with this technique. A disadvantage is that the examiner, sitting beside the patient, is less able to check the patient's fixation. The blind spot should therefore be charted first to confirm reliability.

b. **Color fields.** When charting the field to a colored target, the point to be recorded is when the patient recognizes the true color of the target, and not when the object is first seen, a common error.

c. **The results** on the Bjerrum screen examination can be recorded on a simple chart stamped in one corner of the large perimeter field chart to facilitate quick comparison and filing. This also has merit in reducing the volume of the patient's record.

d. **Field defects detected.** The tangent screen test is particularly valuable for analysis of the following types of visual field defects:

   (1) Enlargement of the blind spot (Fig. 12–3C).
   (2) Arcuate scotoma (Fig. 12–3A) and altitudinal defects (Fig. 12–3B).
   (3) Central scotoma (Fig. 12–3D).
   (4) Centrocecal scotoma (Fig. 12–3E).
   (5) Paracentral scotoma.
   (6) Homonymous scotoma abutting fixation.
   (7) Homonymous hemianopia involving the macula (Fig. 12–3F).
   (8) Generalized constriction of the visual field (Fig. 12–3G).
   (9) Nonorganic (hysterical) constriction of the visual field (Fig. 12–3H).

3. **The Amsler grid** is a name given to a boldly cross-hatched paper. Any rectilinear design can be used for the same purpose. A simple grid with a central fixation point can be drawn on hospital record paper at the bedside.

Its principle is the fact that **central retinal lesions often distort geometric patterns causing metamorphopsia.** In contrast, damage to the optic nerve and chiasm produces hazy defects in central acuity that tend to "fog out" without altering the grid pattern or bending its lines. Often the patient can describe a scotoma very accurately if the examiner keeps a piece of paper of this sort around and allows the patient to look at it in bright illumination fixing on a central spot. The patient can usually outline or draw the affected area quite adequately. With reading glasses on, if needed, each eye is tested in turn. This technique tests only the central 10 degrees of vision.

4. **The hemispheric projection perimeter (Goldmann perimeter)** is a precision instrument used for testing both peripheral and central fields. It is the most popular perimeter in use because it affords a remarkable speed of operation for kinetic perimetry and luminance of the hemispheric background can be kept precisely controlled to keep retinal light-adaptation constant. The patient is positioned on the hemisphere-shaped machine with the chin on a chin rest and the uncovered eye is aligned with the central fixation point. Fixation is monitored by the perimetrist through a telescope. Projected test spots of constant size and fixed contrast are moved from the periphery in toward the center. The patient presses an electric buzzer when the target is in view. The same stimulus spot is moved into the visual field along different meridians, and an **isopter,** i.e., a line of equal sensitivity to light contrast, is charted. (An isopter is analogous to a contour line on a map of uneven terrain.) Selection of the speed of the test spot depends on the reaction time of each patient. Five degrees/second gives reproducible results. An orderly rhythmic presentation of the test spot minimizes fatigue. At least two isopters should be charted, one to a large well-visualized spot to aid in training the patient and the second to the smallest dimmest target he or she can reliably see to permit detection of early defects. Recording several isopters also ensures that all regions of the field are tested in addition to helping to define the **slope** of the borders of a defect. Steep slopes (isopters crowded together) usually indicate the defect is caused by an acute lesion (frequently vascular), gradual slopes by a progressive one (tumor). Unfortunately, the Goldmann perimeter is a large, expensive machine and clearly unsuitable for every examining room. Because of the remarkable reproducibility of the field examination by different examiners, however, the perimeter is essential for use by ophthalmologists who are responsible for the serial evaluation of the visual fields.

5. **Automated static perimetry (Humphrey, Octopus)** is recognized to be a sensitive technique to detect nerve fiber bundle defects in the monocular central 30% visual field. For neuroophthalmic cases, the Octopus 2000 perimeter and program #34, which presents 72 points, have been used. The method is straightforward and similar to kinetic perimetry. The patient is asked to fix on a central target in a hemisphere with a homogenous white background, while a nonmoving light of fixed size and brightness is presented at various points in the hemisphere. Brightness is increased until the patient recognizes the presence of the stimulus above background. Thus, static perimetry measures brightness sensitivity at various retinal points. Serial static visual fields can be subjected to computer analysis using the DELTA program to determine progression or resolution.

E. **Visual field pathology**

1. **The retina.** Retinal lesions cause visual field defects that may correspond to the pattern of the retinal nerve fibers or to the area of supply of the retinal blood vessels. The defects produced do **not respect the vertical meridian.** Frequently, they correspond to areas of infarction or inflammation or to degenerative lesions seen with the ophthalmoscope. Retinal lesions may thus produce isolated scotomas or extensive altitudinal defects. **Macular lesions** produce central scotomas. **Retinitis pigmentosa** produces constricted fields and equatorial ring scotomas.

2. **Papilla and optic nerve.** Lesions of the optic nerve produce four basic

patterns of visual field loss: arcuate scotoma, centrocecal scotoma, generalized constriction, and junctional scotoma.

    a. Arcuate scotomas are located in the central portion of the visual field. They appear as annular or cuneate-shaped scotomas. Most paracentral scotomas are actually arcuate. Characteristically, the apex of the scotoma points directly toward or emanates from the blind spot (see Fig. 12-3A). Intact field usually surrounds the involved area on all sides, but sometimes the scotoma breaks out into the periphery and produces an **altitudinal defect** (see Fig. 12-3B). Arcuate defects have a sharp border on the horizontal meridian. After entering the optic disk, the arcuate nerve fibers remain separate throughout their course in the optic nerve and into the anterior portion of the chiasm. Discrete lesions, frequently ischemic, anywhere along this pathway may produce arcuate field defects. Such lesions include ischemic optic neuropathy, glaucoma, and optic atrophy secondary to papilledema. Rarely, the causal lesion may even be situated as far back as the optic chiasm, i.e., meningioma of the dorsum sellae, pituitary adenoma, or opticochiasmatic arachnoiditis. Careful perimetry of these cases will uncover clear-cut termination of the scotoma at the **vertical** meridian that can be explained anatomically only by a lesion in the anterocentral chiasm where crossing and noncrossing portions of the nerve fiber bundles separate.

    b. Centrocecal scotoma result from damage to axons that run within the central core of the optic nerve from the macular and peripapillary retinal receptor zones. Damage to the former produces a scotoma in the area of central fixation; damage to the latter produces an enlargement of the physiologic blind spot. The composite loss of vision with a lesion that affects these two fiber systems is simply a blend of two scotomas. The resultant field defect extends both to fixation and to the blind spot (see Fig. 12-3E). The centrocecal scotoma is a specific and common sign of optic nerve disease. It occurs in a variety of conditions both intrinsic (demyelination, infiltrative, metabolic-toxic) and compressive in nature.

    c. Generalized constriction is a less specific defect and is less reliable in localizing lesions to the optic nerve **unless it is unilateral.** It rarely occurs without concomitant reduction of central vision; therefore, arcuate or centrocecal scotomas are not uncommonly accompanied by a generalized constriction of the field. **Monocular generalized constriction** of peripheral and central isopters without associated local defects suggests diffuse optic nerve involvement (see Fig. 12-3G). Constriction of central isopters alone suggests early deterioration of central vision. Progressive generalized constriction of peripheral isopters with relative sparing of central vision may be part of the syndrome of perioptic sheath meningioma. Unlike nonorganic "tubular fields," the outer circumference of the field loss in these patients will appear to enlarge in a physiologic manner as the distance between the patient and the test object is increased.

    d. The junctional scotoma is one important exception to the rule that unifocal optic nerve lesions produce strictly monocular visual field defects. At the posterior extremity of the optic nerve, the inferonasal retinal fibers from the opposite eye sweep into the optic nerve for a short distance before crossing back into the optic tract (see Fig. 12-2B). Thus, a **single lesion situated at the junction of nerve and chiasm can produce visual field defects in both eyes**—an ipsilateral centrocecal scotoma along with a contralateral upper temporal quadrantanopia. The combination of perimetric defects, referred to as the **junctional scotoma of Traquair,** is an important localizing sign of **prechiasmal compression.** It thus behooves the perimetrist to search the upper temporal field of the unaffected eye carefully in cases of unexplained loss of monocular vision, since the most common mistake under these circumstances is for the patient to be told that the condition is due to chronic retrobulbar neuritis.

3. The chiasm. Chiasmal lesions cause field defects with three important characteristics. Frequently, they are bitemporal with sharp borders respecting the vertical meridian (tilted disks). Central vision is usually involved. The defects show considerable variability (see Fig. 12-4). The variability is dependent on the position of the chiasm; the varying size, shape, and tilt of the sella; the direction of expansion of the compressing mass; and the distribution of the loops of crossing nasal retinal fibers in the chiasm. The visual field may be monocular or binocular.

a. **Monocular visual field defects** include monocular scotoma, arcuate nerve fiber bundle defects that respect the vertical meridian, and temporal hemianopia. When monocular temporal hemianopia occurs, this rare defect is thought to represent the effects of occlusion or stasis in nutrient chiasmal vessels.

b. **Binocular visual defects** have several different patterns (see Fig. 12-4): junctional scotoma, superior bitemporal quadrantanopia, inferior bitemporal quadrantanopia, bitemporal hemianopia, bitemporal hemianopic scotoma, binasal hemianopia, incongruous homonymous hemianopia, and a complete homonymous hemianopia. Each type can provide a clinical clue to the location and type of chiasmal deformation.

c. **In the analysis of topographic localization** of chiasmal field defects, the perimetrist refers to superior, inferior, anterior, and posterior involvement of the chiasm. This classic approach is somewhat oversimplified. A note of caution: Do not neglect the chiasm's tilted orientation and elevated position above the sella. Clearly, "early" vulnerability of the chiasm to compression from "small" pituitary adenomas is a misconception. For practical purposes, the guidelines are as follows:

(1) **Compression of the anterior angle** of the chiasm causes unilateral blindness or a central scotoma plus a contralateral superotemporal defect (junctional scotoma).

(2) **Compression of the median bar** of the chiasm from below (inferiorly) causes a bitemporal superior quadrantanopia or bitemporal hemianopia (see Fig. 12-4A).

(3) **Compression of the median bar** from above (superiorly) produces a bitemporal inferior quadrantanopia (see Fig. 12-4B), e.g., a craniopharyngioma.

(4) **Compression of the posterior chiasm** from above produces bitemporal hemianopic scotomas (see Fig. 12-4D).

(5) **Compression bilaterally of the lateral margin** of the chiasm produces binasal hemianopia; the chiasm actually becomes squeezed and displaced laterally, e.g., an aneurysm.

(6) A mass in the **retrochiasmatic region** impinging on or displacing the optic tract results in homonymous hemianopia of two types: an incongruous homonymous hemianopia or a complete homonymous hemianopia.

d. **Pseudochiasmal defects.** Pseudochiasmal or ocular syndromes mimicking chiasmal lesions include tilted optic disks (see sec. II.A.4), drug (chloroquine) toxicity, sector retinitis pigmentosa, and bilateral retinal detachments.

4. The optic tract. An anterior optic tract lesion produces an incongruous homonymous hemianopia (Fig. 12-5D), decreased visual acuity, afferent pupil defect **(Wernicke's hemianopic pupil)** and atrophy of the optic disks with characteristic bow-tie atrophy in the contralateral eye. A complete homonymous hemianopia results from a lesion of the posterior optic tract (see Fig. 12-5E).

5. Lateral geniculate body. Lesions of the lateral geniculate body are extremely rare. They produce highly incongruous homonymous hemianopias that may correspond to the laminal organization of the cell layers.

6. **The optic radiation.** Damage to the optic radiations produces a homony-mous hemianopia (Fig. 12–5E). Important considerations are congruity, macular sparing, visual attentiveness, and associated oculomotor signs.
   a. **Congruity** is said to be present when the edge of the field defect in each eye is identical in shape. Field changes due to lesions of the anterior optic radiation tend to be **incongruous**. Those due to damage to the radiations close to the visual cortex are **congruous**. Depending on its site, the lesion may involve only the upper or lower fibers of the radia-tion and thus cause a lower or upper quadrantanopia in the opposite half-field; e.g., temporal lobe radiation lesion causes "pie in the sky" (see Fig. 12–5A), and parietal lobe radiation lesion causes "pie on the floor" (see Fig. 12–5C).
   b. **The edges of the field defects** are **steep** or vertical at the onset if the lesion is due to ischemic infarction, and **shelving** if the lesion is sec-ondary to compression. The more rapid the growth of a tumor, the more gradual the slope of the margin of the defect.
   c. **Macular sparing** in lesions of the optic radiations probably occurs be-cause the macula has such a large area of representation; therefore, destruction of all the macular fibers is uncommon.
   d. **A complete hemianopic defect to attention** may occur in lesions of the parietal area. The monocular confrontation test with double si-multaneous stimulation of the two half-fields by finger movement is a good method of demonstrating the **extinction phenomenon**.
      (1) **Left temporoparietal lesions** cause defective recognition of visual symbols, alexia, and agraphia.
      (2) **Lesions of the right temporoparietal area** cause impaired judg-ment of spatial relationships, as in topographic agnosia and con-structional apraxia.
   e. **Ocular motility signs** are also associated with parietooccipital lesions. In this situation a complete homonymous hemianopia is accompanied by **absent optokinetic nystagmus** when the stripes of the drum are rotated horizontally to the side of the cerebral lesion. On **forced eye closure**, the eyes deviate conjugately upward and laterally to the side opposite the cerebral lesion. An examination for these motor signs is essential in the evaluation of the patient with a homonymous hemi-anopic field defect. The ophthalmologist may then be able to site the lesion along the course of the optic radiations and guide the selection of noninvasive and cerebral angiographic studies.
7. **The visual cortex.** Destruction of the visual cortex of one occipital lobe produces a **contralateral congruous homonymous hemianopia.** This is the most common type of cortical field defect seen and frequently is the result of embolic occlusion of the posterior cerebral artery; however, other patterns of visual loss also occur. These defects permit precise localization. They include congruous homonymous hemianopic scotoma, bilateral alti-tudinal scotoma, congruous homonymous hemianopia sparing the temporal crescent, or, rarely, a monocular field defect due to loss of the temporal crescent, bilateral homonymous hemianopia, cortical blindness, and tunnel or keyhole vision.
   a. **Congruous homonymous hemianopic scotomas** tend to be sector-shaped, filling a triangular area within a quadrant. The apex points toward fixation (see Fig. 12–5F). Such a defect indicates damage to the occipital pole. The most common cause is trauma or infarction second-ary to embolic occlusion.
   b. **Altitudinal scotomas** result from gunshot wounds or contusion of the occipital lobe following a depressed skull fracture. A bullet produces the defect by passing horizontally through both occipital lobes. Inferior al-titudinal defects are more common than superior altitudinal defects, presumably because trauma below the occipital lobe tends to involve the venous sinuses or brainstem or both and results in death. At initial

examination after the trauma, the visual field defect is frequently very extensive; the prognosis for recovery is usually good, however, although not always complete. A guarded prognosis in the early stages is wise.

c. **Sparing of the temporal crescent** in the presence of a congruous homonymous hemianopia permits exact localization of the site of the lesion to the contralateral visual cortex, with sparing of the most medial group of optic radiation fibers projecting to the most anterior end of the visual cortex. Preservation of a homonymous crescent is not found in the nasal half-field of the opposite eye because the temporal field is larger than the nasal field. In rare instances the uniocular temporal crescentic area disappears.

d. **Bilateral homonymous hemianopia** results from bilateral, usually ischemic, lesions of the visual cortex. One occipital lobe is usually infected before the other. The interval between the two strokes may be weeks, months, or years. Prognosis or complete recovery is poor, although there may be a gradual return of vision to light and then to hand movement.

(1) **Cortical blindness.** In severe cases, when the patient remains blind, the patient may deny that he or she is blind. This condition, cortical blindness or **Anton's syndrome,** is characterized by four important features: bilateral blindness, denial of blindness, normal pupil reflexes, and bilateral occipitocortical lesions.

(2) **Tunnel vision** results after bilateral occulusion of the posterior cerebral arteries and infarction of the occipital lobes but with sparing of a small central island of vision. The peripheral fields are severely constricted (see also sec. **8**), but visual acuity is preserved. This situation occurs if the infarction involves only the visual cortex anterior to the posterior pole, preserving a **central keyhole of vision,** or when the middle cerebral artery, which anastomoses with the posterior cerebral artery, provides a vascular supply to the posterior (macular) tip of the cortex.

8. **Nonorganic field defects.** In the absence of optic disk swelling, optic atrophy, and retinal degeneration, bilateral or unilateral constricted fields are often nonorganic. They can be due to patient fatigue, lack of attention, misunderstanding, malingering, or hysteria. Spiral or corkscrew fields are also common in hysteria (see Fig. 12–3H).

F. **Final analysis of visual field testing.** The task of the ophthalmologist in the evaluation of visual field defects is not over when perimetry and field testing are complete. Two additional steps are mandatory. Step one is to identify the anatomic localization of the site of the lesion by interpretation of the visual field defect. Step two is to determine the nature of the lesion.

1. **Step one** can be facilitated only by an ophthalmologist with a thorough knowledge of the anatomy of the anterior visual pathways.

2. **Step two** usually requires the prompt referral of the patient to a neuroophthalmologist or neurologist for a neurologic examination and neuroimaging. A contrast **CT scan** of the orbits with coronal views is still one of the best radiologic techniques to study the intraorbital segment of the optic nerves and the orbit contents. A CT scan with bone windows is required to study the base of the brain. **Magnetic resonance imaging** (MRI) of the brain, in axial, sagittal, and coronal planes with T1- and T2-weighted images, with and without gadolinium, is beginning to replace the conventional CT scan for the detection of cerebral lesions. The MRI is particularly sensitive in detecting small white matter lesions (plaques) of demyelination seen in cases of idiopathic optic neuritis and multiple sclerosis. MRI studies may also help distinguish between a mass due to a tumor or aneurysm. New advances, still in the research phase of development, include MRI angiography, which permits visualization of the carotid vessels in the neck and intracerebral circulation by a specialized computer-assisted MRI technique. Although the study is called an angiogram, it is a noninvasive procedure and requires no arterial injections of dye or the use of contrast.

II. The optic nerve head

   A. Congenital optic disk anomalies are classified in five groups: optic nerve colobomas, pits, optic nerve dysplasia or hypoplasia, tilted disk (dysversion), and pseudopapilledema. The importance of disk anomalies in neuroophthalmology and pediatric ophthalmology, in particular, cannot be overemphasized. Large disks of the dysplastic type have been associated with congenital forebrain abnormalities, including basal encephaloceles. Small disks of the hypoplastic type have been associated with visual loss, nystagmus, and major concomitant CNS anomalies. Congenital dysversion is associated with visual field defects, and anomalous disk elevation with the diagnostic dilemma of pseudopapilledema versus papilledema. Such possibilities must be kept in mind by ophthalmologists concerned with the evaluation of the child with poor vision.

      1. Colobomas and pits. Large anomalous disks are common. They may represent colobomas of the disk contained within peripapillary staphylomas or retinochoroidal colobomas.

         a. Colobomas are bilateral in more than 60% of cases. Bilateral colobomas may be inherited. The transmission is as an autosomal dominant, the gene varying considerably in its penetrance so that sometimes one or more generations are missed. Congenital colobomatous anomalies if associated with hypertelorism or other midline facial anomalies are considered evidence of basal encephalocele until proved otherwise (see Chap. 10, secs. **IX.C** and **D**).

         b. Optic nerve pits, or craterlike holes in the disks, are a peculiar and relatively rare finding. They occur in association with moderate enlargement and irregularity of the disk and are usually unilateral. There is no evidence of a hereditary pattern. The majority of pits are located in the lower temporal quadrant of the papilla, touching the edge of the disk. The size and depth of the pit vary widely. Often vessels can be observed diving into the pit and emerging to continue their normal course.

            (1) Visual acuity. A wide variation in the effect on visual acuity is also noted. Approximately 40% of eyes have good vision, 35% diminished vision, and 25% poor vision.

            (2) Visual field defects. The characteristic field defect is an arcuate bundle scotoma or central scotoma (present in 60% of cases). Pits are of great significance in the pathogenesis of central serous retinopathy. There appears to be a selective involvement of the papillomacular bundle in the hole-forming process. Both conditions are observed in combination in about 30% of cases.

      2. Optic nerve dysplasia. Other forms of optic nerve dysplasia illustrate the spectrum of large anomalous disk malformations. For example, the disk may appear enlarged and elevated, enlarged and flat (megalopapilla), or enlarged and excavated with radial vessel array ("morning-glory" syndrome).

      3. Optic nerve hypoplasia. Small anomalous disks due to congenital **optic disk hypoplasia** may be unilateral or bilateral and vary in the degree of severity. When hypoplasia is borderline or minimum, good vision is preserved; when hypoplasia is pronounced and the disk is pale, severe impairment of vision is the rule. In one-third of these cases, major concomitant CNS anomalies have been recognized. One of these anomalies, **septooptic dysplasia (de Mosier's syndrome),** is characterized by the clinical triad of shortness of stature, nystagmus, and optic nerve hypoplasia. Neurologically, there is absence of the septum pellucidum. This forebrain dysplasia is also accompanied by a deficiency of growth hormone and even by diabetes insipidus. Early recognition permits correction of the hormonal imbalance and a chance for the child to achieve normal growth and stature.

      4. Tilted disk, congenital dysversions. The characteristics of the tilted disk syndrome are the tilted appearance (situs inversus) and the small size of the optic disks. In 80% of cases the condition is bilateral, with or without a congenital conus. An inferior conus is the most common variety, with hypopigmentation of the inferonasal fundus contiguous to the crescent.

a. Visual acuity. Refraction shows myopic astigmatism with an oblique axis.

b. Visual field examination shows bitemporal depression with, usually, superotemporal quadrantic defects that fail to respect the vertical meridian and that fail to progress. Occasionally, the field shows an altitudinal defect.

5. **Pseudopapilledema** is a nonspecific term used to describe elevation of the disk similar in appearance to papilledema. When possible, a diagnosis should be made, for example, intrapapillary drusen, hypermetropia, or persistent hyaloid tissue. Medullated nerve fibers, a congenital anomaly, can also be confused with papilledema.

a. **Optic disk drusen** is an important cause of pseudopapilledema and is the entity that creates the most difficulty clinically in the evaluation of the swollen disk.

(1) **Pathogenesis.** Drusen or hyaline bodies of the optic disk are thought to be a congenital excess of immature neuroglia that undergo degeneration and calcification. Disk drusen are inherited as an autosomal irregular dominant trait.

(2) **Tempo of evolution.** Optic disk drusen are not visible at birth and have rarely been observed in children under the age of 11 years. They erupt on the disk surface in the second or third decade. With increasing age they become more visible and recognizable.

(3) **Ophthalmoscopy.** The ophthalmoscopic appearance of **disk drusen in the child** is atypical. In early life, hyaline bodies remain deep in the nerve (but always anterior to the lamina cribrosa) and not visible with the ophthalmoscope. When they lie just beneath the surface of the disk, they may be seen partially or not at all. Drusen embedded beneath the surface produce a fullness of the papilla, mild elevation, and blurring of the disk. There may also be an abnormal number of vessels on the disk. Intrapapillary drusen account for 75% of diagnostically troublesome elevated disk anomalies in young children. By the second or third decade, when disk drusen become visible, the condition is less likely to be confused with papilledema. The **ophthalmoscopic appearance in the adult is usually diagnostic.** Both disks are involved in 73% of cases, but an asymmetry in appearance is common. Drusen are recognized on the disk as a small, mulberrylike mass or as a waxy tumor composed of a conglomerate of smaller masses. They may enlarge the nerve head, obliterate the physiologic cup, and give the edge of the disk a crenated appearance. Illumination along the disk margin frequently causes drusen to glow, and red-free light (the green filter on the ophthalmoscope) is often helpful. To retroilluminate drusen the slit beam of a halogen ophthalmoscope can be used. The color of the disk is gray-yellow and unlike hyperemia of papilledema. Drusen, when pronounced, show autofluorescence. Ultrasonography and fundic fluorescein angiography may be helpful in identifying buried drusen.

Overt disk drusen may be seen ophthalmoscopically in parents of children with anomalously elevated disks without visible drusen. Examination of family members is mandatory if the distinction between true papilledema and pseudopapilledema in the child is in doubt. Failure to take this simple step is a major cause of misdirected diagnostic studies, including emergency invasive neuroradiologic procedures. When difficulty in fundic diagnosis persists and the patient is otherwise symptom-free and healthy, observe the patient. Reexamine the eyes, reinquire for neurologic symptoms of diplopia, headache, nausea, vomiting, or drowsiness, and arrange for serial fundic photographs. This conservative approach is strongly recommended.

(4) Visual acuity. The majority of cases of disk drusen are harmless and remain asymptomatic. There is no associated refractive error. As a rule central vision is intact.

(5) Visual field defects. Three patterns of field defects are found: enlargement of the blind spot (60% of cases); arcuate or nerve fiber bundle defects producing sector cuts, ring scotomas, paracentral scotomas, and Bjerrum scotomas; or irregular peripheral contractions. Constriction of the lower nasal field is the most characteristic defect. Typically, the defects progress very slowly.

(6) Spontaneous hemorrhage occurring **with disk drusen** may present as peripapillary flame-shaped hemorrhages, intravitreous hemorrhage, or subretinal hemorrhage around the disk that may extend under the macula. Only in this situation should loss of visual acuity and central field be attributed to disk drusen. Blindness is a rare complication. Hemorrhage with optic disk drusen may occur in children.

B. Acquired elevation of the optic disk occurs in papilledema, papillitis, optic disk drusen, infiltration of the nerve head by malignant cells, hypotony, and many other ocular conditions. Only papilledema and papillitis will be discussed.

1. Papilledema is a term that should be reserved strictly for optic disk swelling due to elevation of the intracranial cerebrospinal fluid (CSF) pressure.

a. Pathogenesis. The precise pathogenesis of papilledema is not entirely understood, but it seems clear from experimental autoradiographic and electron microscopic studies that **intraaxonal swelling** with accumulation of mitochondria and **not** extracellular extravasation of fluid is the principal early mechanism due to raised intraneural pressure. This results in swelling of prelaminar nerve axons, and early papilledema is due simply to axoplasmic stasis at the nerve head. The vascular changes, i.e., hyperemia, venous congestion, and hemorrhage, are secondary. In chronic papilledema, in addition to swollen axons there is extracellular accumulation of fluid (edema), vascular engorgement, and ischemia.

Papilledema is nearly always bilateral, although the degree of severity is often asymmetric. Two ocular conditions protect the eye from papilledema: **high myopia** (5–10 diopters [d]) and **optic** atrophy. Therefore, if present, no papilledema can develop in the eye.

b. Tempo of evolution and recovery. Papilledema develops quickly and subsides slowly.

(1) Evolution. Papilledema takes **1–5 days to appear** after the intracranial CSF pressure rises. The exception to this is following an acute intracranial hemorrhage, for example, a subarachnoid bleed. In this situation, papilledema with or without subhyaloid hemorrhages may develop rapidly within 2–8 hours of the catastrophic event. One might anticipate that there would be a delay in the appearance of papilledema in very young children due to the distensibility of the skull. While such a delay undoubtedly exists, severe papilledema is found frequently in children, largely due to the frequency of posterior fossa tumors in childhood (cerebellar astrocytoma, ependymoma, and medulloblastoma).

(2) Recovery from fully developed papilledema takes 6–8 weeks from the time the CSF pressure has returned to normal. Sudden lowering of CSF pressure produces no immediate fundoscopic change.

c. Ophthalmoscopy

(1) Early signs of papilledema are the accentuation of the nerve fiber striations of the disk margins (first upper and lower poles, then nasal, lastly temporal), **hyperemia of the disk,** and **capillary dilation.** A reliable and important first sign is **obscuration of the**

wall of a vessel crossing the disk margin by swelling of the nerve fiber layer.

(2) **Fully developed and late papilledema** is characterized by elevation of the disk (3 d is equal to approximately 1 mm of swelling) with partial or complete obliteration of the physiologic cup. Other characteristics are hemorrhage on or near to the disk to form flame-shaped (nerve fiber layer), punctate (outer nuclear layer), or small splinter hemorrhages. Cotton-wool exudate (cystoid bodies) on and around the disk may also occur. **Macular changes** are visible, with edema and star formation and retinal stress lines (concentric striae about the base of the swollen disk). **Spontaneous venous pulsations,** present in 81% of all eyes (being unilateral in 18%), are obliterated. As a general rule, the presence of unequivocal spontaneous venous pulsations on the disk indicates that papilledema is not present (the intracranial pressure is below 180–190 mm H_2O). This is not an absolute rule, however, since venous pulsation may occasionally persist even though papilledema is pronounced and the intracranial pressure is high.

It should also be noted that increased venous pressure, as well as increased intracranial CSF pressure, prevents pulsation. When optic disk changes are suspicious for early papilledema, a CT brain scan should always be obtained prior to the performance of a lumbar puncture to measure the intracranial pressure.

(3) **Long-term changes** of chronic papilledema are the development of **gliosis** surrounding the disk, sheathing of vessels, and progressive optic atrophy. Complete optic atrophy takes 6–8 months to develop, but it can occur as early as 4 weeks. Recovery from papilledema takes about 6–8 weeks.

d. **The associated ocular symptoms and signs** are transient visual obscurations with preservation of normal visual acuity and diplopia. Chronic papilledema can cause permanent loss of vision and visual field.

(1) **Transient visual obscurations** occur in 25% of patients. The attacks last less than 1 minute, usually 10–30 seconds. They are characterized by sudden blurred vision, like a veil, with simultaneous impairment of color vision, or sudden complete darkness or actual blindness. Chronic papilledema accompanied by frequent visual obscurations may portend a poor visual prognosis.

(2) **Diplopia** may be the presenting ocular symptom of raised intracranial pressure, attributable to a unilateral sixth nerve palsy or, occasionally, with a posterior fossa lesion, to a skew deviation.

(3) **Visual acuity loss** develops slowly in some cases of chronic papilledema with optic atrophy. In fact, in the early stages, papilledema is distinguishable from papillitis by the preservation of normal vision. Rarely, acute loss of vision occurs with papilledema due to infarction of the severely swollen nerve head.

(4) **Visual field defects** associated with papilledema are enlargement of the blind spot and constriction of the peripheral field. With a 2-mm white target at 2 m, the blind spot width is 7.5 degrees and its height is 9.5 degrees. An increased blind spot size greater than 1 degree is abnormal. Horizontal enlargement is most important. An inferior binasal quadrant field cut is the characteristic early peripheral field defect. In the late stage of papilledema with optic atrophy, the peripheral field is severely restricted to a small temporal island around the blind spot.

(5) **Pupil** size and reactivity are vital signs both to observe and preserve in cases of papilledema. In some instances, however, the diagnosis of papilledema is not easy without inspection of the dilatated fundus. If the fundus must be dilated, short-acting mydriatic eye drops must be selected and their use documented in the patient's record.

e. **The associated neurologic symptom** of major importance is **head-ache.** The headache may be acute or chronic, lateralized or generalized, and mild, moderate, or severe. Characteristically, it is worse on waking in the morning and aggravated by coughing, sneezing, and straining. The condition is particularly serious when accompanied by nausea and vomiting.

f. **The differential diagnosis** involves the important distinction of pap-illedema from pseudopapilledema, papillitis, optic disk vasculitis, jux-tapapillary chorioretinitis, sarcoid of the disk, syphilitic optic perineu-ritis, uveitis, malignant hypertensive retinopathy, central retinal vein occlusion, and other causes of disk swelling.

g. **Treatment. Papilledema** indicates raised intracranial pressure and a neurologic emergency. The patient requires **immediate admission to a hospital.**

2. **Papillitis** is the term used to describe disk swelling associated with visual loss due to inflammation, infiltration, or vascular disorders of the nerve head. Two types will be discussed: optic neuritis and ischemic optic neuropathy.

a. **Optic neuritis** results from inflammation or demyelination of the optic nerves. Much confusion exists as to nomenclature. The multiplicity of titles is largely due to efforts to indicate the site or extent of the nerve involvement. **Retrobulbar** neuritis refers to lesions of the nerve that show no abnormality in the fundus. **Papillitis** refers to anterior lesions in which the disk is swollen and hyperemic. Fine opacities in the vit-reous and venous sheathing may be associated. **Neuroretinitis** has the same connotation as papillitis but indicates that the process extends farther into the adjacent retina and uvea. These clinical terms should not necessarily imply an inflammatory process.

(1) **Pathogenesis.** The etiology of idiopathic optic neuritis is not known. In demyelination the lesion of the optic nerve is character-ized pathologically by a focal plaque of myelin destruction with relative preservation of axon continuity. **Lyme disease** and **neu-rosyphilis** are specific infectious causes (see Chap. 5, sec. **IV.L**). Characteristically, idiopathic optic neuritis affects young women (mean age, 31 years) more often than men and one eye only. Si-multaneous bilateral optic neuritis in adults is not common (23% of cases). In contrast, bilateral involvement is the rule in children. In adult cases of idiopathic optic neuritis, the risk of developing multiple sclerosis is approximately 50%. The incidence of multiple sclerosis is greatest within a 2-year period following the attack of optic neuritis.

(2) **Tempo of evolution and recovery**

(a) **Evolution.** Typically, visual acuity is lost progressively over 2–5 days concomitant with loss of color vision and depth per-ception. Chronic progressive visual loss should not be attrib-uted to chronic optic neuritis, a common error. A treatable compressive lesion must be ruled out in every case.

(b) **Visual recovery** usually commences within 1–4 weeks. In some patients it may be delayed as long as several months, partic-ularly if severe visual loss is present. Prognosis for full visual recovery should be guarded, even though some improvement in vision is to be expected in 75% of cases. **Serial** ophthal-mologic **examinations** should be carried out for a minimum of 8 months. In one patient series, follow-up showed the visual acuity was 20/30 or better after 7 months in 48% of the cases; in another series, 20/60 or better after 7 months in 55% of the cases. Two years is the longest period of visual recovery re-ported.

The **final level of visual acuity** attained is unaffected by the sex of the patient, by unilateral or bilateral involvement, by the site of the lesion (papillitis versus retrobulbar optic neuritis), by the presence or absence of pain, or by treatment with parenteral, oral, or retrobulbar corticosteroids.

(3) Ophthalmoscopy

(a) Early changes. Papillitis is present in 38% of cases. The optic disk is normal in 44% of cases. **Temporal pallor,** indicative of a previous optic nerve lesion in the same eye, is observed in as many as 18% of patients at the time of the initial examination. **Early papillitis** is characterized by blurring of the disk margins and by mild hyperemia.

(b) Fully developed papillitis is often impossible to tell from papilledema ophthalmoscopically, as there is marked swelling (up to 3 d), obliteration of the physiologic cup, hyperemia, and splinter hemorrhages. Venous sheathing is rarely seen. A slit-lamp examination for vitreous cells is valuable.

(c) Late changes. In retrobulbar optic neuritis, the disk may remain normal in appearance for as long as 4-6 weeks, at which time pallor develops. Following papillitis there sometimes develops what is described as "secondary optic atrophy." In this condition the disk margins may be indistinct, there may be glial tissue formation on the disk, and temporal disk pallor. Almost invariably, pallor of the nerve head marks the end stage of optic neuritis. At this stage, nerve fiber atrophy may be observed in the retina with the aid of red-free light.

(4) Associated ocular symptoms and signs

(a) Pain occurs as the presenting symptom in 63% of cases. It may be mild or quite severe. It is experienced as a dull retroorbital ache or as sharp eye pain provoked by eye movement or by palpation of the globe. In 19% of patients pain may precede loss of vision by 7 days. More commonly, it occurs only 24-48 hours before or simultaneous with visual loss. Pain rarely persists longer than 10-14 days. If it does, the diagnosis should be reconsidered. No correlation has been noted between the presence of pain and the severity of the visual loss or the appearance of the fundus (papillitis versus retrobulbar optic neuritis). It is of little prognostic significance. Pain possibly originates from distention of the optic nerve and stretching of the nerve sheath.

(b) Transient blurring of vision lasting minutes to a few hours is also experienced in optic neuritis. Factors recognized to produce this symptom include an affective disturbance (16%), exercise—Uhthoff's syndrome (29%), temperature change (8%), menstruation (8%), increased illumination (3%), eating (2%), and smoking (0.8%).

Uhthoff's syndrome appears to be more common in patients who go on to have recurrent optic neuritis. There is also a correlation with an increased incidence of multiple sclerosis. It must be remembered, however, that the Uhthoff's phenomenon of blurring of vision with exertion is not pathognomonic of demyelinating optic neuritis. It has been reported in a patient with a craniopharyngioma and in another with a pituitary adenoma compressing the visual system.

(c) Visual loss may be mild (20/30 or better), moderate (20/60 or better), or severe (20/70 or less). Vision can even be reduced to light perception. The patient complains of misty or blurred vision, difficulty in reading, a blind spot, a subjective difference in the brightness of light, impaired color perception, loss of depth perception, or transient blurring of vision. In the author's series, 65% of patients had a visual acuity of 20/100 or less at the onset. This high incidence of cases with severe visual loss may reflect the confidence the ophthalmologist feels in following mildly affected patients in the office rather than in the hospital.

(d) Visual field defects. A centrocecal scotoma (56%) is the most common type of visual defect. Many other types of field losses are reported, including a paracentral nerve fiber bundle defect (20%), a nerve fiber bundle defect extending to the periphery (9%), a nerve fiber bundle defect involving fixation and the periphery (11%), and a peripheral defect only (4%).

With recovery a centrocecal scotoma gradually shrinks in size and a peripheral field cut or constriction gradually enlarges. After 7 months, 51% of cases may be expected to have normal visual fields.

(e) Pupil size is equal in unilateral optic neuritis even when the eye is blind. Invariably, however, an **afferent pupil defect**, characterized by a sluggish or absent constriction to direct light, is present in the ipsilateral eye. The swinging flashlight test is a simple method of detecting the defect. The consensual light reflex and near response is intact. Since the afferent pupil defect can be observed in an optic nerve lesion even in an eye **with 20/15 vision, absence** of this sign in cases of monocular blindness should alert the examiner to the possibility of **nonorganic visual loss.**

(5) Associated CNS symptoms and signs. The examiner should inquire for existing or preceding transient CNS symptoms, specifically episodic numbness, paresthesias, burning discomfort, lack of dexterity, weakness, or incoordination of the limbs, as well as any sensory disturbance on the trunk or sphincter difficulties. Attacks of vertigo or trigeminal neuralgia or a psychiatric illness may be significant. Additionally, a history of trauma, drug abuse, toxic exposure, or alcoholism is important.

(6) Family history. Multiple sclerosis may be familial. The examiner should inquire for CNS disease in the family and also for a history of eye disease.

(7) Differential diagnosis. Unilateral optic neuritis must be differentiated from hysterical visual loss (stereopsis intact), optic disk vasculitis, papilledema, juxtapapillary chorioretinitis, uveitis, syphilitic optic perineuritis, lactation neuritis, ischemic optic neuropathy, optic disk drusen, other causes of disk swelling, and other optic nerve lesions, notably, a compressive neuropathy. The examiner should have a **high index of suspicion of a compressive lesion if the patient** is **over 40** years, if **optic atrophy** is present yet the history is short, if the **field defect respects** the **vertical meridian,** if the **tempo of evolution** of visual loss is inappropriate, if there is **no recovery,** and if a careful history reveals other leads, such as headache, amenorrhea, sinus disease, or trauma.

(a) Neuromyelitis optica is an important condition to consider in the differential diagnosis of bilateral optic neuritis. Either the optic neuritis or transverse myelitis may appear first. Usually both eyes are affected within hours or a day of each other, and then as long as a week or more may elapse before the transverse myelitis develops, or vice versa. The optic neuritis of the myelitis can recur.

(b) Bilateral loss of vision without myelitis may well represent alcohol-nutrition amblyopia, drug toxicity, metabolic disease, syphilitic optic perineuritis, hereditary optic atrophy, cone dysfunction, or one of the rarer forms of optic neuropathy. A treatable compressive lesion must not be overlooked.

(c) **Leber's hereditary optic neuropathy.** Sequential visual loss due to demyelination must be distinguished from Leber's hereditary optic neuropathy.

This condition affects males primarily, and is transmitted via female carriers through cytoplasmic DNA in the ovum (mitochondrial). It is characterized by rapid loss of central vision caused by neuroretinal degeneration occurring during early adult life (mean age at onset 20–24 years). Both eyes are affected either simultaneously or sequentially. The visual fields contain scotomas that are initially central and rapidly become centrocecal in location. In acute Leber's optic neuropathy, the ophthalmoscopic findings are (1) circumpapillary telangiectatic microangiopathy; (2) swelling of the nerve fiber layer around the disk; and (3) absence of leakage from the disk or papillary region on fluorescein angiography with arteriovenous shunting present in the area of the telangiectatic vessels. In chronic Leber's optic neuropathy, the optic disk is atrophic. About 15% of patients recover useful vision in one or both eyes many years after the ictus. Cardiac dysrhythmias are also a frequent manifestation. Leber's hereditary optic neuropathy is transmitted by maternal inheritance. No case of paternal transmission has ever been documented. The maternal inheritance is explained by the mitochondrial origin of the disease. Analysis of the sequence of mitochondrial DNA has indicated that a single nucleotide change at position 11778 is associated with this disease. This specific point mutation in the mitochondrial DNA that results in Leber's hereditary optic neuropathy converts the 340th amino acid of NADH dehydrogenase subunit 4 from an arginine to a histidine and eliminates an SfaNI endonuclease restriction site. Whole blood samples are required for mitochondrial DNA testing. The specific point mutation is not found in all cases of Leber's optic neuropathy, however. Currently, 60% of cases are reported to be positive and 40% negative.

(8) **Management and investigation.** Most patients with unilateral optic neuritis can be followed in the ophthalmologist's office, without treatment or additional investigations over a minimum period of 8 months. If severe visual loss is followed by complete recovery, the diagnosis can be made with reasonable certainty.

Patients with progressive visual loss, severe visual loss without sign of recovery, atypical persistent pain and bilateral involvement, or exophthalmus should be referred to a neuroophthalmologist or neurologist (or both) for additional studies. **Investigations** are usually limited to a lumbar puncture and visual evoked potential and a brain MRI with gadolinium.

(a) **The CSF** may be expected to show an elevated protein (N < 40 mg/dl) in 42%, an increased cell count (N < 5 cells) in 47%, or an elevated gamma globulin level (N < 10 mg/dl) and oligoclonal bands in 15% of optic neuritis patients.

(b) **The visual evoked potential test** can provide solid evidence for the existence of abnormality but not for its pathologic nature. The role of evoked potentials is essentially that of detecting subclinical second lesions in patients in whom the diagnosis is not yet clinically definite. The greatest usefulness of the visual evoked response is in **detecting damage to the optic nerve when the acuity and the disk are normal.** The results must be interpreted in light of the clinical picture.

(c) **Neuroimaging.** Imaging of plaques with MRI has revealed multifocal white matter lesions in 90–98% of patients with clinical definite multiple sclerosis and 50–70% of adult patients with isolated optic neuritis. In optic neuritis, the MRI findings meet the criteria for a diagnosis of laboratory-supported definite multiple sclerosis, provided that a very conservative approach to the interpretation of the MRI is adopted to ensure that false-positive diagnoses are avoided and an MRI diagnostic scale analogous to the clinical diagnostic classification for multiple sclerosis is utilized.

(i) MRI strongly suggestive of multiple sclerosis: (a) four lesions present, or (b) three lesions present, one periventricular.

(ii) MRI suggestive of multiple sclerosis: (a) three lesions present or (b) two lesions present, one periventricular.

(iii) MRI indicating possible multiple sclerosis: (a) two lesions present or (b) one lesion present in a periventricular location.

(iv) MRI excluding multiple sclerosis: (a) one lesion only, not periventricular, (b) normal scan, or (c) other diagnoses.

(9) **Treatment.** There is no effective treatment for idiopathic optic neuritis. **Corticosteroids** (adrenocorticotropic hormone [ACTH] or prednisone) do **not**, in themselves, cure the disease. The most they can do is to suppress the inflammation or immune reaction, shorten the period of blindness, or relieve pain. There is currently a clinical trial comparing oral prednisone with IV methylprednisolone followed by oral prednisolone designed to determine whether one or both of these therapies increase the speed of recovery and/or reduce the residual visual deficit and whether there is any difference in efficacy between the two therapeutic modes. At the moment, however, there is no evidence that steroid therapy of optic neuritis influences the ultimate level of visual recovery (2-year follow-up) or prevents a second attack.

(a) **Contraindications.** Steroid treatment is contraindicated in optic neuritis when the condition is mild or moderately severe, when signs of spontaneous recovery of vision are already evident, when vision is stable and the condition is burnt out, with the presence of optic atrophy, or in Uhthoff's syndrome.

(b) **Indications** for the use of steroids in the treatment of optic neuritis are controversial because of the tendency toward spontaneous improvement from episodes of demyelination. Circumstances in which the patient may be encouraged to undergo steroid therapy include **when the disease includes both eyes simultaneously or sequentially within hours or days of each other;** when **only the good eye is affected;** in the rare case, when the **tempo** of the disease is **unusual** and **slow progressive visual loss** continues to occur in the absence of a compressive lesion; or when there is a history of **previous episodes that recovered well** during or after corticosteroid therapy, particularly in instances of severe loss of vision such as loss of light perception. A less clear-cut indication for steroids is the unilateral case of optic neuritis with a visual acuity of 20/60 or less. **The decision to treat or not to treat is best assisted by the hospital-based neuroophthalmologist** or neurologist, since these specialists are frequently more familiar with the use and risks of corticosteroids and they are able to provide the very close medical supervision required by a steroid-treated patient.

(c) **Dosage regimen.** Those patients who are treated should receive clearance from their internist before starting a regimen that is commonly 80 mg prednisone PO for 3 days followed by 60 mg PO for 3 days and then 40 mg PO for 1 week before discontinuing therapy. An alternative, more gradual tapering dosage is not required if treatment is to be less than 2 weeks. Patients should take their steroids in the morning after a meal and supplement their diet with potassium.

b. Ischemic optic neuropathy results from infarction of the prelaminar anterior optic nerve.

(1) **Pathogenesis.** Infarction is due to occlusion of the two main posterior ciliary arteries that supply the optic nerve and choroid. Three causes are giant-cell arteritis (temporal arteritis), nonarteritic arteriosclerosis, and emboli to the ciliary circulation.

(a) Approximately 10% of patients with ischemic optic neuritis have **giant-cell arteritis.** This is a disease of the elderly, with onset characteristically over the age of 60 years. Women are more frequently affected than men.

(b) **Arteriosclerotic ischemic optic neuropathy** tends to occur at a younger age, 46–65 years, and the condition is somewhat more prevalent in men. A history of or signs of systemic vascular disease are frequently present (mild hypertension, diabetes mellitus, narrow retinal arteries). Other risk factors include hyperlipidemia.

(c) Attention has also been called to a form of **ischemic optic neuropathy following uncomplicated cataract extraction** with sudden visual loss from 4 weeks to 15 months postoperatively.

(d) **Embolic anterior ischemic optic neuropathy** is a recognized complication of a coronary bypass procedure and may be bilateral.

(2) **Tempo of evolution and recovery**

(a) **Evolution.** Loss of vision is abrupt. It rarely progresses for more than 1 or 2 days.

(i) In **giant-cell arteritis** visual loss usually occurs between 3 and 12 weeks after the first manifestation of this systemic disease. Both optic nerves may be involved simultaneously or sequentially. The interval between involvement varies from a few hours to a few days up to several weeks.

(ii) In **nonarteritic arteriosclerotic ischemic optic neuritis,** both optic nerves are involved simultaneously in 19% and eventually in 49% of cases. The interval between involvement varies between 2 weeks and 17 years, the average being 42 months.

(b) **Recovery.** Visual prognosis is poor in ischemic optic neuritis but better in nonarteritic ischemic optic neuritis than in giant-cell arteritis. When acuity is impaired it may eventually improve in 33% of cases, especially when the defect in the visual field is a central scotoma or small altitudinal scotoma.

(3) **Ophthalmoscopy**

(a) **Early changes.** Ischemic papillitis (the most frequent form of ocular involvement in giant-cell arteritis [60% of cases]) is characterized by pallor and swelling of the nerve head with small nerve fiber layer hemorrhages in the peripapillary area. Frequently, segmental infarction and swelling of the disk are present. The retinal arteries may appear attenuated. Similar changes are seen in arteriosclerotic ischemic papillitis. In other cases, microinfarction of the retina occurs with cotton-wool patches due to focal ischemia of the nerve fiber layer.

(b) Late changes. Optic disk cupping similar to that seen in glaucomatous cupping may develop in eyes with ischemic optic neuritis secondary to giant-cell arteritis or arteriosclerosis. Pallor and optic atrophy are usually more severe in these cases than in patients with glaucoma.

The ophthalmoscopic picture of the **pseudo–Foster Kennedy syndrome** may be seen in this condition, that is, ischemic **papillitis in one eye** and **optic atrophy in the other.** The clinical setting of acute visual loss in the second eye should help distinguish the case from the Foster-Kennedy syndrome.

(4) Associated ocular symptoms and signs

   (a) Pain is not a prominent symptom. Pain on eye motion does not usually occur.

   (b) Transient monocular visual loss, amaurosis fugax, is a prominent symptom in giant-cell arteritis. Characteristically, amaurosis fugax is sudden in onset and short in duration. The typical attack persists for 2–3 minutes and rarely longer than 5–30 minutes. The patient describes the episode frequently as momentary blurred vision or obscuration of vision by a gray cloud. Less commonly, the patient describes a window shade appearing to be drawn down or across the vision of the affected eye (more typical of amaurosis fugax in extracranial occlusive carotid artery disease). Monocular amaurosis fugax that alternates between the two eyes must be considered as due to giant-cell arteritis until proved otherwise. Amaurosis fugax is due to transient retinal ischemia. It is one of the most important warning symptoms of impending blindness. **If the diagnosis is missed, 40–50% of all untreated cases will develop blindness or severe visual loss.**

   (c) Visual loss. Decreased vision is the presenting complaint. As a rule, loss of vision in giant-cell arteritis is profound. In arteriosclerotic ischemic optic neuritis, 42% of cases have a visual acuity of 20/100 or less. In 35% the vision may remain normal.

   (d) Visual field defects. Any type of visual field defect characteristic of an optic nerve lesion is seen. In giant-cell arteritis, usually the whole visual field is depressed. In arteriosclerotic ischemic optic neuritis, frequently the defect is an inferior altitudinal defect or arcuate scotoma.

   (e) Pupil. An afferent pupil defect is present in an eye with severe ischemic papillitis or central retinal artery occlusion. Dilation and paralysis of the pupillary sphincter may indicate severe ischemia of the eye or ciliary ganglion. Tonic pupil may be present.

   (f) Diplopia. Occasionally, diplopia is the presenting symptom of giant-cell arteritis (12% of cases). In patients with diplopia, 50% are due to sixth nerve palsy and 50% are due to a third nerve palsy with pupil sparing. One pathologic study on a patient who died from giant-cell arteritis with bilateral ophthalmoplegia showed, however, that extraocular muscle ischemia was the mechanism responsible for the ophthalmoplegia.

(5) Associated systemic symptoms and signs.

   (a) The systemic symptoms of **giant-cell arteritis,** in order of decreasing frequency, are temporal pain or headache, jaw claudication, tender temporal arteries, swelling in the temples, fatigue, muscle ache or stiffness, neck pain, anorexia, fever, and weight loss. Some of the symptoms are related to involvement of cranial arteries, and there appears to be a close correlation between the susceptibility to giant-cell arteritis and the amount of elastic tissue in the media and adventitia of the individual arteries of the head and neck. The arteries most commonly affected in 75–100% of patients are the superficial temporal, the vertebral (outside the dura), the ophthalmic, and the posterior ciliary arteries. The intracranial arteries are rarely involved. These classic symptoms may be present or absent with the ocular phase.

(b) In contrast, in **nonarteritic arteriosclerotic ischemic optic neuropathy,** symptoms and signs of systemic vascular disease and hypertension are frequently present.

(6) **Management and investigation. Always suspect the diagnosis of giant-cell arteritis in every elderly patient with amaurosis fugax, ischemic optic neuropathy, central retinal artery occlusion, or suggestive systemic symptomatology.**

(a) **Act immediately.** The steps are as follows:

Step 1. **Obtain a stat Westergren sedimentation rate** (normal 35–40 mm/hour); 5–10% of these may be normal.

Step 2. **Get the results,** whenever possible, **before the patient leaves the office.**

Step 3. **Start high-dose oral steroids if the sedimentation rate is elevated** or if patient must return home before the result is known. Telephone patient to further instruct.

Step 4. **Plan a temporal artery biopsy.**

Step 5. **Refer the patient for an emergency consultation** to a physician in internal medicine for consideration of emergency admission to the hospital.

(b) **Hospital admission** may be advisable because blindness may ensue despite adequate steroid treatment, and the initial dose of prednisone may not be adequate to relieve symptoms immediately and drop the level of the sedimentation rate. Some elderly patients also show visual loss related to postural changes. Most important, however, any patient on steroids in this age group should be seen and followed by an internist.

(c) Some **additional laboratory results** are also of value. An elevation of the fibrinogen level (normal, 200–400 mg/dl in plasma) correlates with the increased sedimentation rate. Serum protein electrophoresis may show a marked increase in alpha$_2$ globulin fraction and beta globulins. The white blood count is often increased in association with fever. Fifty percent of patients with giant-cell arteritis show some degree of normocytic hypochromic anemia, which may be responsive to iron, folic acid, and vitamin B$_{12}$.

(d) **Biopsy of the temporal artery,** occasionally the facial artery, or a superficial posterior occipital artery to the scalp is necessary to confirm the clinical diagnosis. Palpation of the temporal artery, characteristically tender, nonpulsate, and nodular, was normal in more than 50% of positive biopsies in one series of 46 patients. **Skip areas,** though occasionally found, are uncommon if an artery is carefully sectioned serially and if a long (3–7 cm) segment is excised. A Doppler ultrasound flow detector can be helpful in selecting the side of the artery biopsy. Biopsy, if done early after steroid therapy, will still show histologic changes of giant-cell arteritis. Though not often reported, patients with classic giant-cell arteritis and elevated sedimentation rates have negative temporal artery biopsies. Nevertheless, a patient with elevated sedimentation rate and symptoms of giant-cell arteritis should have a temporal artery biopsy. A high index of suspicion should be maintained even if the patient's sedimentation rate is normal.

(7) Treatment

(a) Giant-cell arteritis. Prednisone, 60–80 mg PO or IM, should be started immediately. After the initial period of treatment with large doses of steroids, the prednisone dose should be tapered to a maintenance dose of 20 mg qd or less. The appropriate **maintenance dose** is **titrated against** the **sedimentation rate**, the fibrinogen level, and the patient's **symptoms.** It must be adequate to keep the sedimentation rate in the normal range or at a stable baseline level and to abolish symptoms. **Treatment is continued for at least 6 months.** Once steroids are stopped, the sedimentation rate should be measured at 2-week intervals for 6 weeks to check that it is stable, and the patient should be seen in follow-up by an internist. A few patients may not be in full remission after 6 months of steroid therapy. These patients will develop a high sedimentation rate and/or clinical symptoms off steroids, and they will need to go back on steroid therapy. Many elderly patients may show a rising sedimentation rate off steroids due to arthritis. In selected cases, a repeat temporal artery biopsy may be required to identify those patients with active temporal arteritis.

Adverse side effects of steroids occur in 40–50% of cases of giant-cell arteritis. They include a cushingoid appearance (40%), symptomatic vertebral compression fractures (26%), proximal muscle weakness (17%), subcapsular cataracts (5%), and increased insulin requirements (2%). In untreated cases, the **mortality** is 12%.

(b) Nonarteritic arteriosclerotic ischemic optic neuritis. Steroids are of questionable value in arteriosclerotic ischemic optic neuritis, but they should be prescribed pending the results of a temporal artery biopsy to rule out giant-cell arteritis. When the diagnosis of giant-cell arteritis is not confirmed, steroids can be tapered fairly abruptly and stopped. Hypertension, diabetes mellitus, anemia, and glaucoma should all be controlled. Precipitous drops in systemic blood pressure must be avoided by internists treating hypertension, since this may cause further ischemic optic nerve damage. Elective surgery should be avoided in these patients until the ocular disease is stable and until hypertension is under satisfactory control.

c. Optic atrophy

(1) Pathogenesis. Three major etiologic types are recognized: heredofamilial optic atrophy, consecutive optic atrophy consequent on death of retinal ganglion cells and axons, and secondary optic atrophy that follows papillitis and chronic papilledema. This classification, while not complete, affords a simple guide.

(a) Heredofamilial optic atrophy, which includes a number of important entities, must be considered in the evaluation of insidious visual loss and disk pallor in childhood (see Chap. 10). Table 12–1 documents the major features of **Kjer's dominant optic atrophy** and the recessive forms called simple, complicated, and juvenile optic atrophy with diabetes mellitus and deafness. **Leber's hereditary optic neuropathy** is discussed in sec. **II.B.2.a.(7)(c).**

(b) Consecutive optic atrophy, the most frequent form of optic atrophy, includes all diseases that cause **retinal ganglion** injury and **death.** Rare examples are the lipid storage diseases (Tay-Sachs disease), adrenoleukodystrophy, and Menkes' kinky hair syndrome (see Chap. 10, sec. **VII**). Consecutive optic atrophy also follows more common conditions, such as degenera-

Table 12-1. Heredofamilial optic atrophies

	Dominant		Recessive		Indeterminate
	Kjer's juvenile (infantile)	Early infantile (congenital); simple	Behr's type; complicated[a]	Juvenile with diabetes mellitus; with or without deafness	Leber's hereditary optic neuropathy
Age at onset	Childhood (4–8 years)	Early childhood[b] (3–4 years)	Childhood (1–9 years)	Childhood (6–14 years)	Early adulthood (18–30 years; up to sixth decade)
Visual impairment	Mild to moderate (20/40–20/200)	Severe (20/200–HM)	Moderate (20/200)	Severe (20/400–FC)	Moderate to severe (20/200–FC)
Nystagmus	Rare[c]	Usual	In 50%	Absent	Absent
Optic disk	Mild temporal pallor (with or without temporal excavation)[a]	Marked diffuse pallor (with or without arteriolar attenuation)[a]	Mild temporal pallor	Marked diffuse pallor	Moderate diffuse pallor; disk swelling in acute phase
Color vision	Blue-yellow dyschromatopsia	Severe dyschromatopsia or achromatopsia	Moderate to severe dyschromatopsia	Severe dyschromatopsia	Dense central scrotoma for colors
Course	Variable, slight progression	Stable	Stable	Progressive	Acute visual loss, then usually stable; may improve or worsen

HM = hand motions; FC = finger counting.

[a] See discussion of heredodegenerative neurologic syndromes (Secs. VII and VIII and Chap. 10).

[b] Difficult to assess in infancy, but visual impairment usually manifests by age 4 years.

[c] Presence of nystagmus with poor vision and earlier onset suggests separate congenital or infantile form.

[d] Distinguished from tapetoretinal degenerations by normal electroretinogram.

Source: Modified from J. S. Glaser, Heredofamilial Disorders of the Optic Nerve. In M.F. Goldberg (ed.), *Genetic and Metabolic Eye Disease.* Boston: Little, Brown, 1974. With permission.

tive, vascular, and toxic lesions, including tobacco-alcohol amblyopia; ethambutol, chloroquine, ethchlorvynol (Placidyl), and other drug-induced neuropathies; and many other conditions associated with loss of optic nerve axons and retrograde degeneration of retinal ganglion cells, including ischemia, trauma, demyelination, and compressive lesions of the anterior visual pathway.

Nutritional deficiency alcohol amblyopia is mentioned particularly because it is a **potentially reversible** cause of optic atrophy. It is, however, insidious in onset and frequently undetected in the early stage. Small bilateral **paracentral scotomas** develop between fixation and the blind spot and are initially detectable by response to color targets. Progression leads to loss of color perception, impaired visual acuity, and **bilateral central** or **centrocecal scotoma.** Nerve fiber bundle defects do not occur. As a rule, the fundus is normal. Prognosis for recovery is excellent at this stage but poor in the chronic case with optic atrophy. **Treatment** consists of a well-balanced diet, B-complex vitamin supplement, and abstinence from alcohol. IM thiamine may be used. Prevention is the key. Every effort should be made to rehabilitate the alcoholic.

- (c) **Secondary optic atrophy** follows papillitis and chronic papilledema.
- (d) **Lyme disease** and **tertiary syphilis** may cause numerous neurophthalmic disorders including optic atrophy (see chap. 5, sec. **IV.L**).

- (2) **Ophthalmoscopy.** Optic atrophy may be difficult to establish by ophthalmoscopic criteria alone. Serial examinations aided by fundus photography are often necessary, as well as screening for signs of optic nerve dysfunction such as reduced visual acuity, field changes, diminished color perception, or sluggish pupil to light.

  To evaluate the pale disk, the examiner inspects the retina for attrition of ganglion cells and nerve fibers. (The green filter on the ophthalmoscope provides red-free light.) The disk should be inspected for vascularity (Kestenbaum capillary count) and sector pallor. The pattern of insertion of retinal nerve fibers at the nerve head is important. Sector pallor of the disk should be correlated with an area of retinal nerve fiber atrophy and with the type and extent of the visual field defect. A specific example is illustrated by **bow-tie atrophy,** a horizontal band of pallor of the disk in the eye contralateral to an optic tract lesion.

III. **The pupil.*** The pupil is an aperture in the eye formed by the muscles and pigmented stroma of the anterior uveal tract. The muscles are of two types: a circumferential **sphincter** found in the margin of the iris, innervated by the parasympathetic nervous system, and **radial dilator** muscles, which run from the iris margin to the root of the iris, innervated by the sympathetic nervous system.

A. **Afferent limb of the pupillary arc**
  1. **Parasympathetic anatomy**
     a. **The afferent limb** of the pupillary light reflex begins in the retina with axons from retinal ganglion cells. No specialization of the retina into "pupil-specific" ganglion cells is known. The **fibers** from each eye **decussate at the chiasm** with **54% of the fibers crossing and 47% remaining ipsilateral.** Fibers destined for midbrain connections separate from the optic tract and enter the pretectal nucleus, where they synapse. It is not known whether the axons that subverse pupillary light responses are from their own ganglion cells or are branches of axons. The

---

* Reprinted from Special Course No. 12, 1979, Neuroophthalmology, American Academy of Neurology, by permission of the author, James J. Corbett.

fibers from the pretectal nuclei hemidecussate via the posterior commissure and synapse in the **Edinger-Westphal nucleus.** The efferent output from the Edinger-Westphal nucleus is cholinergic and receives equal drive from both optic nerves, as a result of the midbrain hemidecussation. The pupilloconstrictor fibers (iris sphincter) are driven by light and near responses. The near reaction has diffuse cortical inputs and projects directly to the Edinger-Westphal nucleus. The **near reaction** consists of accommodation and convergence as well as constriction of the pupil. Both light and near efferents are carried in the parasympathetic Edinger-Westphal outflow.

- b. **Efferent fibers** from the Edinger-Westphal nucleus are carried in the superficial layer of the **oculomotor nerve** and eventually end in its inferior division, where it passes through the superior orbital fissure and synapses in the ciliary ganglion. **Postganglionic fibers,** the short ciliary nerves, enter the globe near the optic nerve and supply the ciliary body and iris sphincter. There is a topographic relationship between cells in the Edinger-Westphal nucleus and sectors of the iris sphincter. For every axon that leaves the ciliary ganglion to supply the light response, 30 axons serve the near response. This 30:1 ratio is important as the **basis for light-near dissociation.** The iris sphincter is smooth muscle and has acetylcholine receptors, as does the ciliary body.

2. **Relative afferent pupil defect (Marcus Gunn pupil).** Since the irides in both eyes respond to light with an equal change in the size of the pupils, this sensory or afferent limb of the reflex arc can provide evidence for impaired function of the retina or optic nerve.

   - a. **Testing of the pupillary light response** should be done in dim illumination. The patient should be instructed to look into the distance. Using a bright, preferably filament-free light, the examiner shines the light in one eye and then quickly in the other. The normal pupil responds to light with a brief constriction and then slight release to a relatively constant pupil diameter. The light should be alternated from eye to eye, the examiner looking for enlargement of the pupil on the affected ipsilateral side when the light is shone in the affected eye and constriction of the ipsilateral pupil when the light is shown in the non-affected contralateral eye. In persons with no damage to the retina or optic nerve, the response will be symmetric and there will be no change of pupil size from side to side. **When there is a relative afferent pupil defect, both pupils will be larger as the light is directed into the affected eye and smaller as the light is directed into the unaffected eye.** This **sign is present** when the **sensory retina or optic nerve is damaged** but is not seen when visual loss is due to corneal, lenticular, vitreous, refractive, or emotional causes.

     The test may occasionally be difficult to interpret in those patients who have large-amplitude physiologic swings in pupil size known as **hippus.** It may require more than one attempt at different times to establish clearly whether or not there truly is a relative afferent pupil defect. Hippus has no pathologic significance.

   - b. **The pupillary afferent defect can be roughly quantified** by the use of **graded neutral density filters.** By placing a neutral filter in front of the normal eye, the examiner can effectively eliminate the relative afferent defect by "balancing" the visual loss in the two eyes. The filter density needed to balance the pupil defect is a measure of the loss of input to the affected eye and can be compared to earlier measurements for evidence of progression of a disease process.

3. **Light-near dissociation.** In normal patients the amplitude of the pupil response to light is essentially equal to the response to near. When the **afferent** pupil **fibers are disrupted** in the **pretectal region,** the **response** of the pupil to light may be diminished or lost, whereas the reaction to near is preserved. This phenomenon is termed **light-near dissociation.** The pu-

pils tend to be midsized or enlarged, and frequently unequal. This condition has been reported in midbrain lesions in isolation or in association with Parinaud's syndrome, with convergence-retraction nystagmus, and limited up gaze.

4. **Argyll Robertson pupil.** Another form of **light-near dissociation** is the Argyll Robertson pupil. Here, the pupils are **small** and **respond poorly** or not at all to light, but have a prompt response to near. **Both pupils** are almost invariably involved, and these pupils **respond poorly to pupil-dilating agents.** This abnormality is probably due to a lesion in the midbrain light reflex path. While it has been seen in diabetes mellitus and other diseases, the Argyll Robertson pupil should be considered presumptive evidence of neurosyphilis until proved otherwise. In the presence of this sign, a standard serologic test for syphilis as well as a fluorescent treponemal antibody absorption (FTA-Abs) test should be performed (Table 12-2).

B. **Efferent cholinergic pupil defects and Horner's syndrome**
   1. **Pupilloconstrictor dysfunction**
      a. **Compression** of the pupilloconstrictor fibers in the subarachnoid space, in the cavernous sinus, or in the orbit may produce a pupil that is unable to constrict to light or near with or without other elements of a third nerve palsy. The relatively peripheral location of the parasympathetic efferent pupilloconstrictor fibers on the **third nerve** makes them particularly vulnerable to compression. This abnormality is produced with some frequency by posterior communicating artery aneurysms and internal carotid artery aneurysms, as well as the classic uncal herniation syndrome.
      b. **The tonic pupil (Adie's topic pupil)** results from damage to the **ciliary ganglion** or **postganglion fibers** of the **short posterior ciliary nerves.**
         (1) **Dilated pupil.** When these structures are damaged, the pupil becomes enlarged and denervated (usually in a segmental fashion). Because the ratio of cells and fibers that serve the near response is so much greater as compared to those that serve the light response (30:1), the pupil reacts poorly to light but well to near. Furthermore, the **response to near is tonic.** When the patient looks at near and then refixates at distance, the pupil very slowly redilates. In the early phase, observation of a tonic pupil in bright light will accentuate the anisocoria, since the tonic pupil will fail to constrict. Bright light frequently bothers these patients.
         (2) **Denervation sensitivity.** The most characteristic part of the tonic pupil is the phenomenon of denervation supersensitivity of the sphincter of the pupil. Use of 1 or 2 drops **0.12% pilocarpine** will provide intense constriction of the pupil if there is denervation supersensitivity. (Table 12-2).
         (3) **Accommodation.** In addition to the light-near dissociation, large pupil, and denervation supersensitivity, accommodation is frequently affected with blurred vision at near. Although the pupil rarely recovers much light function following damage to the ciliary ganglion, the high proportion of accommodative fibers ensures reinnervation of the ciliary body.
         (4) **Adie's syndrome.** The combination of a **tonic pupil** and **areflexia** is known as Adie's syndrome. This condition is the most common cause of a tonic pupil, but a multitude of other conditions can damage the ciliary ganglion or short ciliary nerves, resulting in a tonic pupil. After a tonic pupil has been present for years, it becomes smaller and may even be the smaller of the two pupils.
   2. **Pupillodilator dysfunction (Horner's syndrome)**
      a. **Anatomy.** The pupillodilator fibers are under the control of the sympathetic nervous system. This neural arc consists of three neurons, beginning in the **posterolateral hypothalamus.** Fibers originating in these areas course caudally through the brainstem in a roughly but diffusely

Table 12-2. Differentiating common pupillary anomalies

Syndrome	Appearance	Size	Light reaction	Near reaction	Comments and special tests
Tonic pupil (Adie's tonic pupil)	Dark / Light / Near / Pilocarpine 0.12%	Large except when old, then small	Vermiform, trace or segmental; best seen under slit lamp	Strong, slow and tonic	Pilocarpine 0.12% reveals denervation supersensitivity; Adie's syndrome tonic pupil plus areflexia
Horner's syndrome	Dark / Light / Near	Small	Normal	Normal	Ptosis, upside-down ptosis, anhidrosis and early hypotony with conjunctival injection; cocaine 10% positive in first-, second-, and third-neuron damage
First- or second-neuron Horner's	Cocaine 10%				
Third-neuron Horner's	Paredrine 1%				Paredrine 1% fails to dilate third-neuron Horner's
Argyll Robertson pupil	Dark / Light / Near	Small	Trace or absent	Brisk	VDRL FTA-Abs Pupils may be irregular

VDRL = Venereal Disease Research Lab (test); FTA-Abs = fluorescent treponemal antibody absorption (test).

dorsolateral location. These first-order axons synapse in the intermediolateral portion of the C8–T2 level of spinal cord known as the **ciliospinal center of Budge.** Second-order axons emerge from the spinal cord at the T1 level in the **ventral root.** They ascend to cross the apex of the lung, course through (without synapse) the stellate ganglion, the inferior cervical ganglion, around the subclavian artery (anterior loop of the ansa subclavia), and through the middle cervical ganglion. At the level of the angle of the mandible (bifurcation of the carotid, C3–C4), these second-order fibers synapse in the **superior cervical ganglion.** From the superior cervical ganglion the third-order neurons form the final common pathway to the pupillodilator muscles. These nerve fibers follow the carotid into the cavernous sinus where they attach to the **ophthalmic division of the trigeminal nerve** and emerge from the cavernous sinus with the **nasociliary branch** and the **long ciliary nerves to the iris.** The neurotransmitter released at the pupillodilator muscle fiber is norepinephrine.

b. **Diagnosis of Horner's syndrome.** Since any dysfunction or damage to the sympathetic chain will decrease the output of norepinephrine in the synaptic cleft of the pupillodilator fiber, the differentiation of Horner's syndrome purely by its clinical effects is not always possible. All patients with Horner's syndrome have **ptosis** and a **miotic pupil** that **reacts equally to light and near.** Early they may have ocular hypotony and conjunctival erythema, and they may also have upside-down ptosis or elevation of the lower lid. **Facial anhidrosis** is less easily identified today due to air conditioning, which eliminates the profuse diaphoresis that helped to identify this sign. Three tests are useful in helping to confirm the diagnosis of Horner's syndrome and in identifying the level of damage.

(1) **The cocaine test.** A drop of **cocaine 5–10%** ophthalmic is placed in either eye and repeated in 1 minute. Sympathetic damage resulting in a Horner's syndrome, no matter at what level, will result in a pupil that dilates poorly to cocaine, which acts to block reuptake of norepinephrine at the synaptic cleft. **The cocaine test confirms or denies the presence of a Horner's syndrome. Without it, the diagnosis on clinical criteria alone is presumptive.** Damage to any neuron of the arc will give a positive cocaine test (Table 12–2).

(2) **The Paredrine test. Hydroxyamphetamine 1% (Paredrine)** ophthalmic drops release packets of **norepinephrine** into the synaptic cleft. If the first or second neurons of the oculosympathetic system have been damaged and the final common pathway is intact, the third-order neurons are able to produce, transport, and store norepinephrine. When Paredrine is instilled, the pupils dilate because norepinephrine is released. When the **third-order** neuron (superior cervical ganglion or postganglionic fibers) is damaged, there is no production, transport, or storage of norepinephrine, and when Paredrine is instilled in the affected eye no pupil dilation occurs. Thus, the cocaine test tells whether or not there is a Horner's syndrome, and the **Paredrine test can separate a third-neuron Horner's syndrome from first- and second-neuron syndromes.** There is no pharmacologic test that can differentiate a first- and second-neuron Horner's syndrome. These must be identified clinically by the associated brainstem (first neuron) or spinal cord and lung apex (second neuron) symptoms and signs (Table 12–2).

(3) **Dilation lag.** Recently, a simple, elegant observation has aided in the identification of Horner's syndrome. Since the pupillodilator muscle actively dilates the pupil in darkness, damage to the sympathetic nerve supply will result in only passive release of the sphincter rather than active dilation. Thus, the affected pupil will

dilate less rapidly in dark as compared to the unaffected side. This is called dilation lag. It is best appreciated in photographs taken at 5 and 15 seconds after turning out the lights, using a flash camera with a close-up attachment. Clinically, it can be appreciated in dim lighting in persons with lightly colored irides.

C. **Simple anisocoria.** About 25% of the normal population will have greater than 0.3 mm of anisocoria from time to time that may even alternate sides. The pupils are otherwise entirely normal and have no light-near dissociation or pharmacologic abnormalities, and they do not demonstrate dilation lag. Since small degrees of ptosis and miosis due to simple anisocoria may occur in the same eye, it becomes all the more important to use formal pharmacologic testing to diagnose Horner's syndrome.

D. **The fixed dilated pupil.** Pharmacologic blockage may be a real diagnostic dilemma and the fixed dilated pupil can be resolved by history and pharmacologic testing. Accidental or factitious instillation of drugs that cause pupillary dilation is seen most commonly in persons in medical settings. Nurses, doctors, and other paramedic people with access to those drugs may inadvertently rub them into their eyes, producing a dilated pupil. **Pilocarpine 1%** will constrict a pupil that is dilated due to compression but will not overcome pharmacologic blockade. **If the pupil fails to respond to pilocarpine 1% and direct obvious trauma is not the cause of the mydriasis, factitious or accidental mydriasis can be assumed.**

Refractive Errors and Clinical Optics

George Edw. Garcia and
Deborah Pavan-Langston

I. **Physical optics affecting vision and correction of visual refractive errors**
  A. **Wavelength of light.** Electromagnetic radiation exists in many forms. The characteristic of the radiation that determines the form in which it is encountered is the wavelength. Long wavelengths are encountered as radio transmissions or radar, and the short wavelengths as cosmic rays and x rays. The visible portion of the electromagnetic radiation spectrum occurs between the ultraviolet and infrared portions, from 380 nm at the violet end of the spectrum to 760 nm at the red end.
  B. **Frequency of light waves.** The frequency of electromagnetic radiation is the number of times a particular position on the wave passes a fixed point in a fixed interval of time. It is inversely related to the wavelength. For example, radio waves have a frequency of 10^4–10^8 cycles per second (cps), while the visible part of the spectrum is in the 10^{14}–10^{15} cps range.
  C. **Velocity of light waves.** Electromagnetic radiation travels at a speed of 3×10^{10} cm/second (186,000 miles/second) in vacuo.
  D. **Index of refraction.** Although the frequency of light does not vary with the density of the medium in which it is traveling, the speed is reduced in a dense medium. The ratio of the velocity in vacuo to the velocity in a particular medium (n/n') is referred to as the index of refraction for that medium. Since the frequency of radiation does not vary with the medium and the speed does, it follows that the wavelength in a dense medium is less than it is in air and is proportional to the change in speed. Each medium, therefore, has a different refractive index for each wavelength. Short wavelengths, or blue light, are slowed down or refracted more than long wavelengths, or red light. This accounts for the **chromatic aberration** present in the eye or in single-element lens systems.
  E. **Quanta or photons.** The energy in electromagnetic radiation is measured in units called *quanta* or *photons*. The energy of an individual photon is proportional to the frequency or inversely proportional to the wavelengths; therefore, the energy of a photon at 400 nm is twice as great as that of a photon at 800 nm. For example, red light is innocuous, ultraviolet light produces burns, and x rays produce severe damage to tissues.
  F. **Loss of light by reflection or absorption.** The light incident on the retina from a light source is decreased by loss from reflection at the cornea, lens, and retinal surfaces. Although the cornea is quite transparent from 400–1200 nm, the crystalline lens does absorb some of the radiant energy, particularly short wavelengths. This absorption at the blue end of the spectrum increases with age as xanthochromic (yellow-brown) proteins accumulate in the lens. Some of the short wavelength radiation is also absorbed by the yellow pigment in the macular region of the retina.
  G. **Color of light.** The physical stimulus that is responsible for the sensation of color is the wavelength of the radiation. Wavelength in the region around 430 nm produces a violet sensation, around 460 nm blue, around 520 nm green, around 575 nm yellow, around 600 nm orange, and around 650 nm red. A mixture of wavelengths such as occurs in sunlight produces a white sensation.
  H. **Reflection.** When light waves strike a smooth surface they may bounce off the surface, or be reflected, rather than pass through. Reflection from polished

surfaces, referred to as "regular" or "specular" reflection, does not occur randomly but follows a simple rule—the angle of reflection is equal to the angle of incidence and lies in the same plane. The angle of reflection and the angle of incidence are measured relative to a perpendicular to the surface at the point of impact. A plane or flat mirror reverses the direction of the light rays only and does not effect vergence, so no magnification or minification or image inversion occurs. Convex or concave reflective surfaces can change the vergence of light rays and focus them, resulting in alterations in the image produced. This has practical significance in that reflections from the ocular surfaces of corrective lenses can produce virtual images near the far point plane of the eye that can be annoying to the patient. These images can be eliminated by **tilting the lenses** slightly or by using an **antireflective coating** if necessary. Using the cornea as a reflective surface can also be employed in **keratometry** to measure the curvature of the cornea for contact lens fitting or for diagnosing keratoconus by comparing object and image sizes produced by an instrument referred to as a keratometer. The cornea is also employed as a reflecting surface when checking it for irregularity with a **keratoscope,** by examining for distortion the reflected images of a series of concentric circles. It is also worth noting that objects appear a particular color because they preferentially reflect wavelengths of that color and absorb the other wavelengths.

I. **Refraction of light.** When rays of light traveling through air enter a denser transparent medium, the speed of the light is reduced and the light rays proceed at a different angle, i.e., they are refracted. The one exception is when the rays are incident perpendicular to the surface, in which case the speed of the light is reduced but the direction of the light is unchanged.

1. **Snell's law of refraction** ($n \sin - n' \sin'$) indicates that the angle of incidence and the angle of refraction are related to the density of the medium for a specific wavelength. When light passes from a medium of low density to a medium of high density, Snell's law predicts that the light ray will be bent toward the normal, a line perpendicular to the surface at the point of impact (Fig. 13-1). In other words, the angle of refraction is less than the angle of incidence when going from a low-density to a high-density medium. Conversely, when light passes from a high-density to a low-density medium (such as out of a tank of water into air), the angle of refraction is greater than the angle of incidence. By bending the surface of a transparent medium that has a high density, such as the cornea or a piece of glass, the angle of incidence can be altered, and by employing Snell's law, the deviation of light rays by this altered surface can be predicted. All light rays from real objects diverge from one another; when these rays encounter a medium of high density, they can be made less divergent, parallel to one another, or convergent, depending on the shape of the refracting element or lens. By using simple formulas, the point at which the redirected rays come to a focus can be calculated quite easily.

2. **Measurement of lens power.** Lenses are measured in **diopters** (d). The power of a lens in diopters is the reciprocal of its focal length (f) in meters: $d = 1/f$. For example, a lens that focuses light from an object at infinity (parallel light rays or 0 vergence) at a plane 1 m beyond the lens is a 1-d lens (Fig. 13-2A). If it focuses the light at a plane 0.5 m beyond the lens, it is a 2-d lens: $2 = 1/0.5$ (Fig. 13-2B).

II. **Types of corrective lenses**

A. **Spherical lenses** have equal curvature in all meridians.

1. **Convex or plus lenses.** By convention, high-density optical surfaces that are convex are referred to as **plus lenses.** They refract light rays so as to make them more convergent (or less divergent). Plus lenses of the same power can be made in a variety of shapes, since it is the relationship of the two surfaces of a spectacle correcting lens that determines the power of the lens (Fig. 13-3A). A **meniscus form,** in which the front surface is more convex than the back surface is concave, results in the most desirable lens

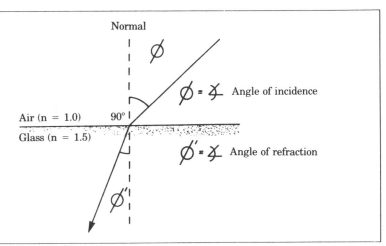

Fig. 13-1. Refraction of light is the change in direction in passage of light between media of different densities.

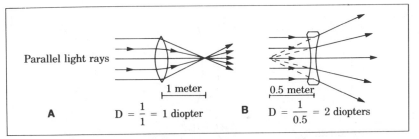

Fig. 13-2. Measurement of lens-focusing power in diopters by plus **(A)** and minus **(B)** lenses.

form for spectacles because there is less aberration over a wider area of the lens. Plus lenses are used for the correction of **hyperopia, presbyopia,** and **aphakia.** When a nearby object is viewed through a plus lens, the object looks larger. If the lens is moved slightly from side to side, the object appears to move in the direction **opposite** to the movement of the lens. Plus lenses can also be identified by their physical characteristics, as they are thicker in the middle and thinner at the edges.

2. **Concave or minus lenses.** High-density optical surfaces that are concave are referred to as **minus lenses.** They refract light rays so as to make them more divergent (or less convergent). As stated previously, it is the relationship of the two surfaces that determines the resultant power, and minus lenses can also be made in many forms (Fig. 13–3B). The most common design used in minus spectacle lenses is the **meniscus,** wherein the back or ocular surface is more concave than the front surface is convex. **Myodisc** lenses (biconcave) are used on patients who need very strong minus lenses. They have less peripheral distortion but a smaller focused central field than the meniscus lens. High-density glass or plastic (polycarbonate) lenses with a higher refractive index than crown glass may be used to reduce the thickness of high minus lenses or regular glass lenses. Minus lenses are used for the correction of **myopia.** When a nearby object is viewed through a minus

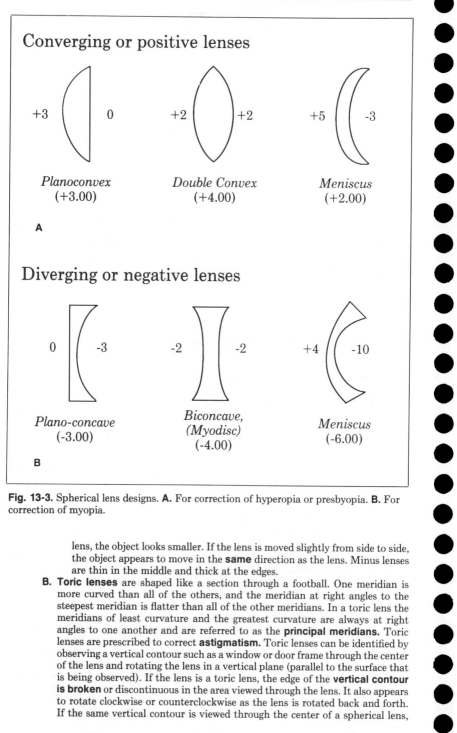

Fig. 13-3. Spherical lens designs. **A.** For correction of hyperopia or presbyopia. **B.** For correction of myopia.

lens, the object looks smaller. If the lens is moved slightly from side to side, the object appears to move in the **same** direction as the lens. Minus lenses are thin in the middle and thick at the edges.

B. **Toric lenses** are shaped like a section through a football. One meridian is more curved than all of the others, and the meridian at right angles to the steepest meridian is flatter than all of the other meridians. In a toric lens the meridians of least curvature and the greatest curvature are always at right angles to one another and are referred to as the **principal meridians.** Toric lenses are prescribed to correct **astigmatism.** Toric lenses can be identified by observing a vertical contour such as a window or door frame through the center of the lens and rotating the lens in a vertical plane (parallel to the surface that is being observed). If the lens is a toric lens, the edge of the **vertical contour is broken** or discontinuous in the area viewed through the lens. It also appears to rotate clockwise or counterclockwise as the lens is rotated back and forth. If the same vertical contour is viewed through the center of a spherical lens,

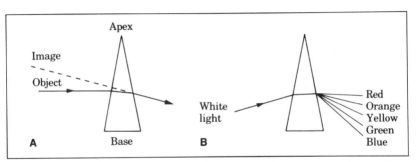

Fig. 13-4. Prism effects. **A.** Prismatic displacement of image for assistance in muscle balance problems. **B.** Chromatic aberration through varying degrees of refraction of lights of differing wavelength (color).

   it remains continuous when viewed within and outside the borders of the lens and does not appear to rotate when the lens is rotated. Toric lenses can be plus lenses, minus lenses, one principal meridian plus and the other minus, meniscus lenses, or they can be fabricated in a planocylinder form in which one principal meridian has zero optical power. Toric lenses are also referred to as **spherocylinders.**

C. **Prisms.** A prism is an optical device composed of two refracting surfaces that are inclined toward one another so they are not parallel. The line at which the two surfaces intersect is the apex of the prism. The greater the angle formed at the apex, the stronger the prismatic effect (Fig. 13-4A). Since the two surfaces of a prism are usually flat, they alter the direction of the light rays but not their vergence. An object viewed through a prism appears to be **displaced in the direction of the prism apex,** but the focus is not altered and no magnification or minification occurs. Prisms are usually prescribed to assist a patient with an **extraocular muscle imbalance,** which results in a deviation of one visual axis relative to the other, so that the patient may achieve single binocular vision or do so more comfortably. They may be oriented in the spectacle correction so as to produce horizontal, vertical, or both horizontal and vertical displacement, as needed. The strength of a prism is measured in **prism diopters,** each prism diopter displacing a ray of light 1 cm at a distance of 1 m. Two prism diopters of displacement are approximately equal to 1 degree of arc. See Chap. 11 for prescribing prisms.

D. **Lensometers** are precision instruments used to measure the spherical power, cylindrical (toxic) power and its axis (astigmatism correction), and prism power, if present, of a spectacle or contact lens.

   1. **Technique.** After the lens to be measured is placed on the lensometer stage, the **power wheel** is turned until the target mires are in focus. The mires cross each other at right angles, usually having three lines in one meridian and one or two in the other. If the mires all focus simultaneously at a given power, no cylinder is present and the lens is completely spherical. The power is read directly off the power wheel. The second wheel on the lensometer is an **axis wheel,** which can be rotated to turn the mires until they are lined up along the principal meridians of a lens containing a cylinder. Alignment is correct when the crossing lines are perfectly straight (not broken). The power wheel is then turned to focus the strongest plus power of the lens of the single or double line meridian focused at the greater plus power (or less minus power), and that power is recorded. The power wheel is turned again to bring the weaker (more minus) meridian into focus with the three line target and the power noted as well as the axis of that meridian, which is read directly from the axis wheel or on the reticule of the eyepiece. The lens prescription is the strongest plus power minus the **difference** in power

between the two settings, and the axis of the cylinder is that of the more minus meridian in the eyepiece reticule or indicated on the axis of the wheel.

2. **Example of *lensometer* calculations**
   a. Strongest plus meridian reading: +4.00
      Weaker plus meridian reading: +2.50
      Axis of weaker meridian: 80 degrees
      Final power: +4.00 − 1.50 × 80 degrees
   b. Strongest plus (weakest minus) meridian reading: −2.00
      Weaker plus (stronger minus) meridian reading: −3.00
      Axis of weaker plus meridian: 40 degrees
      Final power: −2.00 − 1.00 × 40 degrees

3. **Plus cylinder prescriptions** are less convenient and less frequently used but may be done by reversing the above technique, for example:
   Weakest plus meridian: +1.00
   Strongest plus meridian: +2.50
   Axis of strongest plus meridian: 50 degrees
   Final power: +1.00 + 1.50 × 50 degrees

4. **Conversion of minus cylinder prescriptions** to plus or the opposite is carried out by reversing the sign of the cylinder, adding the difference between the two lenses and 90 degrees to its axis, e.g., +3.00 −2.00 × 20 degrees converts to +1.00 + 2.00 × 110 degrees.

5. **Prism** power is measured by reading the amount of decentration of the cross mires directly from the number on the circle or lines on the eyepiece reticule, e.g., 1, 2, 2.5 base in if moved to the nasal side of the lens, base out if temporal.

III. **Refraction techniques.** *Refraction* is the term applied to the various testing procedures employed to measure the refractive errors of the eye in order to provide the proper correction. **Refractive error is by far the most common cause of poor vision.** Fortunately, it is generally the easiest to treat.

A. **Retinoscopy.** A retinoscope is a handheld instrument that the examiner uses to shine a light through the pupil to observe the reflex created by the light reflected from the retina. This is accomplished by using a mirror to reflect the light along the line connecting the examiner's and the patient's pupils and by creating a small aperture in the mirror that allows the examiner to view the patient's illuminated pupil. The light reflected from the patient's retina is refracted by the ocular media and focused at the far point of the patient's eye. By placing plus or minus lenses in front of the patient's eye, the patient's focal point can be altered until it is brought to the examiner's pupil, which produces a visible end point. This process involves moving the light back and forth across a series of lenses held in front of the patient's pupil, resulting in a linear light reflex moving in the same (hyperopia) or opposite direction (myopia) as the light. The filling of the entire pupil with light that does not move indicates neutralization of the refractive error in that meridian and is the end point reading for that meridian. In the case of astigmatism, the retinoscope linear light must be empirically lined up along a principal meridian (the clearest light streak as the retinoscope light is rotated) and plus or minus lenses put up until movement of light in that meridian is neutralized and the lens power recorded. This is repeated in the meridian 90 degrees away for the second lens and axis. By knowing how far the examiner is from the patient and what lenses are required, it is a simple matter to calculate the amount of ametropia. This technique is highly accurate and useful when used by a skilled retinoscopist, with a pupil of reasonable diameter and clear media. Opacities of the media, tiny pupils, poor fixation by the patient, or distortion of the light reflex can all be troublesome, however. Prescribing lenses on the basis of retinoscopic findings alone can too often result in a prescription that is not well tolerated by the patient.

B. **Subjective refraction** requires patient cooperation in obtaining the estimation of refractive error. Retinoscopy findings may be the starting guide or simply starting with a plus or minus 1- to 2-d lens before the patient's eye and asking if the visual acuity chart set at best uncorrected vision is better or worse. In the absence of astigmatism, the refraction is simply a matter of adding more plus or minus until the patient is at the best possible comfortable correction. In the presence of **astigmatism,** and to test for it, the **fogging technique** is very effective (see sec. **VI.B.3.e**). Both retinoscopic and subjective refractions involving astigmatism may be refined by the **Jackson cross-cylinder technique** (see sec. **VI.B.3.f.**).

C. **Automated refraction.** In recent years electronic microcircuitry and computer technology have combined to develop sophisticated instruments for refracting patients. Currently, these instruments cost between $5,000 and $25,000 and require a technician to operate them. The standard to which these instruments are compared is retinoscopy or subjective refraction or both. In general, automated refractometers are reasonably accurate. In order to provide reliable and valid data, however, the instrument must be properly in line with the patient's visual axis, accommodation must be relaxed, the pupil must be of satisfactory size, and the media must be sufficiently clear. There is no evidence that indicates that automated refraction is better than, and there is considerable controversy as to whether it is as good as, retinoscopy and subjective refraction. The primary role for these instruments at this time would appear to be increasing the efficiency with which eye care can be delivered by indicating the approximate refractive error, which should then be manually refined by the refractionist to give the patient most satisfactory vision. For example, an automated refractor may indicate a cylinder axis of 15 degrees, but the patient has been wearing one at axis 10 degrees without discomfort. It is wiser to give the axis 10 degrees with perhaps some sacrifice of visual clarity than axis 15 degrees, which is clear but feels "uncomfortable."

D. **Cycloplegic refraction.** Cycloplegia is the employment of pharmaceutic agents such as atropine, tropicamide, or cyclopentolate to paralyze the ciliary muscle temporarily in order to stabilize the refraction of the eye so that a definitive end point may be measured. It is useful in young patients with highly active accommodation to ensure complete relaxation of that accommodation so that all of the ametropia can be measured in young hyperopes, thereby avoiding overcorrection. **Methods of inducing cycloplegia** include 1% cyclopentolate or tropicamide, 1 drop q5min for 2 or 3 applications in the office just before refraction, or atropine 1%, 1 drop tid for 3 days prior to the refraction.

IV. **Aberrations.** Optical systems generally contain imperfections referred to as *aberrations.* The important aberrations in the visual system and spectacle lenses are chromatic aberration, spherical aberration, radial astigmatism, and distortion.

A. **Chromatic aberration.** The index of refraction for any transparent medium varies with the wavelength of the incident light. This variation is such that blue light is refracted more than red light (Fig. 13-4B). This accounts for the chromatic dispersion that occurs when white light is passed through a prism and a rainbow effect is produced. In a convex or plus lens, blue light is focused slightly closer to the lens than red light. The same is true of the human eye, in which blue light is focused slightly in front of red light.

B. **Spherical aberration.** In most discussions of optics, certain assumptions are made for the sake of simplicity. Higher order optics become quite complex and contribute little to the understanding of the visual system or to measuring and prescribing for refractive errors. So far it has been assumed that all light rays from an object that pass through a lens come to focus at a single image point. A closer analysis reveals that this is true only for light rays that are paraxial, i.e., that pass through the center of the lens. Those light rays that are parallel to the axis but that pass through the periphery of the lens are usually refracted more than the paraxial rays (Fig. 13-5A). Every object point on the axis of the lens will then be represented by a blur circle rather than a point focus. The size of this blur circle can be reduced by restricting the passage of light through the lens to the central portion, as is done when an object is viewed through a pinhole aperture. This same effect accounts for the increased depth of focus

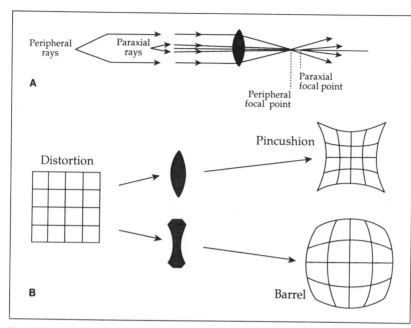

Fig. 13-5. A. Spherical aberration induced by varying degrees of light refraction from center of lens to edge. **B.** Distortion resulting from differential magnification of light between central and more peripheral focusing of rays.

obtained when the iris diaphragm of a camera is reduced in size or when the pupil of the eye is constricted.

C. **Radial astigmatism** occurs when light rays pass through a lens obliquely. Instead of focusing a point of light as a point image, two linear images form at right angles to one another with a "circle of least confusion" between them. This form of aberration is of no great significance in the eye; however, it can create considerable blurring of the image formed by spectacle lenses.

D. **Distortion** is the result of differential magnification in an optical system. This occurs because light from some parts of the object are focused by the central portion of the lens while other parts are focused by peripheral portions of the lens (Fig. 13–5B). In other words, the shape of the image formed does not correspond exactly to the shape of the object. For practical purposes, this is not a problem in the eye, but it can be troublesome in higher powered spectacle lenses. High plus lenses produce "pincushion" distortion, and high minus lenses result in "barrel" distortion.

V. **The eye as an optical instrument.** The analogy of the eye and the camera is a useful one. The focusing elements of the eye are the cornea and the crystalline lens, and the "film" is the retina. To simplify discussions of the eye as an optical instrument, we use some approximations and resort to the schematic or reduced eye, wherein all light rays are assumed to be paraxial and all elements perfectly aligned on the visual axis.

A. **The cornea** contributes approximately two-thirds of the refracting power of the eye. This is true because more deflection of light rays occurs at the air-cornea interface, due to the large difference in index of refraction between these two media. The crystalline lens is in fact a more powerful lens in air since it is biconvex and each of its surfaces is more convex than the cornea. The lens, however, is in the aqueous-vitreous medium, and the difference in refractive index at the aqueous-lens and lens-vitreous interfaces is much less. The cornea has an index of refraction of 1.376 and contributes **+43 d** to the eye.

B. **The crystalline lens** has an index of refraction that increases from the cortex to the nucleus but averages 1.41 with a power of **+20 d.** Since these two lens elements are separated, the **total power of the eye** is not their sum but the equivalent power of **+58.7 d.**

C. **The pupil** is also a significant component of the eye's optical system, reducing the amount of light that enters the eye and aberrations and increasing the depth of focus when it constricts. This accounts for the ability of many people who require reading glasses to get along without them when the illumination is good.

D. **The retina** is a unique kind of film. It contains the "coarse grain" but highly sensitive rods for registering images at very low levels of illumination and the "fine grain" color-sensitive cones for high resolution and discrimination at high levels of illumination. Only one or two quanta of light energy are required to activate the rods. On the other hand, rapid neural adaptation and the more gradual process of adjusting the steady state between bleaching and regeneration of retinal visual pigments enable the retina to function perfectly at extremely high levels of illumination. What other film functions so well both in moonlight and at high noon? The manner in which visual images are formed, transmitted to the visual cortex, and interpreted is a fascinating story but not appropriate to this discussion.

VI. **Refractive errors of the eye**

A. **Emmetropia.** The eye is considered to be emmetropic if parallel light rays, from an object more than 6 m away, are focused at the plane of the retina when the eye is in a completely relaxed state. An emmetropic eye will have a clear image of a distant object without any internal adjustment of its optics (Fig. 13-6). While most emmetropic rays are approximately 24 mm in length, a larger eye can be emmetropic if its optical components are weaker, and a smaller eye can be emmetropic if its optical components are stronger.

B. **Ametropias**

1. **Hyperopia.** When the focused image is formed behind the plane of the retina in ametropia, the eye is "too short" and is considered hyperopic. This is also referred to as *farsightedness.* Near images are usually blurred unless there is sufficient accommodation, as in a child. Unless the optical system of the eye is actively altered to produce an increase in its power, hyperopic eyes will eventually have blurred images for distant objects also, as any elderly hyperope will confirm. Most children are born about +3 d hyperopic, but this usually resolves by age 12.

a. **Structural hyperopia** is based on the anatomic configuration of the eye.

(1) In **axial hyperopia,** the eye is shorter than normal in its anteroposterior diameter, although the refracting portions (e.g., lens, cornea) are normal. These eyes are more prone to develop **angle-closure glaucoma** because of the shorter anterior segment with crowding of the filtration angle. The optic nerves are also smaller and more densely packed, as they are crowded at the disk. Physiologic cupping is uncommon, and **pseudopapilledema** may be noted. The latter is characterized as seen in eyes with greater than +4 d of hyperopia, a normal blind spot on field testing, no venous congestion, and a disk that seems "swollen."

(2) **Curvature hyperopia** results when either the crystalline lens or the cornea has a weaker than normal curvature and consequently lower refractive power.

(3) **Index of refraction hyperopia** is the result of decreased index of refraction due to decreased density in some or several parts of the optic system of the eye, thus lowering the refractive power of the eye.

b. **Accommodation in hyperopia** is of greater importance than the structural factors leading to it because accommodation is a key dynamic

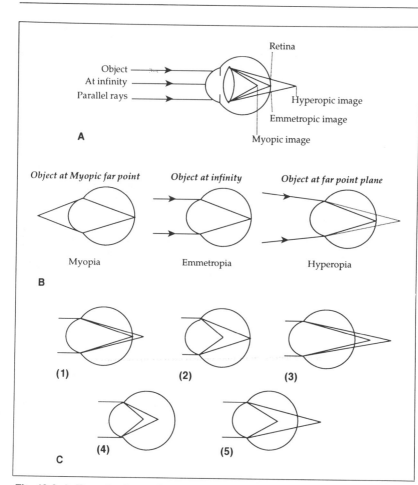

Fig. 13-6. A. Far point (image distance focused on retina in accommodatively relaxed eye) in myopia, emmetropia, and hyperopia. **B.** Focal points of myopic, emmetropic, and hyperopic eye with reference to the retinal plane. **C.** Focal points of astigmatic principal meridians (objects at infinity). **(1)** Simple hyperopic astigmatism: emmetropia/hyperopia. **(2)** Simple myopic astigmatism: emmetropia/myopia. **(3)** Compound hyperopic astigmatism: hyperopia/hyperopia. **(4)** Compound myopic astigmatism: myopia/myopia. **(5)** Mixed astigmatism: hyperopia/myopia.

factor in correcting at least part of the refractive error. It is defined as latent, manifest facultative, and manifest absolute hyperopia.

(1) **Latent hyperopia** is that part of the refractive error completely corrected by accommodation. It is measurable not by manifest refraction but only with paralysis of accommodation via cycloplegic refraction. Latent hyperopia is the difference in measurement between manifest hyperopia and the results of the cycloplegic refraction, which reveals total hyperopia, latent and manifest.

(2) **Manifest facultative hyperopia** is that portion of hyperopia that may be corrected by the patient's own powers of accommodation, by corrective lenses, or both. Vision is normal with or without cor-

rective plus lenses, but accommodation is not relaxed without the glasses.

   (3) Manifest absolute hyperopia is that part of the refractive error that cannot be compensated for by the patient's accommodation. Distance vision is still blurred no matter how much accommodative power the patient puts in. These patients readily accept the aid of plus lenses.

  c. The effect of aging on hyperopia results from progressive loss of accommodative power, thus moving the eye from latent and facultative hyperopia to greater degrees of absolute hyperopia.

  d. Symptoms of hyperopia

   (1) Frontal headaches worsening as the day progresses and aggravated by prolonged use of near vision.

   (2) "Uncomfortable" vision (asthenopia) when the patient must focus at a fixed distance for prolonged periods, e.g., a televised baseball game. Accommodation tires more quickly when held in a fixed level of tension.

   (3) Blurred distance vision with refractive errors greater than 3–4 d or in older patients with decreasing amplitude of accommodation.

   (4) Near visual acuity blurs at a younger age than in the emmetrope, e.g., in the late 30s. This is aggravated when the patient is tired, printing indistinct, or lighting conditions suboptimal.

   (5) Light sensitivity is common in hyperopes, is of unknown etiology, and is relieved by correcting the hyperopia without needing to tint the lenses.

   (6) Intermittent sudden blurring of vision is due to **spasm of accommodation** (SOA) and induces a pseudomyopia. Vision clears with minus lenses. SOA may be detected by cycloplegic refraction, which will reveal the underlying hyperopia.

   (7) "Crossed-eyes" sensation without diplopia is also due to excessive accommodation in a patient with an esophoria that is being pushed by the accommodation-convergence reflex into a symptom-producing state that "the eyes are crossing."

  e. Treatment of hyperopia is usually most satisfactory when slightly less power (1d) than the total of facultative and absolute hyperopia is given in a patient with no extraocular muscle imbalance. If there is accommodative esotropia (convergence), the full correction should be given. In exophoria, the hyperopia should be undercorrected by 1 to 2 d (see Chap. 11). If the total manifest refractive error is small, e.g., 1 d or less, correction is given only if the patient is symptomatic.

2. Myopia. When the focused image is formed in front of the plane of the retina in ametropia, the eye is "too long" and is considered myopic. This is referred to as *nearsightedness,* since there is a point less than 6 m in front of the eye that will be coincident with the retina when the optical system of the eye is relaxed. The term *nearsighted* has relevance; the term *farsighted* does not.

  a. Types of myopia

   (1) In **axial myopia,** the anteroposterior diameter of the eye is longer than normal although the corneal and lens curvatures are normal and the lens is in the normal anatomic position. In this form of myopia may be found pseudoproptosis due to the abnormally large anterior segment, peripapillary myopic crescent from an exaggerated scleral ring, and a posterior staphyloma.

   (2) In **curvature myopia** the eye has a normal anteroposterior diameter, but the curvature of the cornea is steeper than average, e.g., congenitally or in keratoconus, or the lens curvature is increased as in moderate to severe hyperglycemia, which causes lens intumescence.

(3) **Increased index of refraction** in the lens due to onset of early to moderate nuclear sclerotic cataracts is a common cause of myopia in the elderly. The sclerotic change increases the index of refraction, thus making the eye myopic. Many people find themselves ultimately able to read without glasses or having gained "second sight." They may usually be given normal distance vision for years simply by increasing the minus power in their corrective lenses, thus avoiding unnecessary surgery.

(4) **Anterior movement of the lens** is often seen after glaucoma surgery and will increase the myopic error in the eye.

b. **Clinical course.** Myopia is rarely present at birth but often begins to develop as the child grows. It is usually detected by age 9 or 10 in the school vision tests and will increase during the years of growth until stabilizing around the mid-teens, usually at about 5 d.

(1) **Progressive myopia** is a rare form of myopia that increases by as much as 4 d yearly and is associated with vitreous floaters and liquefaction and chorioretinal changes. The refractive changes usually stabilize at about age 20 but occasionally may progress until the mid-30s and frequently results in degrees of myopia of 10–20 d.

(2) **Congenital high myopia** is usually a refractive error of −10 d or greater and is detected in infants who seem to be unaware of a visual world beyond their immediate surroundings but who, fortunately, usually develop normal vision focusing on small objects held an inch or two from their eyes. This myopia is not generally progressive but should be corrected as soon as discovered to help the child develop normal distance vision and perception of the world.

c. **Symptoms of myopia**

(1) **Blurred distance vision**

(2) **Squinting** to sharpen distance vision by attempting a pinhole effect through narrowing of the palpebral fissures.

(3) **Headaches** are rare but may be seen in patients with uncorrected low myopic errors.

d. **Treatment of myopia**

(1) **Children** should be fully corrected and, if under 8 years of age, instructed to wear their glasses constantly both to avoid developing the habit of squinting and to enhance developing a normal accommodation-convergence reflex (see sec. **5**). If the refractive error is low, the child may wear the glasses intermittently as needed, e.g., at school.

(2) **Adults** under the age of 30 are usually comfortable with their full myopic correction. Patients over 30 may not be able to tolerate a full correction over 3 d if they have never worn glasses before and may need a weaker than full correction with resulting undercorrected distance vision but clear reading vision. The patient should be told that full correction may be given in the future if desired. Wearing full correction in a trial frame for about 30 minutes both reading and looking at distance in the waiting room may answer the question of whether to give full correction.

(3) **Undercorrection of myopia** in childhood may result in an adult who has never developed a normal amount of accommodation for near focus. This person will be uncomfortable in full correction and complain that the glasses are too strong and "pull" his or her eyes.

3. **Astigmatism.** The optical systems thus far discussed are spherical, that is, all the meridians of the lenses are of equal curvature, resulting in a surface that resembles a section through a spheroid. Many optical systems, however, are toric surfaces, in which the curvature varies in different meridians, thus refracting light unequally in those meridians and creating the condition known as astigmatism (see sec. **II.B**). Light rays passing through a steep meridian are thus deflected more than those passing through a flatter me-

ridian. This results in the formation of a more complicated image, referred to as the "conoid of Sturm," wherein a point source of light is represented by an image consisting of two lines that are at right angles to one another with a circle of least confusion in a plane midway between them (Fig. 13-7). The steepest and flattest meridians of the eye are usually at right angles to one another, resulting in regular astigmatism. This is fortunate, since technology makes it possible to generate regular astigmatic surfaces in ophthalmic lenses easily so that astigmatism can be corrected economically.

a. **Types of astigmatism**
   (1) **Corneal toricity** accounts for most of the astigmatism of the eye. If the **vertical meridian is steeper** it is referred to as astigmatism **"with the rule,"** and if the **horizontal meridian is steeper** it is referred to as astigmatism **"against the rule."** One meridian may be emmetropic and the other hyperopic or myopic, both may be hyperopic or myopic, or one may be hyperopic and the other myopic. In spherical ametropia only one number is necessary to designate the power of the corrective lens, but in astigmatic corrections three numbers are required to indicate the power needed in each principal meridian plus the axis to provide the correct orientation of the lens in front of the eye (e.g., $+2.00 - 1.00 \times 180$ is a corrective lens prescription for "with the rule" astigmatism).
   (2) **Regular astigmatism** has principal meridians 90 degrees apart and **oblique astigmatism** has them more than 20 degrees from the horizontal or vertical meridians.
   (3) **Irregular astigmatism** is due to an unevenness of the corneal surface such as in corneal scarring or keratoconus. The principal meridians are not 90 degrees and are so irregular that they cannot be completely corrected with ordinary toric lenses (cylinders). The **diagnosis** can be made by shining a light into the eye and observing any irregularity of the pupillary reflex with the ophthalmoscope or retinoscope, by the use of a keratometer that measures the corneal curvature, by examination with a slit lamp, or by observing the corneal reflex with either a keratoscope or **Placido's disk,** both of which contain concentric circles that are reflected by the surface of the cornea and that appear distorted in cases of irregular corneal astigmatism. Irregular astigmatism cannot be corrected with spectacle lenses but can frequently be corrected by contact lenses.
   (4) **Symmetric astigmatism** has principal meridians in each eye with similar but opposite axes, e.g., 20 degrees OD and 160 degrees OS, which together add up to 180 degrees (± 15 degrees).

b. **Symptoms of higher astigmatism** (> 1.00 d) include
   (1) **Blurred vision.**
   (2) **Tilting** of the head for oblique astigmatism.
   (3) **Turning** of the head (rare).
   (4) **Squinting** to achieve "pinhole" vision clarity.
   (5) **Reading** material held **close to eyes** to achieve large (as in myopia) but blurred retinal image.

c. **Symptoms of lower astigmatism** (< 1.00 d) include
   (1) **Asthenopia** ("tired eyes") especially when doing precise work at a fixed distance. With-the-rule astigmatism produces more symptoms but clearer vision than the same amount of against-the-rule astigmatism.
   (2) **Transient blurred vision** relieved by closing or rubbing the eyes (as in hyperopia) when doing precise work at a fixed distance.
   (3) **Frontal headaches** with long periods of visual concentration on a task.

d. **Treating astigmatism** depends on the patient's visual needs and symptoms as noted above in terms of whether glasses are worn constantly or intermittently. It is not within the scope of this book to discuss in detail

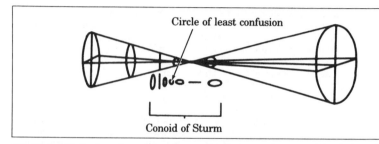

Fig. 13-7. Effect of regular astigmatism on focal planes of eye, resulting in least blur (conoid of Sturm).

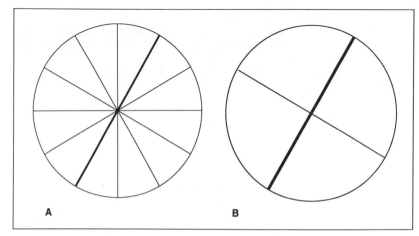

Fig. 13-8. A. Clock dial as seen by "fogged" patient with astigmatic error; 1–7 axis appears darker. **B.** Two-line rotating dial is set at 1–7 position. Axis of correcting **minus** cylinder is 30 degrees (1 × 30). Minus cylinders are placed at 120 degrees (30 degrees + 90 degrees) until all lines appear equal, thus indicating cylinder power and axis needed to correct astigmatic error. Patient is then "defogged."

the many methods of measuring astigmatism for corrective lenses such as plus cylinders, Lancaster-Regan charts, or crossed cylinders, but the fogging technique followed by refinement with the Jackson cross-cylinder is a common method for **measuring regular astigmatic correction** using the clock dial and minus cylinders.

e. **Fogging technique.** Make the patient **artificially myopic (fogged)** to about 20/50 by putting enough plus sphere before the eye to pull all meridians anterior to the retina, e.g., to bring forward compound hyperopic, simple, or mixed astigmatism meridians where both (the former) or one (the latter two) focal plane is posterior to the retina (Fig. 13-8). By making all meridians myopic, the refractionist **inhibits accommodation,** thus stabilizing the error of the eye, and may use minus cylinders to determine the principal meridians.

(1) Have the patient **identify** the **darkest, most distinct line** on the spokes of the astigmatic dial clock, e.g., the 1 to 7 o'clock line, and multiply the lower number by 30 degrees to get the axis of the correcting cylinder.

(2) Switch to a two-line rotating chart with one line oriented along one principal meridian, e.g., 1–7 o'clock. As these lines cross perpendicularly, the other line will be on the opposite principal meridian.

(3) Place **increasing strength minus cylinders** before the eye at an axis 90 degrees from the blackest line, e.g., 4–10 o'clock or 120 degrees (30 + 90 degrees). Add one −0.25- to 0.50-d cylinder at a time until both lines are equal in darkness and distinctness. They will still be blurred. For each −0.50 d of cylinder added after the original −0.75 cylinder is in, add +0.25 sphere to keep the patient artificially myopic.

(4) Switch to a **distance vision chart** and reduce plus spheres until patient achieves maximum clarity of vision.

(5) Example
(a) +2.00 fogs to 20/50.
(b) 4–10 line is darkest.
(c) 4 × 30 degrees = 120 degrees (axis of correcting cylinder).
(d) −1.00 × 30 degrees evens out darkness of the two-line chart.
(e) Reducing plus lenses to +0.25 gives sharpest vision on distant reading chart.
(f) Final prescription: +0.25 − 1.00 × 120.

(6) If axis falls between hours on the clock, multiply by the lowest number plus half, i.e., between 1 and 2 o'clock = 1.5 × 30 degrees = 45 degrees is correcting cylinder.

(7) Refine the final prescription by using the Jackson cross-cylinder. If the final cylinder correction is greater than 3 d and the patient has never worn glasses before, giving one-half to two-thirds of the correction may be prudent to avoid intolerance and discomfort from an initial full correction.

f. The Jackson cross-cylinder (JCC) is a lens of equal-power plus (white dot) and minus (red dot) plano cylinders with axes 90 degrees apart. Lens powers range from ±0.12 to ±1.00 cyl. To test if the patient's **lens axis is correct,** place the JCC before the eye with its handle parallel to the axis of the cylinder in the trial frame. Rotate the handle of the JCC in one direction and then turn it over to the other side, thus changing the combined cylinder axes. Turn the trial frame axis in the direction toward the JCC axis that gives better vision on the distance chart and repeat the test. The end point is when rotating the JCC handle over makes no change in vision. To ascertain if the **cylinder strength is correct,** place the JCC with its handle at 45 degrees with the axis of the trial frame cylinder such that one axis of the JCC will be parallel to and the other 90 degrees from the trial frame cylinder. If vision is better when similar axes are parallel, e.g., minus over minus, the trial frame cylinder needs to be made stronger and vice versa. If rotating the JCC before the trial frame is equally bad in both directions, the cylinder is correct.

4. Anisometropia is a state in which there is a difference in the refractive errors of the two eyes, i.e., one eye is myopic and the other hyperopic or both hyperopic or myopic but to different degrees. This condition may be congenital or acquired due to asymmetric age changes or disease.

a. In anisometropia, the patient may be made visually uncomfortable by
(1) Visual acuity differences between the two eyes.
(2) Aniseikonia: difference in size of the ocular image in each eye (possibly causing retinal rivalry).
(3) Anisophoria: varying heterophoria (muscle imbalance) in different fields of gaze depending on the eye used for fixation.
(4) Suppression scotoma, amblyopia, or **strabismus,** which may develop in young anisometropes. This may be mitigated by the proper refractive correction or even aggravated by the spectacle correction

Table 13-1. Amplitude of accommodation (diopters)*

Age (years)	Duane Monocular Near Point		Donders Binocular Near Point
	Average	Range	Average
10	13	11–16	14
20	11	9–13	10
30	9	7–11	7
40	6	3–8	5
50	2	1–3	3
60	1	1–2	1

* Rounded off to nearest whole diopter.

by inducing obstacles to fusion such as anisophoria and aniseikonia or anisophoria.

b. Treatment

(1) In **children,** both eyes should receive the best visual correction and any muscle imbalance identified and corrected with prisms or surgically.

(2) **Adults** should receive the best correction that will not result in ocular discomfort. Usually the more ametropic (poorer) eye is undercorrected.

5. Accommodation. The cornea is a static or fixed surface. The crystalline lens, however, is capable of increasing its plus power. This is referred to as *focusing,* or *accommodation.* The lens is suspended in the eye by thousands of chemical strands, called *zonules,* that are attached to the ciliary body at one end and the lens capsule at the opposite end. When the ciliary muscle is relaxed, the zonules maintain a slight tension on the capsule. Since the ciliary muscle is a circular sphincterlike muscle, constriction results in a slight decrease in the diameter of the circle. This reduces the tension of the zonules on the lens capsule, which is elastic, and squeezes the lens fibers in such a way that the anterior pole, and to a lesser extent the posterior pole, becomes more convex, thereby increasing the power of the lens. This change in power is called *accommodation.* An emmetrope who wants to view a nearby object contracts the ciliary muscle, which results in an increase of power or accommodation to focus the image back to the plane of the retina (see also Chaps. 6 and 8).

a. Amplitude of accommodation is the range of plus power the lens can produce. This varies with age and is a critical factor in the correction of hyperopia and presbyopia. Table 13-1 indicates a few of the Duane monocular and Donders binocular near point averages of accommodative power at various ages. It is useful to memorize at least the low, middle, and high range figures.

b. The **near point** or **punctum proximum (PP)** is the nearest point at which a person can see clearly. In the unaided (no glasses) emmetropic eye, the PP and retina are in conjugate foci, and the amplitude of accommodation may be measured directly using this distance as it is unaltered by a refractive error. For example, a 20-year-old emmetrope is able to focus clearly at 10 cm, thus indicating a total accommodative power of 10 d by the formula d = focal length (cm). If this patient were a 2-d myope, his total focal length would be 8.3 cm due to his 12-d focal point (10 d accommodation plus 2 d myopic error). A 2-d hyperope would focus at 12.5 cm (10 d accommodation minus 2 d hyperope error =8 d focal length).

    c. The **far point** or **punctum remotum (PR)** is the farthest point at which a patient can see clearly. In emmetropia, the retina is focused at (conjugate with) infinity. In myopia, the focal point is anterior to the retina; in hyperopia, it is behind the retina, i.e., beyond infinity.

    d. **Determining the amplitude of accommodation** may be done by several methods: minus sphere test, Lebensohn target, cycloplegic testing. The simplest method is the **push up method** where, with a distance correction before the eyes (if needed), a fine-print target is gradually moved toward the patient's eyes until the patient notes onset of blurred vision. This test is done monocularly in each eye in the young because of possible extraocular muscle balance effect on the blur distance. The distance at which the blur begins is converted to diopters of accommodative power (d = focal distance [cm]).

    e. **Symptoms of decreased accommodative powers** are presbyopia (see sec. **6**) in patients over 40 and inability to read or do close work for prolonged periods of time because of blurring of vision and "tiring" of the eyes. Intermittent diplopia at near may develop due to the interrelationship between accommodation and convergence. All symptoms are aggravated by fatigue, illness, fever, or other debilitating conditions and may clear completely as the patient recovers and accommodative powers recompensate.

6. Presbyopia is a physiologic decrease in the amplitude of accommodation associated with aging. With time, changes occur in the crystalloids of the lens that result in a decreased elasticity of the lens fibers or a hardening of the lens. When the eye attempts to accommodate, there is less of a change in the curvature of the lens for each unit of contraction. By the early forties, accommodative amplitude has usually decreased to less than 5 d, and objects less than 20 cm away cannot be brought into focus.

    a. **Symptoms of presbyopia** develop when the amount of accommodation needed to focus at near **exceeds more than half of the total amplitude of the eye.** A 48-year-old emmetropic patient with only 5 d of accommodative amplitude will experience presbyopic symptoms when attempting to read at 33 cm (about 14 inches), as he is using 3 d (60%) of his total 5 d to focus. An uncorrected hyperope and a chronically undercorrected myope who, as a result of the undercorrection, never developed full accommodative powers will both develop presbyopic symptoms earlier than an emmetropic patient. The hyperope must use excess accommodation to overcome the hyperopia, thus reducing the available reserve for the early presbyopia. Symptoms of presbyopia include

    (1) Longer reading distance required.
    (2) Inability to focus on close work.
    (3) Excessive illumination required for close work.
    (4) Greater difficulty with close work **as the day goes on.**

    b. **Testing for presbyopia** is done monocularly and binocularly. The latter often indicates a weaker correction; this is the more comfortable one to give. The patient holds a reading card at the distance desired for work, e.g., typing or closer reading, and the weakest additional plus sphere that will give the patient clear small newsprint or footnote vision is determined. Cards commonly used are the **Snellen, Jaeger,** or **Rosenbaum.** The vision obtained should be recorded for future reference. Visual efficiency may also be calculated based on the best corrected near vision, e.g., J-2 is 95% efficient (Table 13-2).

    c. **Correcting presbyopia** is done through supplementing accommodation with plus lenses that do part of the focusing for the eye. The difference between the distance correction and the strength needed for clear near vision is called the **add.** An effective physiologic rule for prescribing the near correction is to give the add that will leave half the amplitude of accommodation in reserve.

Table 13-2. Equivalent visual acuity notations for near

Visual Angle (minutes)	Snellen Equivalent	A.M.A. Notation	Decimal Notation	Jaeger Notation[a]	Meter Notation (m)[b]	Central Visual Efficiency for Near (%)[c]
5.00	20/20	14/14	1.00	J1	0.37	100
6.25	20/25	14/17	0.80	J1−	0.43	100
7.50	20/30	14/21	0.66	J2	0.50	95
10.00	20/40	14/28	0.50	J4	0.75	90
12.50	20/50	14/35	0.40	J6	0.87	50
15.00	20/60	14/42	0.33	J8	1.00	40
20.00	20/80	14/56	0.25	J10	1.50	20
25.00	20/100	14/70	0.20	J11	1.75	15
50.00	20/200	14/140	0.10	J17	3.50	2

[a] Type sizes used in successive editions of Jaeger test cards have not been constant. They were not duplicated in the early Vienna editions of 1857, 1860, and 1865, and the New York series of 1868 showed still further variations. The size of Jaeger letters used here is taken from N.M. Black, N.S. Gradle, J. Patterson, and A.C. Snell, Report of the Committee for Eye Injuries. *Trans. Sec. Ophthalmol.*, *A.M.A.* 1927, p. 370; 1932, p. 365; 1933, pp. 311–313. It is also recognized that it is usually easier to read words printed in Jaeger type than individual Snellen letters of the same size. For this reason, a direct comparison between Jaeger and Snellen acuity cannot be made accurately. Nevertheless, in regard to angular size of letters this table is adequate for clinical purposes.

[b] The m stands for meter. The reading cards originally designed by Snellen (1862) presented type sizes subtending an angle of 5° at the given metric distances. D has been used on some cards instead of m. It was intended to mean *distance in meters* but has sometimes been erroneously interpreted as *diopter*.

[c] These figures were revised and subsequently approved and accepted by the Executive Committee of the Section on Ophthalmology of the A.M.A., June, 1955. It should be noted that these revised figures weigh near visual acuity disability more heavily than the 1940 A.M.A. table (Special reports. Estimation of loss of visual efficiency. *A.M.A. Arch. Ophthalmol.* 54:462, 1955).

Source: Bureau of Visual Science, American Optical Corporation, *The AO Nearpoint Rotochart Manual*, 1956.

(1) The average eyeglass adds for various age levels
- **(a)** 45 years: + 1.00 d to + 1.25 d.
- **(b)** 50 years: + 1.50 d to + 1.75 d.
- **(c)** 55 years: + 2.00 d to + 2.25 d.
- **(d)** 60 years: + 2.50 d to + 3.00 d.

(2) Adjustments for work distance. The strength of the adds must be adjusted up or down depending on whether the patient wants a longer or shorter working distance. For a patient in his or her late 40s with only 3 d total amplitude left, the following adds give varying work distance and leave a comfortable (50%) amount of accommodation in reserve. (See Table 13-3 for range of adds, working distances, and amplitude reserve).
- **(a)** +2.50 : 10 inches.
- **(b)** +1.50 : 13 inches.
- **(c)** +1.00 : 16 inches.
- **(d)** +0.50 : 20 inches.

7. **Aphakia.** If the crystalline lens becomes sufficiently opaque to interfere with vision, it must be removed by **cataract surgery** so that light may reach the retina. Removal of the lens produces a condition referred to as *aphakia* and results in an eye with one of its major optical elements missing. The eye in this state is extremely farsighted and lacks any accommodation.

   a. **Correction of aphakia** is accomplished by prescribing strong plus (convex) lenses. Unfortunately, removing the crystalline lens from within the eye and replacing it with a spectacle lens positioned in front of the eye results in considerable **magnification of the retinal image,** usually 25–30%. The aphake is required to make a considerable adaptation to the visual environment because the larger image of a familiar object is interpreted as indicating that the object is much closer than it really is. In the case of **monocular aphakia** the difference in the size of the aphakic and phakic images precludes combining them in the visual cortex to achieve single binocular vision and results in double vision due to the different image sizes. In addition, strong plus lenses result in a significant increase in lens aberrations that can be very annoying and can limit visual efficiency. It is for these reasons that aphakic contact lenses and even more frequently secondary intraocular lenses are being placed in eyes that did not receive them as part of the primary procedure (see Chap. 6).

   b. **Refraction technique in aphakia** may be by retinoscopy (see sec. III.A.) or by a simple **subjective test** as follows:

   (1) Check potential visual acuity on the distance chart with the pinhole test before starting. If no maculopathy or keratopathy is present, the refractionist should be able to achieve approximately the same vision with lenses as by pinhole.

   (2) Place a +12 d before the eye (trial frame or phoropter), making sure the patient's visual axis passes perpendicularly through the plane of the correcting lenses. If the patient preoperatively was a high hyperope, a +14 to +16 d might be a better starting lens; if a high myope, use a +8 to +10 d to start.

   (3) Place a − 2d cylinder in front of the plus lens and rotate the cylinder slowly until the axis that gives the patient the clearest vision on the distance chart is reached. If no letters are visible, increase or decrease the plus lens power until some letters are seen, and rotate the cylinder again until they are at their clearest.

   (4) Increase or decrease the amount of cylinder at the clearest axis found until the patient again feels the vision is clearest.

   (5) Increase or decrease the amount of plus sphere, keeping 90% of the plus power closest to the eye, i.e., rear cell of the trial frame, until vision is best.

Table 13-3. Necessary add for near-point distances*

Total Amplitude of Accommodation	Amplitude of Accommodation in Reserve	Add for 10 in. (4.00 D)	Add for 13 in. (3.00 D)	Add for 16 in. (2.50 D)	Add for 20 in. (2.00 D)	Add for 26 in. (1.50 D)
6.00	3.00	1.00	—	—	—	—
5.00	2.50	1.50	0.50	—	—	—
4.00	2.00	2.00	1.00	0.50	—	—
3.00	1.50	2.50	1.50	1.00	0.50	—
2.00	1.00	3.00	2.00	1.50	1.00	0.50
1.00	0.50	3.50	2.50	2.00	1.50	1.00
0.50	0.25	3.75	2.75	2.25	1.75	1.25

* Figures in diopters (D).
Source: Garcia, G. *Handbook of Refraction* (4th ed.). Boston: Little, Brown, 1989. P. 81. With permission.

(6) Refinement of plus and cylinders may be done with a Jackson cross-cylinder (see sec. **VI.B.3**).

(7) Note the prescription and the vertex distance (distance between most posterior plus lens and cornea in mm) and record both. Vertex distance will be used to calculate the final spherical lens strength by the optician.

c. Aphakic contact lenses and monocular aphakia correction. One alternative to the spectacle correction of aphakia is the use of **contact lenses.** By placing the lens element on the surface of the cornea, which is closer to the original site of the crystalline lens, magnification is reduced to between 5 and 10%, and this is usually compatible with fusion of the images in the visual cortex in the monocular aphakic. This results in less alteration of the visual environment by magnification and also eliminates most of the aberrations of aphakic spectacles, since the lenses can be made much thinner and much smaller. Peripheral vision is also restored.

d. Intraocular lenses (IOLs) are now by far the most common means of correcting surgical aphakia with approximately 95% of all cataract surgery today including their implantation. A well-placed IOL has the visual advantages of the original crystalline lens but, as with any surgical device, may also cause complications. These are seen far less frequently now with improved lens design and materials. IOLs are discussed further in Chap. 6.

VII. Glasses in correction of ametropia. Most forms of ametropia can be corrected by spectacles. Plus (convex) lenses are used to correct hyperopia, presbyopia, and aphakia. Minus (concave) lenses are used to correct myopia. Toric lenses are employed for the correction of regular astigmatism. Most corrective lenses are made in meniscus form to reduce aberrations and to provide a better cosmetic effect.

A. Safety factors. Lenses are generally made impact resistant; that is, they must withstand the impact of a 1.5-cm steel ball dropped from a height of 127 cm. Industrial safety glasses must withstand a greater impact and are tested with a 2.9-cm steel ball dropped from a height of 127 cm. Glass lenses are generally made of crown glass with an index of refraction of 1.523, with a minimum thickness of 2 mm, and they are heat treated or chemically altered to make them shatterproof. Plastic lenses are naturally shatterproof and lighter in weight but tend to scratch more easily. Because most plastic resins have a density less than that of crown glass, they may be a little thicker than the same diameter glass lens of equal power. Glass and plastic are equally satisfactory for the correction of ametropia but, depending on the power required and the frame style, one may have advantages over the other in certain circumstances.

B. Lens shapes in extreme corrections. In high minus lenses a myodisk form may be used to reduce the weight by grinding the peripheral portion of the lens surfaces parallel to one another so that only the central portion is corrective. This reduces the edge thickness. High plus lenses can be made in a **lenticular form,** wherein only the central portion is corrective and the peripheral surfaces are parallel to one another. Both can be identified by the "fried egg" or "bull's eye" appearance of the lens. High plus aphakic lenses are also made in an **aspheric form** by modifying the lens curvature peripherally to **reduce aberrations and provide better peripheral vision.**

C. Tinted lenses. Lenses may be tinted for comfort, for safety, or for cosmetic effect. Sunglasses are generally tinted green or gray, according to individual preference. In order to be effective, they should be dark enough to absorb 60–80% of the incident light in the visible part of the spectrum and almost all of the ultraviolet and infrared. Both glass and plastic absorb **ultraviolet** very effectively, but glass lenses are more effective in the infrared range. **Photochromic lenses** that alter their absorptive characteristics according to the amount of ultraviolet exposure are available. It is important to bear in mind that it is ultraviolet exposure that alters the absorption, since ordinary glass absorbs considerable ultraviolet. **Photochromic lenses will not function as**

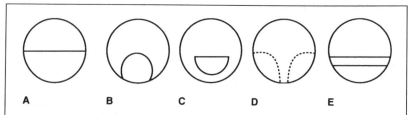

Fig. 13-9. Bifocal styles with segment (reading add) insets in distance correction. **A.** Executive (wide close work field). **B** and **C.** Insets allowing more inferior peripheral vision than A. **D.** Progressive multifocal lens (dotted lines not visible; denote power channel add of increasing strength inferiorly. **E.** Executive trifocal (may be done in B and C styles also) gives intermediate and close focal lengths in mid and lowest add respectively.

efficiently indoors or in an automobile. Also, the darkening process occurs quite rapidly, but the lightening process is much slower, requiring 1 minute and 20 minutes, respectively, for a 75% alteration in transmission. **Photogray** lenses have a minimum absorption of 15% and a maximum of approximately 45%, while **Photosun** lenses have a minimum absorption of 35% and a maximum of 80%. Photogray is not fully effective as a sunglass, therefore, and both, but especially Photosun, should not be worn for night driving. Tinted lenses for **industrial applications** are usually highly absorptive and are especially constructed to eliminate ultraviolet and infrared in order to provide maximum protection for welders, glassblowers, steel processing attendants, and so forth. Light tints for cosmetic effect are not adequate for protection in bright sunlight. If the tints are too dark, they can reduce visual efficiency under conditions of low illumination. **Yellow lenses** absorb all of the ultraviolet and most of the blue light but none of the infrared. These lenses are designed to improve visual efficiency on hazy, bright, or overcast days but are not effective as sunglasses and should not be used to improve night vision. **Polaroid** lenses are helpful where there is a great deal of reflected glare, such as on the water. In **aphakia,** lightly tinted lenses and ultraviolet absorption are helpful since removal of the crystalline lens results in increased sensitivity to light and decreased ultraviolet absorption.

D. **Single and multiple power lenses**
1. **Single-vision** corrective lenses that have the same correction over the entire surface are referred to as *single-vision lenses* and are used to correct hyperopia, myopia, astigmatism, presbyopia, or aphakia.
2. **Multifocals.** Lenses can be made with more than one corrective power. If one portion of the lens corrects the distance vision and the other corrects the near vision, as in presbyopia, it is referred to as a **bifocal** lens (Fig. 13-9). If an additional portion is added for intermediate range vision, it is referred to as a **trifocal** lens. The strength of the middle segment of the trifocal is usually 50% that of the near add (see sec. **VI.B.6**). Bifocals and trifocals can be manufactured by altering the curvature of the surface to make a one-piece multifocal, or by fusing a smaller piece of higher density glass into the crown portion to make a fused multifocal lens. Special occupational multifocal lenses are available.
3. **Progressive lenses** are multifocal lenses with no visible line of an add and no image jump. Although increasingly popular among middle-aged patients, they are visually less satisfactory than bifocals or plain reading lenses because of the progressively narrower field of view as the eye moves down to look through stronger parts of the lens. Because of this restrictive channel, the lenses must be aligned with the eyes with great precision. This still does not prevent the distortion of vision if the patient's eyes move to the right

or left of the channel and may result in a lateral head movement rather than normal eye movement while reading (see Fig. 13-9).

E. **Prescribing spectacles.** It is important to understand that although prescribing spectacles involves writing a series of numbers on a piece of paper, arriving at the most appropriate set of numbers for a particular patient is not a mathematical certainty. **The amount of ametropia measured and what the patient will tolerate with comfort are frequently not the same.** For example, the young hyperope frequently cannot fully relax accommodation and will not tolerate full correction. The patient with astigmatism that has previously been uncorrected may be uncomfortable if all of his or her astigmatism is corrected at once. Presbyopes of the same age have different body configurations, visual habits, and work requirements, all of which will affect the appropriate amount of reading correction. The effect of the spectacle correction on extraocular muscle balance via CNS mechanisms may determine the amount of correction the physician wishes to prescribe. In higher degrees of ametropia, if the distance at which the spectacle lens is going to rest in front of the cornea varies from the distance at which the ametropia was measured, an adjustment has to be made. In some patients, particularly high myopes and astigmats, altering the form or shape of the corrective spectacle lens, even though the power remains the same, can result in spatial aberrations that can be very annoying. Safety considerations, the use of appropriate tints, occupational considerations, and appropriate frame design for the patient's physiognomy must also be taken into consideration. Cosmesis is important but should not override functional considerations. The dispensing optician or optometrist should be skilled in advising patients with regard to these latter aspects of the prescription in addition to ensuring that the prescription is filled accurately.

VIII. **Contact lenses** rest on the surface of the cornea. The same principles of refraction and optics apply to contact lenses as apply to spectacle lenses. They correct the amount of ametropia present by replacing the corneal curvature with a contact lens surface that is calculated to correct the degree of myopia or hyperopia. Since most astigmatism is a result of the toricity of the front corneal surface, **rigid (hard) contact lenses will usually eliminate that astigmatism.** In the case of **soft lenses,** which mold to the surface of the cornea, however, the front surface of the soft lens also becomes toric and the **astigmatism will persist.** This is referred to as **residual astigmatism.** Residual astigmatism is occasionally found with rigid lenses also, especially when the astigmatism is due to toricity in surfaces other than the front surface of the cornea. It is possible to manufacture contact lenses with toric surfaces to correct residual astigmatism, but since contact lenses tend to rotate on the surface of the eye it is not a totally satisfactory solution, even when special designs are used to reduce the rotation. In the correction of myopia, the contact lens is further away from the far point and is slightly weaker than a spectacle prescription for the same patient. In hyperopia and aphakia, the contact lens is closer to the far point (see sec. **VI.B.1, 5,** and **7**) and consequently has to be stronger than the spectacle lens correction. In the past several years there has been a gradual evolution in contact lens technology that has introduced new materials and designs that have increased the lenses' usefulness considerably.

A. **Advantages.** Contact lenses may have optical advantages for some patients in addition to the cosmetic benefit and the convenience of not having to wear glasses. In high degrees of ametropia, peripheral distortions are reduced with contact lenses due to their small diameter and thinness. In monocular aphakia, reduction of the image size with contact lenses generally allows the patient to enjoy the benefits of binocular vision again. Even binocular aphakics enjoy the better peripheral vision, minimum distortion, and reduced magnification that they get with contact lenses. A patient with keratoconus or an irregular cornea for some other reason can frequently achieve satisfactory vision with contact lenses when little or no improvement can be obtained with spectacles. The advantages for those engaged in athletics or with special occupational needs are obvious.

B. **Disadvantages.** Contact lenses are expensive and easily lost or destroyed. Rigid lenses are initially uncomfortable and require a period of adaptation. Soft lenses are more comfortable, but they are still not well tolerated by some patients and frequently do not provide satisfactory correction of vision due to residual astigmatism. With the exception of extended-wear lenses, which are cleaned every 7 days, the care and cleaning of daily-wear contact lenses are important and must be done on a daily basis. Wearing time may be limited by physiologic factors, and the patient may still have to wear glasses part of the time. A superficial ocular infection becomes more significant in the contact lens patient. Corneal ulcers may occur with contact lenses; they never occur as a result of wearing spectacles. Foreign bodies may become entrapped under a contact lens instead of being immediately washed out by tears. This can result in significant discomfort for a period of time, or it may require removal of the lens at a highly inconvenient time. In general, provided there are no medical contraindications, it is safe to wear contact lenses for correction of ametropia, but patients should be aware of their limitations as well as their advantages.

C. **Hard lenses** are made of polymethyl methacrylate (PMMA) and are either lathed or molded. They are relatively rigid and durable, are easy to clean, may be stored wet or dry, and provide satisfactory correction of vision for the vast majority of patients. The curvatures on the corneal surfaces must be properly blended and the edge properly designed and polished to allow adequate exchange of tears between the lens and cornea and to minimize discomfort. Since corneal epithelium has a high metabolic rate and since oxygen solubility in tears is limited, a satisfactory flow of tears must be maintained to prevent corneal epithelial decompensation and the resulting **overwearing syndrome,** consisting of blurred vision, injection, and severe pain a short time after removal of the lenses following several hours of continuous wear. The incidence of **infectious ulcerative keratitis** is 2/10,000 hard lens wearers and 4/10,000 for rigid gas-permeable lenses.

D. **Daily-wear soft lenses** are made of hydroxyethyl methacrylate (HEMA) or related polymers and have the unique characteristic of retaining a large volume of water but still retaining their shape. The water content, which may vary from 30–85% with different polymers, makes them relatively comfortable, easy to adapt to, and useful for intermittent wear. This same quality limits their usefulness in patients with astigmatism. Even patients without astigmatism are sometimes annoyed by slight changes in vision associated with alteration of the lens surface produced by lid movements or changes in hydration. Soft lenses are more difficult to clean and sterilize and have much more of a tendency to accumulate mucus or precipitates. Since they are larger and tend to move less than hard lenses, foreign bodies are generally not much of a problem. They are also less apt to be displaced on the eye or to fall out occasionally. Oxygenation of the cornea is less of a problem with soft lenses but still limits the amount of time they may be worn continuously. So-called thin lenses help to minimize problems with oxygenation, but they are more difficult to handle and are more fragile. In some patients, mechanical compression of the blood vessels at the corneoscleral junction results in congestion of the limbal vessels and a tendency to **corneal vascularization.**

E. **Gas-permeable lenses.** Recently, new materials, such as cellulose acetate butyrate (CAB), silicone, silicone cross-linked with PMMA, and others, have been introduced into contact lens manufacturing. These materials exhibit varying degrees of oxygen permeability and interfere less with corneal epithelial metabolism. They result in little or no corneal edema and few instances of the overwearing syndrome, and in selected cases they can be worn for several days or weeks without being removed, although this is not usually advised. While this represents a significant and exciting new development in contact lenses, there are still problems that need to be solved, and the ultimate material for prolonged, continuous wear of contact lenses is still to be identified. (See sec. **C** regarding ulcerative keratitis incidence.)

F. **Extended-wear contact lenses.** The concept of wearing contact lenses continuously, that is, 24 hours a day, has received a great deal of publicity and has achieved some popularity. This approach to wearing contact lenses originally developed in response to the needs of **aphakic patients.** Visual rehabilitation of aphakic patients is greatly enhanced by using contact lenses instead of spectacles (see sec. **VI.B.7.c**). In many aphakic patients the limiting factors in prescribing contact lenses are the patients' inability to insert, to remove, and to care for their lenses unassisted. Contact lenses made of materials that are sufficiently gas permeable to deliver adequate amounts of oxygen to the corneal surface and that also permit adequate tear exchange reduce or eliminate these handling problems.

1. Materials used to manufacture contacts with these characteristics fall into three categories: (a) 55–80% "high water content" soft lenses, (b) CAB or PMMA-silicone copolymer rigid lenses, and (c) semisoft pure silicone lenses. Although in vitro studies indicate considerable variation in oxygen permeability for these materials, clinical studies indicate that correctly fitted lenses of each type are **successful in approximately 75–85% of properly selected patients** fitted for extended wear. Patients with **certain types of corneal diseases,** dry eyes, chronic lid or ocular infections, or who do not have immediate access to medical care **should not be fitted** with continuous-wear lenses, and every patient considering this mode of wear should be evaluated by an ophthalmologist for the presence of any medical contraindications. Selection of the appropriate type of gas-permeable lens for a particular patient depends on the patient and on the fitter's preference.

2. **Ulcerative keratitis** has proved to be the most vision-threatening disadvantage to cosmetic extended-wear contact lenses. The annual incidence of bacterial keratitis is approximately 20/10,000 persons using extended-wear lenses as opposed to only 4/10,000 persons using daily-wear lenses. Additionally, the risk of developing ulcerative keratitis was 10 to 15 times greater in extended-wear users who kept them in overnight compared to daily-wear users who did not wear the lenses overnight. As a result of these recent data, the FDA has changed its recommendation for extended-wear contact lens use to their being removed and cleaned once weekly as opposed to the originally recommended once monthly regimen.

3. Problems encountered with continuous-wear contact lenses include corneal edema, corneal molding, corneal vascularization, corneal infections, and iritis. All have been reported with continuous wear, along with a "tight lens" syndrome combining many of these findings. While most of these changes are reversible, they occur with sufficient frequency and are severe enough to cause concern among ophthalmologists and patients alike. The buildup of proteinaceous or mineral deposits on the surface of continuously worn lenses (especially the soft and silicone lenses) occurs with varying frequency and can necessitate rather frequent replacements, as can the problem of lost lenses. Although the initial impetus for the use of continuous-wear lenses centered around the needs of aphakic patients, the increasing safety and success of IOLs have diminished this need considerably, since 75–80% of cataract patients currently have an IOL implanted at the time of surgery (see Chap. 6).

4. **Phakic patients and extended-wear lenses.** A tremendous advertising and marketing effort is underway to encourage the use of continuous-wear lenses in phakic patients. In most instances this mode of wear is primarily for purposes of convenience, although some phakic patients experience great difficulty handling their lenses, and some with high degrees of ametropia experience additional benefits. The medical risk-benefit ratio and the justification of the higher costs associated with this mode of wear are not as favorable for these patients as for the aphakic patients. The success rate appears to be about the same overall.

G. **Toric soft lenses.** As previously indicated, astigmatism is not usually a problem when fitting rigid contact lenses. Toric soft lenses are being developed in an attempt to correct this problem for soft lenses. Truncation or ballast is used alone or in combination to design soft lenses that will not rotate on the cornea. Truncation results in an asymmetric shape, and ballast results in asymmetric weight distribution. These efforts have met with only limited success. They work best for low to moderate degrees of astigmatism that are oriented near the 90- to 180-degree meridians. Fitting fees and replacement costs for these lenses are significantly higher than for spherical conventional lenses.

H. **Bifocal contact lenses.** Bifocal contact lenses have been available for many years in hard contact lenses. They have met with very limited success and acceptance. Soft bifocal contact lenses have recently been introduced, also with limited success and acceptance to date. Bifocal contact lenses are based on two designs. One design has a central area to correct far vision and a peripheral concentric area to correct near vision. The second design has an annular or semicircular area along one edge, with the near correction similar to bifocal spectacles. The latter design utilizes truncation or ballast to stabilize the lens and to maintain the proper orientation of the bifocal segment. The major **problems** with both types of lenses are stability of vision and maintaining the proper position of the lens for the visual task at hand, since blinking and eye movements alter the relationship of the visual axis and the different optical zones of the lens. Fitting fees and replacement costs for these lenses are significantly higher than those for conventional single-vision lenses. Many presbyopic patients also benefit from a different approach, referred to as monovision, where the dominant eye is corrected for distance vision and the nondominant eye is corrected for near vision with conventional single-vision contact lenses.

IX. **Subnormal vision aids.** Many patients have eye diseases that result in subnormal vision that cannot be corrected medically or surgically. In some cases, these patients can be helped by the use of subnormal vision aids. These aids function by enlarging the retinal image and are of benefit primarily in patients with **macular diseases.** In these patients, the resolving power of the retina is decreased centrally. Enlarging the image causes it to fall on adjacent, normally functioning areas. Since the resolving power of paramacular areas is relatively low, this is not a substitute for macular vision, but it does allow these patients to perform some visual functions, such as reading, they would not otherwise be able to perform. Since magnification of the visual image reduces the size of the visual field, some loss of visual efficiency occurs, particularly for distance vision. These devices usually have no value for patients who have normal visual acuity but suffer loss of peripheral vision, such as in advanced glaucoma.

A. **Physical magnification.** If an object is brought closer to the eye, the angle that it subtends at the nodal point of the eye is increased, and the image that falls on the retina is similarly increased. For example, an object 2 mm long when viewed at a distance of 50 cm produces a retinal image of 0.06 mm. The same 2-mm object viewed at a distance of 5 cm produces a retinal image of 0.6 mm, a magnification of $10\times$. This method of magnification is particularly useful in young patients with a large amplitude of accommodation. It also contributes to the value of **high plus lenses.** These may range from +4 to +20 d with progressively shorter reading distance and smaller visual field. To a person motivated to read, these disadvantages are tolerable.

B. **Optical magnification.** A wide variety of **telescopic devices** have been developed to aid patients with subnormal vision. Telescopic systems generally have two lenses and are of the terrestrial type to avoid the image inversion that occurs with celestial telescopes. Lens systems of this type are limited by practical considerations to about 2.2 magnifications. Beyond this point the separation of the two lens elements becomes impractical, and reduction of the visual field becomes excessive. Telescopic systems are primarily used to improve distance vision, since high plus single-lens magnifiers are more efficient and provide greater magnification for near vision. For example, a +20-d magnifying lens produces a magnification of $5\times$. In addition, a single-element **magnifier** held close to the eye results in a better field of view. The field size varies directly with the diameter of the magnifying lens and inversely with the distance the lens is held from the eye. For this reason, high-magnification lenses are usually designed as loupes or as special lenses to be held close to the eye rather than at a normal reading distance. Magnification with loupes or high plus lenses is also greatest when the object to be viewed is held just inside the anterior focal point of the lens. Although this is not always the most comfortable reading distance, it does permit the patient to read print he or she would not otherwise be able to see. A **projection system** or television extends the range of magnification available, but these systems are not very portable and are usually quite expensive. Although other highly expensive and sophisticated optical systems are available as subnormal visual aids, they seldom result in improved visual efficiency, and it is only rarely that the expense is justified.

X. **Orthokeratology** is a technique for modifying the refractive error, principally in myopes, by purposely fitting hard contact lenses that are flatter than the corneal curvature in order to induce flattening of the cornea and thereby decrease the amount of myopia. When successful, it is frequently necessary for the patient to wear retaining lenses part of the time to maintain the induced change. The amount of change that can be produced is limited. Many ophthalmologists feel that there are significant risks involved in the application of this technique for the periods of time necessary to achieve the desired effect, and that, since the **effect is transient** and merely reduces the spectacle correction without curing the myopia, it is unwarranted. Because of the frequency of follow-up examinations and the multiple changes in contact lenses required, orthokeratology is also quite expensive. It is not widely accepted as a safe or routine procedure at this time.

XI. **Surgical correction of refractive errors**

A. **Epikeratophakia** is a surgical procedure for the correction of aphakia, keratoconus, and myopia in which a "lens" made of lathed human corneal stroma with intact Bowman's membrane is sutured to the anterior surface of the recipient cornea. The resulting change in the anterior curvature alters the refractive properties of the cornea to correct the preexisting refractive error.

B. **Keratomileusis** and **keratophakia** are both lamellar refractive keratoplasty techniques from which epikeratophakia evolved. In keratomileusis a lamellar section is removed from the anterior cornea, frozen, lathed to a new shape, and replaced on the donor eye. For myopia more tissue is removed from the center of the lamellar section, and in aphakia more tissue is lathed from the periphery of the tissue, thus creating "minus and plus lenses" of stromal tissue to be sutured to their own corneas. In keratophakia a lamellar section is removed from the patient's cornea using a microtome, and a prelathed donor corneal stroma "plus lens" is placed on the corneal bed and the original lamellar section is sutured over it. This or keratomileusis may be used in the correction of aphakia in eyes not able to tolerate intraocular lenses. Recent studies indicate preliminary success using synthetic hydrogel implants rather than lathed stroma.

C. **Radial keratotomy** is an elective surgical procedure on an anatomically normal organ and is designed for the correction of myopia and astigmatism. Patient motivation for having the procedure is usually to be rid of dependence on glasses or contact lenses; others may need it for occupational or athletic purposes. Data collection and evaluation are still ongoing in the National Eye Institute–supported PERK (Prospective Evaluation of Radial Keratotomy) study. At 3 years time the following information is available.

1. Radial keratotomy is most effective in patients with -2 to -5 d of spherical equivalent myopia.

2. Most surgeons now use eight or four radial cuts (bicycle spoke pattern) for myopia, with a variety of peripheral cornea tangential cuts for astigmatic correction.

3. Uncorrected visual acuity of 20/40 or better was achieved overall in 76% of patients, with 91% of low, 81% of medium, and 60% of high myopes falling into this favorable outcome group.

4. The outcome cannot be predicted in about 25% of patients. Some are over-responders and some underresponders.
5. More common undesirable side effects or outcomes include
   a. Undercorrection, overcorrection or premature presbyopia.
   b. Asymmetric correction with resulting symptoms of aniseikoria.
   c. Fluctuating vision during the day.
   d. Glare, usually nondisabling.
   e. Inclusions in incisions and stellate epithelial iron line deposition.
   f. Reduction in achievement of best visual acuity.
   g. Increased difficulty fitting contact lenses.
   h. Regular or irregular astigmatism.
   i. Possible long-term endothelial cell loss (none yet noted).
      In brief, radial keratotomy is a useful refractive surgical procedure being done more frequently in this country with increasingly favorable results. It is not yet, however, a mature procedure but one that needs further refinement to be completely noncontroversial.

Ocular Manifestations of Systemic Disease

Gilbert K. Yamamoto and
Deborah Pavan-Langston

I. **Use of tabulated information.** The eyes are frequently involved in diseases affecting the rest of the body. Ocular manifestations in certain multisystem disorders may offer diagnostic clues to aid in identifying the systemic disease. In other instances, the eye involvement may be subtle enough to avoid detection unless the clinician knows to look for it. Once the diagnosis is made, the major element in therapy of the ophthalmic aspect of the systemic disease is often the treatment and cure of the primary disease itself. This is not always the case, however, and an ophthalmic diagnosis may be necessary to determine the cause of local eye involvement, which may require a different kind of management. This chapter provides the clinician with a quick reference for symptoms and signs of ocular disorders associated with common systemic diseases. Each disease entity, as it affects the eye, has been listed in the Index and has been discussed in detail in the appropriate chapters. When dealing with cases in which patients have eye symptoms without a known systemic disease, the clinician should refer those individuals to ophthalmologists for a specific ocular diagnosis. Evaluations can then be made for the presence or absence of systemic disease. On the other hand, if the patient's systemic disease is known, that individual may be referred to an ophthalmologist mainly for confirmation of the diagnosis and treatment of the ocular component. This chapter is divided into two parts:

The first part outlines major ocular regions affected by systemic diseases and lists the specific diseases affecting each region.

The second part is a series of tables, each devoted to a major systemic disease. The specific disease entities are listed within the larger classification with their ocular manifestations. Diagnostic clinical and laboratory tests are indicated for each condition, and recommendations are made for referral to a specialist.

II. **Ocular regions related to systemic diseases**

    A. **Cornea.** The cornea provides a unique opportunity for observation and diagnosis of systemic diseases and abnormal metabolic processes. It is useful to consider the physical and morphologic properties of the cornea in order to understand how systemic diseases can affect the cornea and conjunctiva.

        1. **Diseases of the skin and mucous membranes.** The corneal epithelium is of ectodermal embryologic origin. Systemic skin and mucous membrane disorders also affect the cornea. Corneal and conjunctival bullae, severe inflammation, and sloughing of the epithelium may occur in the following diseases:

           a. Atopic dermatitis.

           b. Cicatricial pemphigoid.

           c. Epidermolysis bullosa.

           d. Erythema multiforme (Stevens-Johnson syndrome).

           e. Ichthyosis.

           f. Pemphigus.

           g. Phacomatoses.

           h. Xeroderma pigmentosa.

        2. **Disorders of collagen metabolism.** The rest of the cornea is of mesodermal embryologic origin. Disorders of collagen metabolism may affect

the cornea, possibly inducing keratoconus changes. Two disorders of collagen that may affect the cornea are

    a. Ehlers-Danlos syndrome.

    b. Marfan's syndrome.

  3. Collagen diseases. Much of the cornea is made of collagen and mucopolysaccharide ground substance. Systemic diseases affecting collagen may indirectly affect the cornea by way of autoantibodies in the circulation. Marked limbal and marginal corneal ulceration may result. Three systemic diseases affecting collagen that commonly involve the cornea are

    a. Periarteritis nodosa.

    b. Rheumatoid arthritis.

    c. Wegener's granulomatosis.

  4. Metabolic diseases. The cornea stores materials made in excess by the body. Damage to the cornea may occur indirectly by accumulation of metabolic products. Systemic metabolic diseases that produce elevated levels of certain precursors and that may opacify the cornea, producing band keratopathy or lipid keratopathy, are

    a. Amyloidosis.

    b. Cystinosis.

    c. Glycogen storage disease.

    d. Gout.

    e. Hyperlipidemia.

    f. Mucopolysaccharidoses.

    g. Hypervitaminosis D.

    h. Wilson's disease.

  5. Environmentally caused disorders. The cornea is the most anterior part of the eye, exposed to environmental harm. Exposure keratitis and infections may occur where there is poor protective function of the cornea. Environmental hazards include

    a. Exposure (drying, radiant and ionizing energy).

    b. Infectious agents (bacteria, viruses, fungi, and parasites).

B. Cataracts. Cataracts are associated with many systemic diseases. Lens fibers opacify as a response to alterations of the physical and chemical milieu within the semipermeable lens capsule. The exact type of cataract that forms may be distinct from the usual senile lens opacities and may be characteristic for the specific disease entity. Cataracts may be associated with the following systemic diseases:

  1. Chromosomal disorders

    a. Alport's syndrome.

    b. Cri-du-chat syndrome.

    c. Conradi's syndrome.

    d. Crouzon's syndrome.

    e. Myotonia dystrophica.

    f. Patau's syndrome.

    g. Schmid-Fraccaro syndrome.

    h. Trisomy 18 (Edwards' syndrome).

    i. Turner's syndrome.

  2. Diseases of the skin and mucous membranes

    a. Atopic dermatitis.

    b. Basal-cell nevus syndrome.

    c. Ichthyosis.

    d. Pemphigus

  3. Metabolic and nutrition diseases

    a. Aminoaciduria (Lowe's syndrome).

    b. Diabetes mellitus.

    c. Fabry's disease.

    d. Galactosemia.

    e. Homocystinuria.

    f. Hypervitaminosis D.

      g. Hypoparathyroidism.
      h. Hypothyroidism.
      i. Mucopolysaccharidoses.
      j. Wilson's disease.
  4. Infectious diseases
    a. Congenital
      (1) Congenital herpes simplex.
      (2) Congenital syphilis.
      (3) Cytomegalic inclusion disease.
      (4) Rubella.
    b. Others
      (1) Cysticercosis.
      (2) Leprosy.
      (3) Onchocerciasis.
      (4) Toxoplasmosis.
  5. Toxic substances introduced systemically
    a. Corticosteroids.
    b. Haloperidol.
    c. Miotics.
    d. Triparanol (MER/29).
C. Glaucoma is not exclusively the result of a hereditary predisposition (as in primary glaucoma). Secondary glaucomas may arise as complications of the systemic disease itself or from its therapy. Systemic diseases that may cause glaucoma are
  1. Hematologic and cardiovascular diseases
    a. Carotid-cavernous fistulas.
    b. Leukemia.
    c. Sickle cell disease.
    d. Waldenström's macroglobulinemia.
  2. Collagen diseases
    a. Ankylosing spondylitis.
    b. Rheumatoid arthritis.
    c. Sarcoidosis.
  3. Diseases of skin and mucous membranes
    a. Atopic diseases (corticosteroid use).
    b. Nevus of Ota.
  4. Infectious diseases
    a. Congenital rubella.
    b. Onchocerciasis.
  5. Metabolic diseases
    a. Amyloidosis.
    b. Marchesani's syndrome.
  6. Musculoskeletal diseases
    a. Conradi's syndrome.
    b. Osteogenesis imperfecta.
  7. Neoplastic diseases: metastasis to the trabecular meshwork
  8. Phacomatoses
    a. Neurofibromatosis.
    b. Sturge-Weber syndrome.
  9. Pulmonary diseases: asthma and emphysema (corticosteroid use)
  10. Renal diseases
    a. Lowe's syndrome (aminoaciduria).
    b. Wilms' tumor.
    c. Renal transplantation (corticosteroid use).
  11. Toxic substances (see Chap. 15)
    a. Amphetamines.
    b. Anticholinergics.
    c. Corticosteroids.
    d. Hexamethonium.

   e. Reserpine.
   f. Tricyclic antidepressants.
D. Uveitis resulting from systemic diseases presents a difficult diagnostic problem. Inflammation of the iris, ciliary body, and choroid may be caused by a wide variety of diseases, catalogued below.
   1. Systemic allergic diseases: hay fever.
   2. Cardiovascular diseases: endocarditis (subacute bacterial).
   3. Collagen diseases
      a. Ankylosing spondylitis.
      b. Periarteritis nodosa.
      c. Reiter's syndrome.
      d. Rheumatoid arthritis.
      e. Sarcoidosis.
      f. Systemic lupus erythematosus.
      g. Wegener's granulomatosis.
   4. Diseases of skin and mucous membranes
      a. Acne rosacea.
      b. Behçet's disease.
      c. Erythema multiforme (Stevens-Johnson syndrome).
      d. Vogt-Koyanagi-Harada syndrome.
   5. Metabolic diseases
      a. Amyloidosis.
      b. Gout.
   6. Gastrointestinal and nutritional diseases
      a. Regional enteritis.
      b. Peptic ulcer disease.
      c. Ulcerative colitis.
   7. Neoplastic disease
      a. Lymphoma.
      b. Reticulum cell sarcoma.
   8. Toxic substances (see Chap. 15)
      a. Sulfonamides.
      b. Reserpine.
   9. Infectious diseases
      a. Brucellosis.
      b. Gonorrhea.
      c. Leprosy.
      d. Onchocerciasis.
      e. Tuberculosis.
      f. Toxoplasmosis.
      g. Viral infections.
E. Retina. The retina is vulnerable to systemic diseases that affect specific retinal tissue elements such as retinal vessels, choroid (microaneurysms, hemorrhages, exudates, hemangiomas, choroiditis), neural tissue (retinitis, exudative retinal detachment, selective rod and cone destruction), and retinal pigment epithelium (loss of pigment, accumulation of toxic substances). The systemic diseases affecting the retina are
   1. Cardiovascular diseases
      a. Aortic arch syndrome (Takayasu's syndrome).
      b. Endocarditis.
      c. Hereditary telangiectasia (Rendu-Osler-Weber).
      d. Hypertension and toxemia of pregnancy.
      e. Occlusive vascular disease.
   2. Collagen diseases
      a. Dermatomyositis.
      b. Periarteritis nodosa.
      c. Reiter's syndrome.
      d. Sarcoidosis.
      e. Systemic lupus erythematosus.

    f. Temporal arteritis.
    g. Wegener's granulomatosis.
  3. Chromosomal disorders
    a. Cri-du-chat syndrome.
    b. Schmid-Fraccaro syndrome.
    c. Turner's syndrome.
    d. Trisomy 18 (Edwards' syndrome).
    e. Deletion of chromosome 18.
    f. Trisomy 13 (Patau's syndrome).
    g. Ring-D chromosome.
  4. Endocrine diseases
    a. Diabetes mellitus.
    b. Cushing's syndrome.
    c. Hyperthyroidism.
    d. Hypothyroidism.
    e. Hypoparathyroidism.
  5. Diseases of the skin and mucous membranes
    a. Behçet's disease.
    b. Ichthyosis.
    c. Incontinentia pigmenti.
    d. Pseudoxanthoma elasticum.
    e. Vogt-Koyanagi-Harada syndrome.
  6. Gastrointestinal and nutritional diseases
    a. Regional enteritis.
    b. Vitamin A deficiency.
  7. Hematologic diseases
    a. Anemias.
    b. Leukemias.
    c. Polycythemia vera.
    d. Sickle cell disease.
    e. Thrombocytopenia.
    f. Waldenström's macroglobulinemia.
  8. Infectious diseases
    a. *Candida* retinitis.
    b. Histoplasmosis.
    c. Parasites.
    d. Septicemia.
    e. Viral infections.
    f. Tuberculosis.
  9. Phacomatoses: Most affect the retina.
 10. Pulmonary diseases
    a. Bronchiectasis.
    b. Cystic fibrosis.
    c. Pneumonia.
 11. Renal diseases
    a. Alport's syndrome.
    b. Medullary cystic disease.
    c. Nephrotic syndrome.
 12. Metabolic diseases
    a. Albinism.
    b. Amyloidosis.
    c. Cystinosis.
    d. Fabry's disease.
    e. Gaucher's disease.
    f. Niemann-Pick disease.
    g. Lipidoses.
 13. Neoplastic diseases: Most can affect the retina.
III. Specific systemic diseases and their ocular manifestations. Tables 14-1 through 14-17 list several systemic disorders that may affect the eye, their clinical ocular

manifestations, the clinical and laboratory tests indicated to detect suspected underlying systemic disease, differential diagnosis, and indications for referral to a specialist. **In previous editions of this book, several systemic diseases were included in this section that are now discussed in the text in sufficient detail to warrant removal from the tables. Their text location is listed in the footnotes of each pertinent table. These systemic conditions, along with many others not included in the tables, are also listed in the index for rapid text page location.** The systemic diseases that may affect the eye are

A. Systemic allergic diseases. See Chap. 5, sec. VII for atopic eczema, atopic keratoconjunctivitis (hay fever), vernal conjunctivitis, urticaria, and asthma.

B. Diseases of the skin and mucous membranes (Table 14-1).

C. Phacomatoses. See Chap. 7, sec. III for angiomatosis retinae (von Hippel's disease) and Chap. 10, sec. VIII for angiomatosis retinae (von Hippel's disease), ataxia-telangiectasia (Louis-Bar syndrome), encephalotrigeminal angiomatosis (Sturge-Weber syndrome), neurofibromatosis (von Recklinghausen disease), tuberous sclerosis (Bourneville disease), and Wyburn-Mason syndrome.

D. Collagen diseases (Table 14-2).

E. Systemic viral infections (Table 14-3).

F. Systemic bacterial infections (Table 14-4).

G. Systemic chlamydial and protozoal infections (Table 14-5).

H. Systemic fungal infections (Table 14-6).

I. Systemic cestode and nematode infections (Table 14-7).

J. Chromosomal disorders (Table 14-8).

K. Hematologic diseases (Table 14-9).

L. Cardiovascular diseases (Table 14-10).

M. Endocrine diseases (Table 14-11).

N. Gastrointestinal and nutritional disorders (Table 14-12).

O. Metabolic diseases (Table 14-13).

P. Musculoskeletal diseases (Table 14-14).

Q. Pulmonary diseases (Table 14-15).

R. Renal diseases (Table 14-16).

S. Neoplastic diseases with ocular metastases (Table 14-17).

Table 14-1. Diseases of the skin and mucous membranes*

Clinical entity	Significant ocular findings	Orbit, motility, extraocular muscles	Lids, sclera, conjunctiva	Cornea, uvea	Lens, vitreous	Retina, optic nerve	Diagnostic tests	Differential diagnosis, referral to whom?
Atopic dermatitis	Bilateral cataracts		Conjunctivitis	Keratoconus	Cataract (posterior subcapsular)			Dermatologist Ophthalmologist
Epidermolysis bullosa	Lid bullae Lacrimal duct stenosis Conjunctival vessels		Blepharitis Hypertrichosis	Subepithelial bullous keratitis Corneal erosion Corneal perforation			Family history Clinical diagnosis Skin biopsy	Dermatologist Ophthalmologist
Xeroderma pigmentosum	Malignant lid lesions		Symblepharon	Keratitis			Skin malignancies Skin biopsies	Dermatologist

FA = fluorescent antibody.

* See also
  Chap. 5: atopic eczema, atopic keratoconjunctivitis, vernal conjunctivitis, urticaria, hay fever, acne rosacea, erythema multiforme, cicatricial pemphigoid (Stevens-Johnson syndrome) (secs. **VI** and **VII**).
  Chap. 8: psoriasis, Kawasaki disease, ischemic ocular syndrome (sec. **VIII**); Behçet's disease, Vogt-Koyanagi-Harada syndrome (**XVI**).
  Chap. 10: erythema multiforme (sec. **IV**); albinism, Ehlers-Danlos syndrome, pseudoxanthoma elasticum (**VII**).

Table 14-2. Collagen diseases*

Clinical entity	Significant ocular findings	Orbit, motility, extraocular muscles	Lids, sclera, conjunctiva	Cornea, uvea	Lens, vitreous	Retina, optic nerve	Diagnostic tests	Differential diagnosis, referral to whom?
Dermatomyositis	Diplopia Extraocular muscle palsy Retinal hemorrhage	Diplopia Extraocular muscle palsy	Lid redness Lid edema			Retinal hemorrhage Exudates	Elevated ESR Elevated CPK EMG studies useful	Scleroderma Systemic lupus erythematosus Dermatologist Internist
Periarteritis nodosa	Episcleritis Retinal hemorrhage	Nystagmus Ocular muscle palsy	Episcleritis Nodular scleritis Ptosis	Marginal corneal ulcer Iritis Uveitis		Retinal hemorrhage Papilledema	Fever of unknown etiology Arteritis in a male Vessel biopsy	Wegener's disease Internist
Scleroderma	Scarred lids Keratitis Retinopathy		Lid margin scarring and loss	Keratitis with marginal ulceration	Cataract		Skin tense and leathery	Systemic lupus erythematosus Dermatomyositis Dermatologist
Systemic lupus erythematosus	Retinopathy		Diskoid skin lesions Episcleritis Conjunctival hyperemia	Keratitis Iridocyclitis		Soft exudates Retinal hemorrhage Retinal edema Papilledema	ANA LE cell preparation Renal biopsy to show antigen antibody complexes	
Wegener's granulomatosis	Orbital necrosis Corneal marginal degeneration	Necrotizing granulomatous lesions of the orbit		Corneal marginal ulceration Uveitis		Narrowed retinal arterioles Cotton-wool spots Retinal hemorrhage Papilledema	Biopsies showing necrotizing granulomatous lesions Renal involvement	Internist Ophthalmologist

ESR = erythrocyte sedimentation rate; CPK = creatine phosphokinase; EMG = electromyography; RA = rheumatoid arthritis; ANA = antinuclear antibody; LE = lupus erythematosus.
* See also
Chap. 5: **rheumatoid arthritis, lupus erythematosus, pemphigoid, erythema multiforme (Stevens-Johnson syndrome), scleroderma, periarteritis nodosa, Wegener's granulomatosis (secs. VI and VII).**
Chap. 8: **ankylosing spondylitis, Reiter's syndrome, juvenile rheumatoid arthritis (sec. VIII); sarcoidosts (sec. XI).**
Chap. 12: **temporal arteritis (giant-cell arteritis) (sec. II).**

Table 14-3. Systemic viral infections*

Clinical entity	Significant ocular findings	Orbit, motility, extraocular muscles	Lids, sclera, conjunctiva	Cornea, uvea	Lens, vitreous	Retina, optic nerve	Diagnostic tests	Differential diagnosis, referral to whom?
Rubeola (measles)	Koplik's spot on conjunctiva Conjunctivitis Photophobia		Catarrhal conjunctivitis Lesion on caruncle and conjunctiva	Keratitis with multiple epithelial erosions causing photophobia Iritis Uveitis (rare)		Optic neuritis Retinitis	Clinical diagnosis Koplik's spots Multinucleated giant cells in scrapings 14-day incubation period	May develop subacute sclerosing panencephalitis Ophthalmologist Pediatrician
Rubella (German measles)	Microphthalmus Cataract Glaucoma, congenital	Strabismus Nystagmus Nasolacrimal duct	Follicular conjunctivitis (postnatal cases)	Corneal edema Corneal clouding Iris atrophy Iridocyclitis Aniridia	Cataract, unclear	Chorioretinitis Optic atrophy	Clinical history Rash and lymphadenopathy Other associated cardiac, hearing, GU disorders	Cytomegalic inclusion disease Ophthalmologist Pediatrician
Variola (smallpox)	Lid lesions most common Primary smallpox of the eye is rare Iritis	Enlarged periauricular nodes	Pustular lid eruptions Trichiasis Conjunctivitis Symblepharon Ankyloblepharon	Severe keratitis Leukoma Iritis, patchy iris atrophy	Vitreous opacity, rare	Choroiditis Optic neuritis	Cytoplasmic inclusion bodies on scrapings EM studies of virus Fluorescent antibody	Vaccinia Chickenpox Vaccinia immune globulin may be useful Ophthalmologist Internist
Mumps	Conjunctivitis Keratitis Optic neuritis	Dacryoadenitis Ocular palsy associated with encephalitis	Episcleritis Scleritis Conjunctivitis	Unilateral keratitis Interstitial keratitis Iritis		Optic neuritis	Clinical diagnosis	Pediatrician
Infectious mononucleosis	Regional lymphadenopathy Uveitis Dacryocystitis Retinal periphlebitis Papillitis	Dacryocystitis	Eyelid edema Conjunctivitis	Uveitis Nummular keratitis	Vitritis	Retinal periphlebitis Papillitis	Clinical diagnosis Lymphadenopathy Sore throat Lymphocytosis Heterophil test Ophthalmoscopy	Internist Ophthalmologist

397

Table 14-3. (continued)

Clinical entity	Significant ocular findings	Orbit, motility, extraocular muscles	Lids, sclera, conjunctiva	Cornea, uvea	Lens, vitreous	Retina, optic nerve	Diagnostic tests	Differential diagnosis, referral to whom?
Influenza	Extraocular muscle myalgia	Extraocular muscle myalgia Oculopalsy		Mild keratitis Uveitis		Retinal hemorrhage and edema, rare Optic neuritis	Clinical diagnosis	

GU = genitourinary; EM = electron microscopy.

* See also
Chap. 5: adenovirus, AIDS, herpes simplex, herpes zoster, vaccinia, varicella (sec. IV).
Chap. 8: AIDS, cytomegalovirus, herpes simplex, herpes zoster, Epstein-Barr virus (sec. X).
Chap. 10: cytomegalovirus, *Chlamydia*, rubella, herpes simplex (sec. II); subacute sclerosing panencephalitis (sec. III).

Table 14-4. Systemic bacterial infections*

Clinical entity	Significant ocular findings	Orbit, motility, extraocular muscles	Lids, sclera, conjunctiva	Cornea, uvea	Lens, vitreous	Retina, optic nerve	Diagnostic tests	Differential diagnosis, referral to whom?
Brucellosis	Iritis Choroiditis	Dacryocystitis		Nodular iritis with keratic precipitates		Choroiditis Optic neuritis	Positive blood cultures and serologic hemagglutinins	Internist
Diphtheria	Pseudomembranous or membranous conjunctivitis		Lid edema	Corneal ulcer (*Corynebacterium diphtheria* can penetrate intact epithelium)			Enlarged regional nodes Positive smears and cultures	Hemolytic *Streptococcus* Adenovirus Internist
Septicemia bacterial metastatic endophthalmitis	Iritis Endophthalmitis Retinal hemorrhage, Roth's spots		Conjunctival hemorrhage	Iritis Iridocyclitis	Endophthalmitis	Retinal hemorrhage Chorioretinitis	Positive blood cultures	Fungal and protozoal organisms Internist

* See also
Chap 5: gonorrhea, ophthalmia neonatorum (sec **III**); leprosy, Lyme disease, tuberculosis (sec. **IV**).
Chap 8: Tuberculosis (sec. **XI**).
Chap 10: gonorrhea, *Chlamydia*, syphilis (sec. **II**).

Table 14-5. Systemic chlamydial and protozoal infections*

Clinical entity	Significant ocular findings	Orbit, motility, extraocular muscles	Lids, sclera, conjunctiva	Cornea, uvea	Lens, vitreous	Retina, optic nerve	Diagnostic tests	Differential diagnosis, referral to whom?
Lymphogranuloma venereum (chlamydial)	Rare ocular findings Conjunctivitis with preauricular adenopathy		Elephantiasis of lid from lymphatic obstruction Conjunctivitis	Keratitis with superficial vascularization		Retinal vessel dilation, venous Peripapillary	Isolation of organism on cultures, animal inoculation Complement-fixation tests Positive Frei test	Other venereal diseases Internist
Malaria	Ocular involvement (rare)		Conjunctivitis	Keratitis Iritis		Optic neuritis, may be associated with antimalarial drug therapy	Thick blood smears Clinical diagnosis	Parasitologist Internist

* See also
  Chap. 5: *Chlamydia* (sec. **IV**).
  Chap. 8: *Toxoplasma, Toxocara,* other parasites (sec. **XI**).
  Chap. 10: *Chlamydia, Toxoplasma* (sec. **II**).

Table 14-6. Systemic fungal infections*

Clinical entity	Significant ocular findings	Orbit, motility, extraocular muscles	Lids, sclera, conjunctiva	Cornea, uvea	Lens, vitreous	Retina, optic nerve	Diagnostic tests	Differential diagnosis, referral to whom?
Coccidioidomycosis	Rarely causes conjunctivitis Usually occurs as spread from lung lesion		Phlyctenular conjunctivitis Lid skin more commonly affected			Optic neuritis	Chest x ray Complement-fixation tests (over 1 : 16 is significant)	Pulmonary medicine
Cryptococcus infections (yeast form)	Central nervous system predilection Meningitis Eye involved secondarily		Brow lesions		Endophthalmitis, rare	Retinitis Papilledema Retinal hemorrhage Retinal detachment, rare	Difficult to diagnose for ophthalmologist India-ink smears to demonstrate capsule of fungus	Associated with Hodgkin's disease Internist Neurosurgeon Ophthalmologist

* See also
Chap. 3: *Actinomyces, Streptothrix* (sec. II).
Chap. 5: *Candida, Actinomyces, Streptothrix* (sec. IV).
Chap. 8: *Candida,* histoplasmosis (sec. XI).

Table 14-7. Systemic cestode and nematode infections*

Clinical entity	Significant ocular findings	Orbit, motility, extraocular muscles	Lids, sclera, conjunctiva	Cornea, uvea	Lens, vitreous	Retina, optic nerve	Diagnostic tests	Differential diagnosis, referral to whom?
Cysticercosis (tapeworm)	Vitreous hemorrhage Retinal detachment			Iritis	Cataract Vitreous hemorrhage Vitreous cyst	Retinitis Retinal detachment (rare)	Clinical history Geographic locale Eosinophilia	Ophthalmologist Surgery may be required
Echinococcosis (hydatid cyst)	Ocular involvement is usual, but retina and vitreous may be involved	Proptosis related to cyst in orbit		Iritis	Vitreous cyst	Retinal cyst	Clinical history Geographic locale Eosinophilia	Ophthalmologist Surgery may be required
Trichinosis (Trichinella)	Periorbital edema Painful eye movements	Periorbital edema	Conjunctival chemosis				Eosinophilia Skin tests Serologic tests Biopsy of deltoid, gastrocnemius muscles	Internist
Onchocerciasis	Microfilarial invasion of ocular tissue Keratitis Cataract Secondary glaucoma		Conjunctivitis	Superficial punctate and deep keratitis Iritis	Cataract	Chorioretinitis Optic atrophy (rare)	Tissue biopsy Eosinophilia Clinical history Geographic locale	Ophthalmologist Parasitologist
Loiasis (*Loa loa*)	Microfilarial migration in superficial ocular tissues		Conjunctivitis	Keratitis Iritis			Eosinophilia Parasite may be seen in thick blood smear or occasionally in conjunctiva	Internist Ophthalmologist

* See also
  Chap. 8: *Toxocara* (sec. XI).
  Chap. 10: *Toxocara* (sec. III).

Table 14-8. Chromosomal disorders*

Clinical entity	Significant ocular findings	Orbit, motility, extraocular muscles	Lids, sclera, conjunctiva	Cornea, uvea	Lens, vitreous	Retina, optic nerve	Diagnostic tests	Differential diagnosis, referral to whom?
Schmid-Fraccaro syndrome	Microphthalmus Strabismus Coloboma of the iris and retina	Hypertelorism Strabismus	Antimongoloid palpebral fissures	Iris coloboma	Cataract	Choroidal coloboma	Karyotyping	Ophthalmologist Pediatrician
Ring-D chromosome	Microphthalmus Hypertelorism	Hypertelorism Strabismus	Epicanthus Ptosis	Retrocorneal membrane Iris coloboma		Optic disk hypoplasia	Karyotyping	Ophthalmologist Pediatrician
Monosomy-G syndrome	Ptosis Epicanthus	Hypertelorism Strabismus	Ptosis Epicanthus Blepharochalasis		Cataract		Karyotyping	Ophthalmologist Pediatrician
Deletion of long arm of chromosome 13	Hypertelorism	Hypertelorism	Ptosis	Iris coloboma			Karyotyping	Ophthalmologist Pediatrician
Deletion of chromosome 18	Microphthalmus Congenital glaucoma (long arm)	Hypertelorism	Ptosis	Posterior keratoconus (short arm) Corneal opacity	Cataract (long arm)	Retinal degeneration (long arm) Optic atrophy (long arm)	Karyotyping	Ophthalmologist Pediatrician

* See also
Chap. 10: cri-du-chat syndrome, DeGrouchy syndrome, Turner syndrome, trisomies 13, 18, and 21 (sec. **VI**).

Table 14-9. Hematologic diseases

Clinical entity	Significant ocular findings	Orbit, motility, extraocular muscles	Lids, sclera, conjunctiva	Cornea, uvea	Lens, vitreous	Retina, optic nerve	Diagnostic tests	Differential diagnosis, referral to whom?
Anemias	Subconjunctival hemorrhages Dilatated retinal veins Retinal edema and exudates		Subconjunctival hemorrhage			Flame-shaped retinal hemorrhage Dilatated retinal veins Retinal edema and exudates	CBC, Hgb conc. less than 0.5 normal Folate levels B_{12} deficiency RBC indices Marrow biopsy	Pernicious Hemolytic Blood loss Hematologist
Leukemias	Orbital infiltration	Proptosis Exophthalmus				Retinal edema Retinal hemorrhage Papillitis Dilatated tortuous retinal vessels	WBC Blood smear	Lymphoma Hematologist
Lymphomas	Exophthalmus	Proptosis Ocular palsy	Painless lid swelling	Uveitis	Vitritis		Node biopsy Blood smear CBC, WBC X rays	Leukemia Hematologist
Multiple myeloma	Crystals in conjunctiva and cornea		Crystals in the conjunctiva	Crystals in cornea Cysts in iris and ciliary body		Pars plana cysts Dilatated retinal veins Retinal hemorrhage Papilledema	Urinary Bence-Jones proteins Immunoglobulin electrophoresis	Hematologist Internist
Polycythemia vera	Amaurosis fugax Dilatated retinal vessels Vascular congestion					Dilatated retinal vessels Hemorrhages Disk hyperemia Papilledema	RBC count over 6 million/μl Hemoglobin, red cell indices	Hematologist

Sickle cell disease	Capillary dropout in peripheral retina		Comma-shaped conjunctival vessels	Vitreous hemorrhage	Microcirculatory occlusive disorder Papilledema "Black sunburst" ischemic chorioretinal scars	Hemoglobin electrophoresis RBC morphology in low O_2	S disease versus SC trait Internist Ophthalmologist
Thalassemia	Epicanthal folds					RBC morphology Family history	Major versus minor Hematologist
Thrombocytopenia	Retinal hemorrhage Ocular palsy	Orbital hemorrhage Ocular palsy			Retinal edema and exudates	Intracranial hemorrhage Platelet count, marrow biopsy	ITP, TTP Hematologist
Waldenström's macroglobulinemia	Sludging of conjunctival blood flow Retinal vessel occlusion Papilledema				Dilated, tortuous retinal veins Retinal hemorrhage Cotton-wool exudate Retinal detachment	Elevated IgM levels Immunoglobulin electrophoresis	Hematologist

CBC = complete blood count; Hgb conc. = hemoglobin concentration; RBC = red blood count; WBC = white blood count; ITP = idiopathic thrombocytopenic purpura; TTP = thrombotic thrombocytopenic purpura; IgM = immunoglobulin M.

Table 14-10. Cardiovascular diseases[a]

Clinical entity	Significant ocular findings	Orbit, cornea, iris, conjunctiva	Retina, optic nerve	Diagnostic aids, referrals to whom?
Cardiovascular diseases Arteriosclerosis	Arcus senilis Lipid keratopathy Copper- and silver-wire appearances of retinal vessels	Arcus senilis of the peripheral cornea Lipid keratopathy, rarely	Retinal vessel tortuosity Dilation of retinal arterioles AV crossing changes Copper-wire appearance to arterioles Silver-wire appearance to arterioles	Clinical diagnosis Ophthalmoscopy Chest x ray (aortic knob) ECG Renal angiography Fluorescein angiography
Hypertension Chronic Malignant Toxemia of pregnancy	Arcus senilis Lipid keratopathy Tortuous vessels Retinal hemorrhage Papilledema	Arcus senilis	Retinal vessels with abnormal light reflexes (copper or silver wire) AV crossing changes Retinal edema Retinal hemorrhage Hard exudates Papilledema	Clinical diagnosis BP Ophthalmoscopy ECG Chest x ray Fluorescein angiography Fundic photography (documentation)
Occlusive vascular disease (sudden) Emboli and thrombi[b] Central retinal artery occlusion[b] Cardiac myxoma Cranial arteritis[b] Sickle cell attack[b]	Amaurosis fugax Homonymous hemianopia Anisocoria Cherry-red spot	Anisocoria, unusual	Cholesterol plaques in retinal arterioles (Hollenhorst) Cherry-red spot (CRA occlusions) of the macula	Ophthalmoscopy Visual fields Fluorescein angiography Elevated ESR (cranial arteritis)
Occlusive vascular disease (slow, progressive) Carotid artery disease Arterial spasm (TIA) Diabetes mellitus Collagen diseases	Conjunctival vessel dilation Iritis Retinal vessel dilation; hemorrhage Cotton-wool exudates Stasis retinopathy	Engorged conjunctival vessels Iritis (ischemic ocular inflammation) AC reaction Rubeosis iridis Horner's syndrome (affected side), unusual	Arteriolar distention Cotton-wool exudates Venous stasis retinopathy (punctate hemorrhage, retinal edema) Unilateral retinopathy, ipsilateral Unilateral arcus, contralateral	Clinical diagnosis Carotid bruits Visual fields Ophthalmodynamometry Fluorescein angiography Thermography and Doppler sonography Internist or vascular surgeon

Table 14-10. (continued)

Clinical entity	Significant ocular findings	Orbit, motility, extraocular muscles	Lids, sclera, conjunctiva	Cornea, uvea	Lens, vitreous	Retina, optic nerve	Diagnostic tests	Differential diagnosis, referral to whom?
Venous occlusive disease Thrombosis Oral contraceptive use	Rubeosis iridis Retinal venous congestion Branch-vein occlusion			Rubeosis iridis		Retinal venous congestion Branch-vein occlusion Hemorrhage, blotchy	Ophthalmoscopy Visual fields Fluorescein angiography	
Endocarditis	Roth's spots Retinal hemorrhage, exudates Papillitis	Diplopia Ocular palsies Nystagmus Anisocoria	Conjunctival petechiae	Iritis	Metastatic endophthalmitis	Retinal hemorrhages Cotton-wool exudates Roth's spots in retina Papillitis	Blood cultures Clinical signs— fever, anemia, heart murmur, splenomegaly	CVA Hemiplegias Ophthalmologist Cardiologist Neurologist
Myxoma	Retinal vascular emboli Cherry-red spot of macula					Retinal artery emboli Cherry-red spot	ECG Chest x ray Echocardiography Clinical suspicion	Cardiologist
Aortic arch syndrome (Takayasu)	Dilated retinal vessels Retinal hemorrhages Retinal exudates Papilledema Glaucoma			Folds in cornea Descemet's membrane Mild AC reaction Rubeosis iridis	Cataracts Vitreous hemorrhage	Retinal neovascularization Retinal detachment	Clinical diagnosis Angiography Fluorescein angiography	Cardiologist
Toxemia of pregnancy	Altered acuity Retinal hemorrhages Exudates Papilledema	Periorbital edema				Narrowing of retinal arterioles Hemorrhages, exudates Papilledema Exudative retinal detachment	Clinical diagnosis BP elevation Proteinuria Edema	Obstetrician Ophthalmologist
Thromboangiitis obliterans	Not common to have ocular findings Retinal perivasculitis					Retinal perivasculitis	Clinical diagnosis Smokers Jews Raynaud's phenomenon of upper extremities	Collagen vasculitides Internist

Table 14-10. (continued)

Clinical entity	Significant ocular findings	Orbit, motility, extraocular muscles	Lids, sclera, conjunctiva	Cornea, uvea	Lens, vitreous	Retina, optic nerve	Diagnostic tests	Differential diagnosis, referral to whom?
Hereditary telangiectasia Rendu-Osler-Weber (autosomal dominant)	Conjunctival vascular lesions		Dilatated, conjunctival vascular lesions		Vitreous hemorrhages (rare)	Retinal hemorrhages Dilatated veins Disk neovascularization (rare)	Family history Clinical diagnosis Telangiectasia of vessels of face, hands, oral and nasal mucosa	Diabetes mellitus Hypertension Phacomatosis Pediatrician Ophthalmologist

AV = arteriovenous; ECG = electrocardiogram; BP = blood pressure; CRA = central retinal artery; ESR = erythrocyte sedimentation rate; TIA = transient ischemic attack; AC = anterior chamber; CVA = cerebrovascular accident.

^aSee also Chap. 7: hypertensive retinopathy (sec. III).
^bOphthalmic emergency; requires immediate referral to ophthalmologist with telephone call ahead denoting emergency.

Table 14-11. Endocrine diseases*

Clinical entity	Significant ocular findings	Orbit, motility, extraocular muscles	Lids, sclera, conjunctiva	Cornea, uvea	Lens, vitreous	Retina, optic nerve	Diagnostic tests	Differential diagnosis, referral to whom?
Adrenals, Cushing's disease	Exophthalmus Hypertensive retinopathy Papilledema					Hypertensive retinopathy Tortuous, dilatated retinal vessels Hemorrhage and exudates	High levels of endogenous glucocorticoids Clinical diagnosis	Internist
Addison's disease	Hyperpigmentation of skin of lids, conjunctiva Papilledema Optic atrophy		Pigmentation of lids, conjunctiva			Papilledema Optic atrophy		Internist
Diabetes mellitus	Fluctuations in refractive error Diplopia Optic neuritis Optic atrophy	Third nerve palsy, sparring pupil	Xanthelasma	Wrinkles in BM of the cornea Rubeosis iridis Loss of iris pigment Ectropion uvea	Cataract, snowflake Asteroid hyalosis Vitreous hemorrhage Proliferation of new vessels	Dot-blot hemorrhage Microaneurysm Hard exudate Neovascularization of the nerve head Lipemia retinalis	FBS/GTT Fluorescein angiography	Internist Ophthalmologist
Hyperparathyroidism	Band keratopathy		Conjunctival calcification	Corneal opacity Band keratopathy			Elevation of serum calcium levels	Endocrinologist
Hypoparathyroidism	Photophobia Cataract		Lid twitching Conjunctivitis	Keratitis	Polychromatic subcapsular and cortical cataract	Papilledema	Tetany Low serum calcium levels	Endocrinologist Internist
Hyperthyroidism	Exophthalmus	Orbital puffiness	Lid retraction Lid lag	Exposure keratitis Superior limbic keratoconjunctivitis		Optic atrophy Papilledema	RAIU T_3, T_4 Werner suppression test Exophthalmometry Ophthalmoscopy Ultrasonography	Orbital tumor Ophthalmologist Coordinate care with internist, endocrinologist

Table 14-11. (continued)

Clinical entity	Significant ocular findings	Orbit, motility, extraocular muscles	Lids, sclera, conjunctiva	Cornea, uvea	Lens, vitreous	Retina, optic nerve	Diagnostic tests	Differential diagnosis, referral to whom?
Hypothyroidism	Photophobia Cataract	Periorbital edema Loss of brows, lateral one-third	Eyelid edema		Cortical lens opacities, mild	Optic neuritis Optic atrophy	Clinical diagnosis Cretinism Myxedema Dry hair, skin Low T_3, T_4	Endocrinologist Internist

BM = basement membrane; FBS/GTT = fasting blood sugar/glucose tolerance test; RAIU = radioiodine uptake; T_3 = triiodothyronine; T_4 = thyroxine.

* See also Chap. 7: diabetic retinopathy (sec. **III**).

Table 14-12. Gastrointestinal and nutritional disorders

Clinical entity	Significant ocular findings	Orbit, motility, extraocular muscles	Lids, sclera, conjunctiva	Cornea, uvea	Lens, vitreous	Retina, optic nerve	Diagnostic tests	Differential diagnosis, referral to whom?
Alcoholism (see Vitamin B deficiency)	Optic neuritis	Nystagmus Third and sixth nerve palsies Impaired conjugate gaze	Ptosis	Iridoplegia		Optic neuritis	Wernicke's encephalopathy Vitamin B levels Add vitamin B to diet to observe effect	Methyl alcohol toxicity Internist
Liver disease (nutritional)	Scleral icterus Night blindness Color vision impairment Dry eye		Scleral icterus	Keratitis sicca	Cataract?	Night blindness Color vision impairment Optic atrophy	Clinical diagnosis Liver enzymes Vitamin levels Abnormal ERG	Internist Ophthalmologist
Malnutrition	Xerophthalmia Night blindness		Lid edema Chemosis	Keratopathy			Vitamin levels Schirmer testing Abnormal ERG	Internist
Peptic ulcer disease (see Vitamin B deficiency)	Iritis Glaucomatocyclitic crisis			Iritis			Males Clinical diagnosis Gastroscopy	Internist
Pancreatic disease	Glaucoma secondary to therapy with anticholinergic drugs					Fat emboli in retinal vessels Cotton-wool exudates Retinal hemorrhages	Elevation of serum pancreatic enzymes	Internist
Regional enteritis or ulcerative colitis	Episcleritis Conjunctivitis Iritis Optic neuritis		Episcleritis Conjunctivitis	Uveitis Iritis		Retinitis Macular edema Exudative retinal detachment Optic neuritis	Clinical diagnosis Arthritis	Internist

Table 14-12. (continued)

Clinical entity	Significant ocular findings	Orbit, motility, extraocular muscles	Lids, sclera, conjunctiva	Cornea, uvea	Lens, vitreous	Retina, optic nerve	Diagnostic tests	Differential diagnosis, referral to whom?
Vitamin A deficiency	Xerophthalmia Keratomalacia		Bitot's spot in conjunctiva Xerosis of conjunctiva	Dry cornea Corneal perforation		Perivasculitis Degeneration of rod outer segments	Vitamin A levels Dary adaptometry ERG Conjunctival scraping for xerosis bacillus	Internist Ophthalmologist
Vitamin B deficiency	Xerosis of cornea and conjunctiva Optic neuritis					Central scotoma Retrobulbar neuritis	Vitamin B levels Visual fields Color vision	Internist Ophthalmologist
Vitamin C deficiency	Subconjunctival hemorrhage					Retinal hemorrhage in severe cases	Serum vitamin C levels	Scurvy Internist
Hypervitaminosis A, B, and D	Increased intracranial pressure (A) Decreased vision (B)	Exophthalmus (A) Diplopia (A)	Crystalline calcium deposits in conjunctiva (D)	Band keratopathy (D)	Zonular cataract (D)	Cystoid macular edema (B) Papilledema (A)	Serum levels of these vitamins	Internist
Whipple's disease	Intraocular inflammation Vitreous opacity	Ophthalmoplegias			Vitritis Vitreous opacity	Papilledema	Bacillary bodies seen on EM studies Clinical diagnosis Fever, cough, arthritis, intestinal malabsorption	Internist

ERG = electroretinogram; EM = electron microscopy.

Table 14-13. Metabolic diseases*

Clinical entity	Significant ocular findings	Orbit, motility, extraocular muscles	Lids, sclera, conjunctiva	Cornea, uvea	Lens, vitreous	Retina, optic nerve	Diagnostic tests	Differential diagnosis, referral to whom?
Alkaptonuria (ochronosis, autosomal recessive)	Dark pigmentation of sclera, conjunctiva, and cornea		Dark scleral pigmentation Tarsal plate and conjunctival pigmentation	Corneal pigmentation			Metabolic screening tests, urine Enzyme assays	Geneticist
Amyloidosis (autosomal dominant and recessive)	Amyloid deposits in various tissues Glaucoma	Proptosis Ocular muscle palsy	Ptosis Amyloid nodules in lids and conjunctiva	Corneal amyloid deposits, opacities in stroma Iritis, pupillary abnormalities	Vitreous opacity	Retinal hemorrhage Amyloids in the optic nerve	Immunoglobulin electrophoresis	Internist Ophthalmologist
Chédiak-Higashi syndrome (autosomal recessive)	Photophobia Partial ocular albinism	Nystagmus	Light-colored lashes	Light-colored iris		Albinotic fundus	Peripheral blood smear with PMNs having large abnormal granules Hepatosplenomegaly, lymphadenopathy	Ocular albinism Internist Pediatrician
Cystinosis (autosomal recessive)	Corneal and conjunctival crystals Photophobia Slight reduction in acuity		Crystals in the conjunctiva	Corneal crystals (anterior stroma)		Pigmentary disturbance in peripheral retina	Renal complications Short stature Conjunctival biopsy Polarizing light to examine crystals	Pediatrician
Fabry's disease (X-linked)	Corneal opacity Cataract Tortuous retinal vessels		Tortuous conjunctival vessels	Corneal epithelial opacities, vortex pattern	Posterior subcapsular cataract	Dilatated, tortuous retinal vessels Retinal hemorrhage Perimacular edema	Enzyme assays Cultured fibroblasts Prenatal diagnosis possible	Genetic counsel Internist Ophthalmologist
Galactosemia (autosomal recessive)	Cataract			Cataract, nuclear or zonular (reversible)			Galactose intolerance Enzymatic tests Cultured fibroblasts	Ophthalmologist Pediatrician

413

Table 14-13. (continued)

Clinical entity	Significant ocular findings	Orbit, motility, extraocular muscles	Lids, sclera, conjunctiva	Cornea, uvea	Lens, vitreous	Retina, optic nerve	Diagnostic tests	Differential diagnosis, referral to whom?
Gout	Corneal crystals Iridocyclitis		Episcleritis Scleritis	Uric acid crystals in cornea Iridocyclitis			Serum uric acid Clinical diagnosis	Internist
Hemochromatosis	Brown pigment on conjunctiva					Diabetic changes in retina	Iron content in blood; CBC Diabetes and liver cirrhosis may be present	Polycythemia vera Diabetes Wilson's disease Internist
Histiocytosis	Exophthalmus	Exophthalmus Infiltrative lesions of the bone (eosinophilic granuloma)					Clinical diagnosis	Pediatrician
Homocystinuria (autosomal recessive)	Lens discoloration				Lens dislocation, downward		Clinical diagnosis Mental retardation Plasma homocystine and methionine elevated	Marchesani's syndrome Marfan's syndrome Internist—vascular occlusive disease common
Lipidoses	Arcus senilis or juvenilis		Xanthelasma	Arcus Lipid keratopathy		Lipemia retinalis	Lipid electrophoresis Serum lipid assay	Internist— cardiovascular disease common
Marchesani's syndrome	Cataract Secondary glaucoma				Small lens Dislocation or subluxation common		Clinical diagnosis Short, stocky person Subluxed lenses	Marfan's homocystinuria Internist Ophthalmologist

PMN = polymorphonuclear cells; CBC = complete blood count.
* See also Chap 10: albinism, Gaucher disease, Marfan syndrome, mucopolysaccharidoses, Niemann-Pick disease, osteogenesis imperfecta, Wilson's disease (sec. **VII**); other inherited metabolic disorders (sec. **VII**); developmental disorders (secs. **IX** and **XI**); tumors of childhood (sec. **XI**); retinopathy of prematurity (sec. **XII**).

Table 14-14. Musculoskeletal diseases*

Clinical entity	Significant ocular findings	Orbit, motility, extraocular muscles	Lids, sclera, conjunctiva	Cornea, uvea	Lens, vitreous	Retina, optic nerve	Diagnostic tests	Differential diagnosis, referral to whom?
Albright's disease (fibrous dysplasia of bone)	Proptosis	Proptosis Strabismus	Chemosis	Corneal exposure		Optic atrophy	Early epiphyseal closure Café au lait spots X-ray diagnosis	Endocrinologist
Apert's disease	Proptosis	Proptosis	Antimongoloid slant of lids	Exposure keratitis Keratoconus		Optic atrophy Chronic papilledema	Clinical diagnosis Cranial malformation Syndactyly	Ophthalmologist Pediatrician
Conradi's syndrome (autosomal recessive)	Hypertelorism Bilateral cataracts Glaucoma	Hypertelorism		Heterochromia Iris hypoplasia	Dense bilateral cataracts	Optic atrophy	Clinical diagnosis Mental retardation Short stature Micromelia	Ophthalmologist Pediatrician
Craniofacial syndromes	Coloboma Exophthalmos	Exophthalmus Nystagmus Exotropia		Exposure keratitis		Papilledema Optic atrophy Myelinated nerve fibers	Clinical diagnosis Skull x rays	Crouzon's syndrome Platybasia Hypertelorism Pediatrician
Facial deformity syndromes	Coloboma of lower lids Antimongoloid slant of lids Microphthalmus	Preauricular appendages (Goldenhar's syndrome) Nystagmus Strabismus		Epibulbar dermoids (Goldenhar's syndrome)	Cataract		Clinical diagnosis Skull x rays	Goldenhar's syndrome Treacher Collins syndrome Pierre Robin syndrome Hallermann-Streiff-François syndrome Ophthalmologist Pediatrician
Muscular dystrophy disorders	Cataract Ptosis External ophthalmoplegia Dry eye	Ptosis			Cataract, polychromatic subcapsular	Pigmentary retinopathy	Clinical diagnosis EMG studies	Duchenne's syndrome Limb-girdle dystrophy Pediatrician

Table 14-14. (continued)

Clinical entity	Significant ocular findings	Orbit, motility, extraocular muscles	Lids, sclera, conjunctiva	Cornea, uvea	Lens, vitreous	Retina, optic nerve	Diagnostic tests	Differential diagnosis, referral to whom?
Myasthenia gravis	Ptosis Diplopia	Ptosis Diplopia		Pupillary abnormalities			History Tensilon test Lid twitch sign	Ocular myasthenia Thymoma Thyroid and diabetes Neurologist
Paget's disease	Choroidal sclerosis Angioid streaks Extraocular muscle palsies	Extraocular muscle palsies			Cataract?	Angioid streaks Optic atrophy Choroidal sclerosis	X-ray diagnosis Elevated serum alkaline phosphatase	Internist

EMG = electromyography.
* See also Chap. 10: osteogenesis imperfecta (sec. **VII**).

Table 14-15. Pulmonary diseases[*]

Clinical entity	Significant ocular findings	Orbit, motility, extraocular muscles	Lids, sclera, conjunctiva	Cornea, uvea	Lens, vitreous	Retina, optic nerve	Diagnostic tests	Differential diagnosis, referral to whom?
Asthma	Cataract[a] Secondary glaucoma[a]				Posterior subcapsular cataract[a]		Clinical diagnosis Family history	Internist
Bronchogenic carcinoma (see Table 14-17)	Metastasis to choroid and retina Metastatic lesions to iris			Metastasis to iris		Metastasis to choroid	Chest x ray Bronchoscopy and mediastinoscopy	Ocular metastasis Internist Ophthalmologist
Bronchiectasis						Dilatated tortuous retinal vessels Retinal edema Retinal hemorrhage	Chest x ray	Internist
Cystic fibrosis of the pancreas	Retinal vascular dilation Hemorrhage Papilledema Optic neuritis					Dilatated tortuous retinal vessels Retinal edema Retinal hemorrhage Macular holes	Sweat chloride Pancreatic enzymes Stool fats	Pediatrician
Emphysema	Cataract[a] Secondary glaucoma[b]				Posterior subcapsular cataract[a]	Papilledema Optic neuritis[b]	History of smoking Chest x ray Blood gases Spirometry	Internist
Pneumonias	(See Table 14-4)					Septic retinitis Roth's spots	Culture of sputums Blood cultures	Internist

[*] See also Chap. 8: tuberculosis (see **XI.A**).
[a] Resulting from treatment with corticosteroids.
[b] Resulting from long-term treatment with chloramphenicol.

417

Table 14-16. Renal diseases

Clinical entity	Significant ocular findings	Orbit, motility, extraocular muscles	Lids, sclera, conjunctiva	Cornea, uvea	Lens, vitreous	Retina, optic nerve	Diagnostic tests	Differential diagnosis, referral to whom?
Alport's syndrome (autosomal dominant)	Anterior lenticonus Anterior polar cataract				Anterior lenticonus Anterior polar cataract	White retinal dots Drusen of the optic nerve head	Clinical diagnosis Nerve deafness Proteinuria Hypertension Abnormal ERG	Nephrologist
Azotemia (acute and chronic pyelonephritis)	Retinal edema Retinal hemorrhage Cotton-wool exudates					Papilledema, severe Renal retinopathy Retinal detachment, nonrhegmatogenous	High BUN Renin levels Hypertension	Nephrotic syndrome Nephrologist
Lowe's syndrome (recessive X-linked)	Congenital cataract Congenital glaucoma				Small, thin lenses Posterior lenticonus		Aminoaciduria	Nephrologist Ophthalmologist
Medullary cystic disease (dominant or recessive)	Decreased vision Retinitis pigmentosa	Nystagmus				Retinitis pigmentosa Rod and cone degeneration		Nephrologist Ophthalmologist
Nephrotic syndrome (acute glomerulonephritis, diabetic kidney, systemic lupus erythematosus)	Mild retinopathy					Retinopathy, mild Retinal edema, mild Mild papilledema	No rise in BUN No hypertension Proteinuria present	Nephrologist
Renal transplantation	Cataract Glaucoma (Eye findings related to use of heavy doses of corticosteroids)				Posterior subcapsular cataract		Cushingoid appearance	Reduce amount of corticosteroids Ophthalmologist
Wilms' tumor (nephroblastoma)	Aniridia	Orbital mass		Aniridia			Flat plate of abdomen	Nephrologist Ophthalmologist

ERG = electroretinogram; BUN = blood urea nitrogen.

Table 14-17. Neoplastic diseases with ocular metastases

Carcinomas and sites of primary lesions	Ocular symptoms[a]	Orbit	Anterior segment	Posterior segment	Clinical appearance of eye lesion[b]	Diagnostic examinations
Blood Leukemia Lymphoma		Orbital infiltration common (lymphoma, granulocytic leukemia)	Uveitis with reticulum cell sarcomeres Cells in the vitreous	Nerve fiber layer hemorrhage Roth's spots Macular hemorrhage Vascular lesions		Ultrasonography Photos of the fundus Fluorescein angiography Phosphorus-32 uptake studies Cytologies on aqueous aspirates
Breast (high incidence of ocular metastasis)		Orbital metastasis frequent	Iris or angle metastasis common	Choroidal lesions common		
Colon		Unusual	Unusual	Choroidal and retinal metastasis		
Kidney		Unusual	Unusual	Choroidal and retinal metastasis		
Lung (high incidence of ocular metastasis)		Orbital metastasis frequent	Iris or angle metastasis common	Choroidal and retinal metastasis		Surgeon
Genital organs Ovary or cervix Testis or prostate		Unusual	Unusual	Choroidal and retinal metastasis		Urologist
Skin Melanoma (ocular metastasis unusual)		Rarely exophthalmus, ocular palsies	Rarely hyphema	Rarely		Cytologies on vitreous aspirates Dermatologist
Gut Stomach Pancreas	Blurred vision Loss of vision	Unusual	Unusual	Choroidal and retinal metastasis		Surgeon

Table 14-17. (continued)

Carcinomas and sites of primary lesions	Ocular symptoms[a]	Orbit	Anterior segment	Posterior segment	Clinical appearance of eye lesion[b]	Diagnostic examinations
Thyroid (infrequently metastasis to eye)	Loss of field		May occur	Unusual choroidal and retinal metastasis		Endocrinologist Surgeon

[a]All of the following are likely with metastatic lesions of the ocular structures: visible mass; pain; redness; hyphema; exophthalmus; ocular palsies; blurred vision; loss of field.
[b]All metastatic lesions in the eye share these clinical characteristics: pale gray or yellow color; flatness (not usually elevated); faster growth rate than primary malignant melanoma; poor ocular prognosis.

Ocular Drug Toxicity

Gilbert K. Yamamoto

I. **General considerations.** Many undesired side effects on the ocular tissues have been reported involving various drugs used for both the treatment of systemic medical disorders and for local ophthalmic problems. The types of adverse effects of drugs on the eye may be mild and transient, such as temporary decreased visual acuity, impairment of accommodation, abnormal pupillary responses, and color vision disturbances. Other effects, such as eye movement abnormalities, glaucoma, cataracts, and retinal damage, may seriously reduce ocular function. In order to recognize and prevent vision-threatening complications from adverse effects of drug reactions, it is necessary for the clinician to obtain a careful history, with particular attention to specific medications used. The clinician must then be aware of certain oculotoxic drugs and their side effects to recognize the drug-related eye disorder.

II. **Pretreatment examination.** For certain drugs with potential ocular toxicity, a careful pretreatment examination should be performed before the drug is administered, particularly if (1) the drug will be used for a long period of time (isoniazid, streptomycin, quinine, and indomethacin), or (2) it is known to have severe toxic effects (ethambutol, Plaquenil, and thioridazine). Patients taking drugs that are not as toxic may not require the complete baseline examination prior to therapy, but they should undergo frequent monitoring examinations so that if symptoms do arise the drug can be withdrawn immediately. Reversible effects can likewise be observed while the patient is off the drug, and later, after resolution of the effects, the drug regimen may be judiciously reinstituted at a lower dose. The pretreatment examination should include the following:

   A. **Visual acuity with glasses.** Drugs that may alter the visual acuity during the course of therapy include

   Allopurinol
   Chlorambucil
   Chloramphenicol
   Chloroquine
   Corticosteroids
   Digitalis drugs
   Diiodohydroxyquin
   Ethambutol
   Ethchlorvynol
   Ethionamide
   Hydroxychloroquine
   Ibuprofen
   Indomethacin
   Iodochlorhydroxyquin
   Isoniazid
   Monoamine oxidase (MAO) inhibitors
   Nicotinic acid
   Piperazine
   Tetracycline
   Thioridazine
   Tryparsamide
   Vitamin A

Patients who are about to use these drugs should have acuity screening at near and distance with and without pinhole testing.

B. Pupillary responses. Drugs that may alter pupillary responses during the course of therapy include

Amitriptyline (antidepressants)
Amphetamines (CNS stimulants)
Antianxiety agents
Antihistamines
Anticholinergics
Chloral hydrate
Chlorpromazine
Chlorpropamide
Haloperidol
Hexamethonium
Indomethacin
L-Dopa
Morphine (opiates)
Reserpine
Salicylates

Patients who are about to use these drugs should have pupil size, briskness of reactions (direct and consensual) to light, and convergence reflex tested.

C. Ocular motility examination. Drugs that may affect eye movements during the course of therapy include

Alcohol
Antianxiety agents
Antidepressants
Barbiturates
Chlordiazepoxide (Librium)
Chlorpromazine
Diazepam (Valium)
Ethchlorvynol
Gold salts
Nalidixic acid
Phenytoin (Dilantin)
Piperazine
Salicylates
Tetracycline
Vitamin A

Patients who are about to use these drugs should have a complete motility examination in all fields of gaze with ductions, versions, and convergence.

D. Intraocular pressures. Drugs that may alter the eye pressure during the course of therapy include

Anticholinergics
Amphetamines
Corticosteroids
Hexamethonium
Reserpine
Tricyclic antidepressants (amitriptyline)

Periodic tonometry should be performed.

E. Slit-lamp examination (biomicroscopy). Drugs that may affect the **conjunctiva, cornea,** and **lens** during the course of therapy include

Amiodarone
Antimalarials
Allopurinol
Chloroquine

Chlorpromazine
Corticosteroids
Gold salts
Hydroxychloroquine
Indomethacin
Isotretinoin
Practolol
Psoralens
Tetracycline
Vitamin D

Loupe or slit-lamp examination is indicated.

F. Ophthalmoscopy (retinoscopy). Drugs that may cause changes in the **retina** and the **optic nerve** include

Allopurinol
Anticoagulants
Antimalarials
Chlorambucil
Chloramphenicol
Chloroquine
Chlorpromazine
Contraceptives, oral
Corticosteroids
Digitalis
Diiodohydroxyquin
Ethambutol
Ethionamide
Hydroxychloroquine
Indomethacin
Iodochlorhydroxyquin
Isoniazid
MAO inhibitors
Nalidixic acid
Nicotinic acid
Quinine
Salicylates
Tamoxifen
Tetracycline
Thioridazine
Tryparsamide
Vitamin A

Patients who are about to use these drugs should have ophthalmoscopy performed, with dilation, if possible.

G. Special examinations for retinal function. Other tests may be performed to provide supplemental data on retinal function prior to the use of drugs listed in **F.** These examinations include

1. Photography of the fundus.

2. Electroretinography.

3. Visual fields.

4. Color vision tests.

III. Repeat eye examinations. The tests listed in **II.A, E,** and **F** should be repeated frequently if there is any clinical change noted during the course of the patient's therapy. Tests **II.B, C, D,** and **G** could be added at the discretion of the ophthalmologist consultant. Routine frequency of follow-up eye examinations for each specific drug is listed in Tables 15-1 through 15-7.

IV. Ocular manifestations of drug toxicity

A. Reduced visual acuity may result from transient changes in refractive errors induced by antibiotics, carbonic anhydrase inhibitors, and chlorothiazide diuretics. Cholinergic drugs and sedative-hypnotic agents may also bring about disturbing temporary changes in a patient's refractive error.

B. Blurred vision may be caused by dilated pupils (mydriasis) and impairment of accommodation (cycloplegia) resulting from anticholinergic agents, antihistamines, and other drugs used systemically, e.g., amphetamines, hexamethonium, L-dopa, and tricyclic antidepressants.

C. Color vision disturbances can be brought about by the digitalis preparations, trimethadione, chlorothiazide diuretics, and cannabis.

D. Ocular motility abnormalities such as paralytic strabismus, diplopia, and oculogyric crisis can be caused by agents such as anti-infective drugs (e.g., sulfonamides, piperazine), quinine preparations (e.g., chloroquine, quinine), and psychotropic drugs (e.g., haloperidol, diazepam, and ethchlorvynol).

E. Severe **conjunctival inflammation** and **corneal opacification** have occurred from the use of practolol (a beta blocker), sulfonamides, butazolidin, and gold.

F. Glaucoma may occur in those individuals with shallow anterior chamber angles who use anticholinergics (atropine, belladonna), reserpine, corticosteroids, tricyclic antidepressants (amitriptyline), amphetamines, and hexamethonium.

G. More serious are those adverse drug effects that occur in the crystalline **lens** and the **optic nerve.** Cataracts can be caused by corticosteroids and adrenocorticotropic hormone (ACTH) when these are used for a prolonged period of time. Optic neuritis is a serious complication that may result from the use of chloramphenicol, streptomycin, sulfa drugs, isoniazid, ethambutol, chlorpropamide (Diabinese), nicotinic acid, and tryparsamide.

H. There are still other oculotoxic conditions, such as **exophthalmus** (corticosteroids, vitamin A), **retinal** hemorrhages (chlorothiazides, anticoagulants, salicylates), retinal pigment epitheliopathy and **macular** edema (hydroxychloroquine, chloroquine, quinine, nicotinc acid), and retinal vein thrombosis (oral contraceptive agents).

V. Drugs and their ocular toxicity. Tables 15-1 through 15-7 represent major drug classifications under which are listed specific drugs and their potential adverse ocular side effects. Also tabulated are associated symptoms and signs according to specific ocular structures, pertinent ocular examinations, recommended pretreatment examination, and frequency of follow-up ocular examinations while the patient is using the particular drug.

For a more extensive listing, see D. Pavan-Langston and E. Dunkel, *Handbook of Ocular Drug Therapy and Ocular Side Effects of Systemic Drugs* (Boston: Little, Brown, 1991).

Table 15-1. Adverse effects of central nervous system drugs

Drug	Significant adverse ocular effects and symptoms	Orbit, motility, extraocular muscles	Lids, sclera, conjunctiva	Cornea, uvea	Lens, vitreous	Retina, optic nerve	Pertinent ocular examinations	Pretreatment examination, frequency of follow-up examinations
Barbiturates	Ptosis Ocular hypotony Color vision disturbance	Diplopia Nystagmus	Ptosis Dermatitis of skin of lids Conjunctivitis	Mydriasis Miosis		Optic atrophy Papillitis Retinal vessel constriction (all rare)	Visual acuity Color vision Eye movement examination Pupil examination Ophthalmoscopy	Not necessary Every 6-12 months
Chloral hydrate	Miosis Ptosis Tearing	Diplopia	Ptosis Conjunctivitis				Visual acuity Slit-lamp examination Ophthalmoscopy	Not necessary If symptoms arise
Chlorpromazine (Thorazine)	Oculogyric crises Miosis Elevation of IOP possible but very rare		Hyperpigmentation of skin of lids, conjunctiva, and cornea	Corneal pigment deposition—deep stromal location near DM	Pigment deposition on lens	Hyperpigmentation of retina—RPE disturbance Optic atrophy	Visual acuity Eye movement examination Slit-lamp examination Ophthalmoscopy Pressure check ERG testing	Complete eye examination Every 3-6 months
Phenytoin (Dilantin)	Blurred vision Conjunctivitis	Diplopia (rare) Nystagmus Ophthalmoplegias	Ptosis Allergic conjunctivitis				Visual acuity Eye movement examination Slit-lamp examination	Not necessary Annually
Ethchlorvynol	Optic neuritis	Nystagmus, from overdosage				Optic neuritis	Visual acuity Eye movement examination Color vision Visual fields Ophthalmoscopy	Complete eye examination 6 months to 1 year

Table 15-1. (continued)

Drug	Significant adverse ocular effects and symptoms	Orbit, motility, extraocular muscles	Lids, sclera, conjunctiva	Cornea, uvea	Lens, vitreous	Retina, optic nerve	Pertinent ocular examinations	Pretreatment examination, frequency of follow-up examinations
Haloperidol (Haldol)	Blurred vision from mydriasis Cycloplegia Slight lowering of IOP	Oculogyric crises			Lens opacities possible		Visual acuity, near vision Eye movement examination Slit-lamp examination Pressure check	Not necessary If symptoms arise
L-Dopa (Levodopa)	Mydriasis		Eyelid retraction with discomfort				Pupil examination	Not necessary When necessary
MAO inhibitors	Vision disturbances Visual field changes			Mydriasis		Color vision changes Optic neuritis	Visual acuity Color vision Visual fields Ophthalmoscopy	Complete eye examination 3–6 months
Morphine	Miosis Blurred vision Transient myopia Weakness of convergence						Pupil examination Visual acuity Refraction Eye movement examination	Not necessary If symptoms arise Every 6 months
Perphenazine	Oculogyric crises Optic neuritis (rare)	Oculogyric crises				Optic neuritis	Visual acuity Eye movement examination Color vision and ophthalmoscopy if optic neuritis is suspected	Not necessary If symptoms arise
Prochlorperazine	Oculogyric crises Transient myopia Blurred vision	Oculogyric crises					Eye movement examination Vision and refraction	Not necessary If symptoms arise

Drug	Visual effects	Ocular motility	External/conjunctival signs	Fundus signs	Examination	Recommendations
Thioridazine (Mellaril)	Reduced vision Pigmentary retinopathy			Black pigmentary stippling in central fundus	Visual acuity Ophthalmoscopy Color vision Visual field examination Fundic photography ERG testing	Complete examination recommended Patients taking over 800 mg/day seen at 2 to 6-month intervals
Tricyclic antidepressants (Elavil)	Possible narrow-angle glaucoma Cycloplegia Mydriasis				Visual acuity Refraction Pupil examination Ophthalmoscopy Pressure check	Screen patient for narrow angles If symptoms arise pressure check every 6 months
Trimethadione (anticonvulsant)	Sensitivity to bright lights Faded colors	Diplopia (rare) Nystagmus (rare)	Conjunctivitis	Retinal functional changes	Visual acuity Color vision ERG testing if symptoms are severe	Not necessary 6 to 12-month intervals if symptoms arise
Diazepam (Valium)	Blurred vision Blink suppression, probably centrally mediated	Diplopia Nystagmus from overdosage			Visual acuity Eye movement examination Pupil examination	Not necessary When necessary
Amphetamines	Mydriasis Blurring of vision Rise in IOP	Oculogyric crises (rare)	Widened lid fissures		Visual acuity Pupil examination Refraction Eye movement examination Pressure test	Screen angles and chamber depth 6-12 months
Cannabis (marijuana)	Visual disturbances (mainly related to CNS effects) Color perception Lowering of IOP	Diplopia	Conjunctival vessel dilation		Visual acuity Pressure check	Not necessary Glaucoma examination every 12 months

IOP = intraocular pressure; DM = Descemet's membrane; RPE = retinal pigment epithelium; ERG = electroretinogram; MAO = monoamine oxidase; CNS = central nervous system.

Table 15-2. Adverse effects of cholinergic and anticholinergic drugs

Drug	Significant adverse ocular effects and symptoms	Orbit, motility, extraocular muscles	Lids, sclera, conjunctiva	Cornea, uvea	Lens, vitreous	Retina, optic nerve	Pertinent ocular examinations	Pretreatment examination, frequency of follow-up examinations
Neostigmine (myasthenia gravis)	Miosis Lowering of IOP	Nystagmus	Conjunctival hyperemia	Iris cysts (rare)			Pupil examination Visual acuity Pressure check Ophthalmoscopy	Not necessary 3–6 months
Carbachol	Miosis Lowering of IOP Increase in tearing					Retinal detachments (rare)	Pupil examination Visual acuity Pressure check Ophthalmoscopy	Usually under care of ophthalmologist
Atropine (GI medication, iritis)	Mydriasis Blurred vision Acute angle-closure glaucoma possible	Diplopia	Decreased lacrimation				Pupil examination Refraction Pressure check Slit-lamp examination Eye movement examination	Usually under care of ophthalmologist Screen angles and chamber depth

IOP = intraocular pressure; GI = gastrointestinal.

Table 15-3. Adverse effects of anti-infective drugs

Drug	Significant adverse ocular effects and symptoms	Orbit, motility, extraocular muscles	Lids, sclera, conjunctiva	Cornea, uvea	Lens, vitreous	Retina, optic nerve	Pertinent ocular examinations	Pretreatment examination, frequency of follow-up examinations
Chloramphenicol (antibacterial)	Blurred vision Central scotoma Optic neuritis					Optic neuritis	Visual acuity Visual fields Color vision Ophthalmoscopy	For aplastic anemia and bone marrow depression
Chloroquine (Aralen) (antimalarial, systemic lupus erythematosus, rheumatoid arthritis)	Retinal pigment epithelial damage Corneal deposits	Ocular palsies	Whitening of eyelashes Ptosis	Corneal subepithelial deposition (vortex pattern) Corneal edema Decreased corneal sensitivity		Atypical retinitis pigmentosa— vessel narrowing, macular bull's-eye lesion Optic atrophy	Visual acuity Ophthalmoscopy Slit-lamp examination EOM examination Fundic photography	Complete eye examination Acuity checks every 3–6 months Fundic examination
Ethambutol: safe dose = 15 mg/kg/day (tuberculosis)	Optic neuritis Decreased vision and faulty red or green color vision					Optic neuritis (axial and periaxial)	Visual acuity Color vision Ophthalmoscopy Visual fields	Complete eye examination Monthly visual acuity tests for first 6 months
Ethionamide (tuberculosis)	Optic neuritis (rare)					Optic neuritis (rare)	Visual acuity Color vision Ophthalmoscopy Visual fields	Complete eye examination Acuity check and color vision screen every 3–6 months
Hydroxychloroquine (Plaquenil)	Pigmentary retinopathy Corneal deposits			Corneal subepithelial deposition (vortex pattern)		Retinal pigment dispersion "Bull's-eye" maculopathy	Visual acuity Slit-lamp examination Ophthalmoscopy Fundic photography	Complete eye examination Retinal examination Visual acuity every 3–6 months depending on dose

Table 15-3. (continued)

Drug	Significant adverse ocular effects and symptoms	Orbit, motility, extraocular muscles	Lids, sclera, conjunctiva	Cornea, uvea	Lens, vitreous	Retina, optic nerve	Pertinent ocular examinations	Pretreatment examination, frequency of follow-up examinations
Iodochlorhydroxyquin; diiodohydroxyquin	Subacute myelooptic neuropathy Optic atrophy					Optic atrophy	Visual acuity Ophthalmoscopy Visual fields	Monthly acuity and ophthalmoscopy examinations during first 6 months
Isoniazid	Optic neuritis Keratitis						Visual acuity Slit-lamp examination Ophthalmoscopy Visual fields	Complete eye examination Visual acuity and color vision 3–6 months
Nalidixic acid	Blurred vision Papilledema	Sixth nerve palsy				Papilledema	Visual acuity Eye movement examination Ophthalmoscopy	Visual acuity and ophthalmoscopy monthly
Piperazine (anthelmintic)	Vague visual disturbances	Paralytic strabismus (rare)					Visual acuity Refraction Eye movement examination Color vision	Not necessary Monthly if symptoms arise
Quinine (antimalarial, myotonia)	Diplopia Loss of vision— transient, reversible Central scotoma Optic atrophy	Diplopia		Iris atrophy		Optic atrophy Retinal pigment epitheliopathy? Bipolar and ganglion layer damage Retinal vessels narrow	Visual acuity Eye movement examination Visual fields ERG testing Ophthalmoscopy Slit-lamp examination	Complete eye examination Monthly examinations if symptoms arise

Streptomycin (tuberculosis)	Optic neuritis		Optic neuritis	Visual acuity Color vision Visual fields Ophthalmoscopy	Complete eye examination 6 to 12-month examinations
Sulfonamides (antibiotics)	Exudative conjunctivitis Transient myopia	Ocular palsies Iritis	Optic neuritis Retinal hemorrhage or edema or both	Visual acuity Eye movement examination Slit-lamp examination Color vision Ophthalmoscopy	Not necessary Examine monthly if symptoms arise
Tetracycline (antibiotic)	Blurred vision Papilledema		Papilledema associated with benign intracranial hypertension	Visual acuity Refraction Ophthalmoscopy	Not necessary 3–6 months for those on long-term therapy
Tryparsamide (syphilis, trypanosomiasis)	Optic neuritis		Optic neuritis Constriction of fields	Visual acuity Color vision Visual fields Ophthalmoscopy	Complete eye examination 6-month examinations

EOM = extraocular muscle; ERG = electroretinogram.

Table 15-4. Adverse effects of cardiovascular drugs

Drug	Significant adverse ocular effects and symptoms	Orbit, motility, extraocular muscles	Lids, sclera, conjunctiva	Cornea, uvea	Lens, vitreous	Retina, optic nerve	Pertinent ocular examinations	Pretreatment examination, frequency of follow-up examinations
Carbonic anhydrase inhibitors Acetazolamide (Diamox)	Transient myopia Ocular hypotony Retinal hemorrhages					Retinal edema Retinal hemorrhages	Visual acuity Refraction Intraocular pressure check Ophthalmoscopy	Not necessary 6–12 months
Chlorothiazides (Diuril)	Xanthopsia— yellow vision Transient myopia Retinal hemorrhages					Retinal hemorrhages	Color vision Refraction Ophthalmoscopy	Not necessary 6–12 months Frequency depends on symptoms and dosages
Diazoxide	Increased tearing Oculogyric symptoms	Eyes rolling upward	Increased tearing				Eye movement examination	Not necessary
Digitalis preparations (digoxin)	Color vision disturbances Xanthopsia Scotomas	Ocular palsies	Conjunctivitis				Visual acuity Color vision Eye movement examination Slit-lamp examination Ophthalmoscopy	Not necessary Annually
Guanethidine	Ptosis Conjunctival injection and hyperemia		Ptosis Conjunctival hyperemia				Lid examination Slit-lamp examination	Not necessary Annually
Hexamethonium	Mydriasis Cycloplegia Risk of glaucoma Dry eye Optic neuritis					Optic neuritis Optic atrophy Retinal hemorrhage and macular edema (rare)	Visual acuity Pupil examination Pressure check Slit-lamp examination Ophthalmoscopy	Screen angle and chamber depth 6–12 months if symptoms arise

Drug	Effects	Rare effects	Examination	Follow-up
Furosemide (Lasix)	Color vision disturbance Slight lowering of IOP		Visual acuity Color vision Pressure check	Not necessary Annual examination
Practolol	Dry eye Conjunctival damage Decreased vision Conjunctivitis Symblepharon Entropion Keratitis sicca Corneal thinning, opacification, scarring and ulceration		Visual acuity Slit-lamp examination Schirmer and rose bengal testing	Complete eye examination Monthly examination—change drug if symptoms arise
Quinidine	Optic neuritis—quinine-type (rare) Visual disturbances	Optic neuritis (rare)	Visual acuity Refraction Color vision Ophthalmoscopy	Not necessary If symptoms arise, 6–12 months
Reserpine	Miosis Conjunctival hyperemia Glaucoma Ocular palsies (rare) Conjunctival injection and hyperemia	Iritis (rare)	Slit-lamp examination Pressure check Eye movement examination	Not necessary 3–6 months

IOP = intraocular pressure.

Table 15-5. Adverse effects of antirheumatoid drugs

Drug	Significant adverse ocular effects and symptoms	Orbit, motility, extraocular muscles	Lids, sclera, conjunctiva	Cornea, uvea	Lens, vitreous	Retina, optic nerve	Pertinent ocular examinations	Pretreatment examination, frequency of follow-up examinations
Butazolidin (rheumatoid arthritis, gout)	Conjunctivitis Dry eye	Ocular muscle palsies (rare)	Conjunctivitis	Corneal erosion, ulcerative keratitis (rare)		Optic neuritis (rare) Retinal hemorrhages	Visual acuity Slit-lamp examination Ophthalmoscopy	Not required Follow-up every 3–6 months
Gold salts	Lid dermatitis Corneal deposits	Nystagmus (rare) Ocular palsies, secondary to encephalitis	Exfoliative dermatitis of lids Conjunctivitis	Ulcerative keratitis Gold deposits in deep stroma			Slit-lamp examination Eye movement examination Ophthalmoscopy	Not necessary Examine every 6–12 months
Ibuprofen	Color vision disturbance Blurred vision—reversible					Color vision disturbance in cones?	Visual acuity Color vision Ophthalmoscopy	Not necessary Periodic examinations if symptoms arise
Indomethacin (Indocin)	Corneal deposits Mydriasis	Diplopia		Corneal deposits (vortex pattern) in corneal stroma		Various retinal findings Macular edema Central serous retinopathy (rare)	Visual acuity Slit-lamp examination Ophthalmoscopy	Complete examination helpful but not required Follow-up every 6 months
Salicylates	Retinal hemorrhages Mydriasis Ocular hypotony	Nystagmus	Conjunctivitis			Retinal hemorrhages Optic neuritis	Visual acuity Ophthalmoscopy Pressure check Slit-lamp examination Color vision Visual fields	Not necessary Every 6 months

Table 15-6. Adverse effects of hormonal agents

Drug	Significant adverse ocular effects and symptoms	Orbit, motility, extraocular muscles	Lids, sclera, conjunctiva	Cornea, uvea	Lens, vitreous	Retina, optic nerve	Pertinent ocular examinations	Pretreatment examination, frequency of follow-up examinations
ACTH	Transient myopia				Cataracts— posterior subcapsular (less common than with corticosteroids)	Papilledema	Visual acuity Slit-lamp examination Pressure check Refractive examination Ophthalmoscopy	Complete examination Every 2–3 months
Corticosteroids	Transient myopia	Exophthalmus	Ptosis	Mydriasis	Cataracts— posterior subcapsular	Retinopathy Papilledema with pseudotumor Glaucoma	Visual acuity Slit-lamp examination Ophthalmoscopy	Every 2–3 months
Oral contraceptives	Optic neuritis Scotomas associated with migraine headaches			Alterations in corneal curvature?		Central retinal vein and artery occlusion Retinal perivasculitis Papillitis	Visual acuity Visual fields Ophthalmoscopy Fundic photography Color vision Slit-lamp examination	Complete eye examination Every 3 months; more frequently if symptoms arise

ACTH = adrenocorticotropic hormone.

435

Table 15-7. Adverse effects of other therapeutic agents

Drug	Significant adverse ocular effects and symptoms	Orbit, motility, extraocular muscles	Lids, sclera, conjunctiva	Cornea, uvea	Lens, vitreous	Retina, optic nerve	Pertinent ocular examinations	Pretreatment examination, frequency of follow-up examinations
Allopurinol (Zyloprim)	Cataracts (rare)				Cataracts (rare)	Macular lesions (rare)	Visual acuity Slit-lamp examination Ophthalmoscopy	Not necessary 8 to 12-month examinations
Anticoagulants (Coumadin)	Intraocular hemorrhages (rare)					Retinal hemorrhages	Ophthalmoscopy	Not necessary
Chlorambucil	Corneal epithelial damage (rare) Papilledema			Minor corneal epithelial irregularity associated with exfoliative dermatitis			Slit-lamp examination Ophthalmoscopy	Not necessary, but usually when treatment is for uveitis, Behçet's syndrome
Chlorpropamide (Diabinese)	Mydriasis Refractive errors Diplopia	Diplopia	Conjunctivitis			Optic neuritis	Visual acuity Color vision Slit-lamp examination Refraction and eye muscle examination	Not required Follow-up for diabetic retinopathy

Vitamin A	Ocular palsies Retinal hemorrhages	Exophthalmus Ocular palsies Nystagmus Diplopia	Loss of eyebrows and eyelashes Blepharoconjunctivitis (rare)	Retinal hemorrhages Papilledema	Eye movement examination Ophthalmoscopy Exophthalmometry	Not necessary If symptoms arise, and long duration overdosage occurs
Vitamin D	Band keratopathy		Conjunctival calcium deposits	Corneal calcium deposits Band keratopathy	Slit-lamp examination Visual acuity	Not necessary Follow-up examination every 6–12 months for calcification
Nicotinic acid	Maculopathy (possible) Optic neuritis Retinal edema	Proptosis (rare)		Optic neuritis, maculopathy Cystoid macular edema (Gass)	Visual acuity Color and Amsler tests Ophthalmoscopy Fluorescein angiography	Not necessary If maculopathy develops, refer to ophthalmologist

Appendixes

Formulary and Common Dosages of Topical and Systemic Ophthalmic Drugs

Deborah Pavan-Langston

I. **Antiallergy Solutions** (decongestant-antihistamine)
   Usual dose: qd–qid
   A. Phenylephrine 0.12%, pyrilamine maleate 0.1%, and antipyrine 0.1% (Prefrin).
   B. Phenylephrine HCl 0.12% and pheniramine maleate 0.5% (AK-Vernacon).
   C. Naphazoline HCl 0.025% and pheniramine maleate 0.3% (AK-Con-A, Naphcon-A, Opcon-A).
   D. Naphazoline HCl 0.05% and antazoline PO₄ 0.5% (Albalon-A, Vasocon-A).

II. **Topical anesthetic solutions**
   Usual dose: 1–2 drops for temporary (15–20 minutes) anesthesia to allow ocular examination and manipulation.
   A. Cocaine 1–4%.
   B. Benoxinate 0.4%, with fluorescein (Fluress).
   C. Proparacaine HCl 0.5% (Proparacaine, AK-Taine, Ophthaine, Ophthetic; with fluorescein (Fluorocaine).
   D. Tetracaine HCl 0.5% (Tetracaine, Pontocaine).

III. **Topical antibiotic solutions and ointments** (see also sec. **V** and Appendix B)
   Usual dose: tid or qid for 1–2 weeks.
   A. Bacitracin: ointment, 500 units/gm.
   B. Chloramphenicol: ointment 1%; solution 0.05, 0.16, 0.5, 1.0% (AK-Chlor, Chloroptic, Ophthochlor).
   C. Erythromycin: ointment 0.5% (Ilotycin).
   D. Gentamicin: ointment or solution 0.3% (Garamycin, Genoptic, Gentacidin).
   E. Neomycin, 0.35%; polymyxin B, 10,000 units; and bacitracin, 500 units/gm, ointment (Neosporin, AK-Spore, Ocutricin). Neomycin-polymyxin B-gramicidin 0.0025% solution (AK-Spore, Neosporin, Neotricin).
   F. Polymyxin B, 10,000 units, and bacitracin, 500 units/gm, ointment (AK PolyBac, Polysporin).
   G. Polymyxin B, 10,000 units/ml or gm, and neomycin, 0.35%, solution and ointment (Statrol).
   H. Sulfacetamide: ointment 10%; solution 10%, 15%, or 30% (AK-Sulf, Bleph-10, Sulamyd, Isopto-cetamide); with 0.12% phenylephrine (Vasosulf).
   I. Sulfisoxazole: solution or ointment 4% (Gantrisin).
   J. Tetracycline: ointment 1% (Achromycin). Chlortetracycline 1% (Aureomycin). Oxytetracycline 0.5% and polymyxin B, 10,000 units/gm (Terramycin).
   K. Tobramycin: ointment or solution 0.3% (Tobrex).
   L. Trimethoprim 0.1% and polymyxin B, 10,000 units/ml (Polytrim).

IV. **Topical anti-inflammatory agents: corticosteroids**
   Usual dose: See text on specific disease entity.
   A. Prednisolone:
     1. Acetate suspension 0.12% (Pred Mild, Econopred) or 1.0% (AK-Tate, Econopred Plus, Pred Forte).

Names in parentheses are a partial list of proprietary names of drugs.

Concentrations of drugs in combination antibiotics may vary slightly among manufacturers. Major differences are so indicated.

      2. Sodium phosphate solution 0.12% (AK-Pred, Inflamase Mild), 0.5% (Metreton), or 1% (AK-Pred, Inflamase Forte).
  B. Dexamethasone:
      1. Phosphate solution 0.1% (AK-Dex, Baldex, Decadron).
      2. Suspension 0.1% (Maxidex).
      3. Phosphate ointment 0.05% (AK-Dex, Baldex, Decadron, Maxidex).
  C. Progesterone-like agents:
      1. Medrysone 1.0% (HMS).
      2. Fluorometholone suspension 0.1% (FML), 1% (FML Forte).
  D. Steroid—mydriatic/cycloplegic: prednisolone acetate 0.25% and atropine SO$_4$ 1% (Mydrapred).
V. **Topical anti-inflammatory agents: corticosteroid-antibiotic combinations**
  Usual dose: Based on desired corticosteroid dose; see text on specific disease entity.
  A. Hydrocortisone 0.5% and chloromycetin 2.5% solution.
  B. Hydrocortisone 0.5%, chloramphenicol 0.1%, and polymyxin B, 10,000 units/gm, ointment (Ophthocort).
  C. Hydrocortisone 0.5% and neomycin 0.35% solution (Neo-Cortef).
  D. Hydrocortisone 1%; polymyxin B, 10,000 units/gm; bacitracin, 400 units/gm; and neomycin ointment (Cortisporin); suspension (Cortisporin, Bacticort).
  E. Hydrocortisone 1.5%, with 0.5% oxytetracycline suspension (Terra-Cortril) or 0.35% neomycin (AK-NeoCort).
  F. Prednisolone 0.2% and sulfacetamide 10% solution (Blephamide, Isopto-Cetapred, Vasocidin); with 0.5% prednisolone (Metamyd, Predsulfair, Sulfrin, Vasocidin); ointment with 0.2% prednisolone (Blephamide, Cetapred) or 0.5% prednisolone (AK-Cide, Metamyd, Vasocidin).
  G. Prednisolone 0.5%, neomycin 0.35%, and polymyxin B, 10,000 units/ml, suspension (Polypred).
  H. Prednisolone 1% and gentamicin 0.3% suspension (Pred-G).
  I. Dexamethasone 0.1% with neomycin 0.35% (NeoDecadron); with neomycin 0.35% and polymyxin B, 10,000 units/ml (Dexasporin, AK-Trol, Dexacidin, Maxitrol), suspension or ointment.
  J. Dexamethasone 0.1% and tobramycin 0.3% suspension (TobraDex).
VI. **Topical antifungal agents**
  Usual dose: Every 1 or 2 hours initially; see text on specific disease entity for regimen and systemic doses. Only pimaricin is FDA approved for the eye.
  A. Amphotericin B, 0.075–0.3% in distilled water, or dextrose 5% in water solution (made up by pharmacy).
  B. Clotrimazole 1% solution (made up by pharmacy).
  C. Flucytosine solution 1% (made up by pharmacy).
  D. Miconazole solution 1% (parenteral preparation).
  E. Pimaricin suspension 5% (Natamycin).
VII. **Antiglaucoma agents: solutions, carbonic anhydrase inhibitors, and hyperosmotic agents**
  A. Miotics
      1. Carbachol* solution 0.75, 1.5, 2.25, 3% (Carbacel, Isoptocarbachol).
        Usual dose: bid or tid.
      2. Demecarium* 0.125, 0.25% (Humorsol).
        Usual dose: qd-bid.
      3. Echothiophate iodide (phospholine iodide)* solution 0.06%, 0.03%, 0.125%, 0.25% (Echodide).
        Usual dose: qd-bid.
      4. Isofluorophate* 0.025% (Fluropryl).
        Usual dose: qd-bid.
      5. Pilocarpine HCl* 0.25, 0.5, 1, 2, 3, 4, 6, 10% (Adsorbocarpine, Isoptocarpine, Pilocar, Pilomiotin, PV Carpine, Ocusert P 20 or P 40 insert, Pilopine 4% gel).

* Pupillary constrictor (miotic).

Usual dose: 2–6 times daily.
6. Pilocarpine* (P) varied %, epinephrine 1% (E) solution*: combinations (P_1, E_1 to P_6E_1, E-Pilo 1 to E-Pilo 6).
Usual dose: up to qid.
B. **Sympathomimetics**
1. Apraclonidine 1% (Iopidine) pre- and post-laser; q12h (not established).
2. Dipivalyl epinephrine solution 1%† (Propine).
Usual dose: bid.
3. Epinephrine†; borate, bitartrate, or HCl 0.25, 0.5, 1.2% (E-1, E-2, Epifrin, Eppy 1N, Glaucon).
Usual dose: bid or tid.
C. **Beta blockers**
Usual dose: qd–bid
1. Betaxolol 0.5% (Betoptic).
2. Levobunalol 0.5% (Betagan).
3. Timolol solution 0.25% or 0.5% (Timoptic).
D. **Carbonic anhydrase inhibitors**
1. Acetazolamide, 125- or 250-mg tablets (Diamox).
Usual dose: up to qid.
Acetazolamide, 500-mg capsules (Diamox).
Usual dose: q12h.
Acetazolamide 250–500 mg/5–10 ml in distilled water (Diamox).
Usual dose: 500 mg IV q12h.
2. Dichlorphenamide, 50-mg tablets (Daranide).
Usual dose: up to qid.
3. Methazolamide, 50- or 100-mg tablets (Neptazane).
Usual dose: up to tid.
E. **Hyperosomotic agents**
1. Glycerin 75% (Glynol, Osmoglyn).
Usual dose: 1.0–1.5 gm/kg body weight PO (on ice with juice preferably).
2. Isosorbide 45% (Ismotic).
Usual dose: 1.5 gm/kg body weight PO.
3. Mannitol 20% (Osmitrol).
Usual dose: 1–2 gm/kg body weight IV over 30–60 minutes.
VIII. **Antiviral agents**
A. Acyclovir 3% ointment (Zovirax).
Usual dose: 5 times/day for 14 days.
B. Acyclovir, 200-mg tablet (Zovirax).
Usual dose: 200 mg 5 times/day–800 mg 5 times/day PO for 10 days (see text).
C. Acyclovir IV (Zovirax).
Usual dose: 5 mg/kg q8h for 5–10 days (see text).
D. Azidothymidine (AZT, Retrovir).
Usual dose: 100–200 mg PO q4h to q8h (see text).
E. Ganciclovir (Cytovene).
Usual dose: 2.5 mg/kg IV q8h for 10 days, then 5 mg/kg/day (see text).
F. Idoxuridine, solution 0.1% or ointment 0.5% (Stoxil, Herplex).
Usual dose: Solution—qh during the day, q2h at night for 10–21 days.
Ointment—5 times/day for 10–21 days.
G. Vidarabine ointment 3% (Vira-A).
Usual dose: 5 times/day for 14–21 days.
H. Trifluorothymidine solution 1% (Viroptic).
Usual dose: 9 times/day for 14 days.
IX. **Artificial tears and lubricants for dry eyes** ** (partial listing)
A. Methylcellulose or ethylcellulose base:

* Pupillary constrictor (miotic).
† Mild dilator.
** Commercial names given for simplicity.

1. Celluvisc.*
2. Isopto Tears.
3. Lacril solution or Lacri-Lube ointment.
4. Lyteers.
5. Tearisol.
6. Tears Renewed.
B. Polyvinyl alcohol base solutions:
    1. Akwa Tears.
    2. Hypotears.
    3. Liquifilm.
    4. Liquifilm Forte.
    5. Murine.
    6. Refresh.*
C. Polyvinylpyrrolidone polymer base: Adsorbonac sodium chloride 2% or 5% (hyperosmotic).
D. Ointments:
    1. Akwa Tears.*
    2. Duolube.*
    3. Duratears Naturale.
    4. Hypotears.*
    5. Lacrilube.*
    6. Refresh PM.*

X. **Dilating and cycloplegic agents**
   A. Atropine, ointment 0.5% or 1% or solution 0.5, 1, 2, 3% (Atropine Sulfate, Atropisol, Isopto-Atropine).
     Usual dose: qd–qid, as needed.
   B. Cyclopentolate solution 0.5, 1, 2% (AK-Pentolate, Cyclogel).
     Usual dose: qd–qid.
   C. Homatropine solution 2 or 5% (Homatropine HBr, Isopto Homatropine, AK-Homatropine, Homatrine).
     Usual dose: qd–qid as needed.
   D. Phenylephrine solution 2.5 or 10% (AK-Dilate, Mydfrin, Neo-Synephrine Hydrochloride [Ophthalmic], I-Phrine).
     Usual dose: qd–tid.
   E. Scopolamine solution 0.25% (Isopto Hyoscine).
     Usual dose: qd–qid for 4–7 days.
   F. Tropicamide solution 0.5% or 1% (Mydriacyl, Tropicacyl, Tropicamide).
     Usual dose: qd–qid as needed.

XI. **Miotics (pupillary constrictors).** See sec. **VI.**
XII. **Ocular decongestants for unifected, red eyes** (partial listing)
   A. Ephedrine (Collyrium with ephedrine).
   B. Naphazoline hydrochloride (Ak-Con, Albalon, Clear Eyes, Degest 2, Naphcon, Opcon, Vasoclear, Vasocon Regular).
   C. Phenylephrine hydrochloride (Ak-Nefrin, Isopto Frin, Prefrin Liquifilm).
   D. Tetrahydrozoline hydrochloride (Murine Plus, Soothe, Visine).
   E. Zinc sulfate (Zincfrin).

* Preservative-free.

B

Dosages of Systemic Antimicrobial Drugs Used in Ocular Infections

Deborah Pavan-Langston

Drug	Adults Oral daily dosage	Adults Parenteral daily dosage	Children Oral daily dosage	Children Parenteral daily dosage	Usual divided dose interval
Amikacin		15 mg/kg IM, IV		15 mg/kg IM, IV	q8–12h
Amoxicillin/ clavulanic acid[a]	0.75–1.5 gm[2]		20–40 mg/kg		q8h
Ampicillin	2–4 gm	2–12 gm IM, IV	50–100 mg/kg	100–200 mg/kg IM, IV	q6–8h
Carbenicillin[a]	4–8 tablets (382 mg/tablet)	30–40 gm IM, IV	50–65 mg/kg	100–600 mg/kg IM, IV	q4–6h
Cefaclor (1)[b,c]	0.75–1.5 gm		20–40 mg/kg		q8h
Cefamandole (2)[b,c]		1.5–12 gm IM, IV		50–150 mg/kg IM, IV	q4–8h
Cefazolin (1)[b,c]		1–6 gm IM, IV		25–100 mg/kg IM, IV	q6–8h
Cefotaxime (3)[b,c]		2–12 gm IM, IV		100–200 mg/kg IM, IV	q4–8h
Cefoxitin (2)[b,c]		3–12 gm IM, IV		80–160 mg/kg IM, IV	q4–8h
Ceftizoxime (3)[b,c]		2–12 gm IM, IV		150–200 mg/kg	q6–12h
Ceftriaxone (3)[b,c]		1–4 gm IM, IV		50–100 mg/kg	q12–24h
Cephalexin (1)[b,c]	1–4 gm		25–50 mg/kg		q6h
Chloramphenicol	50–100 mg/kg	50–100 mg/kg IV	50–100 mg/kg	50–100 mg/kg IV	q6h
Ciprofloxacin[a,d]	0.5–1.5 gm				q12h
Clindamycin[d]	0.6–1.8 gm	0.6–3.6 gm IM, IV	10–25 mg/kg	10–40 mg/kg IM, IV	q6–8h
Cloxacillin[a]	2–4 gm		50–100 mg/kg		q6h

Usual maximum dose/day	Newborn (Parenteral)		Organism susceptibility guide
	Up to 1 week	1-4 weeks	
1.5 gm	15 mg/kg/day q12h	15.0-22.5 mg/kg/day q8-12h	*Pseudomonas, Escherichia coli, Herellea (Mima), Enterobacter, Proteus, Klebsiella Serratia marcescens, Staphylococcus aureus, Staphylococcus epidermidis*
1.5 gm	Not recommended	Not recommended	*S. aureus, S. epidermidis, Streptococcus* sp., *Haemophilus influenzae, Haemophilus ducreyi, Neisseria gonorrhoeae, E. coli, Klebsiella*
12 gm	50-100 mg/kg/day q12h	100-200 mg/kg/day q6-8h	*Streptococcus* sp., *Streptococcus pneumoniae, Neisseria, Staphylococcus* sp., *H. influenzae, Salmonella, Shigella, E. coli, Proteus*
40 gm	200-300 mg/kg/day q8h IM, IV	400 mg/kg/day q6h IM, IV	*Pseudomonas, Proteus, Klebsiella, E. coli, Serratia,* non-penicillinase-producing *Staphylococcus, Neisseria* sp., β-hemolytic streptococcus, *S. pneumoniae, Streptococcus faecalis,* anaerobes *(Bacteroides, Clostridium, Peptostreptococcus)*
4 gm			*Staphylococcus* sp. including penicillinase producers, *S. pneumoniae* and *Streptococcus pyogenes* but not *S. faecalis, Haemophilus, Escherichia, Proteus, Klebsiella, N. gonorrhoeae, Propionibacterium, Peptostreptococcus*
12 gm		50-150 mg/kg/day q4-8h IM, IV	*S. aureus, S. epidermidis, Streptococcus* sp. (except enterococci, e.g., *S. faecalis*), *Enterobacter, Haemophilus* sp., *E. coli, Klebsiella, Proteus* sp., *Clostridium, Bacteroides, Peptostreptococcus*
6 gm	30 mg/kg/day q12h IM, IV	30-60 mg/kg/day q8-12h IM, IV	See Cefaclor
12 gm	100 mg/kg/day q12h IM, IV	150 mg/kg/day q8h IM, IV	See Cefamandole
12 gm			
12 gm			See Cefamandole
4 gm			See Cefamandole *Neisseria* meningitidis and *N. gonorrhoeae*
4 gm	Not recommended	Not recommended	See Cefaclor
4 gm	25 mg/kg q24h IV	25-50 mg/kg q12-24h IV	*H. influenzae, Salmonella, S. pneumoniae, Neisseria* sp.
2 gm			*Staphylococcus* sp. (including methicillin-resistant strains), *S. faecalis, Haemophilus, Pseudomonas, Proteus, Escherichia, Klebsiella,* other Enterobacteriaceae, anaerobes, *Legionella, N. gonorrhoeae, Serratia, Chlamydia, Acinetobacter, Bacillus cereus*
4-8 gm	Unknown	Unknown	*S. pneumoniae, S. pyogenes, Streptococcus viridans, S. aureus* except methicillin-resistant strains, Bacteroides, Actinomyces
4 gm	Not recommended	Not recommended	*Staphylococcus, S. pneumoniae, S. pyogenes*

Drug	Adults Oral daily dosage	Adults Parenteral daily dosage	Children Oral daily dosage	Children Parenteral daily dosage	Usual divided dose interval
Dicloxacillin[a]	1–2 gm		12.5–25.0 mg/kg		q6h
Doxycycline[a]	100–200 mg	100–200 mg IV	1–2 mg/kg (over 8 years of age)	1–2 mg/kg IV (over 8 years of age)	q12–24h
Erythromycin	1–2 gm	1–4 gm IV	30–50 mg/kg	15–50 mg/kg IV	q6h
Gentamicin		3–5 mg/kg IM, IV		3.0–7.5 mg/kg IM, IV	q8h
Imipenem[a,e]		1–4 gm IV			q6–8h
Methicillin[a]		4–12 gm IM, IV		100–200 gm IM, IV	q4–6h
Minocycline	100 mg		2 mg/kg		q12h
Nafcillin[a]	2–4 gm	2–9 gm IM, IV	50–100 mg/kg	100–200 mg/kg IM, IV	q6h
Norfloxacin[d]	800 mg				q12h
Oxacillin[a]	2–4 gm	2–12 gm IM, IV	50–100 mg/kg	100–200 mg/kg IM, IV	q6h
Oxytetracycline	1–2 gm	0.75–1.0 gm IM	20–50 mg/kg (over 8 years of age)	10–20 mg/kg IM, IV (over 8 years of age)	q12h
Penicillin G potassium	1–2 gm	1.2–24.0 million units IM, IV: potassium or sodium penicillin IM: procaine or benzathine penicillin	25–50 mg/kg	100,000–250,000 units/kg (See Adults)	q6h
Penicillin V	1–2 gm		25–50 mg/kg		q6h
Piperacillin		12–24 gm IM, IV		200–300 mg/kg IM, IV	q4–6h
Rifampin[f]	0.6 gm	0.6 gm	10–20 mg/kg		q12–24h
Spectinomycin[d]		2 gm IM once		40 mg/kg IM	
Streptomycin		1–2 gm IM		20–30 mg/kg IM	q12h
Sulfisoxazole[a]	1–2 gm		100 mg/kg		q6h

Usual maximum dose/day	Newborn (Parenteral)		Organism susceptibility guide
	Up to 1 week	1–4 weeks	
4 gm	Not recommended	Not recommended	*Staphylococcus, S. pneumoniae, S. pyogenes*
200 mg	Not recommended	Not recommended	Some *Staphylococcus* and *Streptococcus, Escherichia, Enterobacter, Acinetobacter (Mima, Herellea), Haemophilus, Klebsiella, Pasteurella, Rickettsia, Borellia, Bacteroides, Brucella*
4 gm	Not recommended	Not recommended	*Streptococcus*, pneumococcus, *Mycoplasma, Treponema pallidum*
5 mg/kg	5 mg/kg/day q12h IM, IV	7.5 mg/kg/day q8h IM, IV	See Amikacin
4 gm			Methicillin-sensitive *S. aureus, S. pneumoniae, Streptococcus* groups A & B, some *S. faecalis, N. meningitidis, N. gonorrhoeae, H. influenzae, E. coli, Klebsiella, Pseudomonas, Bacillus* sp., *Moraxella, Eikenella, Brucella*
12 gm	50–75 mg/kg/day q8–12h IM, IV	100–150 mg/kg/day q6–8h IM, IV	*Staphylococcus, Streptococcus pneumococciae*, other *Streptococcus* sp., *Neisseria* sp., *Peptostreptococcus*
200 mg	Not recommended	Not recommended	See Doxycycline
12 gm	40 mg/kg/day q12h IM, IV	60–80 mg/kg/day q6–8h	See Methicillin
1600 mg			See Ciprofloxacin
12 gm	50–75 mg/kg/day q8–12h	100–150 mg/kg/day q6–8h	See Methicillin
2 gm	Not recommended	Not recommended	See Doxycycline
24 million units IV 4.8 million units IM	50,000–150,000 units/kg/day q8–12h IV, IM	75,000–250,000 units/kg/day q6–8h IM, IV	*S. pneumoniae, S. pyogenes, S. viridans*, non-penicillinase-producing *S. aureus, N. meningitidis, N. gonorrhoeae, Clostridium*, many *Bacteroides*, Enterobacteriaceae, *Actinomyces, Treponema*
4 gm	Not recommended	Not recommended	See Penicillin G. Less active against *N. gonorrhoeae*
24 gm			See Carbenicillin, especially *Pseudomonas* and *Klebsiella*
0.6 gm			*S. aureus, S. epidermidis, Streptococcus* sp., *N. meningitidis, N. gonorrhoeae, H. influenzae, Legionella, Mycobacterium* sp., *Chlamydia*
4 gm	Not recommended	Not recommended	*N. gonorrhoeae*
2 gm	Not recommended	Not recommended	*Mycobacterium tuberculosis* Some gram-negative bacilli
4 gm	Not recommended	100 mg/kg	*Staphylococcus, S. pyogenes, N. meningitidis, Chlamydia, Toxoplasma, Nocardia*

	Adults		Children		Usual
Drug	Oral daily dosage	Parenteral daily dosage	Oral daily dosage	Parenteral daily dosage	divided dose interval
Tetracycline HCl	1–2 gm	0.75–1.0 gm IM	25–50 mg/kg (over 8 years of age)	10–20 mg/kg IM, IV (over 8 years of age)	
Ticarcillin		200–300 mg/kg IM, IV		200–300 mg/kg IM, IV	q4–6h
Tobramycin		3–5 mg/kg IM, IV		6.0–7.5 mg/kg IM, IV	q8h
Trimethoprim-sulfamethoxazole (TMP-SMX)[a,d]	4 tablets (80 mg TMP + 400 mg SMX/tablet)	8–20 mg/kg (TMP) IV	8–20 mg (TMP)	8–20 mg/kg (TMP) IV	q6–12h
Vancomycin[a,d]	0.5–2 gm	2 gm IV	50 mg/kg	40 mg/kg IV	q6–12h

Usual maximum dose/day	Newborn (Parenteral)		Organism susceptibility guide
	Up to 1 week	1–4 weeks	
2 gm	Not recommended	Not recommended	See Doxycycline
16 gm	150–225 mg/kg/day q8–12h	225–300 mg/kg/day q8h	See Carbenicillin *Bacillus fragilis* but most *Klebsiella*-resistant
5 mg/kg	4 mg/kg/day q12h	6.0–7.5 mg/kg/day q6–8h	See Amikacin
1200 mg TMP with 600 mg SMX, IV	Not recommended	Not recommended	*S. aureus, S. epidermidis, S. pneumoniae, S. viridans, H. influenzae, Bacteroides, E. coli, Enterobacter, Klebsiella, Proteus, Serratia, Pneumocystis*
2 gm	20 mg/kg/day q12h	30 mg/kg/day q8h	*S. aureus,* including methicillin-resistant *S. epidermidis, S. pneumoniae, S. viridans, Corynebacterium diphtheria, Clostridium* sp., enterococci *(S. faecalis)*

aActive against penicillinase-producing staphylococci.
bNumber in parentheses indicates cephalosporin generation.
cSecond- and third-generation cephalosporins are less active than first-generation against staphylococci and streptococci but more active against gram-negative bacilli and anaerobes. *Pseudomonas,* indole-positive *Proteus, Acinetobacter (Mima, Herellea),* and most *Serratia* are resistant to all cephalosporins.
dPenicillin-allergy alternate.
eA beta lactam. Imipenem is the most active drug against all pathogenic bacteria.
fNot FDA approved for ocular disease.
For topical, subconjunctival, and intravitreal dosages see Tables 5-5, 5-6, and 5-7 and Table 8-7.
Source: Adapted in part from M. Abramowicz (ed.), *Handbook of Antimicrobial Therapy.* New Rochelle, NY: Medical Letter, 1990.

Index

The abbreviations *f* and *t* stand for figure and table, respectively.